LUNG
Transplantation

Principles and Practice

LUNG
Transplantation
Principles and Practice

Edited by

Wickii T. Vigneswaran, MD, MBA, FRCSC, FRCS(CTh), FACS
Professor and Chief of Thoracic Surgery
Loyola University Medical Center and Stritch School of Medicine
Chicago (Maywood), Illinois, USA

Edward R. Garrity, Jr., MD, MBA
Professor of Medicine
Vice Chair
Clinical Operations
Associate Director
Transplantation Services
University of Chicago
Chicago, Illinois, USA

John A. Odell, MBChB, FRCS(Ed), FACS
Emeritus Professor of Surgery
Mayo Clinic Florida
Jacksonville, Florida, USA

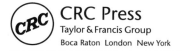
CRC Press
Taylor & Francis Group
Boca Raton London New York

CRC Press is an imprint of the
Taylor & Francis Group, an **informa** business

CRC Press
Taylor & Francis Group
6000 Broken Sound Parkway NW, Suite 300
Boca Raton, FL 33487-2742

First issued in paperback 2020

© 2016 by Taylor & Francis Group, LLC
CRC Press is an imprint of Taylor & Francis Group, an Informa business

No claim to original U.S. Government works

Version Date: 20151009

ISBN 13: 978-0-367-57512-0 (pbk)
ISBN 13: 978-1-4822-3391-9 (hbk)

This book contains information obtained from authentic and highly regarded sources. While all reasonable efforts have been made to publish reliable data and information, neither the author[s] nor the publisher can accept any legal responsibility or liability for any errors or omissions that may be made. The publishers wish to make clear that any views or opinions expressed in this book by individual editors, authors or contributors are personal to them and do not necessarily reflect the views/opinions of the publishers. The information or guidance contained in this book is intended for use by medical, scientific or health-care professionals and is provided strictly as a supplement to the medical or other professional's own judgement, their knowledge of the patient's medical history, relevant manufacturer's instructions and the appropriate best practice guidelines. Because of the rapid advances in medi-cal science, any information or advice on dosages, procedures or diagnoses should be independently verified. The reader is strongly urged to consult the relevant national drug formulary and the drug companies' and device or material manufacturers' printed instructions, and their websites, before administering or utilizing any of the drugs, devices or materials mentioned in this book. This book does not indicate whether a particular treatment is appropriate or suitable for a particular individual. Ultimately it is the sole responsibility of the medical professional to make his or her own professional judgements, so as to advise and treat patients appropriately. The authors and publishers have also attempted to trace the copyright holders of all material reproduced in this publication and apologize to copyright holders if permission to publish in this form has not been obtained. If any copyright material has not been acknowledged please write and let us know so we may rectify in any future reprint.

Except as permitted under U.S. Copyright Law, no part of this book may be reprinted, reproduced, transmitted, or utilized in any form by any electronic, mechanical, or other means, now known or hereafter invented, including photocopying, microfilming, and recording, or in any information storage or retrieval system, without written permission from the publishers.

For permission to photocopy or use material electronically from this work, please access www.copyright.com (http://www.copyright.com/) or contact the Copyright Clearance Center, Inc. (CCC), 222 Rosewood Drive, Danvers, MA 01923, 978-750-8400. CCC is a not-for-profit organization that provides licenses and registration for a variety of users. For organizations that have been granted a photocopy license by the CCC, a separate system of payment has been arranged.

Printed in the UK by Severn, Gloucester on responsibly sourced paper

 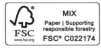

Trademark Notice: Product or corporate names may be trademarks or registered trademarks, and are used only for identification and explanation without intent to infringe.

Visit the Taylor & Francis Web site at
http://www.taylorandfrancis.com

and the CRC Press Web site at
http://www.crcpress.com

Dedication

To all my mentors and teachers for their patience, to my patients whom I had the privilege to serve, and to my wife Rupy and children Yalini, Hari and Janani for their support and the sacrifices they have made.

WTV

To all the patients who have been the real pioneers in this field—thank you for your trust and support of our endeavors. Breathing is good!

And to my wife Linda, who has helped to keep me level and patient-centered throughout.

ERG

To my patients, who had the courage and confidence to accept me as their surgeon and to place their lives in my hands. I would also like to dedicate this to the donors and their families, who have made the lives of others better.

JAO

Contents

PART 4   FUTURE OF LUNG TRANSPLANTATION

Preface

Lung transplantation became a clinical reality just over 30 years ago. The evolution of the process and refinements continue. What used to be individual experience is now becoming evidence-based practice. In 2010 we edited the book *Lung Transplantation* as the 243rd volume of the *Lung Biology in Health and Disease* series. The reception and the feedback for that volume were exceptional. When approached to edit this book, *Lung Transplantation: Principles and Practice*, as an independent entity, we believed that the timing was right for this task. John Odell joined us as co-editor; between the three of us we had close to 80 years of experience in lung transplantation and thought that we could produce a concise and timely state-of-the-art book with international contributors, all experts in this field.

The book is easy to read, containing a combination of personal experiences, consensus, and evidence-based guidelines, with a practical approach to lung transplantation. The book has four sections: General Topics, including history and pre-transplantation considerations; Donor Management; Recipient Management and Outcomes; and finally some thoughts on the Future of Lung Transplantation. Many chapters contain large numbers of references in support of the text and provide additional material for those interested in delving more deeply into the topics presented.

Short- and long-term success in lung transplantation requires a multidisciplinary approach with proper understanding of the process by the entire team. Many patients after lung transplantation are living longer, more productive lives in their community while managed by "non-experts," often the primary care and/or local pulmonary physician, except for issues directly related to transplantation. A clear understanding of lung transplantation is therefore necessary not only for the members of the lung transplantation "team" but also for the broader group of physicians and other healthcare providers in the community. This concise but comprehensive account of contemporary practice will be useful reading and can serve as a quick reference for anyone caring for lung transplant patients.

We believe that this book will appeal to pulmonary physicians, nurses, thoracic surgeons, intensivists, hospitalists, pathologists, social workers, organ donor and transplant coordinators, and transplant administrators. We are confident that providers who may come into contact with potential recipients and lung transplant patients in the community can benefit from this work. We hope that this book will become an essential part of the care of lung transplant recipients seen in medical practice.

Wickii T. Vigneswaran
Edward R. Garrity, Jr
John A. Odell

Acknowledgments

I would like to thank all the authors for their contribution; without them this work would not have been possible. I am indebted to my co-editors, Drs. Garrity and Odell, who were always timely and willing and available to support me in reviewing materials, and for their wise advice. There are several members in the Taylor & Francis family who navigated us through the process. I acknowledge their assistance with gratitude, especially Henry Spielberg, then Senior Editor, and his editorial assistant Nicola Streak, who was instrumental in the birth of this book and initial trouble-shooting with Henry; and Linda Van Pelt, Senior Project Manager, who was very efficient and kept us all on track. I thank our artists at Cenveo Publisher Services for their superb drawings, bringing this book into a class of its own. Finally, I thank Miranda Bromage, who inherited the book from Henry Spielberg, for her support and her final touches, making it even better. I am very proud and privileged to be part of this contribution to lung transplantation.

Wickii T. Vigneswaran

Contributors

Vijayalakshmi Ananthanarayanan, MD
Professor
Department of Pathology
Loyola University Medical Center
Maywood, Illinois, USA

Mara B. Antonoff, MD
University of Texas
MD Anderson Cancer Center
Houston, Texas, USA

Abbas Ardehali, MD
David Geffen School of Medicine
University of California at Los Angeles
Los Angeles, California, USA

Shelly Bansal, MD
Senior Associate Consultant
Department of Surgery
Mayo Clinic Florida
Jacksonville, Florida, USA

Julia B. Becker, MD
Spectrum Health
Grand Rapids, Michigan, USA

Sangeeta M. Bhorade, MD
Associate Professor of Medicine
Section of Pulmonary and Critical Care Medicine
Division of Medicine
Northwestern Memorial Hospital
Chicago, Illinois, USA

Catherine Borders, MD
Division of Cardiovascular Surgery
Department of Surgery
Hospital of the University of Pennsylvania
Philadelphia, Pennsylvania, USA

Jose Luis Campo Cañaveral de la Cruz, MD
Thoracic Surgery and Lung Transplantation
Department
Hospital Universitario de Hierro Majadahonda
Madrid, Spain

Edward M. Cantu III, MD, MSCE
Assistant Professor of Surgery
Hospital of the University of Pennsylvania
Philadelphia, Pennsylvania, USA

Mark A. Chaney, MD
Professor
Director of Cardiac Anesthesia
Program Director, Adult Cardiothoracic Fellowship
Department of Anesthesia and Critical Care
University of Chicago
Chicago, Ilinois, USA

Jason D. Christie, MD, MS
Center for Clinical Epidemiology and Biostatistics
University of Pennsylvania
Philadelphia, Pennsylvania, USA

Stéphane Collaud, MD, MSc
Surgeon
Division of Thoracic Surgery
Toronto Lung Transplant Program
University Health Network
University of Toronto
Toronto, Canada

Daniel Valdivia Concha, MD
Thoracic Surgery and Lung Transplantation Department
Hospital Universitario de Hierro Majadahonda
Madrid, Spain

Joel D. Cooper, MD, FACS, FRCPS
Professor of Surgery
Hospital of the University of Pennsylvania
Philadelphia, Pennsylvania, USA

Joseph Costa, DHSc, PA-C
Instructor of Clinical Surgical Sciences in Surgery
Chief PA Thoracic Surgery & Lung Transplantation
Columbia University College of Physicians and Surgeons
Columbia University Medical Center
New York, New York, USA

Marcelo Cypel, MD, MSc
Canada Research Chair in Lung Transplantation
Thoracic Surgeon
University Health Network
Assistant Professor of Surgery
Division of Thoracic Surgery
University of Toronto
Toronto, Ontario, Canada

Lara Danziger-Isakov, MD, MPH
Professor of Pediatrics
Director
Immunocompromised Host Infectious Disease
Cincinnati Children's Hospital Medical Center
Cincinnati, Ohio, USA

John H. Dark, MB, BS, FRCS
Professor of Cardiothoracic Surgery
Institute of Cellular Medicine
Newcastle University
Newcastle upon Tyne, UK

Hiroshi Date, MD, PhD
Professor
Department of Thoracic Surgery
Kyoto University Graduate School of Medicine
Kyoto, Japan

Jennifer Delacruz, MD
Department of Medicine
University of Chicago Medical Center
Chicago, Illinois, USA

Marc de Perrot, MD, MSc
Division of Thoracic Surgery
Toronto Lung Transplant Program
University Health Network
University of Toronto
Toronto, Canada

Gundeep S. Dhillon, MD, MPH
Pulmonologist
Stanford Health Care
Assistant Professor of Medicine
Division of Pulmonary and Critical Care Medicine
Stanford University Medical Center
Stanford, California, USA

José L. Díaz-Gómez, MD
Chair
Critical Care Medicine
Assistant Professor of Anesthesiology
Mayo Clinic College of Medicine
Consultant
Departments of Critical Care Medicine, Anesthesiology, and Neurology
Mayo Clinic
Jacksonville, Florida, USA

Frank D'Ovidio, MD, PhD
Associate Professor of Surgery
Surgical Director
Lung Transplant Program
Director
Ex-Vivo Lung Perfusion Program
Columbia University College of Physicians and Surgeons
Columbia University Medical Center
New York, New York, USA

Thomas M. Egan, MD, MSc, FACS
Professor of Surgery
University of North Carolina at Chapel Hill
Chapel Hill, North Carolina, USA

John Ellis, MD
Division of Cardiovascular Surgery
Department of Surgery
Hospital of the University of Pennsylvania
Philadelphia, Pennsylvania, USA

Savitri Fedson, MD
Associate Professor of Medicine
The University of Chicago Medicine
Chicago, Illinois, USA

Edward R. Garrity Jr, MD, MBA
Professor of Medicine
Vice Chair
Clinical Operations
Associate Director
Transplantation Services
University of Chicago
Chicago, Illinois, USA

Melissa Gitman, MDCM, MPH
Transplant Infectious Diseases Fellow
Department of Medicine
Division of Infectious Diseases
University Health Network
University of Toronto
Toronto, Ontario, Canada

David Gómez de Antonio, MD
Hospital Universitario de Hierro Majadahonda
Madrid, Spain

Adam S.A. Gracon, MD
Department of Surgery and Center for Immunobiology
Indiana University School of Medicine
Indianapolis, Indiana, USA

Joshua C. Grimm, MD
Halsted Resident
Department of Surgery
The Johns Hopkins Hospital
Baltimore, Maryland, USA

Aliya N. Husain, MD
Professor of Pathology
Residency Program Director
University of Chicago
Chicago, Illinois, USA

Ilhan Inci, MD, FCCP
Professor of Thoracic Surgery
Department of Thoracic Surgery
University Hospital Zürich
Zürich, Switzerland

Cesar A. Keller, MD
Professor of Medicine
Mayo Clinic College of Medicine
Consultant
Department of Transplantation
Division of Transplant Medicine
Mayo Clinic
Jacksonville, Florida, USA

Shaf Keshavjee, MD, FRCSC, FACS
Thoracic Surgery
University of Toronto
Toronto General Hospital
Toronto, Ontario, Canada

Thorsten Krueger, MD
Department of Thoracic and Vascular Surgery
University Hospital of Lausanne
Lausanne, Switzerland

Elizabeth A. Lendermon, MD
Division of Pulmonary, Allergy, and Critical Care
Medicine
Department of Medicine
University of Pittsburgh School of Medicine
Pittsburgh, Pennsylvania, USA

Matthias Loebe, MD, PhD, FCCP, FACC
Director
Thoracic Transplant and Mechanical Support
Professor of Surgery
Miami Transplant Institute
Memorial Jackson Health System
University of Miami
Miami, Florida, USA

Jason M. Long, MD, MPH
Assistant Professor of Surgery
Division of Cardiothoracic Surgery
University of North Carolina at Chapel Hill School of
Medicine
Chapel Hill, North Carolina, USA

Me-Linh Luong, MD, FRCPC
Assistant Professor
Transplant Infectious Disease Specialist
Department of Infectious Diseases and Medical
Microbiology

University of Montreal
St-Luc Hospital
Centre Hospitalier de L'Universite de Montreal (CHUM)
Montreal, Quebec, Canada

Natalie Madoun, BS
Henry Ford Health System
Detroit, Michigan, USA

Oriol Manuel, MD
Infectious Diseases Service and Transplantation Center
University Hospital of Lausanne
Lausanne, Switzerland

David P. Mason, MD
Baylor University Medical Center
Dallas, Texas, USA

Joshua S. Mason, MD
Section of Pulmonary and Critical Care Medicine
University of Chicago Medicine
Chicago, Illinois, USA

John F. McDyer, MD
University of Pittsburgh Medical Center
Pittsburgh, Pennsylvania, USA

Lucas Hoyos Megía, MD
Thoracic Surgery and Lung Transplantation Department
Hospital Universitario Puera de Hierro Majadahonda
Madrid, Spain

Keith C. Meyer, MD, MS
Professor of Medicine
University of Wisconsin Lung Transplant and Advanced
Pulmonary Disease Program
Section of Allergy, Pulmonary and Critical Care Medicine
Department of Medicine
University of Wisconsin School of Medicine and Public
Health
Madison, Wisconsin, USA

Mohammed Minhaj, MD MBA
Vice-Chair Finance and Operations
Associate Chair for Faculty Development
Department of Anesthesia and Critical Care
University of Chicago Medicine
Chicago, Illinois, USA

Nathan M. Mollberg, DO
Bronson Cardiothoracic and Vascular Surgery
Kalamazoo, Michigan, USA

Michael S. Mulligan, MD
Department of Surgery
University of Washington
Seattle, Washington, USA

Hassan Michael Nemeh, MD
Henry Ford Hospital
Detroit, Michigan, USA

John A. Odell, MBChB, FRCS(Ed), FACS
Emeritus Professor of Surgery
Mayo Clinic Florida
Jacksonville, Florida, USA

Miranda A. Paraskeva, MBBS, FRACP
Lung Transplant Service
Alfred Hospital and Monash University
Melbourne, Australia

G. Alexander Patterson, MD
Washington University School of Medicine
St. Louis, Missouri, USA

David Pitrak, MD
Professor of Medicine
Chief of Infectious Diseases and Global Health
University of Chicago
Chicago, Illinois, USA

Kenneth Pursell, MD
Professor of Medicine
University of Chicago Medicine
Chicago, Illinois, USA

Dewei Ren, MD
Attending
Division of Transplantation and Assist Devices
Methodist DeBakey Heart and Vascular Center
J.C. Walter Jr. Transplant Center
Houston, Texas, USA

J. Devin Roberts, MD
Assistant Professor of Anesthesiology
Department of Anesthesiology and Critical Care Medicine
University of Chicago Medical Center
Chicago, Illinois, USA

Susan R. Russell, MD
Assistant Professor in Medicine
Section of Pulmonary and Critical Care Medicine
Feinberg School of Medicine
Northwestern University
Chicago, Illinois, USA

Mark J. Russo, MD, MS
Barnabas Heart Hospital
Newark Beth Israel Medical Center
Newark, New Jersey, USA

Ashish S. Shah, MD
Department of Cardiac Surgery
Vanderbilt University Medical Center
Nashville, Tennessee, USA

Baddr A. Shakhsheer, MD
MacLean Center for Clinical Medical Ethics
University of Chicago
Chicago, Illinois, USA

Mark Siegler, MD, FACP
MacLean Center for Clinical Medical Ethics
University of Chicago
Chicago, Illinois, USA

Leann L. Silhan, MD
Division of Pulmonary and Critical Care Medicine
The Johns Hopkins Hospital
Baltimore, Maryland, USA

Greg I. Snell, MBBS, FRACP, MD
Professor
Lung Transplant Service
Alfred Hospital and Monash University
Melbourne, Australia

Wiebke Sommer, MD
Department of Cardiothoracic, Vascular, and
Transplantation Surgery
Hannover Medical School
Hannover, Germany

Joshua R. Sonett, MD
Chief
General Thoracic Surgery
Edwin C. and Anne K. Weiskopf Professor or Surgical
Oncology
Director
The Price Family Center for Comprehensive Chest Care
Columbia University College of Physicians and
Surgeons
Columbia University Medical Center
New York, New York, USA

Jennifer L. Steinbeck, MD
Fellow, Section of Infectious Diseases
Department of Internal Medicine
University of Chicago Medicine
Chicago, Illinois, USA

Mathew Thomas, MD
Consultant Surgeon
Assistant Professor of Surgery
Division of Cardiothoracic Surgery
Mayo Clinic
Jacksonville, Florida, USA

Bart M. Vanaudenaerde, PhD
KU Leuven - University of Leuven
Department of Clinical and Experimental Medicine
Division of Pneumology
Lung Transplant Unit
Leuven, Belgium

Katherine M. Vandervest, MD
Assistant Professor
Division of Pulmonary Sciences, Critical Care Medicine,
and Lung Transplantation
University of Colorado Hospital
Anschutz Medical Campus
Aurora, Colorado, USA

Andrés Varela de Ugarte, MD, PhD
Thoracic Surgery and Lung Transplantation Department
Hospital Universitario Puerta de Hierro Majadahonda
Madrid, Spain

Geert M. Verleden, MD, PhD
KU Leuven - University of Leuven
Department of Clinical and Experimental Medicine
Division of Pneumology
Lung Transplant Unit
Leuven, Belgium

Stijn E. Verleden, PhD
KU Leuven - University of Leuven
Department of Clinical and Experimental Medicine
Division of Pneumology
Lung Transplant Unit
Leuven, Belgium

Erik Verschuuren, MD
University Medical Center Groningen
University of Groningen
Groningen, The Netherlands

Wickii T. Vigneswaran, MD, MBA, FRCSC, FRCS(CTh), FACS
Professor and Chief of Thoracic Surgery
Department of Thoracic and Cardiovascular Surgery
Loyola University Medical Center and Stritch School of Medicine
Chicago (Maywood), Illinois, USA

Robin Vos, MD, PhD
KU Leuven - University of Leuven
Department of Clinical and Experimental Medicine
Division of Pneumology
Lung Transplant Unit
Leuven, Belgium

Gregor Warnecke, MD
Bereichsleiter Lungen- und
Herzlungentransplantation
Herz-, Thorax-, Transplantations- und Gefäßchirurgie
Medizinische Hochschule Hannover
Hannover, Germany

Walter Weder, MD
Professor of Surgery
Department of Thoracic Surgery
University Hospital Zürich
Zürich, Switzerland

Xiang Wei, MD
Methodist DeBakey Heart and Vascular Center
J.C. Walter Jr. Transplant Center
Houston, Texas, USA

David Weill, MD
Stanford University Medical Center
Stanford, California, USA

Glen P. Westall, MBBS, FRACP, PhD
Associate Professor
Lung Transplant Service
Alfred Hospital and Monash University
Melbourne, Australia

Christopher Wigfield, MD
Section of Cardiac and Thoracic Surgery
Department of Surgery
University of Chicago Medicine
Chicago, Illinois, USA

Sean C. Wightman, MD
MacLean Center for Clinical Medical Ethics
University of Chicago
Chicago, Illinois, USA

David S. Wilkes, MD
Dean
University of Virginia School of Medicine
Charlottesville, Virginia, USA

James J. Yun, MD, PhD
Department of Surgery
Yale School of Medicine
New Haven, Connecticut, USA

Martin R. Zamora, MD
University of Colorado Denver Medical Center
Aurora, Colorado, USA

General Topics

History of lung transplantation

JOEL D. COOPER AND THOMAS M. EGAN

What's past is prologue

William Shakespeare
The Tempest

INTRODUCTION

Shakespeare's aphorism applies to the history of organ transplantation in general and to the history of lung transplantation in particular. The request to prepare this chapter, which came shortly after the 30th anniversary of our initial long-term success with lung transplantation, provided a timely opportunity to reflect not only on the evolution of lung transplantation during the period before clinical success but also on the 30 years since (Table 1.1). It is humbling to reflect on how many investigators have been engaged in this endeavor and how many obstacles had to be overcome. Even now, the definition of what will ultimately be considered true success—and where on the path to that destination we now stand—is unclear. We hope that in the future, when tolerance to donor organs can be induced and decades-long improved quality of life after transplantation becomes the rule, all progress to date will be viewed as but the prologue of the past.

Historical references to the concept of human organ transplantation date back centuries and often cite the third century twin saints Cosmas and Damian, who are credited with the miraculous transplantation of the black leg of a deceased Ethiopian onto the body of a white recipient whose leg required amputation. This legend, which was memorialized by a famous painting, may seem fanciful, but no more so than the actual feat accomplished in the 1940s by the Russian physiologist Demikhov, who transplanted the head of one dog onto the neck of a second dog, with both the host and the donor head remaining alive and active for several days. It was Demikhov as well who experimented with canine pulmonary lobe transplantation and with heart-lung transplantation well before the era of cardiopulmonary bypass.[1] His technical prowess owed much to the prior work of Alexis Carrel, the French physiologist who won the Nobel Prize in 1912 for his pioneering work in developing techniques for end-to-end anastomosis of blood vessels and its use in the transplantation of whole organs.[2] In fact, the first "thoracic" organ transplant was described by Carrel in 1907, when he and his colleague Charles Guthrie performed a heterotopic heart-lung transplant onto the neck of a cat. When the graft died on the third day, Carrel attributed this to technical anastomotic problems, but he was probably witnessing a manifestation of acute rejection.[3]

Table 1.1 Timeline of seminal events in the history of lung transplantation

1907	Guthrie and Carrel—heterotopic heart-lung transplant
1940s–1950s	Demikhov—lobar transplants
1950s	Juvenelle, Metras, Hardy, and Veith—experimental canine lung transplant
1963	Hardy—first human lung transplant
1968	Derom—10-month survival
1981	Reitz et al.—first successful heart-lung transplant
1983	Cooper et al.—first successful single-lung transplant
1986	Cooper et al.—first successful double-lung transplant
1986	Start of Organ Procurement and Transplantation Network (OPTN); United Network for Organ Sharing (UNOS) becomes contractor
1988–1995	Growth of lung transplant programs in the United States and globally
1999	Institute of Medicine report, Final Rule (2000)
2001	Steen—First lung transplant after ex vivo lung perfusion
2005	Introduction of the lung allocation score system in the United States

The final proof that an organ from one human could be transplanted into another with long-term clinical benefit was demonstrated by the first successful human kidney transplant, which was performed by Dr. Joseph Murray and colleagues in 1954.[4] The donor and recipient were identical twins, thus eliminating the unsolved problem of organ rejection. This accomplishment, for which Dr. Murray was awarded the Nobel Prize in 1990, clearly demonstrated the potential for treatment of end-stage disease by means of organ transplantation. Nothing dramatized this potential more than the occasion of the first human heart transplant, conducted by Dr. Christiaan Barnard in December 1967. Although the recipient succumbed to pneumonia 18 days later, postoperative photographs of the recipient looking well and cheerful captivated the attention of the world.

UNIQUE ISSUES ASSOCIATED WITH LUNG TRANSPLANTATION

By 1980, liver and heart transplants had joined renal transplants as accepted options for treating end-stage organ failure. However, progress in lung transplantation lagged, and expectations were dampened by lack of success in the laboratory and in the clinical arena.

It became obvious that lung transplantation posed unique obstacles. The lung is the only organ transplanted without reattachment of its systemic arterial blood supply (the bronchial arteries). Thus, one of the major anastomoses—the bronchial anastomosis—is rendered ischemic; it is also open to the external environment and very prone to infection. In addition, the lung is a fragile organ prone to injury and infection and also significantly more susceptible to rejection than other major organs.

Most experimental lung transplantations were conducted on a canine model. However, the dog, like other subprimate animals, is dependent on the Hering-Breuer reflex to maintain central respiratory control. With total denervation of both lungs, such as would occur with bilateral or unilateral lung transplantation and removal of the opposite lung, the dog cannot survive because of loss of the normal respiratory control mechanism. This problem made it difficult to assess the function of an experimentally transplanted lung when the animal was removed from the ventilator following transplantation. Only in a primate model, a complex and expensive undertaking, can the recipient animal remain alive for days or weeks solely on the function of transplanted lungs. In addition, as the authors can well attest, lung transplantation in a canine model is technically more challenging than in humans, partly because the atrial anastomosis tends to accumulate blood clots if there is any gap in the endothelial-to-endothelial apposition of the atrial anastomosis.

EXPERIMENTAL ANIMAL TRANSPLANTATION

Resection and reimplantation of a lung in a dog was initially reported by Juvenelle and colleagues in 1951. Severing and reconnection of the pulmonary artery, superior and inferior pulmonary veins, and bronchus of the right lung of the dog was undertaken to evaluate the effect of denervation on the postulated pulmonary reflex known as bronchospasm, whose "existence has yet to be proved."[5] In 1950, Metras in Marseilles reported a technique for canine allotransplantation.[6] The technique involved performing the venous anastomosis by using a cuff of atrium surrounding the two pulmonary veins rather than separate individual vein-to-vein anastomoses. This important technical contribution continues to be used. Metras reported survival for a matter of days at best, with death attributed to either infection or rejection.

Early attempts at suppressing rejection included adrenocorticotropic hormone, cortisone, total body irradiation, and splenectomy. Hardy observed that survival in dogs undergoing single-lung transplantation could be prolonged for more than a week with the use of methotrexate and further extended to an average of 29 days when recipient animals were treated with azathioprine and cortisone.[7]

The ability of a transplanted lung to totally support an animal's respiratory requirement was documented in the early 1960s in a model that involved ligation of the contralateral pulmonary artery following lung transplantation. Survival for weeks was accomplished. Other areas of investigation included the role of pulmonary lymphatic interruption as a contributor to posttransplant pulmonary edema and attempts to restore bronchial arterial circulation at the time of transplantation. Reimplantation of the left bronchial artery to the aorta at the time of left lung transplantation led to more normal healing of the bronchial anastomosis than occurred without such reconnection. However, the technique of direct restoration of bronchial circulation is difficult and seldom used, with a few notable exceptions, as recently reviewed[8] and championed by Dr. Pettersson. This leaves only a tenuous blood supply to the proximal donor bronchus, provided by retrograde bronchial arterial flow originating from postcapillary communication between the pulmonary and bronchial circulations.

Veith studied varied techniques for bronchial anastomosis and developed a "telescoping" bronchial anastomosis in an attempt to reduce anastomotic complications.[9] He also emphasized the importance of keeping the donor bronchus as short as possible to reduce the most ischemic segment.

HUMAN LUNG TRANSPLANTATION

After years of laboratory research, Hardy and coworkers performed the first human lung transplant in 1963.[10] The donor lung was harvested postmortem from a patient who had cardiac arrest after a massive myocardial infarction. The recipient of the left lung transplant was a penitentiary inmate with a central carcinoma of the lung and nodal metastases. The patient survived 18 days, with death attributed to renal failure and malnutrition. Immunosuppression consisted of azathioprine, cortisone, and a 5-day course of cobalt irradiation to the mediastinum. Hardy's effort confirmed the technical feasibility of human lung transplantation and established that transplanted lungs in humans could function satisfactorily. Though Hardy's experience initiated the era of human lung transplantation, he was criticized because the recipient was a prisoner, the indication was a central carcinoma with lymph node metastases, and significant confounding comorbid conditions (including renal insufficiency and nephrotic syndrome) were present in the recipient, which reduced the chances of success. Furthermore, at the time, meaningful long-term survival had not been accomplished in an experimental animal model.

THE FIRST 10 YEARS

Over the next 10 years, 34 attempted lung transplants were reported around the world, without much success. Only one of those recipients survived long enough to leave the hospital. He was a young man with silicosis who underwent unilateral lung transplantation by Dr. Derom and colleagues in 1968.[11] The patient survived for 10 months but was hospitalized most of the time.

In 1970, Wildevuur and Benfield reviewed the accumulated world experience with lung transplantation.[12] Twenty-three lung transplants had been performed by 20 surgeons. Only Derom's patient survived longer than 30 days. Three of the recipients each received a lobe; all were subsequently explanted because of rejection. During this time, most of the deaths were attributed to respiratory failure, which was often associated with infection. In the 16 patients who survived longer than 5 days, it was not possible to distinguish pulmonary infection from rejection as the cause of death.

THE SECOND 10 YEARS—SUCCESS REMAINED ELUSIVE

Between 1973 and 1983, only four or five additional lung transplants were performed. Laboratory investigation occurred at a slower pace, undoubtedly as a result of the discouraging lack of clinical success. This contrasted with the increasing success achieved with other organ transplants. At the same time, however, other advances in the field of thoracic surgery and respiratory care ultimately had a positive effect on the development of lung transplantation. Such advances included improvements in ventilatory support, thoracic anesthesia, hemodynamic monitoring, and imaging of the chest, as well as the establishment of extracorporeal membrane oxygenation (ECMO) support. Furthermore, the development of fiberoptic bronchoscopic techniques facilitated visualization of the airway, better diagnosis and treatment of pulmonary infection, and the ability to conduct transbronchial biopsies for assessment of pulmonary pathology, including posttransplant rejection.

In 1968, Dr. F.G. Pearson established a major center for thoracic surgery at the University of Toronto, where laboratory investigation in the area of lung transplantation was a major interest. This, combined with expertise in surgery on the major airways, successful experience with ECMO for patients with acute respiratory failure, and outstanding pulmonary medicine and respiratory care units, prompted that institution's initial attempt at clinical lung transplantation in 1978.[13] That right single-lung transplant was organized by Dr. Bill Nelems, who had spent a year doing lung transplantation research in Holland under Dr. Charles Wildevuur. The recipient was a young man who had inhalation injuries from a house fire 5 months earlier and remained ventilator dependent. Except for his lungs, all his other organ systems were functioning normally. To minimize ischemic time, the donor and recipient were in adjacent operating rooms. ECMO support was used before, during, and for 4 days after the transplant. The recipient was weaned from ventilatory support 7 days after surgery, and supplemental oxygen was not needed by the ninth day. Immunosuppression consisted of methotrexate, azathioprine and prednisone. On the 17th postoperative day, cough, hemoptysis, and dyspnea developed, and the patient died on the 18th postoperative day. Autopsy showed bronchial dehiscence. At autopsy, the donor right main bronchus showed full-thickness necrosis for a distance of 2 cm beyond the suture line. An unanticipated finding was the appearance of the atrial anastomosis, which though intact and normal in appearance, showed no evidence of wound healing between the donor and recipient atria. The suture line looked as though it had been placed hours, not weeks, earlier.

Although the outcome of this initial transplant at the University of Toronto was disappointing, several aspects were encouraging. The experience confirmed that a single transplanted lung could function exceedingly well in the short term, converting a long-term ventilator-dependent patient with pronounced hypercarbia to an individual who could be weaned from the ventilator and become ambulatory in a relatively short period. It also reaffirmed the ability to conduct the procedure without technical complications and the potential usefulness of ECMO support in the perioperative period.

BRONCHIAL ANASTOMOTIC COMPLICATIONS—THE ACHILLES' HEEL

Following this initial attempt, one of us (J.D.C.) reviewed the world experience. The Toronto attempt was approximately the 38th in the world and only the second attempt at human lung transplantation in the previous 5 years. Of the eight patients surviving more than 2 weeks, all recipients had suffered major bronchial complications. It was believed that this complication required a solution if lung transplantation were to ultimately become successful.

In 1981, Reitz and colleagues at Stanford performed a successful heart-lung transplant on a patient with pulmonary hypertension and right-sided heart failure. A subsequent procedure was also successful. The report of these cases emphasized the potential of heart-lung transplants for patients "with pulmonary vascular diseases and certain other intractable cardiopulmonary disorders."[14] The Stanford group attributed much of its success to use of cyclosporine (or Cyclosporin A as it was then known) as an immunosuppressant. Importantly, the group also demonstrated that successful lung transplantation was clearly achievable and gave added impetus to finding a solution to the bronchial anastomosis problem.

A series of animal experiments were initiated in Toronto in 1980 with a primary goal of improving bronchial anastomotic healing in a canine model. Possible causes of failure included infection, rejection, and ischemia resulting from loss of the bronchial arterial supply. Indeed, bronchial ischemia had long been recognized as a potential problem, but its role remained uncertain. Initial experiments were designed to specifically evaluate the effects of immunosuppression on wound healing; they used an autotransplantation model in which the left lung was completely detached and then reattached.

With this model, factors related to rejection could be eliminated, thereby allowing other variables to be studied. Following left lung autotransplantation, animals were randomized to receive either no immunosuppression or immunosuppression with prednisone and azathioprine, as was consistent with clinical practice at the time. Animals receiving no immunosuppression showed primary healing of the bronchial anastomosis. However, they developed substantial anastomotic narrowing localized to the distal side of the bronchial reconnection. On the other hand, in animals receiving immunosuppression, bronchial anastomotic complications were frequent, including disruption, ulceration, and loss of mucosal surface of the reimplanted bronchus. The Toronto group then conducted studies to separately evaluate the effect of either prednisone or azathioprine alone. These studies demonstrated that prednisone alone caused the same adverse wound-healing consequences as the combination of prednisone and azathioprine, whereas azathioprine alone had no apparent adverse effect.[15]

At the time, cyclosporine became available for experimental studies, and Sandoz Pharmaceutical Company provided sufficient material for further experiments. These experiments demonstrated that cyclosporine itself or in combination with azathioprine had no adverse effect on healing of the bronchial anastomosis.[16] This finding was important because it suggested the possibility of delaying high doses of steroids until 2 weeks after transplantation, when bronchial anastomotic healing was well under way.

BRONCHIAL ISCHEMIA

The bronchial anastomotic stenosis observed after autotransplantation in the absence of postoperative immunosuppressive agents was interpreted to be secondary to ischemia of the implanted bronchus. Experiments to address this issue incorporated the use of an omental wrap around the bronchial anastomosis at the time of autotransplantation or allotransplantation. It was found that demonstrable collateral circulation to the distal bronchus occurred within a matter of hours, and further experiments showed that use of the omental wrap in the autotransplant model resulted in excellent bronchial healing without any significant anastomotic narrowing.[17] This encouraging finding was confirmed in a canine allotransplant model.[18]

SUCCESSFUL UNILATERAL LUNG TRANSPLANTATION

The results of laboratory experiments and the subsequent availability of cyclosporine for use in human lung transplants led to resumption of a clinical lung transplant program at the University of Toronto. The initial attempt, in 1982, involved a patient with respiratory failure from accidental Paraquat poisoning. A right lung transplant was successfully performed, but residual Paraquat in the patient's body led to lung damage; 3 weeks later, a left lung transplant was performed. The patient died 3 months later, having required ongoing ventilatory assistance because of Paraquat-induced myopathy. However, the patient had no significant bronchial anastomotic complications.[19] This case reemphasized the importance of appropriate criteria for recipient selection if human lung transplantation was to be successful. By this time, approximately 44 lung transplants had been performed in the world without long-term clinical success.

Although the risk associated with lung transplantation was clearly extremely high, its application as a death-bed rescue attempt in patients who were on a ventilator, often with organ failure, seemed doomed to repeated failure. The Toronto team thought that ideal recipients would be individuals with end-stage lung disease without significant comorbid conditions who were not yet in a hospital on a ventilator. They decided that initial attempts would be limited only to patients with idiopathic pulmonary fibrosis whose clinical course indicated that life expectancy was just a matter of months.

On November 7, 1983, a right lung transplant was performed by the Toronto group using a protocol developed in the laboratory and consisting of an omentopexy placed around the bronchial anastomosis and initial immunosuppression with azathioprine and cyclosporine. Prednisone was added several weeks later. The patient was discharged from the hospital 6 weeks after transplantation. He returned to work and maintained an active life for the next 5 years.[20] He died in the sixth year of complications following a transbronchial lung biopsy.

A year later, the Toronto group performed a subsequent unilateral lung transplant in a patient with pulmonary fibrosis; a third transplant for pulmonary fibrosis was performed a year after that. The latter two patients survived for 5 and 12 years, respectively.

Following the success with single-lung transplantation for pulmonary fibrosis, the combined heart-lung technique was considered for patients with end-stage pulmonary disease who were thought to require a bilateral rather than a unilateral transplant even if cardiac function was satisfactory. This category included patients with cystic fibrosis in whom unilateral transplantation was deemed inappropriate because of the chronic infection present in the opposite lung. It also included patients with chronic obstructive pulmonary disease (COPD) because of the potential imbalance between the distribution of ventilation and perfusion between the transplanted lung and the retained native emphysematous lung. Clearly, however, the use of combined heart-lung transplants for patients who did not require a new heart was problematic because it exposed the recipients to the unnecessary acute and long-term problems associated with cardiac transplantation and denied the use of a suitable donor heart for a more appropriate recipient in need of a heart transplant.

EN BLOC DOUBLE-LUNG TRANSPLANTATION

Cadaver dissections confirmed the feasibility of performing en bloc bilateral lung transplantation with a distal tracheal anastomosis for the airway, pulmonary artery anastomosis at the level of the main pulmonary artery, and venous anastomosis using a cuff of donor left atrium containing all four pulmonary veins. After successful experiments in a primate model, three successful double-lung transplants were performed at the University of Toronto over a 3-month period in patients with end-stage obstructive lung disease.[21] The initial patient died 14 years later of intracranial hemorrhage,

the second patient recently celebrated her 27th posttransplant anniversary and works regularly, and the third patient died of chronic rejection 12 years after transplantation.

SEQUENTIAL BILATERAL LUNG TRANSPLANTATION

Although the combined en bloc double-lung transplant procedure proved successful, it was nonetheless a complex operation from a technical standpoint and required cardiopulmonary bypass as well. It was subsequently demonstrated that replacing each lung separately using the same technique as single-lung transplantation, first on one side and then on the other, was technically simpler and clinically more successful and could usually be accomplished without the need for cardiopulmonary bypass.[22] The procedure used a transverse bilateral thoracosternotomy incision but has also been reported using separate bilateral anterior thoracotomy incisions without sternal division. The ability to perform bilateral lung transplants opened the door to performing transplants on patients with COPD and those with cystic fibrosis.

SUCCESSFUL UNILATERAL LUNG TRANSPLANTATION FOR COPD

Unilateral lung transplantation was thought unsuitable for patients with end-stage COPD because of a theoretical ventilation-perfusion imbalance between the native and transplanted lungs, but in 1989, Mal and colleagues in Paris reported successful single-lung transplants in two such patients.[23] This important contribution greatly extended the application of lung transplantation for patients with COPD.

With increasing experience, earlier postoperative extubation, enhanced lung preservation, and improved diagnosis and management of infection and acute rejection, the incidence of airway complications following lung transplantation rapidly diminished and, within several years, omentopexy was no longer found to be necessary and was generally abandoned in favor of wrapping the bronchial anastomosis with local tissues.

The achievement of successful clinical lung transplantation in the 1980s closed one chapter in the history of lung transplantation and opened the door to many others. With renewed enthusiasm, many centers were able to accelerate progress in the field. Emphasis shifted to important clinical issues, including criteria for selection of donor lungs, selection of appropriate recipients, appropriate timing for transplantation, improved organ preservation, prevention of posttransplant reperfusion injury, diagnosis and treatment of both acute and chronic rejection, improved methods for immunosuppression, technical refinements, improvements in postoperative management, and use of living donor lobes.

GROWTH OF LUNG TRANSPLANTATION

The rapid growth of solid-organ transplantation in the United States led to creation of the Organ Procurement

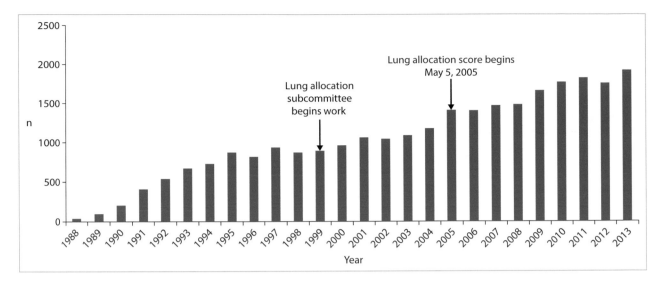

Figure 1.1 Number of isolated lung transplant procedures in the United States reported to the Organ Procurement and Transplantation Network (OPTN) annually since 1988, the first year data were available. The increase since 2005 is associated with the new lung allocation score (LAS) policy without a substantial increase in brain-dead organ donors. (OPTN Web site. http://optn.transplant.hrsa.gov. Accessed June 7, 2014.)

and Transplantation Network (OPTN) in 1986. The OPTN links the solid-organ donation and transplantation system organizations in the United States, including transplant centers, organ procurement organizations (OPOs), and histocompatibility laboratories. The United Network for Organ Sharing (UNOS), a private nonprofit organization, has been under contract with the U.S. Department of Health and Human Services to run the OPTN since its inception. The first isolated lung transplant in the United States was reported in 1987.[24] By 1988, 16 institutions in the United States were reporting lung transplant activity to UNOS; the total peaked in 1996 at 75 centers, before leveling off at 65 centers for the past 10 years. The number of lung transplants performed in the United States also increased, leveling off at about the same time (Figure 1.1).

IMPROVEMENT IN CARE

In the last 3 decades, improvements in the quality of care in intensive care units, ventilator management, and postoperative pain control, as well as early ambulation after major surgery, other quality assurance and improvement strategies, and the development of care pathways, have contributed to better outcomes after major surgery. These advances have all undoubtedly improved early postoperative care and the survival of lung transplant recipients.

Similarly, improved care of brain-injured patients may have contributed to fewer brain-dead organ donors. Earlier recognition of the futility of continuing care in severely brain-injured patients who do not meet the criteria for brain death has led to withdrawal of care and an increase in controlled donation after circulatory determination of death (cDCDD) donors. Some concerns have been raised that this practice, though medically appropriate, has contributed to the decline in brain-dead donors.

ALLOCATION OF DONOR LUNGS

Initially, the OPTN allocated lungs in the United States in the same way as hearts, through policies designed by the UNOS Thoracic Organ Committee. Lungs from brain-dead organ donors were allocated to recipients based on time waiting, first within the donor OPO and then to centers within concentric 500 nautical-mile circles. This policy was based on attempts to minimize cold ischemic time; 500 nautical miles was the distance a Learjet could fly in 1 hour.

By the late 1990s, organ allocation policies had become controversial. The shortage of brain-dead organ donors, and suitable lung donors in particular, led the lung transplant community to recommend strict listing guidelines.[25] In 1998, the Department of Health and Human Services first released the "Final Rule" on organ allocation,[26] which required the OPTN to emphasize broader sharing of organs, reduce the use of waiting time as an allocation criterion, and create equitable organ allocation systems focused on using objective medical criteria and medical urgency for allocation. A 1999 Institute of Medicine report stated that allocation should be based on measures of medical urgency while avoiding futile organ transplants, should minimize the effect of waiting time, and should use broader geographic sharing.[27] In 1999, the Lung Allocation Subcommittee of the OPTN Thoracic Organ Transplantation Committee was created to evaluate the lung allocation system and make recommendations to comply with the Final Rule.* After years of analyses, the OPTN introduced a new system of lung allocation in May 2005. Now, lungs are allocated in the United States based on a lung allocation score (LAS)

* T.M.E. was a member of the Thoracic Organ Committee and the Lung Allocation Subcommittee in 1999, and he chaired the Lung Allocation Subcommittee from 2000 through 2005.

for each potential recipient that is based on two calculated predictions: waiting list survival for the next year without a transplant (a measure of urgency) and transplant benefit, which is based on predicted 1-year survival if a lung transplant were performed minus predicted survival if the recipient continued waiting. The intent of the LAS was to reduce deaths while on the waiting list and offer lungs to those most in need (those most likely to die without a transplant), thereby minimizing wasting of lungs.[28]

Introduction of the LAS was associated with substantial changes in lung transplantation in the United States. More transplant procedures were performed (see Figure 1.1), and fibrotic lung disease became the main indication for lung transplantation instead of COPD. Death while on the waiting list was reduced. Although older and arguably sicker patients were receiving transplants, 1-year posttransplant survival was not reduced.[29] Despite the Institute of Medicine recommendation about broader geographic sharing, lungs are still allocated locally within OPOs first and then in concentric 500 nautical-mile circles. The U.S. lung allocation system has been adopted by Germany and the Netherlands, and it is used by Eurotransplant to allocate lungs between member countries when a match is not made within the donor's country.

INVOLVEMENT OF THE INTERNATIONAL SOCIETY FOR HEART AND LUNG TRANSPLANTATION

Dr. Shumway started the International Society for Heart Transplantation in 1981 to bring together people interested in this new field. In 1992, the society changed its name to the International Society for Heart and Lung Transplantation (ISHLT). Councils were formed in 1993 to facilitate interaction among physicians, surgeons, pathologists, nurses, coordinators, and other transplant professionals. The Pulmonary Council became very active, defining primary graft dysfunction (PGD), modifying classification of chronic graft dysfunction, and listing guidelines (see later).

The ISHLT began a voluntary registry and negotiated data sharing with the OPTN. To this day, almost two thirds of the lung transplant activity reported by the ISHLT Registry is from the United States, but international participation is increasing. Results from the ISHLT Lung Transplant Registry are usually cited as the benchmark for new interventions.

LUNG GRAFT DYSFUNCTION

Bronchiolitis obliterans (BO) was first reported in heart-lung transplant recipients but was soon observed in recipients of isolated lung transplants. The first conference to define chronic post–lung transplantation dysfunction was sponsored by the ISHLT in 1993.[30] It recognized the disconnect between the pathologic finding of BO and the clinical manifestation of chronic allograft dysfunction, defined and classified as changes in forced expiratory volume in the first second of respiration (FEV_1), which led to the new term *bronchiolitis obliterans syndrome* (BOS). As experience with lung transplantation accrued, changes in the original classification system were initiated through the Pulmonary Council of the ISHLT. The classification system was updated in 2001.[31] It has been updated again and is now being circulated before publication. More recently, a restrictive allograft syndrome was identified as another type of chronic lung allograft dysfunction.[32] Groups from the Pulmonary Council defined the criteria and a grading system for early PGD, which was published in 2005.[33] This system is currently undergoing revision by the Pulmonary Council.

IMMUNOSUPPRESSION

Introduction of cyclosporine allowed the widespread development of solid-organ transplantation. Minimizing reliance on high-dose steroids reduced, but did not eliminate, airway complications. Annual reports of the ISHLT Lung Transplant Registry document changes in patterns of immunosuppression over time. "Triple-drug therapy" consisting of a calcineurin inhibitor, steroids, and either azathioprine or mycophenylate mofetil remains the mainstay of immunosuppression following lung transplantation with variable use of a variety of induction strategies.

LUNG PRESERVATION

When the Toronto program first began to perform isolated lung transplants in 1983, preservation consisted simply of atelectatic hypothermic immersion in cold saline. By the mid to late 1980s, most programs were flushing lungs with modified Euro-Collins solution—the same solution that was being used for kidney preservation. The electrolyte composition of this solution mimicked the composition of intracellular fluid with a high potassium level. Using a preservation perfusate with an electrolyte composition similar to that of extracellular fluid, including a low potassium level, and with the addition of phosphate buffer and low-molecular-weight dextran, Fujimura demonstrated successful preservation for 24 hours or longer in a canine lung transplant model.[34] However, this model did not assess the early function of the transplanted lung in terms of gas exchange or pulmonary vascular resistance. Research at the University of Toronto and at Washington University[35-39] confirmed the efficacy of the Fujimura solution (low-potassium dextran [LPD] solution) and further demonstrated that the preserved lung could maintain aerobic metabolism for 12 to 24 hours by using the oxygen stored in the inflated lung during the preservation. It was also demonstrated that the addition of 1% glucose to the perfusate further improved preservation: safe, effective preservation was achieved in canine and baboon lung transplant models by using this LPD-glucose solution for periods of 12 to 24 hours.[38,39]

Steen and coworkers[40] confirmed the efficacy of the LPD-glucose solution in a porcine model and were then successful in having the solution produced commercially and approved for human use. Marketed as Perfadex, the solution is now virtually universally and very successfully used for human lung preservation, thereby greatly reducing the incidence of posttransplant dysfunction and eliminating duration of cold ischemic time as a risk factor for early death after lung transplantation (as based on ISHLT annual reports).

EX VIVO LUNG PERFUSION

Although some would consider isolated ex vivo lung perfusion (EVLP) the future of lung transplantation, not part of its history, the first lung transplant performed after EVLP was reported by Steen in 2001.[41] The procedure involved a Maastricht category II uncontrolled donation after circulatory determination of death donor (uDCDD). Steen used an EVLP system that he developed in pigs, which he later reported,[42] and a proprietary solution that bears his name. Unfortunately for the use of uDCDD, the recipient succumbed, not from graft failure, but from sepsis related to ascending cholangitis from a common bile duct stone 3 weeks after receiving a successful transplant obtained through uDCDD. Steen did not transplant any more lungs recovered from uDCDDs, but he did use his EVLP system to evaluate and "recondition" lungs recovered from brain-dead donors initially judged unsuitable for transplantation.[43]

The University of Toronto group modified the EVLP circuit by reconstructing the left atrium with proprietary cannulas from Vitrolife/XVIVO. This group reported successful lung transplants in 20 recipients using lungs evaluated with their EVLP system.[44] Nine donor lungs were recovered from cDCDD donors and 11 from conventional brain-dead donors initially judged unsuitable for transplant. The 30-day and 1-year survival rates were equivalent to those of recipients who had contemporaneously received transplant from brain-dead donors.*

This experience resulted in the widespread use of EVLP in an effort to increase the number of lungs for transplantation. Three different proprietary EVLP systems are approved for use in Europe. The Food and Drug Administration approved XVIVO's XPS EVLP system with Steen solution after a multicenter U.S. clinical trial. The impact of EVLP on the size of the lung donor pool will be limited by the number of brain-dead and cDCDD donors not affected by aspiration pneumonia and other irreversible lung pathology. EVLP may also be very useful as a therapeutic platform[45] and to evaluate lungs recovered from uDCDD donors.†

ADDITIONAL SOURCES OF DONOR LUNGS

In the mid-1990s, there was some interest in bilateral lower lobe transplants. These transplants required a small recipient and two larger donors who were healthy enough

to undergo a lower lobectomy. Most recipients were small patients with cystic fibrosis. The centers with the most experience in the United States were the University of Southern California and St. Louis Children's Hospital.[46] In most centers, survival after lobar transplants has been shorter than after conventional lung transplants.[47,48] Exceptional results have been achieved in Japan by Date's groups.[49] In the United States, this procedure has been performed rarely since introduction of the lung allocation system, presumably because as patients become ill enough to justify this procedure, a conventional donor lung is offered. In Spain and more recently in France, uDCDD has been used as a source of donor lungs. Such donation may make a larger contribution to the lung donor pool in the future.

SUMMARY

Lung transplantation has become an established therapy for end-stage lung diseases since the first success 30 years ago. Its efficacy remains limited by too few suitable lungs from conventional brain-dead organ donors, early graft failure, and chronic rejection. However, exciting developments in the field are continuing, and there is reason to believe that the progress over the past 30 years is but the prologue for major advances in the future.

ACKNOWLEDGMENT

The authors wish to acknowledge the donors and donor families who make the gift of organ transplant possible; the brave recipients, particularly the early ones whose future was so uncertain; and the surgeons, physicians, nurses, organ procurement staff, ancillary staff, and everyone involved who has made the history of lung transplantation work so relevant today. We also wish to acknowledge the administrative assistance of Melissa Thompson (University of Pennsylvania) and editorial assistance of Margaret Alford Cloud (University of North Carolina).

REFERENCES

1. Demikhov VP. Experimental Transplantation of Vital Organs. New York: Consultants Bureau Enterprises; 1962.
2. Carrel A, Guthrie CC. Anastomosis of blood vessels by the patching method and transplantation of the kidney (classical article reprinted from JAMA 1906;47:1648-51). Yale J Biol Med 2001;74:243-247.
3. Carrel A. The surgery of blood vessels, etc. Bull Johns Hopkins Hosp 1907;18:18-28.
4. Murray JE, Merrill JP. Harrison JH. Kidney transplantation between seven pairs of identical twins. Ann Surg 1958;148:343-357.
5. Juvenelle AA, Citret C, Wiles CE Jr, Stewart JD. Pneumonectomy with replantation of the lung in the dog for physiologic study. J Thorac Surg 1951;21:111-113.

---

* Dr. Cooper served as a consultant for XVIVO.
† T.M.E. is principal investigator of a National Institutes of Health–funded clinical trial to use EVLP to assess suitability of lungs for transplant recovered from uDCDD donors (www.clinicaltrials.gov NCT01615484).

6. Metras H. Note preliminaire sur la greffe totale du poumon chez le chien. C R Acad Sci (Paris). 1950;231:1176-1178.

7. Hardy JD, Eraslan S, Dalton ML. Autotransplantation and homotransplantation of the lung: Further studies. J Thorac Cardiovasc Surg 1963;46:606-615.

8. Tong MZ, Johnston DR, Pettersson GB. Bronchial artery revascularization in lung transplantation: Revival of an abandoned operation. Curr Opin Organ Transplant 2014;19:460-467.

9. Veith FJ, Richards K. Improved technic for canine lung transplantation. Ann Surg 1970;171:553-558.

10. Hardy JD, Webb WR, Dalton ML, Walker GR. Lung homotransplantation in man. JAMA 1963;186:1065-1074.

11. Derom F, Barbier F, Ringoir S, et al. Ten-month survival after lung homotransplantation in man. J Thorac Cardiovasc Surg 1971;61:835-846.

12. Wildevuur CR, Benfield JR. A review of 23 human lung transplantations by 20 surgeons. Ann Thorac Surg 1970;9:489-515.

13. Nelems JM, Duffin J, Glynn FX, et al. Extracorporeal membrane oxygenator support for human lung transplantation. J Thorac Cardiovasc Surg 1978;76:28-32.

14. Reitz BA, Wallwork JL, Hunt SA, et al. Heart-lung transplantation: Successful therapy for patients with pulmonary vascular disease. N Engl J Med 1982;306:557-564.

15. Lima O, Cooper JD, Peters WJ, et al. Effects of methylprednisolone and azathioprine on bronchial healing following lung transplantation. J Thorac Cardiovasc Surg 1981;82:211-215.

16. Goldberg M, Lima O, Morgan E, et al. A comparison between cyclosporin A and methylprednisolone plus azathioprine on bronchial healing following canine lung autotransplantation. J Thorac Cardiovasc Surg 1983;85:821-826.

17. Morgan E, Lima O, Goldberg M, et al. Improved bronchial healing in canine left lung reimplantation using omental pedicle wrap. J Thorac Cardiovasc Surg 1983;85:134-139.

18. Saunders NR, Egan TM, Chamberlain D, Cooper JD. Cyclosporine and bronchial healing in canine lung transplantation. J Thorac Cardiovasc Surg 1984;88:993-999.

19. Toronto Lung Transplant Group. Sequential bilateral lung transplantation for Paraquat poisoning. J Thorac Cardiovasc Surg 1985;89:734-742.

20. Toronto Lung Transplant Group. Unilateral lung transplantation for pulmonary fibrosis. N Engl J Med 1986;314:1140-1145.

21. Cooper JD, Patterson GA, Grossman R, et al. Double-lung transplant for advanced chronic obstructive lung disease. Am Rev Respir Dis 1989;139:303-307.

22. Pasque MK, Cooper JD, Kaiser LR, et al. Improved technique for bilateral lung transplantation: Rationale and initial clinical experience. Ann Thorac Surg 1990;49:785-791.

23. Mal H, Andreassian B, Pamela F, et al. Unilateral lung transplantation in end-stage pulmonary emphysema: Case report. Am Rev Respir Dis 1989;140:797-802.

24. Raju S, Coltharp WH, Gerken MV, et al. Successful single lung transplantation. South Med J 1988;81:931-933.

25. Orens JB, Estenne M, Arcasoy S, et al. International guidelines for the selection of lung transplant candidates: 2006 update—a consensus report from the Pulmonary Scientific Council of the International Society for Heart and Lung Transplantation. J Heart Lung Transplant 2006;25:745-755.

26. Department of Health and Human Services. Organ Procurement and Transplantation Network; Final Rule. In 42 CFR - Part 121: Federal Register, Oct. 20, 1999:56649-56661.

27. Committee on Organ Procurement and Transplantation Policy, Division of Health Sciences Policy, Institute of Medicine. Organ Procurement and Transplantation: Assessing Current Policies and the Potential Impact of the DHHS Final Rule. 1999; Washington, DC: National Academy Press. Available at http://www.nap.edu/openbook/php?isbn=030906578X.

28. Egan TM, Murray S, Bustami RT, et al. Development of the new lung allocation system in the United States (2005 SRTR Report on the State of Transplantation). Am J Transplant 2006;6:1212-1227.

29. Valapour M, Skeans MA, Heubner BM, et al. OPTN/SRTR 2012 annual data report: Lung. Am J Transplant 2014;14(Suppl 1):139-165.

30. Cooper JD, Billingham M, Egan T, et al. A working formulation for the standardization of nomenclature and for clinical staging of chronic dysfunction in lung allografts (consensus document). J Heart Lung Transplant 1993;12:713-716.

31. Estenne M, Maurer JR, Boehler A, et al. Bronchiolitis obliterans syndrome 2001: An update of the diagnostic criteria. J Heart Lung Transplant 2002;21:297-310.

32. Verleden GM, Raghu G, Meyer KC, et al. A new classification system for chronic lung allograft dysfunction. J Heart Lung Transplant 2014;33:127-133.

33. Christie JD, Carby M, Bag R, et al. Report of the ISHLT Working Group on Primary Lung Graft Dysfunction. Part II: Definition. A consensus statement of the International Society for Heart and Lung Transplantation, J Heart Lung Transplant 2005;24:1454-1459.

34. Fujimura S, Handa M, Kondo T, et al. Successful 48-hour simple hypothermic preservation of canine lung transplants. Transplant Proc 1987;19:1334-1336.

35. Jones MT, Hsieh C, Yoshikawa K, et al. A new model for assessment of lung preservation. J Thorac Cardiovasc Surg 1988;96:608-614.

36. Keshavjee SH, Yamazaki F, Cardoso PF, et al. A method for safe twelve-hour pulmonary preservation. J Thorac Cardiovasc Surg 1989;98:529-534.

37. Date H, Matsumura A, Manchester JK, et al. Changes in alveolar oxygen and carbon dioxide concentration and oxygen consumption during lung preservation: The maintenance of aerobic metabolism during lung preservation. J Thorac Cardiovasc Surg 1993;105:492-501.

38. Date H, Matsumura A, Manchester JK, et al. Evaluation of lung metabolism during successful twenty-four-hour canine lung preservation. J Thorac Cardiovasc Surg 1993;105:480-491.

39. Sundaresan S, Lima O, Date H, et al. Lung preservation with low-potassium dextran flush in a primate bilateral transplant model. Ann Thorac Surg 1993;56:1129-1135.

40. Steen S, Sjöberg T, Massa G, et al. Safe pulmonary preservation for 12 hours with low-potassium-dextran solution. Ann Thorac Surg 1993;55:434-440.

41. Steen S, Sjöberg T, Pierre L, et al. Transplantation of lungs from a non–heart beating donor. Lancet 2001;357:825-829.

42. Steen S, Liao Q, Wierup PN, et al. Transplantation of lungs from non–heart-beating donors after functional assessment ex vivo. Ann Thorac Surg 2003;76:244-252.

43. Ingemansson R, Eyjolfsson A, Mared L, et al. Clinical transplantation of initially rejected donor lungs after reconditioning ex vivo. Ann Thorac Surg 2009;87:255-260.

44. Cypel M, Yeung JC, Liu M, et al. Normothermic ex vivo lung perfusion in clinical lung transplantation. N Engl J Med 2011;364:1431-1440.

45. Cypel M, Liu M, Rubacha M, et al. Functional repair of human donor lungs by IL-10 gene therapy. Sci Transl Med 2009;1:4ra9.

46. Data Reports—Center Data. Organ Procurement and Transplantation Network. http://optn.transplant. hrsa.gov/latestData/Step2.asp. Accessed September 2, 2014.

47. Slama A, Ghanim B, Klikovits T, et al. Lobar lung transplantation—is it comparable with standard lung transplantation? Transpl Int 2014;27: 909-916.

48. Starnes VA, Bowdish ME, Woo MS, et al. A Decade of living lobar lung transplantation: Recipient outcomes. J Thorac Cardiovasc Surg 2004;127:114-122.

49. Date H. Update on living-donor lobar lung transplantation. Curr Opin Organ Transplant 2011;16:453-457.

50. Gomez-de-Antonio D, Campo-Canaveral JL, Crowley S, et al. Clinical lung transplantation from uncontrolled non–heart-beating donors revisited. J Heart Lung Transplant 2012;31:349-353.

2

Immunology of lung transplantation

ADAM S.A. GRACON AND DAVID S. WILKES*

INTRODUCTION

Lung transplantation remains the only definitive treatment available for many end-stage pulmonary diseases, including cystic fibrosis, pulmonary fibrosis, and chronic obstructive pulmonary disease. In 1905 Alexis Carrel proclaimed that the surgical challenges of organ transplantation had been overcome, but it was not until the advent of immunosuppression in the 1960s that solid-organ transplantation developed into a viable treatment option for patients.[1,2] Indeed, since the first transplant, many of the significant advances made in transplant medicine have been the result of advances in immunology. Currently, more than 3600 lung transplants are performed annually throughout the world, a dramatic increase from the 5 performed in 1985.[3] However, despite improvements in immunosuppressive regimens, surgical technology and techniques, and coordinated patient care, survival among lung allograft recipients has seen only modest improvement over the past 10 years.[3,4] This finding is largely due to difficulty in abrogating the recipient's innate immune, alloimmune, and autoimmune responses to the allograft. These processes are critical to the development of primary graft dysfunction (PGD) and acute rejection in the early posttransplant period. Additionally, they play a pivotal role in chronic lung allograft dysfunction (CLAD), a more universally inclusive term that accounts for both the restrictive and obstructive patterns that occur as a result of chronic rejection. The clinical impact of these immunologic processes is profound. A recent prospective cohort study by the Lung Transplant Outcomes Group (LTOG)

found that the rate of grade 3 PGD occurring during the first 72 hours after transplantation reached 30.8%.[5] The 2013 annual lung transplantation report from The Registry of the International Society for Heart and Lung Transplantation stated that 30% of recipients experienced an episode of acute rejection within the first year. Furthermore, the 5-year graft survival rate was 50%, primarily because of the development of CLAD.[3] Combined, these processes contribute to lung transplant recipients having the lowest 5-year survival among all solid-organ allograft recipients.[4] This fact highlights the immunology-dependent obstacles that continue to persist in lung transplantation. However, it also illustrates that despite incredible accomplishments, robust opportunities for research and innovation in lung transplant immunology exist and will be critical to improving outcomes in the future. This chapter focuses on describing the recipient's innate, alloimmune, and autoimmune responses to the allograft.

INNATE IMMUNITY

The immune response in transplantation can be divided into innate and adaptive responses. Whereas the adaptive immune response consists of T cells and antibody-producing B cells, the innate immune response includes natural killer (NK) cells, neutrophils, monocytes, innate lymphoid T cells, macrophages, platelets, NK T cells, and γδ cells, as well as pattern recognition receptors, complement proteins, chemokines, and cytokines.[6,7] The innate system serves as

* Dr. Wilkes' Laboratory is funded by National Institutes of Health grants R01 HL096845 and NIAID P01AI084853.

a first responder; it is capable of acting more rapidly than the adaptive component, but with less specificity. In fact, the innate immune system may be activated within minutes of allograft reperfusion.[8] Once activated, the components of the innate system assist in facilitating the more directed response of the adaptive system.[6] A lung with chronic environmental exposure to microbes and significant ischemia-reperfusion injury (IRI) at the time of transplantation may be particularly susceptible to the detrimental inflammatory effects associated with innate activation.

Innate immunity: Pattern recognition receptors

Pattern recognition receptors (PRRs) are a critical component of the innate immune response. The molecular basis for PRR signaling became much clearer with discovery of the Toll-like receptor (TLR) subfamily in 1997.[9] TLRs are expressed on immune cells, including dendritic cells (DCs), macrophages, and neutrophils, as well as on parenchymal tissue.[10] Ligation of PRRs, including TLRs, results in upregulation of chemokines, cytokines, and costimulatory molecules required for initiation of the adaptive immune response.[11] TLR activation has been specifically implicated in IRI in experimental models of transplantation, including the development of PGD.[12] Clinical studies of patients with TLR4 polymorphisms that result in receptor hyporesponsiveness have established an association between TLR4 and both acute rejection and bronchiolitis obliterans syndrome (BOS).[13,14] In addition to TLR, several other families of PRRs have been identified, such as nucleotide-binding oligomerization domain–like (NOD-like) receptors and retinoic acid–inducible gene-like (RIG-like) helicases.[15]

PRRs are activated as a result of interaction with structural components of the microorganism termed *pathogen-associated molecular patterns* (PAMPs) or endogenous molecules referred to as *danger-associated molecular patterns* (DAMPs).[16] DAMPs are molecules that are normally not accessible to the immune system because of their intracellular location or incorporation in the extracellular matrix. However, these molecules are released into the extracellular space following tissue injury, thus enabling their interaction with PRRs.[17] DAMPs specifically implicated in sterile inflammatory processes include high-mobility group box 1, heat shock proteins, adenosine triphosphate, uric acid, haptoglobin, hyaluronan, and heparin sulfate.[6,17]

Innate immunity: Dendritic cells

DCs are the major antigen-presenting cells (APCs) in the lung and are able to prime naïve T cells.[18,19] After transplantation, DCs directly induce the alloimmune response by either activating T cells in the lung or draining lymph nodes (Figure 2.1). Studies have found that depleting DCs significantly reduces acute allograft rejection in both animal models and human kidney transplant patients (reviewed by Solari and Thomson[19]). Studies in a mouse model of

orthotopic lung transplantation also support an essential role for DCs in acute allograft rejection.[20] However, because the mucosal surface of the lung is estimated to have a network of 500 to 750 dendritic cells/mm^2, which is comparable to the network of Langerhans cells found in the skin, depletion of DCs before lung transplantation would be difficult.[21]

The lung has different types of DCs characterized by location, cell surface receptors, and morphology. This confers biologic activity that is unique to the lung.[18] DCs capture antigens from the allograft, as well as from the environment, and as they migrate to the draining lymph nodes, their phenotype matures, thereby leading to upregulation of the costimulatory molecules necessary for effective T-cell activation.[18] The stimuli received by DCs and their particular biology determine the type of T-cell response. T-cell responses differ by the secretion of cytokines, which define different subsets, such as the helper T cells (Th) Th1 (interferon-γ [IFN-γ] and lymphotoxin), Th2 (interleukin-4 [IL-4], IL-5, and IL-13), or the newly recognized Th17 (IL-17 and IL-22).[22] Alternatively, DCs may have a more tolerogenic phenotype that activates regulatory T cells (Tregs), which can suppress other T cells or anergize T cells to make them less responsive. Interestingly, data from studies of patients with allograft tolerance have shown that DCs may be involved in promoting tolerance and may be useful as tolerogenic vaccines.[19] Future studies on the unique biology of lung DCs may offer novel therapies for inducing tolerance to lung alloantigens.

Innate immunity: Macrophages and other innate cells

Although DCs are probably the APCs responsible for initiating the alloimmune response, other innate immune cells in the lung are capable of modifying the adaptive immune response. Macrophages, neutrophils, and NK cells have been specifically implicated in transplant rejection. Macrophages are involved in pathogen defense and inflammatory amplification, and they have been shown to be a source of growth factors thought to mediate the fibroproliferation in OB in humans.[23,24] Depletion of macrophages in an isolated murine lung model has been demonstrated to attenuate the injury associated with IRI, thus suggesting a role in IRI.[25] Furthermore, macrophage depletion in a heterotopic rat tracheal model prevented the development of obliterative airways disease, a lesion that shares many features with OB, thus suggesting that macrophages may play a causative role in OB lesions as well.[26] Another role for macrophages may rely on the link between innate and adaptive immunity. Recent studies highlight the role of Th17 cells in the pathogenesis of OB,[27] and monocytes and macrophages have been suggested to play a key role in the induction of Th17 immunity.[28] In addition, Th1 immune responses were diminished in macrophage-depleted lung allografts.[29]

The role of NK cells in lung transplant rejection remains unclear, but insight gained from transplantation

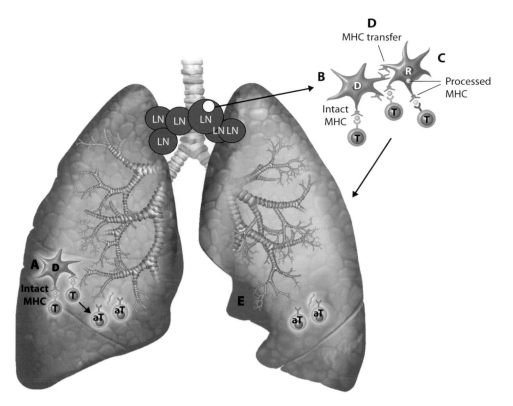

Figure 2.1 Mechanisms of initiation of an alloimmune response. After lung transplantation, allorecognition may occur via direct, indirect, or possibly semidirect antigen presentation to T cells. A, B, Direct allorecognition occurs when donor dendritic cells (DCs) (D, blue) displaying intact donor major histocompatibiltiy complex (MHC)-peptide complexes directly present antigen in the lung to naïve T cells (T) infiltrating the graft from the blood early after engraftment (A) or when donor DCs migrate from the lung allograft to lymph nodes when the lymphatics are restored (B). C, Indrect allorecognition occurs when recipient DCs (R, pink) in the draining lymph nodes activate naïve T cells with complexes of self-MHC and processed donor MHC peptides. D, Semidirect allorecognition may occur when intact donor MHC molecules are transferred from donor to recipient DCs and subsequently presented by recipient DCs to naïve T cells. E, Activated CD4+ and CD8+ T cells (aT) then return to the lung and induce rejection of the allograft.

studies in other solid organs and the lung suggests a role for these cells in the rejection response. For example, NK cells have been found to affect chronic graft vasculopathy in models of cardiac transplantation and have also been implicated in lung transplant rejection in humans.[30–32] In the case of lung transplantation, it has been demonstrated that recipients with CLAD have decreased numbers of activated NK cells in the blood, but increased numbers in the lung. This finding suggests that NK cells undergo activation peripherally with migration to the lung in the setting of CLAD.[32] NK cells are known to be resistant to calcineurin inhibitor–mediated immune suppression. Therefore, major histocompatibility complex (MHC) class I molecules expressed on donor-derived resident NK cells could remain a strong stimulus for immune responses in the immunosuppressed transplant recipient. NK cells may be a future target for therapies to prevent CLAD.[33] Invariant NK cells have also been implicated in IRI. Studies in preclinical models have demonstrated that this subset of NK cells facilitates the ischemia-reperfusion inflammatory response, including neutrophil migration, and that it is IL-17 dependent.[34]

Innate immunity: Complement

The complement system consists of three major pathways referred to as classical, lectin, and alternative. Constituents of the system include a complex array of proteins that are divided into circulating complement produced by the liver and localized complement components produced by cells migrating to or present in tissues.[35] Complement activation results in phagocytic removal or cellular lysis by membrane attack complex formation, as well as in the generation of inflammatory mediators.[36] The most critical components involved in this process are C3 and C5 and their cleavage products. The action of activated complement proteins is subsequently regulated by complement regulatory proteins, including CD55 (also known as decay-accelerating factor [DAF]) and CD46.[37,38]

Complement activation has been demonstrated to be a component of lung injury in preclinical models of IRI.[39] Clinically, the role of complement in IRI was supported by Keshavjee and colleagues, who showed that use of a complement inhibitor facilitated early extubation in transplant recipients.[40] Complement activation has also been implicated in acute transplant rejection, where it facilitates antigen processing, as well as B- and T-cell activation.[35] Obliterative bronchiolitis (OB) has also been associated with complement. Preclinical models have established elevation of C3a and downregulation of complement regulatory proteins associated with OB, a process that was reversed by complement inhibition.[41] Additionally, in contrast to their counterparts with stable graft function, transplant recipients in whom BOS develops have been found to have persistently elevated mannose-binding lectin at 6 and 12 months after transplantation.[42] C3a and C5a were reported to be elevated in bronchoalveolar lavage fluid from lung transplant recipients with histologically proven OB.[41] Complement activation may also enhance adaptive immunity, as shown by studies reporting that C3a and C5a augment alloantigen and autoantigen induction of T-cell–derived IL-17.[41] Additionally, C3a and C5a have been implicated in costimulation leading to T-cell differentiation and proliferation through interaction with their receptors on APCs and T cells.[43]

Greater understanding of the innate immune response in the lung and its impact on IRI, acute rejection, and OB may provide novel therapeutic targets.

ADAPTIVE IMMUNITY

The adaptive immune response includes both cellular and humoral components consisting of T cells and antibody-producing B cells. In contrast to the innate immune system, the adaptive system acts with more specificity and results in the generation of memory.[44,45] Both cell types are produced in the bone marrow; however, T cells undergo further maturation in the thymus, including removal of self-reactive cells. The adaptive immune response has traditionally served as the target of the immunomodulatory therapies used to date. As a result, our understanding of these pathways has been critical to progress in the posttransplant management of allograft recipients.

Adaptive immunity: Cellular and humoral alloimmunity

A critical component of solid-organ rejection is host recognition of non-self donor antigens, or the alloimmune response. After transplantation, the T-cell receptor (TCR) on host T cells recognizes the peptide-MHC (or human leukocyte antigen [HLA]) present on donor cells. However, the TCR lacks intracellular signaling capabilities. Consequently, expression of the TCR occurs in combination with CD3, and together, their protein chains form the TCR complex. The immune response to alloantigens is initiated primarily by T cells, which may then promote a B-cell response, including T-cell–dependent donor-specific B-cell production of anti-donor antibody. Antibodies bind MHC and minor histocompatibility antigens, as well as complement factor C1q, thereby resulting in activation of the complement cascade.[46]

Following the recognition of MHC antigen, T cells require secondary costimulatory signaling. This includes CD80 (B7-1) and CD86 (B7-2) on the surface of APCs binding CD28 on T cells, as well as CD40 on APCs binding CD154 (CD40L) on T cells.[47] MHC antigen recognition in conjunction with adequate costimulation results in T-cell proliferation and differentiation. The primary cell types responsible for ongoing immune reactivity include Th1 and Th17, which act mainly through the release of IFNγ and IL-17, respectively.[47] The Th2 cell and its cytokines have also been implicated in the immune response following transplantation; however, their role in lung transplantation is unclear.[48] These mediators further facilitate amplification of the immune response.[49] Why humans' evolution has included the development of alloreactive T cells is unknown, but it may be a result of the inherent affinity of the TCR for MHC molecules.[50] Additionally, induction of virus-specific memory T cells as a result of viral exposure has been implicated in cross-reaction with allogeneic HLA.[51] Humans all have circulating allogeneic lymphocytes regardless of whether they have been exposed to alloantigens in the past. These mostly naïve cells can be activated after transplantation when they are presented with their cognate antigen in the right context of MHC.

The alloimmune response depends on migration of APCs to secondary lymphoid organs. This includes traveling to the spleen, regional lymph nodes in the lung, and bronchus-associated lymphoid tissue (BALT), where T cells may be activated.[52] T cells may also be stimulated directly by DCs in the lung.[20] It has been established that initiation of T-cell alloreactivity occurs via at least two pathways (see Figure 2.1). In the *direct pathway*, recipient T cells recognize intact donor MHC molecules displayed on the surface of donor cells, either traditional APCs or other nonhematopoietic graft cells.[53,54] Studies have confirmed a role for the direct pathway in the initiation of lung transplant rejection.[20] The *indirect pathway* includes recipient APCs engulfing and processing damaged donor cells and presenting donor-derived MHC peptides to recipient T cells via self-MHC–donor peptide complexes.[55] The direct pathway, characterized by alloreactive T cells with a high precursor frequency and a multitude of receptor specificities capable of recognizing numerous allogeneic MHC molecules, dominates the early posttransplant period when numerous donor APCs are present.[53,54] In contrast, T cells involved in the indirect pathway are aimed at a single or a few principal donor MHC peptides displayed on the surface of recipient MHC molecules.[53,54] The indirect pathway is likely to remain active throughout the life of the allograft as a result of either the infiltration of recipient APCs into the allograft or the continued presence of donor antigens in the lymphoid tissue.[56] As a result, the indirect pathway may be responsible for allorecognition later in the posttransplant period and be critical in the pathogenesis of CLAD.[24,57]

Although indirect allorecognition may dominate the chronic immune response to lung allografts, direct recognition of MHC molecules by T cells can contribute to this process after donor APCs have been depleted.[58,59] CD8+ T cells recognize antigens presented by class I MHC, which exists on all cells—unlike class II MHC (CD4+ T cells), which is primarily expressed by specialized hematopoietic cells. Evidence in murine models suggests that CD8+ T cells with direct class I MHC alloreactivity to the graft persist and participate in the chronic destruction and subsequent airway obliteration of tracheal allograft transplants.[60] Furthermore, following transplantation in a rat model, class II MHC was upregulated on both the epithelium and endothelium of lung allografts.[61] Increased class II MHC on lung allografts has also been implicated in the development of CLAD.[62] Expression of class II MHC on nonhematopoietic cells in an allograft may also provide a means of direct allorecognition for CD4+ T cells, although proof of this in vivo is lacking. Persistent direct allorecognition may also be explained by the proposed *semidirect pathway* of alloantigen presentation (see Figure 2.1).[63] Semidirect allorecognition describes the process by which recipient APCs acquire intact donor MHC-peptide complexes through either cell-cell contact or exosomes.[56] This process may enable recipient APCs to interact with both CD4+ and CD8+ T cells at the same time. It is possible that episodes of acute rejection in human lung transplantation may injure lung epithelium and endothelium, thereby leading to cellular fragments of donor MHC that can be taken up by recipient APCs and presented to alloreactive T cells. However, unlike in the situation with other solid-organ allografts, no direct evidence of the semidirect pathway occurring with lung allografts exists.[24]

Acute rejection after lung transplantation occurs frequently in the first year after transplantation and is characterized by the infiltration of CD4+ and CD8+ T cells and mononuclear cells into the perivascular and peribronchiolar regions of the lung.[64] Interestingly, acute rejection can occur in the immediate postoperative period, when lymphatics are not available to drain donor APCs to secondary lymph nodes (which are thought to be the site of initiation of alloreactivity). In other solid-organ allograft animal models, removal of the lymphatics has been shown to prevent acute allograft rejection.[65] Recently, in a mouse model of orthotopic lung transplantation, Gelman and colleagues demonstrated that secondary lymphoid organs are not necessary for acute allograft rejection.[20] These data suggest that the lung is the primary site of activation of naïve allogeneic T cells (see Figure 2.1) immediately after transplantation, which makes the lung distinct from other solid organs, including the intestine.[65]

Adaptive immunity: Cellular and humoral autoimmunity

One critical pathophysiologic feature that occurs after transplantation is a cycle of repeated injury and repair.[66]

Injury may occur as a result of IRI or innate or adaptive immune responses, and it can result in the release of inflammatory products, matrix metalloproteinases, and other mediators that combine to cause interstitial remodeling. The process of remodeling exposes previously concealed autoantigens that the immune system does not encounter under normal circumstances.[67] Autoimmunity to these antigens has emerged as a significant component of the adaptive immune response. Type V collagen [col(V)], identified as one of the critical self-antigens liberated by this process, is present in the lung's perivascular and peribronchial tissues.[68] It is assembled in the same fibril as type I collagen, which effectively masks its epitopes from the immune system.[69] When the lung undergoes repeated injury, these antigenic proteins are unmasked, thereby allowing for an immune response to autoantigens. Col(V) cellular autoimmunity has been demonstrated in both animal and human studies.[47] An orthotopic rat lung transplant model with autoreactivity to col(V) has been found to exacerbate acute rejection.[70] This model has been used to reveal new-onset T-cell responses to col(V) after the development of OB in allograft recipients—a response not present with other self-antigens or in naïve animals.[71,72] Clinically, col(V)-reactive CD4+ T cells have been associated with a nearly 10-fold increase in risk for BOS after transplantation, which is greater than that associated with acute rejection episodes, HLA mismatch, or anti-HLA antibodies.[27] Cellular immune responses to col(V) are mediated by IL-17A, tumor necrosis factor α (TNF-α), and IL-1β, but not IFN-γ.[27] Whereas DCs are known to be key in initiating cellular immunity, col(V) reactivity appears to be dependent on monocytes (CD14+).[27] More recent work by Sullivan and Burlingham has implicated an ATP receptor, P2X7R, in col(V)-specific Th17 responses to self-antigens.[73] Such findings provide evidence for a new paradigm involving coordination between CD4+ T cells and monocytes that results in an effector response and suggests that autoreactive Th17 cells are mediators of BOS.[47]

The humoral response to autoantigens has included identification of col(V) and K-α1 tubulin (Kα1T) antibodies as a pathophysiologic component of BOS in preclinical models (Figure 2.2).[74,75] K-α1 tubulin is a protein constituent of microtubules that provides cytoskeletal structure as a part of normal cellular function.[76] Kα1T exposure may result from chronic injury to the airway epithelium, and col(V) exposure may result from similar inciting events. Additionally, cell surface expression can occur under certain circumstances. Anti-Kα1T antibody binding to airway epithelial cells results in transcription of the factors involved in fibroproliferation, a hallmark of OB.[74] Clinically, the presence of anti-col(V) and anti-Kα1T after transplantation has been strongly associated with BOS.[77] Furthermore, anti-col(V) and anti- Kα1T have been found in a subset of patients before transplantation, which is probably a result of their end-stage pulmonary disease—which increases the risk for BOS as well.[47,78]

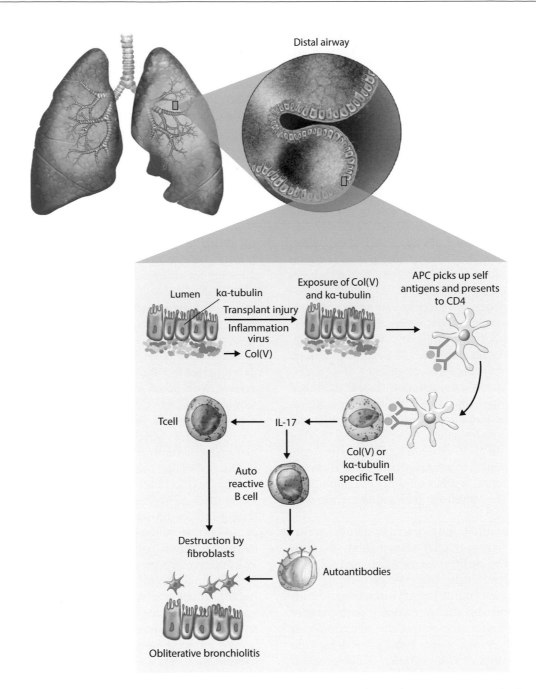

Figure 2.2 Autoimmunity in lung transplantation. After transplantation, unmasking of autoantigens, including collagen type V and K-α1 tubulin, results in both humoral and cell-mediated autoimmune responses. (Revised from Weber DJ, Wilkes DS. The role of autoimmunity in obliterative bronchiolitis after lung transplantation. Am J Physiol Lung Cell Mol Physiol 2013;304:L307-L311.)

IMMUNOLOGY OF CHRONIC ALLOGRAFT DYSFUNCTION

In the past, chronic rejection of lung allografts was diagnosed clinically on the basis of an obstructive ventilatory impairment referred to as BOS. More recently, an awareness of variations in the ventilatory defects that accompany chronic rejection, including restrictive patterns, has resulted in use of the broader term *CLAD*.[79] CLAD incorporates restrictive allograft syndrome, as well as BOS.[79] To date,

most studies have focused on immunology in the context of BOS or OB. As a result, whether other pathologic conditions encompassed by the term *CLAD* are linked to similar immunologic pathways is unknown. Studies in humans with BOS have consistently implicated persistent alloimmunity in the pathogenesis of OB. Clinically, anti-donor HLA antibodies have been demonstrated to confer an increased risk for BOS, as well as decreased survival.[80] This is mechanistically supported by the finding that anti-HLA antibodies induce fibrogenic growth factors, tissue proliferation, and apoptotic death in airway epithelial cells.[81] Anti-donor–specific indirect T-cell responses have also been associated with BOS.[57,82,83] Data from animal models support a role for alloantibodies in promoting the pathogenesis of OB but also indicate that they are not necessary to induce OB.[84,85] An association between oligoclonal expansion of CD4[+] T cells in peripheral blood and the development of BOS has also been found, thus suggesting that specific CD4[+] T cells may expand and contribute to the pathogenesis of OB.[86] Taken together, these studies suggest that the alloimmune response during both acute and chronic rejection involves a limited subset of T cells, as well as B cells and alloantibodies, which may be exploited and targeted by future therapies.[24]

REGULATORY T CELLS AND LUNG TRANSPLANTATION

One hypothesis for why autoimmunity and alloimmunity cannot be as easily suppressed once initiated is that Tregs are decreased in number, absent, or dysfunctional following transplantation.[47] Additionally, calcineurin inhibition, a key component of most recipient immunosuppression regimens, has been shown to abrogate Treg function.[87] A correlation between decreased number of Tregs and the incidence of BOS in lung transplant recipients has been reported.[88] Furthermore, Bharat and colleagues found that T-cell lines reactive to col(V) isolated from lung transplant recipients produced IL-10 and are capable of suppressing proliferation and IFN-γ secretion from autoreactive T cells.[89] However, patients in whom BOS developed had a decline in the frequency of IL-10–producing T-cell clones.[89] These data suggest that lung transplant recipients may be able to lessen the autoimmune response to col(V) through either natural Tregs or adaptive Tregs.[90] Interestingly, a recent study provided evidence that alveolar epithelial cells may induce Tregs specific for endogenous lung antigens during inflammation, thus suggesting that lung epithelium is a major regulator of induced Tregs.[91] The normal homeostasis of the lung may be undermined by immunosuppression and alloimmunity. Strategies to promote immune tolerance to alloantigens, autoantigens such as col(V), or yet-to-be-identified antigens in lung transplantation hold promise to prevent the devastating complication of CLAD.

SUMMARY

The lung can be considered a "lymph node with alveoli" that is highly susceptible to disturbances in local immune homeostasis.[92] The lung has immunocompetent cells within the airways, interstitium, and alveoli, as well as BALT, and they are sufficient to mount local immune responses even without systemic secondary lymphoid tissues.[20,92] The immune response includes both innate and adaptive components that involve alloantigens and autoantigens. T and B cells in the lung can interact with other components of the lung, such as the extracellular matrix, endothelial and epithelial cells, and cells of the innate immune system.

Therefore, the lung is immunologically unique when compared with other solid-organ allografts such as the kidney, heart, pancreas, or liver.[90] The insults encountered by the lung, such as IRI, infection, and acid reflux, induce chemokines that attract lymphoid cells to the lung and facilitate acute and chronic rejection, as well as the development of BALT. BALT may be a site of continued antigen presentation and T- and B-cell proliferation, which perpetuates the alloimmune response and induces an environment that may be susceptible to autoreactivity.[90] The lung has distinct mechanisms for maintaining immunity while avoiding impaired gas exchange, but such mechanisms may be deleterious in the face of chronic immune modulation, such as that seen in lung transplantation. Substantive improvements in the survival of lung transplant recipients are likely to occur only after we are able to fully understand how the distinct interactions between immune and nonimmune cells affect the physiology of the transplanted lung.

REFERENCES

1. Carrel A, Guthrie CC. Functions of a transplanted kidney. Science 1905;22:473.
2. Starzl TE, Marchioro TL, Waddell WR. The reversal of rejection in human renal homografts with subsequent development of homograft tolerance. Surg Gynecol Obstet 1963;117:385-395.
3. Yusen RD, Christie JD, Edwards LB, et al. The Registry of the International Society for Heart and Lung Transplantation: Thirtieth adult lung and heart-lung transplant report—2013; focus theme: Age. J Heart Lung Transplant 2013;32:965-978.
4. Lodhi SA, Lamb KE, Meier-Kriesche HU. Solid organ allograft survival improvement in the United States: The long-term does not mirror the dramatic short-term success. Am J Transplant 2011;11:1226-1235.
5. Diamond JM, Lee JC, Kawut SM, et al. Clinical risk factors for primary graft dysfunction after lung transplantation. Am J Respir Crit Care Med 2013;187:527-534.
6. Kreisel D, Goldstein DR. Innate immunity and organ transplantation: Focus on lung transplantation. Transpl Int 2013;26:2-10.
7. Spahn JH, Li W, Kreisel D. Innate immune cells in transplantation. Curr Opin Organ Transplant 2014;19:14-19.
8. Thierry A, Giraud S, Robin A, et al. The alarmin concept applied to human renal transplantation: Evidence for a differential implication of HMGB1 and IL-33. PLoS One 2014;9:e88742.
9. Medzhitov R, Preston-Hurlburt P, Janeway CA Jr. A human homologue of the Drosophila Toll protein signals activation of adaptive immunity. Nature 1997;388:394-397.
10. Iwasaki A, Medzhitov R. Toll-like receptor control of the adaptive immune responses. Nat Immunol 2004;5:987-995.

11. Xu Y, Tao X, Shen B, et al. Structural basis for signal transduction by the Toll/interleukin-1 receptor domains. Nature 2000;408:111-115.

12. Diamond JM, Wigfield CH. Role of innate immunity in primary graft dysfunction after lung transplantation. Curr Opin Organ Transplant 2013;18(5):518-523.

13. Palmer SM, Burch LH, Davis RD, et al. The role of innate immunity in acute allograft rejection after lung transplantation. Am J Respir Crit Care Med 2003;168:628-632.

14. Palmer SM, Burch LH, Trindade AJ, et al. Innate immunity influences long-term outcomes after human lung transplant. Am J Respir Crit Care Med 2005;171:780-785.

15. Akira S, Uematsu S, Takeuchi O. Pathogen recognition and innate immunity. Cell 2006;124:783-801.

16. Ibrahim ZA, Armour CL, Phipps S, Sukkar MB. RAGE and TLRs: Relatives, friends or neighbours? Mol Immunol 2013;56:739-744.

17. Chen GY, Nunez G. Sterile inflammation: Sensing and reacting to damage. Nat Rev Immunol 2010;10:826-837.

18. Cook DN, Bottomly K. Innate immune control of pulmonary dendritic cell trafficking. Proc Am Thorac Soc 2007;4:234-239.

19. Solari MG, Thomson AW. Human dendritic cells and transplant outcome. Transplantation 2008;85:1513-1522.

20. Gelman AE, Li W, Richardson SB, et al. Cutting edge: Acute lung allograft rejection is independent of secondary lymphoid organs. J Immunol 2009;182:3969-3973.

21. Holt PG. Pulmonary dendritic cells in local immunity to inert and pathogenic antigens in the respiratory tract. Proc Am Thorac Soc 2005;2:116-120.

22. Reinhardt RL, Kang SJ, Liang HE, Locksley RM. T helper cell effector fates—who, how and where? Curr Opin Immunol 2006;18:271-277.

23. Hertz MI, Henke CA, Nakhleh RE, et al. Obliterative bronchiolitis after lung transplantation: A fibroproliferative disorder associated with platelet-derived growth factor. Proc Natl Acad Sci U S A 1992;89:10385-10389.

24. Grossman EJ, Shilling RA. Bronchiolitis obliterans in lung transplantation: The good, the bad, and the future. Transl Res 2009;153:153-165.

25. Zhao M, Fernandez LG, Doctor A, et al. Alveolar macrophage activation is a key initiation signal for acute lung ischemia-reperfusion injury. Am J Physiol Lung Cell Mol Physiol 2006;291:L1018-1026.

26. Oyaizu T, Okada Y, Shoji W, et al. Reduction of recipient macrophages by gadolinium chloride prevents development of obliterative airway disease in a rat model of heterotopic tracheal transplantation. Transplantation 2003;76:1214-1220.

27. Burlingham WJ, Love RB, Jankowska-Gan E, et al. IL-17–dependent cellular immunity to collagen type V predisposes to obliterative bronchiolitis in human lung transplants. J Clin Invest 2007;117:3498-506.

28. Evans HG, Gullick NJ, Kelly S, et al. In vivo activated monocytes from the site of inflammation in humans specifically promote Th17 responses. Proc Natl Acad Sci U S A 2009;106:6232-6237.

29. Sekine Y, Bowen LK, Heidler KM, et al. Role of passenger leukocytes in allograft rejection: Effect of depletion of donor alveolar macrophages on the local production of TNF-alpha, T helper 1/T helper 2 cytokines, IgG subclasses, and pathology in a rat model of lung transplantation. J Immunol 1997;159:4084-4093.

30. Uehara S, Chase CM, Colvin RB, et al. Further evidence that NK cells may contribute to the development of cardiac allograft vasculopathy. Transplant Proc 2005;37:70-71.

31. Uehara S, Chase CM, Kitchens WH, et al. NK cells can trigger allograft vasculopathy: The role of hybrid resistance in solid organ allografts. J Immunol 2005;175:3424-3430.

32. Fildes JE, Yonan N, Tunstall K, et al. Natural killer cells in peripheral blood and lung tissue are associated with chronic rejection after lung transplantation. J Heart Lung Transplant 2008;27:203-207.

33. Fildes JE, Yonan N, Leonard CT. Natural killer cells and lung transplantation, roles in rejection, infection, and tolerance. Transpl Immunol 2008;19:1-11.

34. Sharma AK, LaPar DJ, Zhao Y, et al. Natural killer T cell–derived IL-17 mediates lung ischemia-reperfusion injury. Am J Respir Crit Care Med 2011;183:1539-1549.

35. Chen G, Chen S, Chen X. Role of complement and perspectives for intervention in transplantation. Immunobiology 2013;218:817-827.

36. Sacks SH, Zhou W. The role of complement in the early immune response to transplantation. Nat Rev Immunol 2012;12:431-442.

37. Medof ME, Kinoshita T, Nussenzweig V. Inhibition of complement activation on the surface of cells after incorporation of decay-accelerating factor (DAF) into their membranes. J Exp Med 1984;160:1558-1578.

38. Yu GH, Holers VM, Seya T, et al. Identification of a third component of complement-binding glycoprotein of human platelets. J Clin Invest 1986;78:494-501.

39. Eppinger MJ, Deeb GM, Bolling SF, Ward PA. Mediators of ischemia-reperfusion injury of rat lung. Am J Pathol 1997;150:1773-1784.

40. Keshavjee S, Davis RD, Zamora MR, et al. A randomized, placebo-controlled trial of complement inhibition in ischemia-reperfusion injury after lung transplantation in human beings. J Thorac Cardiovasc Surg 2005;129:423-428.

41. Suzuki H, Lasbury ME, Fan L, et al. Role of complement activation in obliterative bronchiolitis post-lung transplantation. J Immunol 2013;191:4431-4439.

42. Carroll KE, Dean MM, Heatley SL, et al. High levels of mannose-binding lectin are associated with poor outcomes after lung transplantation. Transplantation 2011;91:1044-1049.

43. Strainic MG, Liu J, Huang D, et al. Locally produced complement fragments C5a and C3a provide both costimulatory and survival signals to naive CD4+ T cells. Immunity 2008;28:425-435.

44. Delves PJ, Roitt IM. The immune system. First of two parts. N Engl J Med 2000;343:37-49.

45. Delves PJ, Roitt IM. The immune system. Second of two parts. N Engl J Med 2000;343:108-117.

46. McManigle W, Pavlisko EN, Martinu T. Acute cellular and antibody-mediated allograft rejection. Semin Respir Crit Care Med 2013;34:320-335.

47. Gracon AS, Wilkes DS. Lung transplantation: Chronic allograft dysfunction and establishing immune tolerance. Hum Immunol 2014;75:887-894.

48. Illigens BM, Yamada A, Anosova N, et al. Dual effects of the alloresponse by Th1 and Th2 cells on acute and chronic rejection of allotransplants. Eur J Immunol 2009;39:3000-3009.

49. Derks RA, Jankowska-Gan E, Xu Q, Burlingham WJ. Dendritic cell type determines the mechanism of bystander suppression by adaptive T regulatory cells specific for the minor antigen HA-1. J Immunol 2007;179:3443-3451.

50. Felix NJ, Allen PM. Specificity of T-cell alloreactivity. Nat Rev Immunol 2007;7:942-953.

51. D'Orsogna LJA, Roelen DL, Doxiadis IIN, Claas FHJ. Alloreactivity from human viral specific memory T-cells. Transpl Immunol 2010;23:149-155.

52. Larsen CP, Morris PJ, Austyn JM. Migration of dendritic leukocytes from cardiac allografts into host spleens. A novel pathway for initiation of rejection. J Exp Med 1990;171:307-314.

53. Benichou G. Direct and indirect antigen recognition: The pathways to allograft immune rejection. Front Biosci 1999;4:D476-D480.

54. Game DS, Lechler RI. Pathways of allorecognition: Implications for transplantation tolerance. Transpl Immunol 2002;10:101-108.

55. Lechler RI, Batchelor JR. Restoration of immunogenicity to passenger cell–depleted kidney allografts by the addition of donor strain dendritic cells. J Exp Med 1982;155:31-41.

56. Gokmen MR, Lombardi G, Lechler RI. The importance of the indirect pathway of allorecognition in clinical transplantation. Curr Opin Immunol 2008;20:568-574.

57. Stanford RE, Ahmed S, Hodson M, et al. A role for indirect allorecognition in lung transplant recipients with obliterative bronchiolitis. Am J Transplant 2003;3:736-742.

58. Lee RS, Grusby MJ, Glimcher LH, et al. Indirect recognition by helper cells can induce donor-specific cytotoxic T lymphocytes in vivo. J Exp Med 1994;179:865-872.

59. Smyth LA, Afzali B, Tsang J, et al. Intercellular transfer of MHC and immunological molecules: Molecular mechanisms and biological significance. Am J Transplant 2007;7:1442-1449.

60. Richards DM, Dalheimer SL, Hertz MI, Mueller DL. Trachea allograft class I molecules directly activate and retain CD8+ T cells that cause obliterative airways disease. J Immunol 2003;171:6919-6928.

61. Romaniuk A, Prop J, Petersen AH, et al. Expression of class II major histocompatibility complex antigens by bronchial epithelium in rat lung allografts. Transplantation 1987;44:209-214.

62. Burke CM, Glanville AR, Theodore J, Robin ED. Lung immunogenicity, rejection, and obliterative bronchiolitis. Chest 1987;92:547-549.

63. Herrera OB, Golshayan D, Tibbott R, et al. A novel pathway of alloantigen presentation by dendritic cells. J Immunol 2004;173:4828-4837.

64. Wilkes DS, Egan TM, Reynolds HY. Lung transplantation: Opportunities for research and clinical advancement. Am J Respir Crit Care Med 2005;172:944-955.

65. Wang J, Dong Y, Sun JZ, et al. Donor lymphoid organs are a major site of alloreactive T-cell priming following intestinal transplantation. Am J Transplant 2006;6:2563-2571.

66. Sumpter TL, Wilkes DS. Role of autoimmunity in organ allograft rejection: A focus on immunity to type V collagen in the pathogenesis of lung transplant rejection. Am J Physiol Lung Cell Mol Physiol 2004;286:L1129-L1139.

67. Iwata T, Chiyo M, Yoshida S, et al. Lung transplant ischemia reperfusion injury: Metalloprotease inhibition down-regulates exposure of type V collagen, growth-related oncogene-induced neutrophil chemotaxis, and tumor necrosis factor-alpha expression. Transplantation 2008;85:417-426.

68. Madri JA, Furthmayr H. Isolation and tissue localization of type AB2 collagen from normal lung parenchyma. Am J Pathol 1979;94:323-331.

69. Birk DE, Fitch JM, Babiarz JP, Linsenmayer TF. Collagen type I and type V are present in the same fibril in the avian corneal stroma. J Cell Biol 1988;106:999-1008.

70. Sumpter TL, Wilkes DS. Role of autoimmunity in organ allograft rejection: A focus on immunity to type V collagen in the pathogenesis of lung transplant rejection. Am J Physiol Lung Cell Mol Physiol 2004;286:L1129-L1139.

71. Yasufuku K, Heidler KM, O'Donnell PW, et al. Oral tolerance induction by type V collagen downregulates lung allograft rejection. Am J Respir Cell Mol Biol 2001;25:26-34.

72. Yasufuku K, Heidler KM, Woods KA, et al. Prevention of bronchiolitis obliterans in rat lung allografts by type V collagen-induced oral tolerance. Transplantation 2002;73:500-505.

73. Sullivan JA, Jankowska-Gan E, Shi L, et al. Differential requirement for P2X7R function in IL-17 dependent vs IL-17 independent cellular immune responses. Am J Transplant. 2014; 4:1512-1522.

74. Goers TA, Ramachandran S, Aloush A, et al. De novo production of K-alpha1 tubulin-specific antibodies: Role in chronic lung allograft rejection. J Immunol 2008;180:4487-4494.

75. Haque MA, Mizobuchi T, Yasufuku K, et al. Evidence for immune responses to a self-antigen in lung transplantation: Role of type V collagen–specific T cells in the pathogenesis of lung allograft rejection. J Immunol 2002;169:1542-1549.

76. Yin S, Zeng C, Hari M, Cabral F. Paclitaxel resistance by random mutagenesis of alpha-tubulin. Cytoskeleton (Hoboken) 2013;70:849-862.

77. Saini D, Weber J, Ramachandran S, et al. Alloimmunity-induced autoimmunity as a potential mechanism in the pathogenesis of chronic rejection of human lung allografts. J Heart Lung Transplant 2011;30:624-631.

78. Tiriveedhi V, Gautam B, Sarma NJ, et al. Pre-transplant antibodies to Kalpha1 tubulin and collagen-V in lung transplantation: Clinical correlations. J Heart Lung Transplant 2013;32:807-814.

79. Verleden GM, Raghu G, Meyer KC, et al. A new classification system for chronic lung allograft dysfunction. J Heart Lung Transplant 2014;33:127-133.

80. Palmer SM, Davis RD, Hadjiliadis D, et al. Development of an antibody specific to major histocompatibility antigens detectable by flow cytometry after lung transplant is associated with bronchiolitis obliterans syndrome. Transplantation 2002;74:799-804.

81. Jaramillo A, Smith CR, Maruyama T, et al. Anti–HLA class I antibody binding to airway epithelial cells induces production of fibrogenic growth factors and apoptotic cell death: A possible mechanism for bronchiolitis obliterans syndrome. Hum Immunol 2003;64:521-529.

82. SivaSai KS, Smith MA, Poindexter NJ, et al. Indirect recognition of donor HLA class I peptides in lung transplant recipients with bronchiolitis obliterans syndrome. Transplantation 1999;67:1094-1098.

83. Reznik SI, Jaramillo A, SivaSai KS, et al. Indirect allorecognition of mismatched donor HLA class II peptides in lung transplant recipients with bronchiolitis obliterans syndrome. Am J Transplant 2001;1:228-235.

84. Kuo E, Maruyama T, Fernandez F, Mohanakumar T. Molecular mechanisms of chronic rejection following transplantation. Immunol Res 2005;32:179-185.

85. Higuchi T, Jaramillo A, Kaleem Z, et al. Different kinetics of obliterative airway disease development in heterotopic murine tracheal allografts induced by CD4+ and CD8+ T cells. Transplantation 2002;74:646-651.

86. Duncan SR, Leonard C, Theodore J, et al. Oligoclonal CD4(+) T cell expansions in lung transplant recipients with obliterative bronchiolitis. Am J Respir Crit Care Med 2002;165:1439-1444.

87. Miroux C, Morales O, Ghazal K, et al. In vitro effects of cyclosporine A and tacrolimus on regulatory T-cell proliferation and function. Transplantation 2012;94:123-131.

88. Mamessier E, Lorec AM, Thomas P, et al. T regulatory cells in stable posttransplant bronchiolitis obliterans syndrome. Transplantation 2007;84:908-916.

89. Bharat A, Fields RC, Trulock EP, Patterson GA, Mohanakumar T. Induction of IL-10 suppressors in lung transplant patients by CD4+25+ regulatory T cells through CTLA-4 signaling. J Immunol 2006;177:5631-5638.

90. Shilling RA, Wilkes DS. Immunobiology of chronic lung allograft dysfunction: New insights from the bench and beyond. Am J Transplant 2009;9:1714-1718.

91. Gereke M, Jung S, Buer J, Bruder D. Alveolar type II epithelial cells present antigen to CD4(+) T cells and induce Foxp3(+) regulatory T cells. Am J Respir Crit Care Med 2009;179:344-355.

92. Moyron-Quiroz JE, Rangel-Moreno J, Kusser K, et al. Role of inducible bronchus associated lymphoid tissue (iBALT) in respiratory immunity. Nat Med 2004;10:927-934.

93. Weber DJ, Wilkes DS. The role of autoimmunity in obliterative bronchiolitis after lung transplantation. Am J Physiol Lung Cell Mol Physiol 2013;304:L307-L311.

3

Ethical considerations in transplantation: A focus on lung transplantation

BADDR A. SHAKHSHEER, SEAN C. WIGHTMAN, SAVITRI FEDSON, AND MARK SIEGLER

BACKGROUND OF LUNG TRANSPLANTATION

Even the first-ever reported lung transplant was accompanied by ethical controversy. On April 15, 1963, John Russell, a 58-year-old prisoner at the Mississippi State Penitentiary serving a life sentence for murder, was admitted to the University of Mississippi Medical Center with recurrent pneumonia unresponsive to antibiotics. He had squamous cell carcinoma of his left lung and was also suffering from emphysema and kidney disease. On June 11, 1963, famed surgeon Dr. James D. Hardy performed a lung transplant on this prisoner and published the case as the first reported lung transplant.[1] The patient did well initially but succumbed to complications of renal failure and died 18 days after the operation. In a five-paragraph section titled "The Moral Decision," Hardy stated, "Although the patient was serving a life sentence for a capital offense, there was no discussion with him regarding the possibility of a change in his prison sentence. However, authorities of the state government were contacted privately, and they indicated that a very favorable attitude might be adopted if the patient were to contribute to human progress in this way." The Governor of Mississippi, Ross Barnett, issued a proclamation commuting Russell's prison sentence, stating that the transplant would "alleviate human misery and suffering in years to come."

The last 30 years have seen an increase in the safety and efficacy of lung transplantation. In the 1960s and 1970s, 38 lung transplant surgeries were attempted with minimal long-term success, mostly attributable to a lack of effective postoperative immunosuppressive management.[2] The introduction of cyclosporine into clinical practice in the 1980s, combined with improved operative technique, led to better patient outcomes and wider acceptance of lung transplantation as an efficacious treatment of end-stage lung disease. In the most recent data published by the International Society for Heart and Lung Transplantation (ISHLT), adults undergoing lung transplantation have a median survival of 5.6 years, with an increased life span in the case of bilateral lung transplant recipients.[3] For comparison, median survival after heart transplantation worldwide is 11 years.[4] Indications for transplantation of the lung, in order of frequency, include chronic obstructive pulmonary disease (COPD), interstitial lung disease (including idiopathic pulmonary fibrosis), cystic fibrosis, α_1-antitrypsin deficiency, and pulmonary hypertension.[3] According to the ISHLT Registry, 3640 lung transplants were performed globally in 2011. Most were bilateral transplants. That number has increased significantly since 2005, around the time when the lung allocation score (LAS) was implemented in the United States and Donate Life America implemented its Donor Designation Collaborative to increase the total number of registered donors.

As with all solid-organ transplants, lack of available donor organs is the predominant factor limiting the number of lung transplants performed. The availability of donor lungs is further limited because the lung is especially susceptible to medical complications that arise during a potential donor's hospitalization, thereby often excluding the lungs from transplant eligibility. Such medical complications include aspiration, ventilator-associated lung injury, pneumonia, pulmonary edema, and thoracic trauma. For these reasons, hearts, livers, and kidneys are procured from cadaveric donors in far greater numbers than lungs.

ETHICAL CONSIDERATIONS

The field of solid-organ transplantation raises many ethical concerns. These issues arise because of the scarcity of organs and the subsequent disparity between the number of available organs and the larger number of patients who need these vital organs to survive. Furthermore, the field of transplantation frequently has more than one patient to consider: the potential donor, the potential recipient, and often, other potential recipients and their needs. As immunosuppression and therapies for patients on the waiting list have improved, the number of patients eligible for lung transplants has increased the demand-supply ratio, which has in turn increased the ethical issues related to the field. To best proceed with an ethical analysis of lung transplantation, certain key terms should be defined: *equity* denotes impartiality and a lack of bias, *justice* refers to the principle of distribution of benefits fairly among all participants in the system, and *utility* is a principle that attempts to maximize the benefit of a situation to all participants—donors and recipients.

Access

In the United States, the organ transplant system is managed by the United Network for Organ Sharing (UNOS). For a potential recipient to be considered for lung transplantation, the patient must have access to a transplant center. Because of the medical resources required to optimize performance, lung transplant centers exist only in large tertiary care facilities, which are often located in urban areas. In addition to being limited by geography, patients' access to transplantation can also be limited by their physicians' lack of information (which may hinder patients' timely referral for transplantation as a potential therapy) and by insurance barriers. UNOS has undertaken major education efforts for both health care providers and patients in an effort to maximize the efficacy of timely referral of appropriate patients to transplant centers.

Medical contraindications to a potential transplant include cancer or comorbid conditions that would otherwise limit duration of life after transplantation. The use of advanced age as an exclusionary criterion to lung transplantation is controversial. Since 1985, the median age of lung transplant recipients has increased from 45 to 55 years, with North American transplant centers leading in the trend of performing transplants in older recipients.[3] However, age is still used as an exclusionary criterion that is often justified by the concept of "physiologic age" in conjunction with the presence of other comorbid conditions. It is worth noting that no age limit has been established as an absolute contraindication to lung transplantation.

Lung transplantation is expensive. The cost of the surgery itself is daunting and includes procurement, operative, and postoperative hospitalization costs. These costs are greatly increased by posttransplant care, including immunosuppressive medications, anti-infective medications, and posttransplantation surveillance visits and procedures.

According to the 2008 Milliman research report, hospitalization for a lung transplant in the United States costs $256,600 for a single-lung transplant and $344,700 for a bilateral lung transplant. When physician costs, posttransplant care for the first 180 days, and medications are factored in, these costs increase to $450,400 for a single-lung transplant and to $657,800 for a bilateral lung transplant. For comparison, the cost of an admission for heart transplantation is $486,400 and $787,700 when posttransplant care, physician costs, and medications are factored in. A kidney transplant is far less expensive; it is priced at $92,700 for the hospitalization and $259,000 when the other costs are taken into account. The average cost of a liver transplant is similar to that of a lung transplant: $286,100 for the hospitalization and $523,400 when the adjunctive costs are included.[5] A study of lung transplants performed at Johns Hopkins University Hospital between 2005 and 2009 demonstrated that the sickest patients are the most expensive. The median cost for patients with the lowest LASs was $153,995; the median cost for patients with LASs in the highest quartile was significantly higher: $276,668.[6] Because of the costs associated with transplantation, patients in the United States are routinely excluded from transplantation if they are not insured. The impact of the Patient Protection and Affordable Care Act of 2010 on access to health care and thus on transplant centers has yet to be determined.

Organ allocation

Historically, organ allocation has been based strictly on time on the transplant waiting list. One purported benefit of this system is that it appears to maximize equity because it is blinded to patient factors; on the other hand, it does nothing to address utility arguments, which attempt to maximize the efficacy of transplanted organs. The ideal allocation system should endeavor to benefit the greatest number of patients with the best possible clinical outcomes while optimizing survival for those on the waiting list.

In 2005, the LAS was implemented in the United States to address long waiting list times and subsequent high waiting list mortality.[4] New features of the LAS included a posttransplant survival measure and an urgency measure, thus estimating the time that a patient would be expected to live without a transplant. These measures were calculated by using statistical models based on a potential recipient's clinical and physiologic parameters.[7]

The ethical implications of such a system are important. First, the LAS establishes potential benefit from transplantation as being more important than absolute waiting list time by attempting to place greater emphasis on systemic utility and by relying on predicted outcomes rather than a standard queue. The outcome is complicated: are all lives saved of equal value? Are absolute potential years of life all that should be optimized, or should quality of life or even age of the potential recipient be considered? Potential life extension in number of years may be evaluated because it seems to be the least biased measure of transplant success;

however, it may not provide absolute equity in the system inasmuch as models may be biased toward certain inciting pathologies and may not yield the desired utility because quality of life after transplantation is not evaluated. For instance, since implementation of the LAS, fewer patients with COPD have received transplants.[8] Patients with COPD are more likely than other patients with end-stage lung disease to be better compensated before transplantation, and this results in a lower LAS and thus in a lower likelihood of receiving a transplant. Compounding this, patients with COPD are more likely than patients with other causes of end-stage lung disease to have been former smokers, and a possible bias against former smokers in organ allocation has emerged.

Utility

RECIPIENT FACTORS

In addition to performing physiologic evaluation, transplant centers also assess patients based on psychosocial factors. This approach often includes a multidisciplinary team of psychologists, psychiatrists, and social workers. However, no uniform criteria for evaluating candidacy exist. According to the ISHLT, absolute contraindications to consideration for lung transplantation include "untreatable psychiatric or psychological condition associated with the inability to cooperate or comply with medical therapy" and "absence of a consistent or reliable social support system."[9] Data specific to psychosocial evaluation in lung transplantation are sparse; however, heart transplantation programs in the United States are more apt to perform psychosocial evaluation; they use evaluation in 92% of cases as opposed to 57% of cases in non-U.S. centers.[10]

The goal of psychosocial assessment is to evaluate potential adherence to medical recommendations, to assess coping mechanisms for dealing with the stress associated with transplantation, to ensure understanding of the transplant process and its responsibilities, to investigate potential substance abuse, and to determine social support. In 2008, a consensus conference on nonadherence in the context of immunosuppressive medications differentiated between compliance, in which patient behavior "matches the provider's recommendations," and adherence, in which patient behavior "matches the agreed-upon provider's recommendations," with adherence preferentially highlighted.[11] Adherence implies consideration of systems issues. For instance, a transplant center may endeavor to colocate surgical and medical clinics and coordinate appointment times to ease the burden of patient visits, which can improve adherence.

Nonadherence in both chronic diseases and solid-organ transplantation is well studied, with published rates often reaching 25%. Few studies include lung transplant patients even though the consequences of nonadherence for a lung transplant recipient far outweigh those for a kidney transplant patient inasmuch as there is no equivalent of dialysis for lung failure. A single-institution study from the University of Pittsburgh demonstrated a 13% medication nonadherence rate in lung transplant recipients in the first 2 years after transplantation.[12] In addition, this study cited a 62% rate of nonadherence to spirometry recommendations. A study of pretransplant medication adherence in heart, liver, and lung patients correlated nonadherence with a higher educational level and younger age.[13]

Evaluation of depression and other psychological disorders by assessment instruments is a robust field, and transplant-specific assessments have been developed as well. Tools include the Transplant Evaluation Rating Score,[14] the Psychosocial Assessment of Candidates for Transplantation,[15] and the Pediatric Transplant Rating Instrument.[16] These field-specific assessments focus on stressors specific to transplant patients, including time on the waiting list before transplantation and the posttransplant course.

DONOR FACTORS

The scarcity of solid donor organs is especially acute in lung transplantation. This scarcity may be due to the aforementioned medical factors and to the fact that lungs are especially susceptible to injury during the critical illnesses that often lead to death (e.g., ventilator injury during pneumonia). Many measures have been implemented in an attempt to increase the cadaveric donor supply of solid organs. Such efforts include less strict brain death standards, required request of patients' organ donation status, presumed consent, "expanded criteria" donors, and donation after cardiac death (DCD).

Donation after cardiac death is used much less frequently for lungs than for abdominal organs. Some programs will reintubate DCD donors, thereby raising ethical questions regarding interventions in a deceased donor for the benefit of a recipient. Long-term data on the success of DCD lungs are still pending, but a study from the Netherlands indicated that although up to 28% of DCD lungs may be suitable for procurement, only 5% were procured.[17]

Living donor lung transplantation was first performed in the United States in 1990. Living donation of organs raises many ethical questions, including the potential harm to the donor for no or limited recipient benefit and the possibility of donor coercion.[18] Living donors may benefit psychologically from helping a loved one, but they may also benefit financially in cases in which the recipient is the primary income provider for the family. Because only a single lobe is donated, more than one living donor is often necessary for adequate functioning of the recipient's lung with most conditions. Living donor lung transplants are now rarely performed in the United States; however, countries such as Japan use living donors for up to two thirds of their lung transplants.[19] Because of its limitations, living donor lung transplantation is usually reserved for cases in which the potential recipient is too sick to probably survive the approximate waiting list time required to obtain a cadaveric lung transplant. This fact highlights the complicated relationship between the living donor and the recipient. Because the living donor is usually a relative or close friend, the donor is often under undue pressure in these already stressful circumstances. Here, a potential recipient is too sick to survive the time on the waiting list for donor organs, so the family and friends are subjected to a request to donate. This request almost obligates family members to donate if they want to offer the recipient all potential chances of survival. In such stressful and time-limited circumstances it is essential that extra evaluation of donor motives, risk, and benefits be carefully considered. Therefore, living donor advocates are essential to the transplantation process and are often required by law.

PAYMENT FOR ORGANS

Organ transplantation has always been a field in which demand has surpassed supply. The issue of payment for organs is raised on a regular basis. In 1984, the National Organ Transplant Act was passed and forbade "any person to knowingly acquire, receive, or otherwise transfer any human organ for valuable consideration for use in human transplantation." However, other countries, including India, Turkey, Pakistan, and Iran, have implemented market systems for organs.

Proponents of market exchanges in the United States argue that payment for organ donors will increase the donor pool and ease the supply-demand difference. Compensation has been proposed in both a direct (i.e., cash payment) and indirect (funeral vouchers, health insurance, directed charitable contributions) manner.

Those against payment for organs argue that other methods should be used to increase the donor pool. For instance, the maximum number of potential deceased donors in this country is 13,000 per year, and 60% of them donate; increasing this number could yield an additional 4000 donors per year.[20] Concerns about exploitation of the poor also exist. Data from Iran substantiate this claim: Ghods and colleagues found that 84% of paid kidney donors were poor.[21] Goyal and associates found that 96% of Indian donors sold kidneys to resolve financial debts.[22] Furthermore, the quality of purchased organs is a concern; data from Pakistan show higher rates of hepatitis B and C as well as decreased renal function in vendor donors.[23] Canadian data have confirmed the same problem: worse graft survival and patient outcomes with commercially acquired donors.[24] Finally, some oppose the idea of payment for organs on a philosophical basis and ask the question: should the body be treated as a commodity?

CONTEXTUAL FEATURES

A common approach to reaching clinical ethics decisions is through the four-box model, which uses categories to analyze an ethical case from multiple perspectives.[25] Each category is grounded and supported by the four ethical principles of beneficence, nonmaleficence, respect for autonomy, and justice. Like many surgical ethics cases, those involving lung transplantation also require consideration of the first three boxes of the model: medical indications, patient preference, and quality of life. However, what sets transplantation drastically apart from other surgical ethics scenarios are the components of the fourth box: contextual features. Unlike a typical surgical case, a lung transplantation case must incorporate the issues of scarce health resources, public health, and conflicts of interest.

Organ allocation, mentioned earlier, is especially pertinent to lung transplantation in that a lung is a scarce health resource. For most pathologic conditions, recipients can undergo either single-lung transplantation or bilateral lung transplantation. Bilateral lung transplant recipients have greater individual long-term survival.[3] However, the two organs could be split and given to two potential recipients. Thus the ethical question is raised: should the system favor maximizing the number of patients receiving transplants and accepting a potentially decreased length of life after transplantation, or should we maximize the length of life per transplant recipient? Retransplantation is used when chronic graft dysfunction, bronchiolitis obliterans, and severe airway problems result in failure of the graft. Survival rates for retransplantation are lower than those for initial lung transplants, with 1-year survival rates of 65% versus 85% in the primary transplant group in this publication.[26] Currently, retransplantation is reserved for patients who are ambulatory and meet most of the other criteria for an initial lung transplant. Retransplantation raises questions of justice: why should a patient receive a second organ when so many have yet to receive their first?[18,27] How does the medical community compare these two patient populations clinically and ethically?

Because lungs for transplantation are provided by the public, usually in the form of a deceased individual whose family consented to organ procurement, the public as a whole must be considered when decisions about organ use are made. Systems and procedures, many discussed earlier, have been created and are currently in place to ensure fair, equitable, and timely allotment of the limited supply of lungs. However, these systems and procedures are complicated, and although the goal is to be equitable, we must continue to challenge current standards and protocols and monitor to prevent marginalizing underserved populations.

All patients who receive a lung transplant trade the sequelae of end-stage lung disease for the complications associated with lung transplantation. Accordingly, informed consent should cover these topics in depth so that patients can choose appropriately based on their personal values. Although surgeons are trained to identify appropriate operative candidates and routinely obtain the consent for organ transplantation, they have an innate bias toward surgery. This bias often takes the form of surgeons pushing for the treatment that they believe is best for the patient. Careful evaluation must be performed when explaining the risks associated with this complicated procedure to confirm patient understanding of the procedure and, more importantly, the alternatives. It can be beneficial to have additional parties (family or friends) who also understand the patient's personal beliefs and desires present during the consenting process. These steps are designed to confirm that patients understand the procedure and, more importantly, that the final treatment plan is consistent with the patient's individual life goals. Achieving intentional, meaningful, and informed consent in this process definitely includes surgeon patience and is often accompanied by multiple long visits to ensure that difficult-to-understand health care issues are explained in a satisfactory manner.

The Sarah Murnaghan case

In May 2013, the case of Sarah Murnaghan in Philadelphia, Pennsylvania, garnered national attention. At the time, Sarah was a 10-year-old girl suffering from end-stage lung disease secondary to cystic fibrosis. She had been hospitalized for 3 months and was dependent on a ventilator. Her physicians estimated that without a transplant, she would die within 1 month. Under UNOS rules at the time, children younger than 12 years were allocated lungs based on time spent on the waiting list, whereas older children were included in the adult donor pool, with organ allocation based on individual LASs.[28] The donor pool for children younger than 12 years is far smaller than that for adults; outcomes in this age group versus in adults are controversial. Murnaghan's parents appealed to the Organ Procurement and Transplantation Network (OPTN) for an exception, and their request was denied by the Health and Human Services Secretary Kathleen Sebelius. Sebelius ordered a review of the lung transplant policy, but given Murnaghan's critically ill state, she would not survive to see the results. Therefore, her parents turned to the media and politicians, claiming that the policy was arbitrary and amounted to age discrimination.

The parents' efforts led a federal judge to grant a temporary restraining order allowing Murnaghan to be listed for an adult lung transplant. At the time, Murnaghan's LAS was 91 out of 100, and on June 12, 2013, she underwent double-lung transplantation from an adult donor. The lungs failed within hours, and Murnaghan was placed on an extracorporeal membrane oxygenation (ECMO) circuit and relisted for another transplant. On June 15, 2013, she underwent another transplant and was discharged from the hospital on August 27, 2013.

The case not only raised many medical questions about the data regarding pediatric lung transplantation but also raised questions about equity in how children are allocated lungs and the ethical principles by which Murnaghan received transplantation. This case has resulted in a flurry of publications on these topics and further investigation of the data.[29–31] The data and subsequent policy decisions, including the "under 12 years of age" provision, are currently under review. However, the larger ethical questions remain. Did Kathleen Sebelius properly balance Murnaghan's need for transplantation against the needs of others on the list when she denied the exception? Was the federal judge who issued the temporary restraining order responding to public pressure regarding the case or to the medical facts? Was justice afforded to other patients on the waiting list for lung transplantation?

CONCLUSION

The field of lung transplantation has benefited from better outcomes over the past 35 years. Limitations include organ scarcity and problems with living donor lobar transplantation. Ethical questions accompany the growing field. Does the LAS adequately represent the best method to allocate organs? What should the criteria for lung retransplantation be? Do we ever achieve satisfactory informed consent from recipients? Can we standardize the psychosocial assessment of potential recipients to minimize bias and discrimination? As the field of lung transplantation continues to improve and evolve, the ethical questions raised in this chapter will become even more prevalent and pressing.

REFERENCES

1. Hardy JD, Webb WR, Dalton ML Jr, Walker GR Jr. Lung homotransplantation in man. JAMA 1963;186:1065-1074.
2. Morrison DL, Maurer JR, Grossman RF. Preoperative assessment for lung transplantation. Clin Chest Med 1990;11:207-215.
3. Yusen RD, Christie JD, Edwards LB, et al. The Registry of the International Society for Heart and Lung Transplantation: Thirtieth adult lung and heart-lung transplant report—2013; focus theme: Age. J Heart Lung Transplant 2013;32:965-978.
4. Stehlik J, Edwards LB, Kucheryavaya AY, et al. The Registry of the International Society for Heart and Lung Transplantation: Twenty-eighth Adult Heart Transplant Report—2011. J Heart Lung Transplant 2011;30:1078-1094.
5. Hauboldt RH, Hanson SG, Bernstein GR: 2008 U.S. organ and tissue transplant cost estimates and discussion. http://publications.milliman.com/research/health-rr/pdfs/2008-us-organ-tisse-RR4-1-08.pdf. Accessed May 28, 2014.
6. Arnaoutakis GJ, Allen JG, Merlo CA, et al. Impact of the lung allocation score on resource utilization after lung transplantation in the United States. J Heart Lung Transplant 2011;30:14-21.
7. Davis SQ, Garrity ER Jr. Organ allocation in lung transplant. Chest 2007;132:1646-1651.
8. 2009 Annual Report of the U.S. Organ Procurement and Transplantation Network and the Scientific Registry of Transplant Recipients: Transplant Data 1999-2008. Rockville, MD: U.S. Department of Health and Human Services, Health Resources and Services Administration, Healthcare Systems Bureau, Division of Transplantation.
9. Orens JB, Estenne M, Arcasoy S, et al. International guidelines for the selection of lung transplant candidates: 2006 update—a consensus report from the Pulmonary Scientific Council of the International Society for Heart and Lung Transplantation. J Heart Lung Transplant 2006;25:745-755.

10. Levenson JL, Olbrisch ME. Psychosocial evaluation of organ transplant candidates. A comparative survey of process, criteria, and outcomes in heart, liver, and kidney transplantation. Psychosomatics 1993;34:314-323.

11. Fine RN, Becker Y, De Geest S, et al. Nonadherence consensus conference summary report. Am J Transplant 2009;9:35-41.

12. Dew MA, Dimartini AF, De Vito Dabbs A, et al. Adherence to the medical regimen during the first two years after lung transplantation. Transplantation 2008;85:193-202.

13. Dobbels F, Vanhaecke J, Desmyttere A, et al. Prevalence and correlates of self-reported pretransplant nonadherence with medication in heart, liver, and lung transplant candidates. Transplantation 2005;79:1588-1595.

14. Twillman RK, Manetto C, Wellisch DK, Wolcott DL. The Transplant Evaluation Rating Scale. A revision of the psychosocial levels system for evaluating organ transplant candidates. Psychosomatics 1993;34:144-153.

15. Olbrisch ME, Levenson JL. Psychosocial evaluation of heart transplant candidates: An international survey of process, criteria, and outcomes. J Heart Lung Transplant 1991;10:948-955.

16. Fung E, Shaw RJ. Pediatric Transplant Rating Instrument—a scale for the pretransplant psychiatric evaluation of pediatric organ transplant recipients. Pediatr Transplant 2008;12:57-66.

17. Nijkamp DM, van der Bij W, Verschuuren EA, et al. Non–heart-beating lung donation: How big is the pool? J Heart Lung Transplant 2008;27:1040-1042.

18. Martin D, Singer PA, Siegler M. Ethical considerations in live donor lung transplantation. In Kern J, Kron I, eds. Medical Intelligence Unit. Reduced-Size Lung Transplantation. Austin, TX: RG Landes; 1993:88-97.

19. Shiraishi T, Okada Y, Sekine Y, et al. Registry of the Japanese Society of Lung and Heart-Lung Transplantation: The official Japanese lung transplantation report 2008. Gen Thorac Cardiovasc Surg 2009; 57:395-401.

20. Sheehy E, Conrad SL, Brigham LE, et al. Estimating the number of potential organ donors in the United States. N Engl J Med 2003;349:667-674.

21. Ghods AJ, Shekoufeh S. Iranian model of paid and regulated living-unrelated kidney donation. Clin J Am Soc Nephrol 2006;1:616-625.

22. Goyal M, Mehta R, Schneiderman L, and Sehgal A. Economic and health consequences of selling a kidney in India. JAMA 2002;288:1589-1593.

23. Rizvi S, Naqvi S, Zafar M, et al. Health function and renal function evaluation of kidney vendors: A report from Pakistan. Am J Transplant 2008;8:1444-1450.

24. Prasad RG, Shukla A, Huang M, et al. Outcomes of commercial renal transplantation: A Canadian experience. Transplantation 2006;82:1130-1135.

25. Jonsen AR, Siegler M, Winslade WJ. Clinical Ethics: A Practical Approach to Ethical Decisions in Clinical Medicine, 7th ed. New York: McGraw-Hill Medical; 2010.

26. Kawut SM, Lederer DJ, Keshavjee S, et al. Outcomes after lung retransplantation in the modern era. Am J Respir Crit Care Med 2008;177:114-120.

27. Martin D, Singer PA, Siegler M. Ethical considerations in live donor lung transplantation. In Kern J, Kron I, eds. Medical Intelligence Unit. Reduced-Size Lung Transplantation. Austin, TX: RG Landes; 1993:88-97.

28. Organ Procurement and Transplantation Network. Policy for allocation of thoracic organs. http://optn.transplant.hrsa.gov/policiesandbylaws2/policies/pdfs/policy_9.pdf. Accessed July 6, 2014.

29. Ladin K, Hanto DW. Rationing lung transplants—procedural fairness in allocation and appeals. N Engl J Med 2013;369:599-601.

30. Snyder JJ, Salkowski N, Skeans M, et al. The equitable allocation of deceased donor lungs for transplant in children in the United States. Am J Transplant 2014;14:178-183.

31. Sweet SC, Barr ML. Pediatric lung allocation: The rest of the story. Am J Transplant 2014;14:11-12.

4

Indications for lung transplantation and patient selection

JOSHUA S. MASON, JULIA B. BECKER, AND EDWARD R. GARRITY JR.

In this chapter we discuss general indications for and contraindications to lung transplantation. We review recommended transplantation criteria for the most common disease processes and review the most recent literature that may assist in patient selection.

INDICATIONS

The 31st official lung and heart-lung transplant report of the Registry of the International Society for Heart and Lung Transplantation was released in 2014. Lung transplantation has become an increasingly common procedure, with 3719 transplants performed in 2012; an increasing share of the transplants are bilateral.[1] Chronic obstructive pulmonary disease (COPD) and idiopathic pulmonary fibrosis (IPF) were the leading indications for transplantation, with IPF increasing from 16% in 2000 to 29% in 2008 (Table 4.1).[2]

In 2006 the International Society for Heart and Lung Transplantation (ISHLT) released the most recent guidelines for the selection of lung transplant candidates.[3] Given the current challenge of chronic rejection and the high mortality rate relative to other solid-organ transplants, as well as the limited availability of donor lungs, lung transplantation should be limited to those in whom a survival benefit is expected. Overall median survival in most recent reports is 5.3 years; those who survived at least 1 year had a median survival of 7.5 years.[2,4] Thus, selected patients should have end-stage lung disease and have failed maximum medical therapy with a 50% expected survival of less than 2 to 3 years or have significant symptoms, which the ISHLT has defined by using the New York Heart Association (NYHA) classes for functional status. NYHA functional class III (symptoms with minimal activity) and class IV (symptoms at rest) are considered indications for transplantation.[3] In addition, given the rigors of transplantation, patients must be in relatively good health.

CONTRAINDICATIONS

The ISHLT's 2006 guidelines included absolute contraindications (Table 4.2). Some of these contraindications represent areas of growth in transplantation.

Malignancy

Although malignancy in general is a contraindication, certain subtypes of lung cancer have been proposed as

Table 4.1 Indications for adult lung transplants performed from January 1995 through June 2013

Diagnosis	Total (N = 41,900)
Chronic obstructive pulmonary disease or emphysema	16,015 (38.2%)
Diffuse parenchymal lung disease	11,826 (28.2%)
Cystic fibrosis	6,862 (16.4%)
Pulmonary arterial hypertension	1,599 (3.8%)
Bronchiectasis	1,131 (2.7%)
Sarcoidosis	1,056 (2.5%)
Retransplant	1,123 (2.7%)
Obliterative bronchiolitis	691 (1.6%)
Nonobliterative bronchiolitis	432 (1.0%)
Connective tissue disease	586 (1.4%)
Obliterative bronchiolitis (not retransplant)	456 (1.1%)
Lymphangioleiomyomatosis	440 (1.1%)
Congenital heart disease	267 (0.9%)
Cancer	36 (0.1%)
Other	770 (1.8%)

Source: Modified from Yusen RD, Edwards LB, Kucheryavaya AY, et al. The Registry of the International Society for Heart and Lung Transplantation: Thirty-first lung and heart-lung transplant report—2013; focus theme: Retransplantation. J Heart Lung Transplant 2014;33:1009–1024.

appropriate indications for lung transplantation. The terms *adenocarcinoma in situ* and *minimally invasive adenocarcinoma* of the lung have been adopted in a recent interdisciplinary classification scheme to replace the term *bronchoalveolar cell carcinoma*.[5] Patients with bilateral or multifocal carcinoma of this sort have been treated by lung transplantation without short-term recurrence.[6,7] However, several series of patients who received transplants for advanced minimally invasive adenocarcinoma demonstrated a high rate of recurrence.[8,9]

Patients with end-stage lung disease and stage I non–small cell lung carcinoma have also been treated by lung transplantation, though often unintentionally, with good success. One survey of ISHLT lung transplant centers reported 43 cases of incidentally found primary lung carcinoma in patients who received transplants for other indications; those with stage I carcinoma and minimally invasive adenocarcinoma demonstrated low rates of recurrence or disseminated disease, whereas those with stage II or III non–small cell lung cancer had high rates of death from recurrence of lung cancer.[10] The Cleveland Clinic reported a 2% (4 cases) incidence of undetected lung carcinoma in 214 consecutive transplant patients between 1991 and 2000, with no evidence of recurrence or decreased survival in the 3 patients with stage I disease; of note, this review was conducted before the age of routine computed tomography (CT), and presumably some of those patients would currently be excluded from transplantation.[11]

Table 4.2 Absolute contraindications to lung transplantation

1. Malignancy in the last 2 years, with the exception of cutaneous squamous and basal cell tumors. In general, a 5-year disease-free interval is prudent.
2. Untreatable advanced dysfunction of another major organ system (e.g., heart, liver, or kidney). Coronary artery disease not amenable to percutaneous intervention or bypass grafting or associated with significant impairment of left ventricular function is an absolute contraindication to lung transplantation, but heart-lung transplantation could be considered in highly selected cases.
3. Incurable chronic extrapulmonary infection, including chronic active viral hepatitis B, hepatitis C, and human immunodeficiency virus.
4. Significant chest wall or spinal deformity.
5. Documented nonadherence or inability to follow through with medical therapy or office follow-up, or both.
6. Untreatable psychiatric or psychological condition associated with the inability to cooperate or comply with medical therapy.
7. Absence of a consistent or reliable social support system.
8. Substance addiction (e.g., alcohol, tobacco, or narcotics) that either is active or occurred within the last 6 months.

Source: Modified from Orens JB, Estenne M, Arcasoy S, et al. International guidelines for the selection of lung transplant candidates: 2006 update—a consensus report from the Pulmonary Scientific Council of the International Society for Heart and Lung Transplantation. J Heart Lung Transplant 2006;25:745–755.

Significant chest wall and spinal deformities

Because of mechanical difficulty with surgery, as well as with postoperative mechanical ventilation and pulmonary toilet, thoracic transplantation is rarely performed in patients with significant deformities. A handful of transplant procedures performed on patients with severe scoliosis or chest wall deformities have been reported,[12–14] and in at least one patient, scoliosis contributed to recurrent airway stenosis requiring frequent bronchoscopy and intervention.[15] If transplantation is performed, the surgical approach and donor selection would need to be tailored to thoracic size.[14]

Incurable extrapulmonary infection

Three decades of progress in the treatment of human immunodeficiency virus (HIV) has changed the prognosis to that of a chronic disease. One successful case of an HIV- and hepatitis B virus (HBV)- positive patient receiving a transplant because of cystic fibrosis (CF) and having excellent lung function and no unusual complications 2 years after transplantation has been reported.[16] A review of 170 hepatitis C virus (HCV)-seropositive patients who received lung transplants demonstrated no difference in survival, although most patients were not viremic.[17] A small group of HCV-positive lung transplant recipients at Cleveland Clinic with no evidence of cirrhosis have shown no increased mortality.[18]

Untreatable advanced dysfunction of another major organ system

In general, advanced dysfunction has been a contraindication to lung transplantation. However, a combined organ transplant may be considered. Based on Organ Procurement and Transplantation Network (OPTN) data as of November 10, 2014, 35 kidney-lung, 63 liver-lung, 12 liver-lung-heart, 4 heart-lung-kidney, and 3 pancreas-lung transplants and 1 liver-pancreas-lung transplant had been performed in the United States since 1988.

Lung transplantation in combination with dialysis has been associated with increased 1-year mortality,[2,4] but the small numbers limit the data.

Most of the available data deal with liver-lung transplants, which are typically performed for CF complicated by cirrhosis or for portopulmonary hypertension or hepatopulmonary syndrome complicating cirrhosis. The available series have reported survival no different from that of single-organ transplant patients.[19-26]

Adherence and addiction

Careful assessment of social support and adherence by experienced transplant psychologists and social workers is essential. One available tool is the Transplant Evaluation Rating Scale, which has been used to assess patients before organ and bone marrow transplantation.[27] Nonadherence to immunosuppression, lifestyle, and general medical prescriptions is common in recipients of solid-organ transplants; it is estimated to affect nearly half of patients who received organ transplants, including those who live alone.[28] Pretransplant nonadherence is associated with late acute rejection.[29] Pretransplantation nonadherence to the medication regimen, lower social support, lower personality trait scores for "conscientiousness," and higher educational level have been shown to be predictors of nonadherence to the immunosuppressive regimen at 1 year after transplantation.[29]

Rates of adherence among lung transplant recipients have varied in different studies and with different definitions of adherence.[30,31] Lung transplant patients may exhibit more nonadherent behavior than other solid-organ transplant patients do, in part because of their higher medication needs.[30] Prior tobacco smoking is common in patients who have end-stage lung disease, so interest in smoking behavior is critical. One survey of self-reported rates of smoking

after receiving a lung transplant showed 100% abstinence after transplantation.[32] However, self-reported rates tend to underestimate smoking compared with biologic markers such as urine cotinine,[33] and one can imagine substantial desire among lung transplant recipients to report total abstinence. We suggest that biologic testing, such as urine cotinine testing, be performed in patients considered to be at high risk for smoking recidivism.

RELATIVE CONTRAINDICATIONS

Relative contraindications to transplantation are, not surprisingly, an area of more clinical debate.

Age

Although the 2006 ISHLT guidelines recommend against transplantation in recipients older than 65 years,[3] the practice has been controversial. Registry data indicate that older patients have been receiving transplants with increasing frequency; in 2000, 28 transplants (1.6%) were documented in patients aged 66 or older. In contrast, in the first 6 months of 2010, 182 transplants (12.1%) were performed on recipients in this age group[2] despite increased mortality with advanced age. Results to support a precise upper age limit for transplantation are lacking because the studies used different definitions for older patients. In a matched cohort study from the Toronto group, 42 patients older than 60 years were compared with matched patients younger than 60. Survival at 1, 2, 3, 4, and 5 years was significantly worse in the older cohort because of increased infection-related deaths in the early posttransplant period, followed by increased malignancy-related deaths.[34]

A subsequent retrospective review of more than 8000 patients in the United Network for Organ Sharing (UNOS) database from 1999 to 2006 stratified patients into age quartiles. Age older than 60 years, the highest age quartile, was associated with a 37% increase in risk for death within 1 to 2 years, whereas short-term (30- and 60-day) mortality was no different from that in younger patients. Within the quartile of patients older than 60 years, the oldest patients (age >70) had a substantially increased risk for short-term mortality. Unlike in previous studies, age was thought to be protective against infection and rejection.[35] In a past ISHLT report, patients older than 65 had decreased median survival (3.5 years versus 6.7 years) and decreased long-term survival rates (38% versus 55% to 57% at 5 years) when compared with patients younger than 50 years.[2]

Other studies, many of which report results with carefully selected recipients, have demonstrated that transplantation in older patients with a body mass index (BMI) in the accepted range and absence of obstructive coronary artery disease, peripheral or cerebrovascular disease, renal insufficiency, or debilitation may be performed with mortality similar to that in younger patients.[36-38] A larger series comparing survival rates in patients younger than 60 years, between 60 and 65, and older than 65 between January 2006 and May 2008 found no survival difference but did find that complications differed by age group, with malignancy and drug toxicity more common in patients older than 65 and rejection more common in those aged 60 to 65.[39]

Several series have suggested that single-lung transplantation (SLT) may be tolerated better in the older population, which has led some centers to consider only SLT in older patients. Meyer and colleagues reviewed 2260 recipients of lung transplants for COPD (1835 single-lung and 425 bilateral lung transplants) and found that a mortality benefit existed for bilateral transplantation until the age of 60, after which SLT was associated with improved mortality.[40] A similar review of patients with pulmonary fibrosis who had received transplants demonstrated no benefit for bilateral lung transplantation (BLT) over SLT.[41] However, some contradictory studies exist. Series have shown similar 30-day[42] and 1-, 2-, and 5-year survival in patients older than 60 who undergo BLT as opposed to SLT,[43] and a large review of UNOS data demonstrated no mortality effect of SLT versus BLT in patients older than 60.[44]

Nutritional status

Nutritional status is frequently abnormal in patients with chronic lung disease; in one study, only about half of patients were deemed to have normal nutritional status, with the remainder being underweight or overweight.[45] The ISHLT guidelines recommend against performing transplants on patients with a BMI of 30 kg/m² or higher, although they do not comment on underweight recipients.[3]

A link between increased BMI and mortality is fairly consistent, thus supporting a BMI threshold for transplantation. The Toronto program and others have shown similar deleterious effects of excess weight on outcomes.[46–48] A Spanish study of 256 transplant recipients, including 38 obese patients, was one of the few to find no statistical difference in mortality between BMI groups, although trends toward increased mortality and longer mechanical ventilation in the obese did exist.[49]

Underweight had been suspected as a risk factor for death.[50] More recently, very large reviews of the lung transplant databases have shown effects of BMI at both extremes, with patients stratified into underweight (BMI <18.5), normal weight (BMI = 18.5 to 24.9), overweight (BMI = 25.0 to 29.9), and obese (BMI >30) by World Health Organization categories. Lederer and associates retrospectively reviewed the UNOS registry data on 5978 lung recipients with CF, COPD, or diffuse parenchymal lung disease to evaluate the effect of BMI. A BMI other than normal was associated with increased risk for death overall and at 1 and 5 years, with a hazard ratio for overall mortality of 1.15 to 1.16 for being underweight, 1.14 to 1.17 for being overweight, and 1.20 to 1.25 for being obese.[51] In the largest evaluation, Allen and colleagues reviewed 11,411 lung transplants performed between 1998 and 2008 for which UNOS data adequate to stratify by BMI were available. A small but statistically

significant increase in mortality existed for every BMI strata above or below normal BMI, with odds ratios for death of 1.06 for being overweight, 1.16 for obese, and 1.14 for being underweight in multivariate analysis. The risk for death appeared to involve a short-term increase in mortality that is seen only within the first year for patients who are overweight or obese but is manifested more as later mortality (after 1 year) in underweight patients.[52] We thus suggest that underweight patients undergo aggressive nutritional support before transplantation to bring their weight into normal range and that patients above the BMI threshold of 30 lose weight before listing.

Other medical conditions that have not resulted in end-stage organ damage

CORONARY ARTERY DISEASE

Underlying coronary artery disease has been associated with increased mortality in a univariate analysis of a Brazilian transplant cohort.[53] Intervention for preexisting coronary artery disease may be performed before or at lung transplantation. The UCLA group recently reported a 10-year experience during which 27 patients with discrete coronary lesions and a preserved left ventricular ejection fraction underwent coronary revascularization before lung transplantation and had no difference in survival or causes of death.[54] This finding echoes previous series that showed similar success.[55,56] Of note, all patients demonstrated preserved cardiac function and had discrete (i.e., not diffuse) coronary artery lesions.

DIABETES

Diabetes is a common comorbidity in lung transplant patients, particularly in those patients with CF. Although the number of patients with diabetes in one series was small, Plantier and colleagues found that diabetes before transplantation was independently associated with death from all causes and from cardiovascular causes.[57] Likewise, a small retrospective review of 25 patients who received transplants because of CF demonstrated increased morbidity and mortality in those with pretransplant CF-related diabetes,[58] but interestingly, a larger study suggested no effect of diabetes on survival in patients with CF and improved 1-year survival for those patients with preexisting diabetes.[59] No systematic assessment of the effect of diabetes control on success after transplantation has been conducted, although the experience of Bradbury and colleagues suggests that uncontrolled diabetes played a role in some posttransplant readmissions.[58] We suggest carefully selecting diabetic patients to include those with good control and engaging expert consultation for the management of blood glucose in the perioperative setting.

GASTROESOPHAGEAL REFLUX DISEASE

Gastroesophageal reflux disease (GERD) has been recognized as a cause of allograft dysfunction after lung transplantation, with both increased rates of bronchiolitis obliterans syndrome and acute rejection episodes,[60,61] as well as with worse short-term forced expiratory volume in the first second of respiration (FEV$_1$) and early survival than in patients without reflux.[62] Gastroesophageal reflux is highly prevalent in candidates for lung transplantation and may be asymptomatic, thus requiring invasive testing[63–65]; this condition also worsens after transplantation,[66] perhaps in part in connection with medication-induced gastroparesis.[67] Treatment may require surgical intervention. Proton pump inhibitor therapy alone may affect gastric acid but does not prevent non–acid reflux and gastric aspiration.[68] Fundoplication after transplantation has been associated with improvement in bronchiolitis obliterans.[69] Laparoscopic fundoplication has also been performed successfully in patients before transplantation[70] and may preserve lung function in patients before and after transplantation.[71,72] Thus, we suggest that invasive testing for esophageal reflux be performed on patients before transplantation and surgical management be considered. In patients with severe, symptomatic disease that is refractory to treatment, reflux may be a relative contraindication to transplantation.

Critical or unstable condition

The use of mechanical ventilation and hospitalization at the time of transplantation are associated with increased 1-year risk for mortality. In the most recent ISHLT report, the 390 patients who received transplants while on mechanical ventilation from January 1996 through June 2009 had a relative risk for death at 1 year of 1.57 compared with patients with COPD and a single-lung transplant. Being hospitalized at all, including in an intensive care unit (ICU), also conferred increased risk (RR = 1.70).[2]

In a review of UNOS data from October 1987 to January 2008, 586 transplants were performed on patients maintained on mechanical ventilation and 51 were performed on patients on extracorporeal membrane oxygenation (ECMO) support. Patients undergoing mechanical ventilation and ECMO had significantly lower survival, but at levels suggesting that performing transplants on such supported patients may be feasible. Those on mechanical ventilation had unadjusted survival rates at 1, 6, 12, and 24 months of 83%, 67%, 62%, and 57%, respectively. The corresponding rates for patients undergoing ECMO were 72%, 53%, 50%, and 45%, and those for unsupported patients were 93%, 85%, 79%, and 70%.[73] Patients treated with mechanical ventilation tended to be younger and were more likely to have a diagnosis of CF.[73] Despite these overall numbers, some smaller series have shown no change in survival with select populations, mainly patients with CF,[74–76] whereas another series has shown decreased survival compared with controls.[77] Subsequent studies have had mixed populations and results. Baz and colleagues reported no decrease in 1-year posttransplant survival for nine patients who were mechanically ventilated for at least 13 days and up to 6 years, were able to undergo physical therapy, and had no lower airway colonization with resistant bacteria.[78]

One center reported that transplantation was successful in 15 patients on mechanical ventilation, 5 of whom had been already listed for a transplant; 13 of those 15 patients were alive at 52 months with no survival difference compared with controls.[79] Another series reported higher 1-year mortality for urgent transplantation while patients were on mechanical ventilation.[80] Current minimal experience thus suggests that transplantation in mechanically ventilated patients should be carefully restricted to those with single-organ failure, no airway colonization with antibiotic-resistant bacteria, and the ability to participate in physical therapy and rehabilitation.

Other series have reported small numbers of patients who have received transplants while on ECMO. A 19-year experience at one center included 17 patients maintained on ECMO before transplantation, with a median duration of support of 3.2 days (range = 1 to 49 days). These patients demonstrated higher perioperative mortality but acceptable midterm survival, with a 3-year survival rate of 65% as compared with 62% in the control group.[81] Other smaller series have demonstrated some success with a Novalung venovenous[82,83] and other devices[84] for extracorporeal removal of carbon dioxide in the absence of hypoxemia as bridges to transplantation. ECMO devices, or portable artificial lungs (PALs), placed to allow ambulation and physical therapy performed while the patient is on support have shown promise in early use as bridges to transplantation.[85–89] The experience needed to provide guidelines about when and how to use this technology when bridging to transplant is growing but currently insufficient.

Colonization with highly resistant or highly virulent bacteria, fungi, or mycobacteria

Active infection is a contraindication to transplantation because of concern that it may cause sepsis-related deaths after intense immunosuppression. The suppurative lung diseases (CF and non-CF bronchiectasis) are characterized by colonization with microbes that may become resistant. The specific risk factors for transplant mortality in a non-CF population have not been well described. Airway colonization with CF is described separately in the section of this chapter on specific diseases.

Severe or symptomatic osteoporosis

Osteoporosis and osteopenia are highly prevalent in lung transplant recipients.[90–92] Therapy consisting of bisphosphonates and resistance training has been shown to be effective prophylaxis in lung transplant recipients,[93,94] but those with advanced disease before transplantation are at risk for severe complications inasmuch as osteoporosis routinely worsens after transplantation.[92,95,96] Given the steroid therapy that accompanies lung transplantation, patients with very severe or symptomatic osteoporosis would be at risk for excessive complications after transplantation.

OTHER CONSIDERATIONS

Previous thoracic surgery

Previous thoracic surgery, particularly previous pleural procedures, is associated with increased bleeding in the perioperative period, but it has not been associated with increased mortality[97–99] and should not in general be considered a contraindication to transplantation. However, pleural adhesions are associated with increased technical challenge during transplantation.[100]

Clinical circumstances require adjustment of surgical technique based on surgeon preference because specific scenarios may impart increased risk. In the circumstance of SLT after previous contralateral pneumonectomy, Le Pimpec-Barthes and colleagues reported increased mortality related to mediastinal shift,[101] and Dietrich and colleagues reported bleeding complications requiring right lower lobectomy after a heart and bilateral lung transplant.[102] Kawaguchi and colleagues reported success in performing a heart and unilateral lung transplant in settings in which one pleural space has significant adhesions.[103]

Chronic obstructive pulmonary disease

COPD remains the most common indication for lung transplantation to date.[4] Its heterogeneous course makes prognostication difficult and thus raises challenges for selection of patients for transplantation.

SURVIVAL BENEFIT

Hand in hand with the challenge in prognostication, survival benefit for transplantation with COPD is less clear. In early experience before the current lung allocation method, those with emphysema had improved waiting list survival in comparison to those with other diseases.[104] Thabut and colleagues created a statistical model to predict survival benefit from lung transplantation for COPD; it suggested that some, but not all currently wait-listed patients would benefit from lung transplantation. Pulmonary artery pressure, FEV_1, BMI, exercise capacity, functional status, and need for continuous mechanical ventilation or oxygen were all major determinants of the survival effect of a transplant. Their analysis of the 8182 people on the lung transplant waiting list estimated that 50.1% of those undergoing SLT and 63.7% of those undergoing BLT would have a survival benefit. This model has not yet been validated.[105] An analysis by Charman and associates also supported a survival benefit for transplantation for COPD.[106] Lahzami and coworkers reviewed 54 consecutive lung transplants for COPD and evaluated the pretransplant BODE index (see later) and survival; patients in the subgroup with a BODE index of 7 or higher were found to live longer with a transplant than would have been predicted by the original BODE index cohort (Box 4.1).[107]

BOX 4.1: Guidelines for patients with chronic obstructive pulmonary disease[3]

GUIDELINE FOR REFERRAL

BODE index > 5

GUIDELINES FOR TRANSPLANTATION

Patients with a BODE index of 7 to 10 or at least one of the following:

- History of hospitalization for exacerbation associated with acute hypercapnia (PCO_2 exceeding 50 mm Hg)
- Pulmonary hypertension, cor pulmonale, or both despite oxygen therapy
- Forced expiratory volume in 1 second < 20% and either diffusing capacity of the lungs for carbon monoxide < 20% or homogeneous distribution of emphysema

PROGNOSTICATION

Recent large population studies have demonstrated that progression of COPD is heterogeneous. An observational study of 2163 patients with COPD showed a highly variable decline in FEV_1 over a period of 3 years, with 38% having a decline in FEV_1 of greater than 40 mL/yr, 31% having a decline of 21 to 40 mL/yr, 23% having a change within the range from –20 to +20 mL/yr, and 8% having an increase of greater than 20 mL/yr. Patients with very severe COPD declined less than did those with less severe disease.[108] Many characteristics have been found to be markers for mortality in patients with COPD, including FEV_1, lung hyperinflation, weight loss with low BMI, anemia, exercise capacity, dyspnea, health-related quality of life and activity level, use of oxygen supplementation, distribution of emphysema, and exacerbations.[109–112]

FEV_1

Dating back to the earliest attempts to prognosticate, survival of patients with COPD has been tracked by FEV_1, with Burrows and associates noting an overall 58% mortality for a group of 200 patients over a 7-year period. Patients with an FEV_1 lower than 0.75 L had substantially worse survival than did those with an FEV_1 between 0.75 L and 1.24 L, with the best survival for those with an FEV_1 greater than 1.24 L. It was also noted that FEV_1 dropped a mean of 56 mL/yr but was highly variable.[113] An association between postbronchodilator FEV_1 and mortality was confirmed in observational studies of nonhypoxic patients with COPD who were monitored for 3 years.[114]

EXACERBATIONS

Mortality following hospitalization for acute exacerbations of COPD has long been noted to be high, with a 1-year mortality of 22% to 59% reported in various studies and the highest mortality in those who had a $Paco_2$ of 50 mm Hg or greater (49%)[115] or were admitted to an ICU (59%).[115-118] The link between repeated exacerbations requiring hospitalization and mortality was established by a prospective analysis of 304 patients with COPD who were monitored over a 5-year period. Patients with three or more exacerbations per year had a hazard ratio for death of 4.13, and those with one or two exacerbations had a hazard ratio of 2.0 compared with patients with no exacerbations, a risk that was independent of lung function or age.[110] More recently, large population-based studies confirmed that each exacerbation confers an increased risk for death regardless of other exacerbations and baseline lung function.[119]

PULMONARY HYPERTENSION

Elevated pulmonary artery diastolic pressure has been associated with death on the lung transplant waiting list for patients with emphysema.[120]

COMPOSITE INDEXES

BODE index

In 2004 Celli and colleagues released a landmark prognostication score for COPD known as the BODE index (Table 4.3), which is based on BMI (B), degree of airflow obstruction (O), dyspnea (D), and exercise capacity (E) measured by the 6-minute walk test (6MWT). This index was created by using a base of 207 patients and subsequently validated in a cohort of 625 patients. Patients with higher BODE scores were at higher risk for death, with improved concordance compared with FEV_1.[121] A modification of the BODE score using cardiopulmonary exercise testing with Vo_2max[122] did not improve prognostication, and one replacing the 6MWT with severe exacerbations performed equally well and may simplify scoring.[123]

Extrapolation to a transplant population is limited because the score was validated in a cohort of predominantly elderly patients who were almost entirely male; however, Lahzami and colleagues found that a BODE score of 7 or higher may predict patients expected to have a mortality benefit from transplantation.[107] Martinez and associates, in a review of 609 patients enrolled in the National

Emphysema Treatment Trial, found that increased mortality was independently associated with age, use of supplemental oxygen, anemia, lung hyperinflation (measured by the increase in residual volume percent predicted [RV% predicted]), lower diffusing capacity percent predicted, lower maximum exercise performance on cardiopulmonary exercise testing, greater lower–lung zone emphysema, and higher modified BODE score.[112] This study was limited to patients with severe emphysema ($FEV_1 \leq 45\%$, $RV \geq 150\%$)[124] and, interestingly, found only a weak relationship with the modified BODE score and prognosis.[112] An analysis of the same patient population found that changes in the modified BODE score at 6, 12, and 24 months were predictive of future mortality.[125]

A recent large study prospectively monitored both BODE and FEV_1 over at least three measurements in 751 patients in the United States and Spain from 1997 through 2008. Interestingly, only a small percentage of patients (18%) had a statistically significant decline in FEV_1, only 14% had a statistically significant increase in the BODE index over time, and the correlation between those groups was low. The group with increasing BODE score but stable FEV_1 ($n = 69$) demonstrated higher mortality. Patients who were excluded for having fewer than three measurements also had higher mortality.[126] Of particular note, use of the BODE index, or any index, is not now part of the lung allocation score used for priority rating.

HADO score

The HADO (health status, physical activity, dyspnea scale, and obstruction) score was compared with the BODE scale in a prospective analysis of 543 eligible patients, predominantly men, who were monitored for 3 years. Both the BODE index and HADO score remained good predictors of all-cause and respiratory mortality; however, the BODE index performed better in patients with more severe lung disease ($FEV_1 < 50\%$).[127]

Classification and regression tree analysis

Classification and regression tree (CART) analysis was used to predict mortality risk in a 5-year period with covariates derived from previous prognostic scores: age, FEV_1,

Table 4.3 The BODE index

	Points on the BODE index			
Variables	0	1	2	3
FEV_1 (% predicted)	≥65	50–64	36–49	≤35
6-minute walk test (m)	≥350	250–349	150–249	≤150
Dyspnea (Modified Medical Research Council Dyspnea Scale)	0–1	2	3 (minimal exertion)	4 (at rest)
Body mass (body mass index), kg/m²	>21	≤21	–	–

Source: Celli BR, Cote CG, Marin JM, et al. The body-mass index, airflow obstruction, dyspnea, and exercise capacity index in chronic obstructive pulmonary disease. N Engl J Med 2004;350:1005–1012.

Note: Total of 10 points, with higher scores indicating a worse prognosis and 7 or more points associated with approximately 50% mortality over a 2-year period; FEV_1, forced expiratory volume in the first second of respiration.

dyspnea, physical activity, general health, and number of hospital admissions in the previous 2 years. This represents a different method of prognostication, with physicians tracking their patients down a tree rather than calculating a score, and its use in the lung transplant population has not been described.[128]

BIOMARKERS

Some attempts at using biomarker data such as C-reactive protein to aid in prognostication have been made, but they have not been successful,[111,129] although a recent large-scale trial noted a weak association with level of CC-16 and decline in FEV_1.[108]

LUNG VOLUME REDUCTION SURGERY

Lung volume reduction surgery (LVRS) has been used to improve hyperinflation in patients with heterogeneous emphysema; a series of 150 patients with a mean FEV_1 of 25%, no hypercapnia, and few associated comorbid conditions along with hyperinflation demonstrated excellent 1- and 2-year survival rates (93% and 92%). These patients showed a rise in FEV_1, forced vital capacity (FVC), resting Pao_2, and 6MWT score along with decreasing total lung capacity, forced residual capacity, $Paco_2$, O_2 required at rest and with exercise, and a decrease in patients using continuous corticosteroids.[130] In a randomized controlled trial, LVRS improved mortality in patients with upper lobe–predominant disease and low exercise ability.[131] A modified version of the BODE score showed that surgically treated patients had improvements in the BODE score associated with improved mortality.[125] Successful LVRS has been shown to extend time before a lung transplant is needed without significantly affecting posttransplant morbidity and mortality,[132-136] although patients with unsuccessful LVRS represented a group at increased risk associated with transplantation.[135,136] In one series, 24 of 31 patients were able to be deactivated from the transplant list after LVRS.[132] Patients with an FEV_1 of less than 20%, as well as a diffusing capacity of the lungs for carbon monoxide ($DLCO$) of less than 20% or homogenous emphysema, are at high risk for death with LVRS[135] and are not eligible for this procedure.

CHOICE OF PROCEDURE

Although both SLT and BLT are performed for COPD, bilateral transplants are gaining favor. A review of the ISHLT/UNOS registry from 1991 to 1997 looked at 2260 lung transplant recipients (1835 single-lung transplants and 425 bilateral lung transplants) with COPD and concluded that in those younger than 60 years, a survival benefit existed for BLT; in those older than 60, mortality favored SLT.[40] In 2002 the Washington University group published its experience from 1998 to 2000 with 306 patients who received transplants for emphysema and noted a significant 5-year survival benefit for BLT both in patients with COPD and in those with α_1-antitrypsin deficiency. Five-year survival overall was unchanged between patients with COPD and those with α_1-antitrypsin deficiency and was not different

from that with other diagnoses, and even early hospital survival was unchanged between COPD and α_1-antitrypsin deficiency.[138]

α_1-Antitrypsin deficiency

Emphysema related to α_1-antitrypsin deficiency, a genetic disorder with an autosomal codominant inheritance, is the fourth most common indication for lung transplants and accounted for 7% of the transplants in the most recent ISHLT registry report.[4] It is an underrecognized contributor to obstructive lung disease, with an estimated 59,000 people in the United States having symptomatic emphysema related to α_1-antitrypsin deficiency.[139] It causes accelerated lung disease in young persons; between 1979 and 1991, α_1-antitrypsin deficiency was listed in 2.7% of deaths in persons aged 35 to 44 years with obstructive lung disease.[140] The most common severe deficiency is found in patients homozygous for the ZZ allele, although phenotypes with the SZ and SS combinations of alleles, as well as with the rare null/null genotype, are also described.[139]

PROGNOSIS

The National Heart, Lung, and Blood Institute began a registry for patients with severe α_1-antitrypsin deficiency in 1989, with 1129 patients enrolled between March 1989 and October 1992.[141] Those patients were followed for a mean of 4.4 years (range = 0 to 7.2 years), during which 204 patients died. Those who died were older, had a slightly higher serum α_1-antitrypsin level, had a lower FEV_1, were more likely to have a former or current history of tobacco use, and had a lower educational level. A history of lung or liver transplantation was also more common in the patients who had died. Emphysema was the cause of death of 72% of the patients for whom a cause of death was available.[142] Five-year Kaplan-Meier mortality rates have been found to be significantly related to FEV_1 at baseline, with 30.3% mortality for patients with an FEV_1 of 35% or less, 12.0% for an FEV_1 between 35% and 49%, and 4.3% for patients with an FEV_1 of 50% predicted or higher.[143]

On average, FEV_1 declined 54 mL/yr, with the decline occurring faster in men, patients aged 30 to 44 years, active smokers, those with an FEV_1 of 35% to 79% predicted, and patients who have ever had a bronchodilator response. In patients with an FEV_1 of 35% to 49%, augmentation therapy was associated with a slower decline in FEV_1, and in all patients, augmentation therapy was associated with lower mortality. One hundred twelve of the patients, about 10%, underwent lung transplantation.[142] The Danish registry reported a median life expectancy of 54.5 years, with smoking remaining a major risk factor for death.[144] In a further review of 75 never-smokers with severe disease, emphysema was the major cause of death in 14 of the 21 patients who died.[145] FEV_1 and $DLCO$ have been found to correlate with respiratory mortality, and the CT scan score has been shown to be associated with all-cause mortality and respiratory death.[146,147] For patients in the lowest tercile of FEV_1 values (<37.5% predicted), mortality was substantially increased.[147]

Diffuse parenchymal lung disease

Diffuse parenchymal lung disease is a frequent indication for transplantation. IPF is now the second most common indication for transplantation and represents an increasing proportion of lung transplants performed. The other diffuse parenchymal lung diseases for which transplants are also performed include lymphangioleiomyomatosis (LAM), sarcoidosis, and at times, collagen vascular disease–associated interstitial lung diseases.[1,2,4]

IDIOPATHIC PULMONARY FIBROSIS AND FIBROTIC NONSPECIFIC INTERSTITIAL PNEUMONIA

Prognosis

The American Thoracic Society released an updated classification of idiopathic interstitial pneumonias based primarily on histopathology.[148] IPF, with its pathologic pattern of usual interstitial pneumonia (UIP), has a uniquely poor prognosis when compared with other histopathologic patterns, and diagnosing it appropriately when considering a patient for a transplant is thus crucial. In contrast to patients with desquamative interstitial pneumonia and respiratory bronchiolitis–associated interstitial lung disease (80% 5-year survival rate) and nonspecific interstitial pneumonia (NSIP) (70% survival rate), patients with UIP in one series were found to have a 20% 5-year survival rate.[149] Similarly, a prospective analysis of 315 patients with diffuse parenchymal lung disease demonstrated substantially worse survival for patients with IPF (2-year survival rate = 48.4%, 5-year survival rate = 35.4%) than in those with the other diseases (2-year survival rate = 74.9% to 100%, 5-year survival rate = 69.5% to 91.6%).[150] A survival benefit for patients with IPF who receive transplants has been established in several evaluations.[106,151,152]

Listing and transplantation must be timed with consideration for the patient's prognosis, with the goal being to identify those patients with high short-term mortality for immediate listing and hold off on transplantation for those who may be predicted to have a more indolent course. Such assessment has been made more challenging by the at times rapid and unpredictable decline of patients with IPF.[153] Median survival was previously thought to be 2 to 3 years; however, recognition that the clinical course is variable and may include some patients with much longer survival is increasing.[153] The 2006 ISHLT guidelines for the referral of patients with interstitial lung disease include histologic or radiographic evidence of UIP irrespective of vital capacity or histologic evidence of fibrotic NSIP.[2] Patients with a histologic diagnosis of both UIP and NSIP (discordant biopsies) have been shown to have a prognosis approximately as poor as that for patients with UIP alone and may be considered for transplantation in the same category.[154]

Pulmonary function

Different parameters of vital capacity at baseline have been associated with survival. Assessment of vital capacity at baseline has been related to mortality, although the value at which increased risk is conferred has varied between studies: 60% predicted or lower,[155] and with cutoffs ranging from an FVC of 60% to 83%.[156] More recently, Nathan and colleagues noted that patients divided by FVC (mild, ≥70%; moderate, 55% to 69%; and severe, <55%) had correspondingly worse median survival of 55.6, 38.7, and 27.4 months, respectively.[152] Latsi and coworkers found that patients with high short-term (2-year) mortality had a lower baseline FVC (62.0% versus 78.7%).[157] Longitudinal change in FVC has been noted to be associated with increased mortality in multiple studies,[158–162] and even marginal changes in FVC (5% to 10%) over a 6-month period conferred higher mortality than in patients with stable disease.[159]

Diffusing capacity of the lungs for carbon monoxide

D_{LCO} has been correlated with survival, although like FVC, its predictive value differs in different studies, with ranges from 30% to 45% and with other studies noting a continuous increase in mortality with decreasing D_{LCO} below 50% predicted and the worst outcomes occurring in those with a D_{LCO} less than 20% predicted.[152,156,157,163,164] In a group of 487 patients with IPF who were seen at Mayo Clinic, decreased D_{LCO} was associated with a relative risk of 1.4 for every 10–percentage point decrease[161]; Mogulkoc and colleagues also found that D_{LCO} was significantly associated with survival on multivariate analysis, with the hazard of death increasing by 4% for every 1% decrease in D_{LCO}.[164] In longitudinal analysis, a greater than 20% decline in D_{LCO} at 1 year was found to be significantly correlated with mortality,[162] although lower levels of change in D_{LCO} were not significant in some analyses.[159,165]

Alveolar-arterial oxygen gradient

The results for a decline in the alveolar-arterial oxygen gradient have been mixed, with some suggesting an association with mortality[160] and others finding none.[165]

Pulmonary hypertension

Pulmonary hypertension has been associated with worsening outcomes in patients with IPF[155,163,166] and combined pulmonary fibrosis and emphysema,[167] with 5-year survival declining as mean pulmonary arterial pressure rose above 17 mm Hg.

Exercise tolerance

Performance and longitudinal change in the 6MWT score provide useful prognostic information. A population of 822 patients enrolled in a clinical trial of interferon gamma-1b who completed the 6MWT at screening, baseline, and 24-week intervals were monitored over a 72-week period. Risk for death was more than four times greater in patients whose 6MWT distance decreased by more than 50 m and three times greater in patients whose walk distance declined by 26 to 50 m.[168] A similar value of 29 to 34 m was found in a previous analysis.[169] In an Israeli population awaiting lung transplantation, distance on the 6MWT has been inversely associated with risk for death while wait-listed for a transplant.[170] Likewise, abnormal heart rate recovery 1 and 2 minutes after 6MWT, desaturation, and lowest saturation on climbing or on the 6MWT have also been correlated with a poorer prognosis and may be associated with pulmonary hypertension.[171–173]

Radiology

High-resolution computed tomography (HRCT) characteristics have been reproducibly found to be predictive of mortality in early studies[174] and from a trial of interferon gamma-1b. HRCT was performed on 326 patients at baseline and scored on a standardized form for the presence and extent of ground-glass attenuation, reticulation, honeycombing, decreased attenuation, centrilobular nodules, other nodules, consolidation, and emphysema, with the extent of fibrosis determined on a four-point scale of 0, 1 (1% to 25%), 2 (26% to 50%), 3 (51% to 75%), and 4 (76% to 100%) and further classified by at least two radiologists as typical, atypical, or inconsistent with IPF. The extent of fibrosis was associated with increased risk for death, and patients with more fibrosis were also more likely to have a low DLco and FVC and increased alveolar-arterial oxygen gradient,[175] with the risk for death increasing by 106% for every unit increase in the HRCT fibrosis score.[164] Interestingly, in a review of 660 patients with UIP, the 221 who had coexistent emphysema with a similar degree of fibrosis had improved mortality, with a median survival of 7.5 years in the UIP group versus 8.5 years in the patients with UIP and emphysema.[176]

Symptoms

Six-month and 12-month changes in the dyspnea score, as well as the baseline dyspnea score, are associated with mortality.[160] Nishiyama and colleagues suggested that the Modified Medical Research Council (MMRC) Dyspnea Scale may be used alone to assess prognosis (Table 4.4).

Their study showed that median patient survival with an MMRC grade of 0 or 1 was 66.7 months. When breathlessness increased to grade 2, survival was 30.9 months, and with grade 3 it was 10.2 months.[172] Cough is a predominant symptom of IPF and may be associated with prognosis. Cough was found to be more prevalent in never-smokers and in patients with advanced disease with exertional desaturation and lower FVC, and it predicted progression of disease independent of disease severity.[177] Predictive value is limited by the lack of objective grading criteria for cough.

Biomarkers

Some experimental biomarkers have been associated with decreased survival, although to date none are used routinely in clinical practice. CCL18 levels greater than 150 ng/mL were associated with significantly higher mortality, with a

Table 4.4 Modified medical research council scale for dyspnea

Grade	Description of breathlessness
0	I get breathless only with strenuous exercise
1	I get short of breath when hurrying on level ground or walking up a slight hill
2	On level ground I walk slower than people of the same age because of breathlessness, or I have to stop for breath when walking at my own pace on level ground
3	I stop for breath after walking about 100 yards or after a few minutes on level ground
4	I am too breathless to leave the house, or I am breathless when dressing

Source: Adapted from Launois C, Barbe C, Bertin, et al. The modified Medical Research Council scale for the assessment of dyspnea in daily living in obesity: A pilot study. BMC Pulm Med 2012;12:61.

hazard ratio of 8.0 after adjustment for age, sex, and baseline pulmonary function.[178] In samples from 241 patients with IPF, concentrations of the plasma proteins matrix metalloproteinase-7 (MMP-7), intercellular adhesion molecule 1 (ICAM-1), interleukin-8 (IL-8), vascular cell adhesion molecule 1 (VCAM-1), and S100 calcium-binding protein A12 (S100A12) predicted poor transplant-free survival, with MMP-7, ICAM-1, and IL-8 also predicting poor overall survival.[179] Patients with IPF and both surfactant protein D (SP-D) and KL6/MUC1 have shorter survival and more symptoms than do those who have only SP-D elevated.[180] Patients with elevated circulating fibrocytes (>5% of total blood leukocytes), which is thought to be a marker for disease activity, were found to have substantially reduced mean survival.[181]

Mechanical ventilation

Mortality in patients with IPF who require mechanical ventilation for acute respiratory failure is exceedingly high. Traditionally, patients requiring mechanical ventilation have been excluded from consideration for transplantation.[156] In one retrospective review of 34 patients with IPF and respiratory failure, 15 were placed on invasive mechanical ventilation, with 100% in-house mortality; the 19 patients placed on noninvasive ventilation had a 74% mortality rate. Of the five surviving patients, four died within 6 months of discharge (Box 4.2).[182]

Single-lung versus bilateral lung transplantation

Several analyses have found a survival benefit favoring BLT over SLT despite the initial challenge of longer and more difficult surgery. A review of the UNOS database from 1987 to 2008 found a 1-year conditional survival benefit for BLT over SLT in younger patients.[183] The UNOS data from 2005 to 2007 also demonstrated better 1-year survival after BLT in patients with the highest risk as measured by the highest lung allocation score.[184] In another evaluation of patients with IPF, posttransplant 6MWT and best FEV_1 were better for recipients of bilateral lung transplants, who also had better 1-year, overall, and bronchiolitis obliterans syndrome–free survival rates than did recipients of single-lung transplants; this benefit held despite the significantly higher preoperative mean pulmonary arterial pressure in recipients of bilateral lung transplants.[185]

Other evaluations have shown overall worse 30-day and 1-year survival in patients with IPF than in patients with other diagnoses, as well as no difference between recipients of single-lung transplants and bilateral lung transplants.[41,186]

Other diffuse parenchymal diseases

CONNECTIVE TISSUE DISEASE WITH ASSOCIATED LUNG DISEASE

Transplantation for pulmonary fibrosis associated with connective tissue disease accounts for only 0.8% of transplants,[1] at least partly because of concerns over systemic disease complicating transplantation, as well as a better prognosis than that with IPF.[187] Diffuse lung disease has been associated with multiple connective tissue diseases, including systemic sclerosis, polymyositis and dermatomyositis,

rheumatoid arthritis, mixed connective tissue disease, systemic lupus erythematosus, and Sjögren syndrome.[156] Given the limited experience, no specific recommendations for timing of referral or transplant exist.

SYSTEMIC SCLEROSIS

Pulmonary disease is ubiquitous in patients with systemic sclerosis but progressive in a minority of patients.[188] The prognosis is associated with obstruction, as well as decreased DLCO. Su and colleagues found that patients with systemic sclerosis had better 1-, 3-, and 5-year survival than did those with IPF and other connective tissue disease–associated lung disease, perhaps related to earlier diagnosis.[189] Transplants have been performed on patients with success,[190-193] with one center reporting 14 successful transplants and 1-year survival no different from that in patients with IPF, albeit with more acute rejection seen.[190] In a report from two centers, 29 patients who received transplants for scleroderma had slightly higher 6-month survival but an identical 2-year survival after transplantation when compared with patients with IPF and pulmonary hypertension,[191] and a UNOS database review of patients who received transplants between 1987 and 2004 for scleroderma revealed 1- and 3-year survival rates of 67.6% and 45.9%, which were similar to those of patients who received transplants in the same era.[192]

The systemic problems associated with scleroderma, including skin ulceration, chronic kidney disease, and esophageal dysmotility with aspiration, can be a contraindication of transplantation.[194] Patients to be considered for transplantation for scleroderma should have minimal systemic disease and progressive lung disease.

IDIOPATHIC INFLAMMATORY MYOPATHIES

Polymyositis, dermatomyositis, clinically amyopathic dermatomyositis, and antisynthetase syndrome are associated with interstitial lung disease in 35% to 40% of patients, with some experiencing progressive respiratory decline.[195] The associated muscle weakness may be a contraindication to transplantation[156] because it would preclude rehabilitation and pulmonary clearance. Transplantation may be considered in a patient with progressive lung disease as measured by serial pulmonary function tests and quiescent systemic disease.

RHEUMATOID ARTHRITIS, MIXED CONNECTIVE TISSUE DISEASE, SYSTEMIC LUPUS ERYTHEMATOSUS, AND SJÖGREN SYNDROME

Interstitial lung disease is seen in patients with rheumatoid arthritis with varying frequency, with debilitating pulmonary disease demonstrated in 1% to 4% of patients; severe inflammatory arthritis remains the most important contraindication to transplantation in this group.[156] A UIP pattern on HRCT and on biopsy is seen more frequently in rheumatoid arthritis compared with in other connective tissue disease–associated interstitial lung disease and correspondingly appears to be correlated with a worse prognosis.[196]

Pleural disease is common in those with systemic lupus erythematosus, but progression of overt fibrotic lung disease appears to be rare and the disease most likely progresses slowly; in a small series of 14 patients with interstitial disease and lupus, only 2 died of progressive lung disease.[197,198] In one sequential series of 144 patients with mixed connective tissue disease, 96 (66.6%) had evidence of active interstitial lung disease, most of which resolved after therapy, although in 13 patients some fibrosis remained on HRCT and in 1 honeycombing remained.[199] In patients with mixed connective tissue disease, an association exists between esophageal dilatation and interstitial lung disease,[200] raising concern that this could be an additional contraindication to transplantation. Finally, interstitial lung disease complicates the course of Sjögren syndrome for many patients; in one series it affected 9 of 20 patients.[201]

The approach to transplantation is similar to that with the other connective tissue diseases in that patients with progressive pulmonary disease and minimal systemic disease should be referred to a transplant center.

SARCOIDOSIS

A multisystem disease, sarcoidosis may lead to significant dysfunction of other organs (e.g., heart, liver), which can preclude transplantation. Sarcoidosis currently accounts for 2.6% of the lung transplants performed.[4] Patients with advanced pulmonary sarcoidosis have been shown to have high mortality while on a lung transplant list; of 43 patients with sarcoidosis who were listed for lung transplantation at the University of Pennsylvania Medical Center, 23 (53%) died while listed. Listed patients had a 31% survival rate at 3 years, although the 12 patients who received transplants had a 50% survival rate at 3 years.[202] Waiting list survival has been shown to be similar to that for patients with idiopathic pulmonary fibrosis, although those with sarcoidosis had a higher burden of pulmonary hypertension.[203]

Prognosis

Pulmonary hypertension has emerged as the most important risk factor for mortality in patients with sarcoidosis.[204] In multivariate analysis, right arterial pressure of 15 mm Hg was independently associated with an increased risk for death.[202] In a review of 405 patients listed for transplantation for sarcoidosis in the United States between 1995 and 2000, risk for death was associated with increased pulmonary artery pressure, increased need for supplemental oxygen, and Afro-American race (Box 4.3).[205]

LYMPHANGIOLEIOMYOMATOSIS

LAM, which is the indication for 1.1% of the transplants performed in a recent ISHLT report,[1] is a rare disease that had been thought to occur only in women of childbearing age and to be nearly uniformly fatal within 10 years when it was first described.[206,207] With increased awareness, detection, and the creation of rare disease registries,[208] the full spectrum of the disease is now understood to include older women and some who have a slow and indolent course, with

---

BOX 4.3: Guidelines for patients with sarcoidosis

GUIDELINE FOR REFERRAL

New York Heart Association (NYHA) functional class III or IV

GUIDELINES FOR TRANSPLANTATION

Impairment of exercise tolerance (NYHA functional class III or IV) and any of the following:

- Hypoxemia at rest
- Pulmonary hypertension
- Elevated right atrial pressure >15 mm Hg

10-year survival rates reported to be as high as 91%.[209–212] In a LAM registry that enrolled patients from 1998 until 2001, one third of patients either received or were listed for a lung transplant for LAM.[213]

Transplant concerns

Although survival has been comparable to that with other conditions, disease-specific complications after transplantation have included recurrent pneumothorax and chylothorax requiring intervention, and surgery may be complicated by previous pleural procedures, thus leading to increased bleeding.[99,214–216] Transplantation for LAM has also rarely been complicated by recurrence of disease.[215–217] These risks must be adequately conveyed to a patient during the process of evaluation for transplantation.

Progression

Disease progression has typically been defined as a decrease in FEV_1 and/or D_{LCO}, both of which have been correlated with the extent of disease as determined by CT and histology score.[218,219] The LAM histologic score, which expresses the extent of involvement of both cystic and smooth muscle lesions, has also been associated with survival time and time to transplantation.[220] The declines in FEV_1 and D_{LCO} are highly variable, with the yearly decline in FEV_1 ranging anywhere from none to 285 mL/yr in rapidly progressive disease[218] and with one study averaging a 110-mL loss of FEV_1 per year.[209] The presence of reversible airflow obstruction has been associated with an accelerated decline in lung function.[221,222]

Only one treatment, sirolimus, has proved to have some efficacy in slowing the decline in lung function[223]; its effect on progression to lung transplantation for LAM remains to be seen.

Timing for transplantation

Serial assessment of lung function and functional capacity remains the best way to determine those patients headed for decline who may require transplantation. The 2006 ISHLT guidelines have recommended criteria for referral and listing (Box 4.4).[3]

BOX 4.4: Guidelines for patients with lymphangioleiomyomatosis

GUIDELINE FOR REFERRAL

New York Heart Association (NYHA) functional class III or IV

GUIDELINES FOR TRANSPLANTATION

- Severe impairment in lung function and exercise capacity (e.g., Vo_2max <50% predicted)
- Hypoxemia at rest

If serial lung function measurements demonstrate rapid decline despite therapy, earlier referral should be considered.

BOX 4.5: Guidelines for patients with pulmonary Langerhans cell histiocytosis

GUIDELINE FOR REFERRAL

New York Heart Association (NYHA) functional class III or IV

GUIDELINES FOR TRANSPLANTATION

Impairment of exercise tolerance (NYHA functional class III or IV) and any of the following:

- Severe impairment in lung function and exercise capacity
- Hypoxemia at rest

PULMONARY LANGERHANS CELL HISTIOCYTOSIS (EOSINOPHILIC GRANULOMA)

Transplantation

Pulmonary Langerhans cell histiocytosis is a rare diagnosis for lung transplantation, a reflection of the fact that in many patients the disease may stabilize or regress.[224]

A retrospective review of 39 patients throughout France who received transplants for pulmonary Langerhans cell histiocytosis demonstrated survival rates of 76.9% at 1 year, 63.6% at 2 years, 57.2% at 5 years, and 53.7% at 10 years; an almost 20% recurrence rate was seen and associated with extrapulmonary disease before transplantation.[225]

Prognosis

Median survival in two retrospective studies was similar at 12.5 and 13 years.[226,227] Decreased survival has been associated with older age at diagnosis, lower FEV_1, higher RV, lower ratio of FEV_1 to FVC, higher ratio of RV to total lung capacity, steroid therapy during follow-up, and reduced D_{LCO}.[226,227] Advanced disease is very commonly associated with severe pulmonary hypertension unrelated to the degree of impairment in pulmonary function, with the disease directly causing a pulmonary vasculopathy.[224,225,228–230] Pulmonary hypertension is nearly ubiquitous in such transplant recipients.[225]

Timing for transplantation

As with LAM, serial assessment of lung function and functional capacity is required because no precise prognostic tools exist for this rare disease. Attention to the severity and progression of pulmonary hypertension should be part of consideration when listing. The 2006 ISHLT guidelines have recommended criteria for referral and listing similar to those for LAM (Box 4.5).[3]

CYSTIC FIBROSIS AND OTHER CAUSES OF BRONCHIECTASIS

CF is a major indication for lung transplantation; it accounted for 16% of transplants between 1995 and 2010.[2]

CF is a multisystem disease that affects patients younger than those with diagnoses typically necessitating a transplant. A survival benefit for patients undergoing transplantation for CF has been consistently demonstrated,[106,231–233] and in some analyses it has been the best among transplant diagnoses.[231,232]

Bronchiectasis not associated with CF may occur as a result of a variety of causes, including congenital, related to autoimmune disease or malignancy, related to previous infection, and related to immune deficiency.[234] These disorders have been treated similarly to CF with regard to lung transplantation.[3]

Prognosis

FEV_1

The traditional transplant referral basis of an FEV_1 of 30% predicted came from an early study by Kerem and associates in 1992. In a retrospective study of 673 patients between 1977 and 1989, patients with an FEV_1 less than 30% predicted, Pao_2 less than 55, and Pco greater than 50 had a 2-year mortality rate greater than 50%. The relative risk of death was 2.0 for each 10 percentage points of FEV_1 below predicted.[240] This mortality rate implied an appropriate time for transplantation to confer survival benefit. Worsening FEV_1 has also been associated with death while listed for transplantation; in one series, patients who died while awaiting a transplant had a significantly lower FEV_1 (15% predicted) than did those who received successful transplants (21% predicted), as well as a lower 6MWT distance.[241] FEV_1% predicted has been included in several predictive models for survival for CF.[237,242,243]

As CF survival has improved, more recent studies have suggested that an FEV_1 cutoff of 30% is insufficient as an absolute cutoff for transplantation. Augarten and colleagues evaluated 40 patients with an FEV_1 less than 30% predicted and found a trend for patients who did not receive a transplant to have improved survival.[244]

The mortality rate of 50% at 2 years described by Kerem and colleagues[238] has not been reproduced in follow-up evaluation of patients with severely decreased lung function, thus suggesting that evolution in CF treatment has affected survival. One retrospective review examined 61 patients with a consistent FEV_1 less than 30% predicted at the University of Minnesota. Of 49 deceased patients with an FEV_1 less than 30% predicted, only one third had reached that level within 2 years of death. The remainder lived with this severe reduction in FEV_1 for a range of 2 to 14 years. Survival analysis indicated that the median life span for patients with an FEV_1 less than 30% predicted was 3.9 years.[245] Another series found that 178 patients with an FEV_1 less than 30% predicted had a median survival of 4.6 years, with 25% living more than 9 years in the pretransplant era (1986 to 1990).[246] George and colleagues monitored 276 patients with an FEV_1 less than 30% predicted who were identified between 1990 and 2003 and followed until 2007 at one center in the United Kingdom; they found that median survival improved from 1.2 years in 1990 to 5.3 years in 2003. The largest gain occurred between 1994 and 1997; it was coincident with the availability of DNAse in the United Kingdom, as well as with improved nutritional status for the cohort.[247]

Rate of decline in FEV_1 has also been indicated as a useful parameter to predict mortality and timing for transplantation.[248] For patients who survived less than the median, the rate of decline in FEV_1 was higher (1.8% predicted per year) than that in patients who survived longer than the median (0.73% predicted per year), with the rate of decline in FEV_1 being a significant predictor of death. An increase in the relative risk for death of 1.3 for every increase in the rate of decline by 1% predicted per year was noted.[245] Augarten and colleagues also found that rate of decline in FEV_1 contributed independently to mortality (Box 4.6).[244]

Sex

Female sex has been associated with increased risk for death in many studies,[235,237,249–251] although a handful have also evaluated for sex and not found an effect.[244,245,252] The mechanism of this effect of sex is unclear, and the extent of the disparity is difficult to estimate. Kerem and associates found that female patients had an increased risk for death for any given FEV_1, with a relative risk of 2.2.[240] In another study, female patients were more likely to have frequent exacerbations.[253] Patients in whom CF is diagnosed at an older age may not have such a disparity; retrospective review of the Colorado Cystic Fibrosis Foundation database (1992 to 2008), the Cystic Fibrosis Foundation registry (1992 to 2007), and the Multiple Cause of Death Index (1992 to 2005) demonstrated the existence of sex disparity, particularly for patients in whom CF was diagnosed during childhood. Females with CF diagnosed in childhood had a steeper decline in FEV_1 and were less likely to reach the age of 40, with female patients representing only 35.7% of the patients in the Cystic Fibrosis Foundation registry who reached age 40. Female patients in whom CF was diagnosed in childhood lost the expected survival advantage seen in unaffected people. In contrast, when compared with males, females who were diagnosed in adulthood had an equal decline in FEV_1 and longer survival.[235]

Age

Younger age has been implicated in increased mortality. Age younger than 18 has been associated with shorter survival[245]; in the review by Kerem and colleagues, younger patients (age <18 years) had a relative risk of death of 2.0.[240] A more recent retrospective review of UNOS data on patients receiving a transplant for CF from 1999 to 2007 with follow-up to 2008 stratified patients into age quartiles. Patients in the youngest quartile (age = 7 to 20) had significantly worse long-term survival (with a 5-year cumulative survival rate of 43%) than did those in the oldest quartiles (age = 28 to 34 and >35), who had a 5-year cumulative survival rate of 62%.[239] Interestingly, once they are older than 40 years, patients in whom CF was diagnosed in adulthood (who have delayed clinical symptoms) and patients in whom it was diagnosed in childhood have similar rates of decline in FEV_1 and death from respiratory disease, thus indicating that the disease will progress to end-stage disease requiring transplantation even in those initially seen as adults.[235]

Frequency of exacerbations

Acute exacerbations are associated with worse outcome. Number of admissions has been correlated with mortality,[253] and more severe admissions requiring intensive care are associated with worse outcomes.[254] Ellaffi and colleagues found that patients admitted to the ICU had a 1-year survival rate of 52% versus with 91% for those admitted to a regular floor.[254] A 3-year prospective cohort study monitored 446 patients with CF. When compared with patients with less than one exacerbation per year, those patients with more than two exacerbations per year had an increased risk for decline in FEV_1, as well as an increased risk for lung transplantation or death with an adjusted hazard ratio of 4.0.[255]

Pulmonary hemodynamics

Pulmonary hemodynamics was shown to be important in a series of 45 patients on the lung transplant list at one institution. Patients who died while awaiting transplantation were more likely to have had severe pulmonary hypertension; the patients who died while on the waiting list had worse mean pulmonary arterial pressure, $Paco_2$, and systemic vascular resistance than did those who either received a transplant or were alive and waiting for one. Patients with supplemental oxygen use, an intrapulmonary shunt, lower Pao_2/Fio_2 ratio, systemic vascular resistance, a lower cardiac index, a higher mean pulmonary arterial pressure, and a deranged heart rate trended toward an increased risk for death while on the transplant list.[256] The severity of pulmonary hypertension was also associated with death in a small series of 27 patients,[253] and another review of 146 patients wait-listed for lung transplantation for CF at Barnes Jewish Hospital showed that higher pulmonary artery pressure was an independent risk factor for death while awaiting a transplant.[236]

Predictive model

One predictive model for 5-year survival was proposed in 2001; it was created and validated by using patients in the Cystic Fibrosis Foundation Patient registry. The model included age, FEV_1, sex, weight-for-age z value, pancreatic sufficiency, diabetes, *Staphylococcus aureus* infection, *Burkholderia cepacia* infection, and annual number of acute pulmonary exacerbations. The same researchers found that using their model to identify patients with less than a 30% 5-year survival rate resulted in a survival benefit for that group whereas using only the criterion of FEV_1 less than 30% predicted resulted in an equivocal survival benefit. Groups with higher expected survival by predictive model had either an equivocal or a negative survival effect from transplantation.[257]

This model was applied to Italian patients as a validation cohort and found to be inaccurate; improved prediction with a model consisting of FEV_1, *S. aureus*, *B. cepacia* complex infection, and number of yearly pulmonary exacerbations provided better prediction of survival.[243]

Risk for infection

Airway microbial colonization plus infection is a chronic problem for patients with CF. For this reason, virtually all lung transplants performed for CF are bilateral.

B. cepacia

The microbial milieu of an individual patient has been evaluated for both mortality and risk for the transplant. The presence of *B. cepacia* infection has been associated with an odds ratio for death of 4.12 in the predictive model of Liou and colleagues.[237] Likewise, *B. cepacia* infection has been thought to increase the risk associated with transplantation, and at many centers it is considered a contraindication to transplantation.

Chaparro and colleagues reviewed 53 patients who received transplants for CF, 28 of whom had *B. cepacia* complex colonization. Survival was affected in both the early and later years, with early mortality in the first 3 months contributing to a 1-year survival rate of 67% in *B. cepacia*–infected patients as opposed to a 1-year survival rate of 96% in noninfected patients. Three-year survival rates decreased from 86% to 45%; infections were the predominant cause of death for both early and late mortality.[258]

Aris and colleagues performed a retrospective review of 121 patients who received transplants for CF at the University of North Carolina and found a significant decrease in survival for those infected with *B. cepacia* before transplantation ($n = 21$) in the first 6 and 12 months, with 5 of the 21 dying of *B. cepacia* sepsis. In 1993 to 1998 no transplants were performed in patients infected with *B. cepacia*. All five patients who died of infection had *Burkholderia cenocepacia*, also referred to as genomovar III.[259] Recent analysis has agreed that the increased risk seems peculiar to *B. cenocepacia*, which in one series of 75 transplant patients at Duke was associated with substantially reduced survival when compared with that in both those not infected with *Burkholderia*

and those infected with other *B. cepacia* strains. Uninfected patients had a 5-year survival rate of 63%, patients infected with other *B. cepacia* strains had a 5-year survival rate of 56%, and those infected with *B. cenocepacia* had a 5-year survival rate of 29%.[260] One additional study looking at 216 patients who received transplants for CF beginning in 1989 found that of the 22 patients with preoperative *B. cepacia* infection, the 12 patients with *B. cenocepacia* had decreased survival, with 9 experiencing early mortality from *B. cenocepacia* sepsis. The remaining 10 patients, who were infected with a *Burkholderia* species other than *cenocepacia*, had the same survival as the remainder of the cohort.[261]

Other microbial colonization aside from *Burkholderia* has not demonstrated a significant impact. Liou and associates reported a survival benefit of *S. aureus* colonization in their predictive model.[237] At one center, patients with pan-resistant bacterial infection aside from *B. cepacia* were found to have decreased survival when compared with patients not infected with such bacteria, although their survival compared favorably to the UNOS data. Microbial colonization in that cohort was mostly with resistant *Pseudomonas aeruginosa*, *Stenotrophomonas*, and *Achromobacter*.[262]

Liver disease

Significant liver disease, evolving to cirrhosis in many patients, is common in those with CF; the cumulative incidence of hepatic involvement is thought to be between 27% and 35%. Most frequently it is focal biliary cirrhosis, which in a subset of patients progresses to multilobular cirrhosis and complications of end-stage liver disease.[263] Liver disease has been noted to be an independent risk factor for death or lung transplantation.[264] Successful lung transplants have been performed in patients with well-compensated CF liver disease who had preserved hepatic synthetic function, with no adverse effect on outcomes.[265,266] Those with advanced liver and lung disease may be considered for a combined lung-liver transplant.

Critical illness and mechanical ventilation

As described earlier, mechanical ventilation before transplantation carries an increased risk for death and shorter survival.[1,2,73] Hospitalization in an ICU has also been shown to increase mortality before transplantation in patients with CF.[239] Some small series have reported success in performing transplants on patients with CF who require mechanical ventilation.[75–77] Transplantation should be limited to patients who have single-organ failure, do not have systemic infection, and are still able to participate in physical therapy.[267]

PULMONARY ARTERIAL HYPERTENSION

Pulmonary hypertension, which is a disorder with many different causes,[268] has long been an indication for lung transplantation. Idiopathic pulmonary arterial hypertension has represented a decreasing share of the total number of transplants performed, now representing 3.2% of all transplants since 1995.[2] Patients with idiopathic pulmonary

---

BOX 4.6: Guidelines for patients with cystic fibrosis

GUIDELINES FOR REFERRAL

- Forced expiratory volume in 1 second (FEV_1) <30% predicted or a rapid decline in FEV_1—especially in young female patients
- Exacerbation of pulmonary disease requiring stay in an intensive care unit
- Increasing frequency of exacerbations requiring antibiotic therapy
- Refractory and/or recurrent pneumothorax
- Recurrent hemoptysis not controlled by embolization

GUIDELINES FOR TRANSPLANTATION

- Oxygen-dependent respiratory failure
- Hypercapnia
- Pulmonary hypertension

---

arterial hypertension demonstrate high short-term mortality but good long-term survival when compared with other transplant patients, second only to those with CF. The decreasing percentage of transplants for idiopathic pulmonary arterial hypertension has been influenced by modern therapy, thus leading to an improved prognosis.

Prognosis

Before the current age of therapy, the prognosis was grim for patients with pulmonary arterial hypertension; the survival rate for a group of 57 patients with pulmonary hypertension who did not receive transplants was reported to be 35% at 3 years.[269] Median survival was estimated to be 2.8 years from the National Institutes of Health registry and was negatively affected by mean pulmonary artery pressure (≥85 versus ≤55 mm Hg), mean right atrial pressure (<10 versus ≥20 mm Hg), and mean cardiac index (<2 versus ≥4 L/min/m²).[270]

Subsequent evaluations have confirmed that right-sided heart failure and a right atrial pressure of 12 mm Hg or higher are associated with poor survival at baseline.[271] Even with successful unloading of pulmonary resistance with medical therapy, a progressive decline in right ventricular function may be seen and is associated with a poor prognosis.[272]

Continuous intravenous epoprostenol was tested in a 12-week randomized controlled trial of 81 patients with severe pulmonary hypertension and found to improve exercise capacity, quality of life, and hemodynamics (mean pulmonary artery pressure decreasing 8% in the treatment group and a mean decrease in pulmonary vascular resistance of 21%), and most impressively, it was found to significantly improve survival in the treatment group.[273] Longer-term benefit was confirmed by following the course

of 162 patients receiving intravenous epoprostenol between 1991 and 2001; the observed survival rates at 1, 2, and 3 years were 87.8%, 76.3%, and 62.8%, as compared with the National Institutes of Health registry data of 58.9%, 46.3%, and 35.4%, respectively.[270,274]

Functional class and response to therapy can be predictive of mortality. In one study, 178 patients with pulmonary arterial hypertension were treated with long-term prostacyclin infusion. The overall survival rates of the patients treated were 85% at 1 year, 70% at 2 years, 63% at 3 years, and 55% at 5 years. Patients with NYHA functional class IV when initially seen had a worse survival rate (47% at 3 years) than patients in NYHA class III (71% at 3 years). Although some patients had improvement in functional status, the group of patients who persisted in class III or IV had survival rates of 77% at 1 year, 46% at 2 years, and 33% at 3 years. Patients who did not have improvement in functional class or a 30% decrease in pulmonary resistance had significantly increased mortality.[271]

The 6MWT has been correlated with Vo_2max obtained during cardiopulmonary exercise testing and has been independently related to mortality in a multivariate analysis of 43 patients with pulmonary arterial hypertension. Survival was significantly decreased in patients walking less than 332 m in 6 minutes.[275] The patients enrolled in the randomized controlled trial of epoprostenol who died had significantly lower 6MWT distances as well.[271]

Echocardiography may be of prognostic benefit; in a prospective analysis of 81 patients with pulmonary arterial hypertension, echocardiographic findings of pericardial effusion and an enlarged right atrium were predictors of death or transplantation, along with lower 6MWT score, lower mixed venous oxygen saturation, and treatment randomization to conventional therapy instead of prostacyclin.[276]

Referral

Based on the aforementioned prognostic data, the ISHLT has developed recommendations for referral of patients with pulmonary arterial hypertension (Box 4.7).

Despite the effectiveness of medical therapy, survival of patients with progressive disease remains improved with lung transplantation for patients with severe disease,[277] although waiting list mortality has not been improved by the recently implemented lung allocation score.[278] Serial assessment remains important to identify patients with a declining course who will require surgical therapy.[279] Identification of those who can benefit remains a major challenge facing the lung transplant community because those with severe pulmonary hypertension may be underserved by current allocation.

This chapter has dealt in some detail with the difficulties associated with patient selection for lung transplantation. Updated guidelines will soon be available to supplement the information contained here. In the meantime, the authors encourage readers and learners to explore selection criteria via the references included here.

BOX 4.7: Guidelines for patients with pulmonary arterial hypertension

GUIDELINES FOR REFERRAL

- New York Heart Association (NYHA) functional class III or IV, irrespective of ongoing therapy
- Rapidly progressive disease

GUIDELINES FOR TRANSPLANTATION

- Persistent NYHA class III or IV on maximal medical therapy
- Low (<350 m) or declining 6-minute walk test (6MWT) score
- Failing therapy with intravenous epoprostenol or equivalent
- Cardiac index <2 L/min/m^2
- Right atrial pressure >15 mm Hg

REFERENCES

1. Yusen RD, Edwards LB, Kucheryavaya AY, et al. The Registry of the International Society for Heart and Lung Transplantation: Thirty-first lung and heart-lung transplant report—2013; focus theme: Retransplantation. J Heart Lung Transplant 2014;33:1009-1024.
2. Christie JD, Edwards LB, Kucheryavaya AY, et al. The Registry of the International Society for Heart and Lung Transplantation: Twenty-eighth Adult Lung and Heart-Lung Transplant Report—2011. J Heart Lung Transplant 2011;30:1104-1122.
3. Orens JB, Estenne M, Arcasoy S, et al. International guidelines for the selection of lung transplant candidates: 2006 update—a consensus report from the Pulmonary Scientific Council of the International Society for Heart and Lung Transplantation. J Heart Lung Transplant 2006;25:745-755.
4. Christie JD, Edwards LB, Kucheryavaya AY, et al. The Registry of the International Society for Heart and Lung Transplantation: Twenty-seventh official adult lung and heart-lung transplant report—2010. J Heart Lung Transplant 2010;29:1104-1118.
5. Travis WD, Brambilla E, Noguchi M, et al. International Association for the Study of Lung Cancer/American Thoracic Society/European Respiratory Society International Multidisciplinary Classification of Lung Adenocarcinoma. J Thorac Oncol 2011;6:244-285.
6. Etienne B, Bertocchi M, Gamondes JP, et al. Successful double-lung transplantation for bronchioalveolar carcinoma. Chest 1997;112:1423-1424.
7. Wang Y, Chen J. [Lung transplantation for lung carcinoma: A case report and literature review.] Zhongguo Fei Ai Za Zhi 2011;14:633-636.
8. Zorn GL Jr, McGiffin DC, Young KR Jr, et al. Pulmonary transplantation for advanced bronchioloalveolar carcinoma. J Thorac Cardiovasc Surg 2003;125:45-48.
9. de Perrot M, Chernenko S, Waddell TK, et al. Role of lung transplantation in the treatment of bronchogenic carcinomas for patients with end-stage pulmonary disease. J Clin Oncol 2004;22:4351-4356.
10. de Perrot M, Fischer S, Waddell TK, et al. Management of lung transplant recipients with bronchogenic carcinoma in the native lung. J Heart Lung Transplant 2003;22:87-89.
11. Abrahams NA, Meziane M, Ramalingam P, et al. Incidence of primary neoplasms in explanted lungs: Long-term follow-up from 214 lung transplant patients. Transplant Proc 2004;36:2808-2811.
12. Su JW, Mason DP, Murthy SC, et al. Successful double lung transplantation in 2 patients with severe scoliosis. J Heart Lung Transplant 2008;27:1262-1264.
13. Fukahara K, Minami K, Hansky B, et al. Successful heart-lung transplantation in a patient with kyphoscoliosis. J Heart Lung Transplant 2003;22:468-473.
14. Piotrowski JA, Splittgerber FH, Donovan TJ, et al. Single-lung transplantation in a patient with cystic fibrosis and an asymmetric thorax. Ann Thorac Surg 1997;64:1456-1458; discussion 1458-1459.
15. Garcha PS, Santacruz JF, Machuzak MS, et al. Clinical course after successful double lung transplantation in a patient with severe scoliosis. J Heart Lung Transplant 2011;30:234-235.
16. Bertani A, Grossi P, Vitulo P, et al. Successful lung transplantation in an HIV- and HBV-positive patient with cystic fibrosis. Am J Transplant 2009;9:2190-2196.
17. Fong TL, Cho YW, Hou L, et al. Outcomes after lung transplantation and practices of lung transplant programs in the United States regarding hepatitis C seropositive recipients. Transplantation 2011;91:1293-1296.
18. Sahi H, Zein NN, Mehta AC, et al. Outcomes after lung transplantation in patients with chronic hepatitis C virus infection. J Heart Lung Transplant 2007;26:466-471.
19. Barshes NR, DiBardino DJ, McKenzie ED, et al. Combined lung and liver transplantation: The United States experience. Transplantation 2005;80:1161-1167.
20. Corno V, Dezza MC, Lucianetti A, et al. Combined double lung-liver transplantation for cystic fibrosis without cardio-pulmonary by-pass. Am J Transplant 2007;7:2433-2438.

21. Couetil JP, Houssin DP, Soubrane O, et al. Combined lung and liver transplantation in patients with cystic fibrosis. A 4 1/2-year experience. J Thorac Cardiovasc Surg 1995;110:1415-1422; discussion 1422-1423.

22. Couetil JP, Soubrane O, Houssin DP, et al. Combined heart-lung-liver, double lung-liver, and isolated liver transplantation for cystic fibrosis in children. Transpl Int 1997;10:33-39.

23. Dennis CM, McNeil KD, Dunning J, et al. Heart-lung-liver transplantation. J Heart Lung Transplant 1996;15:536-538.

24. Gandhi SK, Reyes J, Webber SA, et al. Case report of combined pediatric heart-lung-liver transplantation. Transplantation 2002;73:1968-1969.

25. Praseedom RK, McNeil KD, Watson CJ, et al. Combined transplantation of the heart, lung, and liver. Lancet 2001;358:812-813.

26. Wise PE, Wright JK, Chapman WC, et al. Heart-lung-liver transplant for cystic fibrosis. Transplant Proc 2001;33:3568-3571.

27. Erim Y, Beckmann M, Marggraf G, Senf W. Psychosomatic evaluation of patients awaiting lung transplantation. Transplant Proc 2009;41:2595-2598.

28. Germani G, Lazzaro S, Gnoato F, et al. Nonadherent behaviors after solid organ transplantation. Transplant Proc 2011;43:318-323.

29. Dobbels F, Vanhaecke J, Dupont L, et al. Pretransplant predictors of posttransplant adherence and clinical outcome: An evidence base for pretransplant psychosocial screening. Transplantation 2009;87:1497-1504.

30. De Bleser L, Dobbels F, Berben L, et al. The spectrum of nonadherence with medication in heart, liver, and lung tranplant patients assessed in various ways. Transpl Int 2011;24:882-891.

31. Bosma OH, Vermeulen KM, Verschuuren EA, et al. Adherence to immunosuppression in adult lung transplant recipients: Prevalence and risk factors. J Heart Lung Transplant 2011;30:21275-1280.

32. Evon DM, Burker EJ, Sedway JA, et al. Tobacco and alcohol use in lung transplant candidates and recipients. Clin Transplant 2005;19:207-214.

33. Gorber SC, Schofield-Hurwitz S, Hardt J. The accuracy of self-reported smoking: A systematic review of the relationship between self-reported and cotinine-assessed smoking status. Nicotine Tob Res 2009;11:12-24.

34. Gutierrez C, Al-Faifi S, Chaparro C, et al. The effect of recipient's age on lung transplant outcome. Am J Transplant 2007;7:1271-1277.

35. Weiss ES, Allen JG, Merlo CA, et al. Lung allocation score predicts survival in lung transplantation patients with pulmonary fibrosis. Ann Thorac Surg 2009;88:1757-1764.

36. Smith PW, Wang H, Parini V, et al. Lung transplantation in patients 60 years and older: Results, complications, and outcomes. Ann Thorac Surg 2006;82:1835-1841; discussion 1841.

37. Machuca TN, Camargo SM, Schio SM, et al. Lung transplantation for patients older than 65 years: Is it a feasible option? Transplant Proc 2011;43:233-235.

38. Mahidhara R, Bastani S, Ross DJ, et al. Lung transplantation in older patients? J Thorac Cardiovasc Surg 2008;135:412-20.

39. Vadnerkar A, Toyoda Y, Crespo M, et al. Age-specific complications among lung transplant recipients 60 years and older. J Heart Lung Transplant 2011;30:273-281.

40. Meyer DM, Bennett LE, Novick RJ, Hosenpud JD. Single vs bilateral, sequential lung transplantation for end-stage emphysema: Influence of recipient age on survival and secondary end-points. J Heart Lung Transplant 2001;20:935-941.

41. Meyer DM, Edwards LB, Torres F, et al. Impact of recipient age and procedure type on survival after lung transplantation for pulmonary fibrosis. Ann Thorac Surg 2005;79:950-957; discussion 957-958.

42. Minambres E, Llorca J, Suberviola B, et al. Early outcome after single vs bilateral lung transplantation in older recipients. Transplant Proc 2008;40:3088-3089.

43. Palmer SM, Davis RD, Simsir SA, et al. Successful bilateral lung transplant outcomes in recipients 61 years of age and older. Transplantation 2006;81:862-865.

44. Nwakanma LU, Simpkins CE, Williams JA, et al. Impact of bilateral versus single lung transplantation on survival in recipients 60 years of age and older: Analysis of United Network for Organ Sharing database. J Thorac Cardiovasc Surg 2007;133:541-547.

45. Souza SM, Nakasato M, Bruno ML, Macedo A. Nutritional profile of lung transplant candidates. J Bras Pneumol 2009;35:242-247.

46. Madill J, Gutierrez C, Grossman J, et al. Nutritional assessment of the lung transplant patient: Body mass index as a predictor of 90-day mortality following transplantation. J Heart Lung Transplant 2001;20:288-296.

47. Kanasky WF Jr, Anton SD, Rodrigue JR, et al. Impact of body weight on long-term survival after lung transplantation. Chest 2002;121:401-406.

48. Culver DA, Mazzone PJ, Khandwala F, et al. Discordant utility of ideal body weight and body mass index as predictors of mortality in lung transplant recipients. J Heart Lung Transplant 2005;24:137-144.

49. de la Torre MM, Delgado M, Paradela M, et al. Influence of body mass index in the postoperative evolution after lung transplantation. Transplant Proc 2010;42:3026-3028.

50. Plochl W, Pezawas L, Artemiou O, et al. Nutritional status, ICU duration and ICU mortality in lung transplant recipients. Intensive Care Med 1996;22:1179-1185.

51. Lederer DJ, Wilt JS, D'Ovidio F, et al. Obesity and underweight are associated with an increased risk of death after lung transplantation. Am J Respir Crit Care Med 2009;180:887-895.

52. Allen JG, Arnaoutakis GJ, Weiss ES, et al. The impact of recipient body mass index on survival after lung transplantation. J Heart Lung Transplant 2010;29:1026-1033.

53. Machuca TN, Schio SM, Camargo SM, et al. Prognostic factors in lung transplantation: The Santa Casa de Porto Alegre experience. Transplantation 2011;91:1297-1303.

54. Sherman W, Rabkin DG, Ross D, et al. Lung transplantation and coronary artery disease. Ann Thorac Surg 2011;92:303-308.

55. Parekh K, Meyers BF, Patterson GA, et al. Outcome of lung transplantation for patients requiring concomitant cardiac surgery. J Thorac Cardiovasc Surg 2005;130:859-863.

56. Patel VS, Palmer SM, Messier RH, Davis RD. Clinical outcome after coronary artery revascularization and lung transplantation. Ann Thorac Surg 2003;75:372-377; discussion 377.

57. Plantier L, Skhiri N, Biondi G, et al. Impact of previous cardiovascular disease on the outcome of lung transplantation. J Heart Lung Transplant 2010;29:1270-1276.

58. Bradbury RA, Shirkhedkar D, Glanville AR, Campbell LV. Prior diabetes mellitus is associated with increased morbidity in cystic fibrosis patients undergoing bilateral lung transplantation: An 'orphan' area? A retrospective case-control study. Intern Med J 2009;39:384-388.

59. Hofer M, Schmid C, Benden C, et al. Diabetes mellitus and survival in cystic fibrosis patients after lung transplantation. J Cyst Fibros 2011;11:131-136.

60. Palmer SM, Miralles AP, Howell DN, et al. Gastroesophageal reflux as a reversible cause of allograft dysfunction after lung transplantation. Chest 2000;118:1214-1217.

61. Shah N, Force SD, Mitchell PO, et al. Gastroesophageal reflux disease is associated with an increased rate of acute rejection in lung transplant allografts. Transplant Proc 2010;42:2702-2706.

62. Murthy SC, Nowicki ER, Mason DP, et al. Pretransplant gastroesophageal reflux compromises early outcomes after lung transplantation. J Thorac Cardiovasc Surg 2011;142:47-52 e3.

63. Reid KR, McKenzie FN, Menkis AH, et al. Importance of chronic aspiration in recipients of heart-lung transplants. Lancet 1990;336:206-208.

64. Sweet MP, Herbella FA, Leard L, et al. The prevalence of distal and proximal gastroesophageal reflux in patients awaiting lung transplantation. Ann Surg 2006;244:491-497.

65. Fortunato GA, Machado MM, Andrade CF, et al. Prevalence of gastroesophageal reflux in lung transplant candidates with advanced lung disease. J Bras Pneumol 2008;34:772-778.

66. Young LR, Hadjiliadis D, Davis RD, Palmer SM. Lung transplantation exacerbates gastroesophageal reflux disease. Chest 2003;124:1689-1693.

67. D'Ovidio F, Keshavjee S. Gastroesophageal reflux and lung transplantation. Dis Esophagus 2006;19:315-320.

68. Blondeau K, Mertens V, Vanaudenaerde BA, et al. Gastro-oesophageal reflux and gastric aspiration in lung transplant patients with or without chronic rejection. Eur Respir J 2008;31:707-713.

69. Davis RD Jr, Lau CL, Eubanks S, et al. Improved lung allograft function after fundoplication in patients with gastroesophageal reflux disease undergoing lung transplantation. J Thorac Cardiovasc Surg 2003;125:533-542.

70. Gasper WJ, Sweet MP, Hoopes C, et al. Antireflux surgery for patients with end-stage lung disease before and after lung transplantation. Surg Endosc 2008;22:495-500.

71. Hoppo T, Jarido V, Pennathur A, et al. Antireflux surgery preserves lung function in patients with gastroesophageal reflux disease and end-stage lung disease before and after lung transplantation. Arch Surg 2011;146:1041-1047.

72. Hartwig MG, Appel JZ, Davis RD. Antireflux surgery in the setting of lung transplantation: Strategies for treating gastroesophageal reflux disease in a high-risk population. Thorac Surg Clin 2005;15:417-427.

73. Mason DP, Thuita L, Nowicki ER, et al. Should lung transplantation be performed for patients on mechanical respiratory support? The US experience. J Thorac Cardiovasc Surg 2010;139:765-773.

74. Flume PA, Egan TM, Westerman JH, et al. Lung transplantation for mechanically ventilated patients. J Heart Lung Transplant 1994;13:15-21; discussion 22-23.

75. Massard G, Shennib H, Metras D, et al. Double-lung transplantation in mechanically ventilated patients with cystic fibrosis. Ann Thorac Surg 1993;55:1087-1091; discussion 1091-1092.

76. Bartz RR, Love RB, Leverson GE, et al. Pre-transplant mechanical ventilation and outcome in patients with cystic fibrosis. J Heart Lung Transplant 2003;22:433-438.

77. Elizur A, Sweet SC, Huddleston CB, et al. Pre-transplant mechanical ventilation increases short-term morbidity and mortality in pediatric patients with cystic fibrosis. J Heart Lung Transplant 2007;26:127-131.

78. Baz MA, Palmer SM, Staples ED, et al. Lung transplantation after long-term mechanical ventilation: Results and 1-year follow-up. Chest 2001;119:224-227.

79. Vermeijden JW, Zijlstra JG, Erasmus ME, et al. Lung transplantation for ventilator-dependent respiratory failure. J Heart Lung Transplant 2009;28:347-351.

80. Algar FJ, Alvarez A, Lama R, et al. Lung transplantation in patients under mechanical ventilation. Transplant Proc 2003;35:737-738.

81. Bermudez CA, Rocha RV, Zaldonis D, et al. Extracorporeal membrane oxygenation as a bridge to lung transplant: Midterm outcomes. Ann Thorac Surg 2011;92:1226-1231; discussion 1231-1232.

82. Fischer S, Hoeper MM, Tomaszek S, et al. Bridge to lung transplantation with the extracorporeal membrane ventilator Novalung in the veno-venous mode: The initial Hannover experience. ASAIO J 2007;53:168-170.

83. Fischer S, Simon AR, Welte T, et al. Bridge to lung transplantation with the novel pumpless interventional lung assist device NovaLung. J Thorac Cardiovasc Surg 2006;131:719-723.

84. Ricci D, Boffini M, Del Sorbo L, et al. The use of CO_2 removal devices in patients awaiting lung transplantation: An initial experience. Transplant Proc 2010;42:1255-1258.

85. Garcia JP, Iacono A, Kon ZN, Griffith BP. Ambulatory extracorporeal membrane oxygenation: A new approach for bridge-to-lung transplantation. J Thorac Cardiovasc Surg 2010;139:e137-e139.

86. Turner DA, Cheifetz IM, Rehder KJ, et al. Active rehabilitation and physical therapy during extracorporeal membrane oxygenation while awaiting lung transplantation: A practical approach. Crit Care Med 2011;39:2593-2598.

87. Reeb J, Falcoz PE, Santelmo N, Massard G. Double lumen bi-cava cannula for veno-venous extracorporeal membrane oxygenation as bridge to lung transplantation in non-intubated patient. Interact Cardiovasc Thorac Surg 2012;14:125-127.

88. Hayes D Jr, Kukreja J, Tobias JD, et al. Ambulatory venovenous extracorporeal respiratory support as a bridge for cystic fibrosis patients to emergent lung transplantation. J Cyst Fibros 2012;11:40-55.

89. Hammainen P, Schersten H, Lemstrom K, et al. Usefulness of extracorporeal membrane oxygenation as a bridge to lung transplantation: A descriptive study. J Heart Lung Transplant 2011;30:103-107.

90. Lakey WC, Spratt S, Vinson EN, et al. Osteoporosis in lung transplant candidates compared to matched healthy controls. Clin Transplant 2011;25:426-435.

91. Jastrzebski D, Lutogniewska W, Ochman M, et al. Osteoporosis in patients referred for lung transplantation. Eur J Med Res 2010;15(Suppl 2):68-71.

92. Spira A, Gutierrez C, Chaparro C, et al. Osteoporosis and lung transplantation: A prospective study. Chest 2000;117:476-481.

93. Braith RW, Conner JA, Fulton MN, et al. Comparison of alendronate vs alendronate plus mechanical loading as prophylaxis for osteoporosis in lung transplant recipients: A pilot study. J Heart Lung Transplant 2007;26:132-137.

94. Mitchell MJ, Baz MA, Fulton MN, et al. Resistance training prevents vertebral osteoporosis in lung transplant recipients. Transplantation 2003;76:557-562.

95. Seijas R, Ares O, Malik A, Maled I. Bilateral pathological hip fractures in a patient with a bipulmonary transplant: A case report. J Orthop Surg (Hong Kong) 2009;17:240-242.

96. Aris RM, Neuringer IP, Weiner MA, et al. Severe osteoporosis before and after lung transplantation. Chest 1996;109:1176-1183.

97. Detterbeck FC, Egan TM, Mill MR. Lung transplantation after previous thoracic surgical procedures. Ann Thorac Surg 1995;60:139-143.

98. Almoosa KF, Ryu JH, Mendez J, et al. Management of pneumothorax in lymphangioleiomyomatosis: Effects on recurrence and lung transplantation complications. Chest 2006;129:1274-1281.

99. Koulouri S, Woo MS, Horn MV, et al. Previous thoracic surgery does not increase peri-operative mortality in pediatric heart-lung transplant recipients. J Heart Lung Transplant 2004;23:1228-1230.

100. Rolla M, Anile M, Venuta F, et al. Lung transplantation for cystic fibrosis after thoracic surgical procedures. Transplant Proc 2011;43:1162-1163.

101. Le Pimpec-Barthes F, Thomas PA, Bonnette P, et al. Single-lung transplantation in patients with previous contralateral pneumonectomy: Technical aspects and results. Eur J Cardiothorac Surg 2009;36:927-932.

102. Diethrich EB, Bahadir I, Gordon M, et al. Postoperative complications necessitating right lower lobectomy in a heart-lung transplant recipient with previous sternotomy. J Thorac Cardiovasc Surg1987;94:389-392.

103. Kawaguchi A, Gandjbakhch I, Pavie A, et al. Heart and unilateral lung transplantation in patients with end-stage cardiopulmonary disease and previous thoracic operations. J Thorac Cardiovasc Surg 1989;98:343-349.

104. De Meester J, Smits JM, Persijn GG, Haverich A. Listing for lung transplantation: Life expectancy and transplant effect, stratified by type of end-stage lung disease, the Eurotransplant experience. J Heart Lung Transplant 2001;20:518-524.

105. Thabut G, Ravaud P, Christie JD, et al. Determinants of the survival benefit of lung transplantation in patients with chronic obstructive pulmonary disease. Am J Respir Crit Care Med 2008;177:1156-1163.

106. Charman SC, Sharples LD, McNeil KD, Wallwork J. Assessment of survival benefit after lung transplantation by patient diagnosis. J Heart Lung Transplant 2002;21:226-232.

107. Lahzami S, Bridevaux PO, Soccal PM, et al. Survival impact of lung transplantation for COPD. Eur Respir J 2010;36:74-80.

108. Vestbo J, Edwards LD, Scanlon PD, et al. Changes in forced expiratory volume in 1 second over time in COPD. N Engl J Med 2011;365:1184-1192.

109. Celli BR, Cote CG, Lareau SC, Meek PM. Predictors of survival in COPD: More than just the FEV_1. Respir Med 2008;102(Suppl 1):S27-S35.

110. Soler-Cataluna JJ, Martinez-Garcia MA, Roman Sanchez P, et al. Severe acute exacerbations and mortality in patients with chronic obstructive pulmonary disease. Thorax 2005;60:925-931.

111. Celli BR. Predictors of mortality in COPD. Respir Med 2010;104:773-779.

112. Martinez FJ, Foster G, Curtis JL, et al. Predictors of mortality in patients with emphysema and severe airflow obstruction. Am J Respir Crit Care Med 2006;173:1326-1334.

113. Burrows B, Earle RH. Course and prognosis of chronic obstructive lung disease. A prospective study of 200 patients. N Engl J Med 1969;280:397-404.

114. Anthonisen NR, Wright EC, Hodgkin JE. Prognosis in chronic obstructive pulmonary disease. Am Rev Respir Dis 1986;133:14-20.

115. Connors AF Jr, Dawson NV, Thomas C, et al. Outcomes following acute exacerbation of severe chronic obstructive lung disease. The SUPPORT investigators (Study to Understand Prognoses and Preferences for Outcomes and Risks of Treatments). Am J Respir Crit Care Med 1996;154:959-967.

116. Seneff MG, Wagner DP, Wagner RP, et al. Hospital and 1-year survival of patients admitted to intensive care units with acute exacerbation of chronic obstructive pulmonary disease. JAMA 1995;274:1852-1857.

117. Groenewegen KH, Schols AM, Wouters EF. Mortality and mortality-related factors after hospitalization for acute exacerbation of COPD. Chest 2003;124:459-467.

118. Almagro P, Calbo E, Ochoa de Echaguen A, et al. Mortality after hospitalization for COPD. Chest 2002;121:1441-1448.

119. Garcia-Aymerich J, Serra Pons I, Mannino DM, et al. Lung function impairment, COPD hospitalisations and subsequent mortality. Thorax 2011;66:585-590.

120. Egan TM, Bennett LE, Garrity ER, et al. Predictors of death on the UNOS lung transplant waiting list: Results of a multivariate analysis. J Heart Lung Transplant 2001;20:242.

121. Celli BR, Cote CG, Marin JM, et al. The body-mass index, airflow obstruction, dyspnea, and exercise capacity index in chronic obstructive pulmonary disease. N Engl J Med 2004;350:1005-1012.

122. Cote CG, Pinto-Plata VM, Marin JM, et al. The modified BODE index: Validation with mortality in COPD. Eur Respir J 2008;32:1269-1274.

123. Soler-Cataluna JJ, Martinez-Garcia MA, Sanchez LS, et a;. Severe exacerbations and BODE index: Two independent risk factors for death in male COPD patients. Respir Med 2009;103:692-699.

124. Rationale and design of The National Emphysema Treatment Trial: A prospective randomized trial of lung volume reduction surgery. The National Emphysema Treatment Trial Research Group. Chest 1999;116:1750-1761.

125. Martinez FJ, Han MK, Andrei AC, et al. Longitudinal change in the BODE index predicts mortality in severe emphysema. Am J Respir Crit Care Med 2008;178:491-499.

126. Casanova C, de Torres JP, Aguirre-Jaime A, et al. The progression of chronic obstructive pulmonary disease is heterogeneous: The experience of the BODE cohort. Am J Respir Crit Care Med 2011;184:115-121.

127. Esteban C, Quintana JM, Moraza J, et al. BODE-Index vs HADO-score in chronic obstructive pulmonary disease: Which one to use in general practice? BMC Med 2010;8:28.

128. Esteban C, Arostegui I, Moraza J, et al. Development of a decision tree to assess the severity and prognosis of stable COPD. Eur Respir J 2011;38:1294-1300.

129. de Torres JP, Pinto-Plata V, Casanova C, et al. C-reactive protein levels and survival in patients with moderate to very severe COPD. Chest 2008;133:1336-1343.

130. Cooper JD, Patterson GA, Sundaresan RS, et al. Results of 150 consecutive bilateral lung volume reduction procedures in patients with severe emphysema. J Thorac Cardiovasc Surg 1996;112:1319-1329; discussion 1329-1330.

131. Fishman A, Martinez F, Naunheim K, et al. A randomized trial comparing lung-volume-reduction surgery with medical therapy for severe emphysema. N Engl J Med 2003;348:2059-2073.

132. Bavaria JE, Pochettino A, Kotloff RM, et al. Effect of volume reduction on lung transplant timing and selection for chronic obstructive pulmonary disease. J Thorac Cardiovasc Surg 1998;115:9-17; discussion 17-18.

133. Burns KE, Keenan RJ, Grgurich WF, et al. Outcomes of lung volume reduction surgery followed by lung transplantation: A matched cohort study. Ann Thorac Surg 2002;73:1587-1593.

134. Meyers BF, Yusen RD, Guthrie TJ, et al. Outcome of bilateral lung volume reduction in patients with emphysema potentially eligible for lung transplantation. J Thorac Cardiovasc Surg 2001;122:10-17.

135. Senbaklavaci O, Wisser W, Ozpeker C, et al. Successful lung volume reduction surgery brings patients into better condition for later lung transplantation. Eur J Cardiothorac Surg 2002;22:363-367.

136. Wisser W, Deviatko E, Simon-Kupilik N, et al. Lung transplantation following lung volume reduction surgery. J Heart Lung Transplant 2000;19:480-487.

137. National Emphysema Treatment Trial Research Group. Patients at high risk of death after lung-volume-reduction surgery. N Engl J Med 2001;345:1075-1083.

138. Cassivi SD, Meyers BF, Battafarano RJ, et al. Thirteen-year experience in lung transplantation for emphysema. Ann Thorac Surg 2002;74:1663-1669; discussion 1669-1670.

139. Stoller JK, Aboussouan LS. Alpha1-antitrypsin deficiency. Lancet 2005;365:2225-2236.

140. Browne RJ, Mannino DM, Khoury MJ. Alpha 1-antitrypsin deficiency deaths in the United States from 1979-1991. An analysis using multiple-cause mortality data. Chest 1996;110:78-83.

141. McElvaney NG, Stoller JK, Buist AS, et al. Baseline characteristics of enrollees in the National Heart, Lung and Blood Institute Registry of alpha 1-antitrypsin deficiency. Alpha 1-Antitrypsin Deficiency Registry Study Group. Chest 1997;111:394-403.

142. Stoller JK, Tomashefski J Jr, Crystal RG, et al. Mortality in individuals with severe deficiency of alpha1-antitrypsin: Findings from the National Heart, Lung, and Blood Institute Registry. Chest 2005;127:1196-1204.

143. Alpha-1-Antitrypsin Deficiency Registry Study Group. Survival and FEV_1 decline in individuals with severe deficiency of alpha1-antitrypsin. Am J Respir Crit Care Med 1998;158:49-59.

144. Seersholm N, Kok-Jensen A, Dirksen A. Survival of patients with severe alpha 1-antitrypsin deficiency with special reference to non-index cases. Thorax 1994;49:695-698.

145. Seersholm N, Kok-Jensen A. Clinical features and prognosis of life time non-smokers with severe alpha 1-antitrypsin deficiency. Thorax 1998;53:265-268.

146. Dawkins PA, Dowson LJ, Guest PJ, Stockley RA. Predictors of mortality in alpha1-antitrypsin deficiency. Thorax 2003;58:1020-1026.

147. Dawkins P, Wood A, Nightingale P, Stockley R. Mortality in alpha-1-antitrypsin deficiency in the United Kingdom. Respir Med 2009;103:1540-1547.

148. American Thoracic Society/European Respiratory Society International Multidisciplinary Consensus Classification of the Idiopathic Interstitial Pneumonias. This joint statement of the American Thoracic Society (ATS), and the European Respiratory Society (ERS) was adopted by the ATS board of directors, June 2001 and by the ERS Executive Committee, June 2001. Am J Respir Crit Care Med 2002;165:277-304.

149. Bjoraker JA, Ryu JH, Edwin MK, et al. Prognostic significance of histopathologic subsets in idiopathic pulmonary fibrosis. Am J Respir Crit Care Med 1998;157:199-203.

150. Thomeer MJ, Vansteenkiste J, Verbeken EK, Demedts M. Interstitial lung diseases: Characteristics at diagnosis and mortality risk assessment. Respir Med 2004;98:567-573.

151. Thabut G, Mal H, Castier Y, et al. Survival benefit of lung transplantation for patients with idiopathic pulmonary fibrosis. J Thorac Cardiovasc Surg 2003;126:469-475.

152. Nathan SD, Shlobin OA, Weir N, et al. Long-term course and prognosis of idiopathic pulmonary fibrosis in the new millennium. Chest 2011;140:221-229.

153. Raghu G, Collard HR, Egan JJ, et al. An official ATS/ERS/JRS/ALAT statement: Idiopathic pulmonary fibrosis: Evidence-based guidelines for diagnosis and management. Am J Respir Crit Care Med 2011;183:788-824.

154. Monaghan H, Wells AU, Colby TV, et al. Prognostic implications of histologic patterns in multiple surgical lung biopsies from patients with idiopathic interstitial pneumonias. Chest 2004;125:522-526.

155. Jezek V, Fucik J, Michaljanic A, Jezkova L. The prognostic significance of functional tests in cryptogenic fibrosing alveolitis. Bull Eur Physiopathol Respir 1980;16:711-20.

156. Flaherty KR, White ES, Gay SE, et al. Timing of lung transplantation for patients with fibrotic lung diseases. Semin Respir Crit Care Med 2001;22:517-532.

157. Latsi PI, du Bois RM, Nicholson AG, et al. Fibrotic idiopathic interstitial pneumonia: The prognostic value of longitudinal functional trends. Am J Respir Crit Care Med 2003;168:531-537.

158. Taniguchi H, Kondoh Y, Ebina M, et al. The clinical significance of 5% change in vital capacity in patients with idiopathic pulmonary fibrosis: Extended analysis of the pirfenidone trial. Respir Res 2011;12:93.

159. Zappala CJ, Latsi PI, Nicholson AG, et al. Marginal decline in forced vital capacity is associated with a poor outcome in idiopathic pulmonary fibrosis. Eur Respir J 2010;35:830-836.

160. Collard HR, King TE Jr, Bartelson BB, et al. Changes in clinical and physiologic variables predict survival in idiopathic pulmonary fibrosis. Am J Respir Crit Care Med 2003;168:538-542.

161. Douglas WW, Ryu JH, Schroeder DR. Idiopathic pulmonary fibrosis: Impact of oxygen and colchicine, prednisone, or no therapy on survival. Am J Respir Crit Care Med 2000;161:1172-1178.

162. Hanson D, Winterbauer RH, Kirtland SH, Wu R. Changes in pulmonary function test results after 1 year of therapy as predictors of survival in patients with idiopathic pulmonary fibrosis. Chest 1995;108:305-310.

163. Hamada K, Nagai S, Tanaka S, Handa T, et al. Significance of pulmonary arterial pressure and diffusion capacity of the lung as prognosticator in patients with idiopathic pulmonary fibrosis. Chest 2007;131:650-656.

164. Mogulkoc N, Brutsche MH, Bishop PW, et al. Pulmonary function in idiopathic pulmonary fibrosis and referral for lung transplantation. Am J Respir Crit Care Med 2001;164:103-108.

165. King TE Jr, Safrin S, Starko KM, et al. Analyses of efficacy end points in a controlled trial of interferon-gamma1b for idiopathic pulmonary fibrosis. Chest 2005;127:171-177.

166. Nadrous HF, Pellikka PA, Krowka MJ, et al. The impact of pulmonary hypertension on survival in patients with idiopathic pulmonary fibrosis. Chest 2005;128(Suppl 6):616S-617S.

167. Mejia M, Carrillo G, Rojas-Serrano J, et al. Idiopathic pulmonary fibrosis and emphysema: Decreased survival associated with severe pulmonary arterial hypertension. Chest 2009;136:10-15.

168. du Bois RM, Weycker D, Albera C, et al. Six-minute-walk test in idiopathic pulmonary fibrosis: Test validation and minimal clinically important difference. Am J Respir Crit Care Med 2011;183:1231-1237.

169. Holland AE, Hill CJ, Conron M, et al. Small changes in six-minute walk distance are important in diffuse parenchymal lung disease. Respir Med 2009;103:1430-1435.

170. Shitrit D, Gershman Y, Peled N, et al. Risk factors for death while awaiting lung transplantation in Israeli patients: 1997-2006. Eur J Cardiothorac Surg 2008;34:444-448.

171. Swigris JJ, Swick J, Wamboldt FS, et al. Heart rate recovery after 6-min walk test predicts survival in patients with idiopathic pulmonary fibrosis. Chest 2009;136:841-848.

172. Nishiyama O, Taniguchi H, Kondoh Y, et al. A simple assessment of dyspnoea as a prognostic indicator in idiopathic pulmonary fibrosis. Eur Respir J 2010;36:1067-1072.

173. Shitrit D, Rusanov V, Peled N, et al. The 15-step oximetry test: A reliable tool to identify candidates for lung transplantation among patients with idiopathic pulmonary fibrosis. J Heart Lung Transplant 2009;28:328-333.

174. Wells AU, Rubens MB, du Bois RM, Hansell DM. Serial CT in fibrosing alveolitis: Prognostic significance of the initial pattern. AJR Am J Roentgenol 1993;161:1159-1165.

175. Lynch DA, Godwin JD, Safrin S, et al. High-resolution computed tomography in idiopathic pulmonary fibrosis: Diagnosis and prognosis. Am J Respir Crit Care Med 2005;172:488-493.

176. Kurashima K, Takayanagi N, Tsuchiya N, et al. The effect of emphysema on lung function and survival in patients with idiopathic pulmonary fibrosis. Respirology 2010;15:843-848.

177. Ryerson CJ, Abbritti M, Ley B, et al. Cough predicts prognosis in idiopathic pulmonary fibrosis. Respirology 2011;16:969-975.

178. Prasse A, Probst C, Bargagli E, et al. Serum CC-chemokine ligand 18 concentration predicts outcome in idiopathic pulmonary fibrosis. Am J Respir Crit Care Med 2009;179:717-723.

179. Richards TJ, Kaminski N, Baribaud F, et al. Peripheral blood proteins predict mortality in idiopathic pulmonary fibrosis. Am J Respir Crit Care Med 2012;185:67-76.

180. Hisata S, Kimura Y, Shibata N, et al. A normal range of KL-6/MUC1 independent of elevated SP-D indicates a better prognosis in the patients with honeycombing on high-resolution computed tomography. Pulm Med 2011;2011:806014.

181. Moeller A, Gilpin SE, Ask K, et al. Circulating fibrocytes are an indicator of poor prognosis in idiopathic pulmonary fibrosis. Am J Respir Crit Care Med 2009;179:588-594.

182. Mollica C, Paone G, Conti V, et al. Mechanical ventilation in patients with end-stage idiopathic pulmonary fibrosis. Respiration 2010;79:209-215.

183. Force SD, Kilgo P, Neujahr DC, et al. Bilateral lung transplantation offers better long-term survival, compared with single-lung transplantation, for younger patients with idiopathic pulmonary fibrosis. Ann Thorac Surg 2011;91:244-249.

184. Weiss ES, Allen JG, Merlo CA, et al. Survival after single versus bilateral lung transplantation for high-risk patients with pulmonary fibrosis. Ann Thorac Surg 2009;88:1616-1625; discussion 1625-1626.

185. Neurohr C, Huppmann P, Thum D, et al. Potential functional and survival benefit of double over single lung transplantation for selected patients with idiopathic pulmonary fibrosis. Transpl Int 2010;23:887-896.

186. Algar FJ, Espinosa D, Moreno P, et al. Results of lung transplantation in idiopathic pulmonary fibrosis patients. Transplant Proc 2010;42:3211-3213.

187. Navaratnam V, Ali N, Smith CJ, et al. Does the presence of connective tissue disease modify survival in patients with pulmonary fibrosis? Respir Med 2011;105:1925-1930.

188. Greenwald GI, Tashkin DP, Gong H, et al. Longitudinal changes in lung function and respiratory symptoms in progressive systemic sclerosis. Prospective study. Am J Med 1987;83:83-92.

189. Su R, Bennett M, Jacobs S, et al. An analysis of connective tissue disease–associated interstitial lung disease at a US tertiary care center: Better survival in patients with systemic sclerosis. J Rheumatol 2011;38:693-701.

190. Saggar R, Khanna D, Furst DE, et al. Systemic sclerosis and bilateral lung transplantation: A single centre experience. Eur Respir J 2010;36:893-900.

191. Schachna L, Medsger TA Jr, Dauber JH, et al. Lung transplantation in scleroderma compared with idiopathic pulmonary fibrosis and idiopathic pulmonary arterial hypertension. Arthritis Rheum 2006;54:3954-3961.

192. Massad MG, Powell CR, Kpodonu J, et al. Outcomes of lung transplantation in patients with scleroderma. World J Surg 2005;29:1510-1515.

193. Shitrit D, Amital A, Peled N, et al. Lung transplantation in patients with scleroderma: Case series, review of the literature, and criteria for transplantation. Clin Transplant 2009;23:178-183.

194. Rosas V, Conte JV, Yang SC, et al. Lung transplantation and systemic sclerosis. Ann Transplant 2000;5:38-43.

195. Connors GR, Christopher-Stine L, Oddis CV, Danoff SK. Interstitial lung disease associated with the idiopathic inflammatory myopathies: What progress has been made in the past 35 years? Chest 2010;138:1464-1474.

196. Kim EJ, Collard HR, King TE Jr. Rheumatoid arthritis–associated interstitial lung disease: The relevance of histopathologic and radiographic pattern. Chest 2009;136:1397-1405.

197. Weinrib L, Sharma OP, Quismorio FP Jr. A long-term study of interstitial lung disease in systemic lupus erythematosus. Semin Arthritis Rheum 1990;20:48-56.

198. Cheema GS, Quismorio FP Jr. Interstitial lung disease in systemic lupus erythematosus. Curr Opin Pulm Med 2000;6:424-429.

199. Bodolay E, Szekanecz Z, Devenyi K, et al. Evaluation of interstitial lung disease in mixed connective tissue disease (MCTD). Rheumatology (Oxford) 2005;44:656-661.

200. Fagundes MN, Caleiro MT, Navarro-Rodriguez T, et al. Esophageal involvement and interstitial lung disease in mixed connective tissue disease. Respir Med 2009;103:854-860.

201. Deheinzelin D, Capelozzi VL, Kairalla RA, et al. Interstitial lung disease in primary Sjögren's syndrome. Clinical-pathological evaluation and response to treatment. Am J Respir Crit Care Med 1996;154:794-799.

202. Arcasoy SM, Christie JD, Pochettino A, et al. Characteristics and outcomes of patients with sarcoidosis listed for lung transplantation. Chest 2001;120:873-880.

203. Shorr AF, Davies DB, Nathan SD. Outcomes for patients with sarcoidosis awaiting lung transplantation. Chest 2002;122:233-238.

204. Shorr AF, Helman DL, Davies DB, Nathan SD. Pulmonary hypertension in advanced sarcoidosis: Epidemiology and clinical characteristics. Eur Respir J 2005;25:783-788.

205. Shorr AF, Davies DB, Nathan SD. Predicting mortality in patients with sarcoidosis awaiting lung transplantation. Chest 2003;124:922-928.

206. Corrin B, Liebow AA, Friedman PJ. Pulmonary lymphangiomyomatosis. A review. Am J Pathol 1975;79:348-382.

207. Silverstein EF, Ellis K, Wolff M, Jaretzki A 3rd. Pulmonary lymphangiomyomatosis. Am J Roentgenol Radium Ther Nucl Med 1974;120:832-850.

208. Peavy H, Gail D, Kiley J, Shurin S. A National Heart, Lung, and Blood Institute history and perspective on lymphangioleiomyomatosis. Lymphat Res Biol 2010;8:5-8.

209. Cohen MM, Pollock-BarZiv S, Johnson SR. Emerging clinical picture of lymphangioleiomyomatosis. Thorax 2005;60:875-879.

210. Johnson SR, Tattersfield AE. Clinical experience of lymphangioleiomyomatosis in the UK. Thorax 2000;55:1052-1057.

211. Taylor JR, Ryu J, Colby TV, Raffin TA. Lymphangioleiomyomatosis. Clinical course in 32 patients. N Engl J Med 1990;323:1254-1260.

212. Urban T, Lazor R, Lacronique J, et al. Pulmonary lymphangioleiomyomatosis. A study of 69 patients. Groupe d'Etudes et de Recherche sur les Maladies "Orphelines" Pulmonaires (GERM"O"P). Medicine (Baltimore) 1999;78:321-337.

213. Maurer JR, Ryu J, Beck G, et al. Lung transplantation in the management of patients with lymphangioleiomyomatosis: Baseline data from the NHLBI LAM Registry. J Heart Lung Transplant 2007;26:1293-1299.

214. Boehler A. Lung transplantation for cystic lung diseases: Lymphangioleiomyomatosis, histiocytosis x, and sarcoidosis. Semin Respir Crit Care Med 2001;22:509-516.

215. Boehler A, Speich R, Russi EW, Weder W. Lung transplantation for lymphangioleiomyomatosis. N Engl J Med 1996;335:1275-1280.

216. Pechet TT, Meyers BF, Guthrie TJ, et al. Lung transplantation for lymphangioleiomyomatosis. J Heart Lung Transplant 2004;23:301-308.

217. Bittmann I, Dose TB, Muller C, et al. Lymphangioleiomyomatosis: Recurrence after single lung transplantation. Hum Pathol 1997;28:1420-1423.

218. Taveira-DaSilva AM, Pacheco-Rodriguez G, Moss J. The natural history of lymphangioleiomyomatosis: Markers of severity, rate of progression and prognosis. Lymphat Res Biol 2010;8:9-19.

219. Yao J, Avila N, Dwyer A, et al. Computer-aided grading of lymphangioleiomyomatosis (LAM) using HRCT. Proc IAPR Int Conf Pattern Recogn 2008(8-11 Dec 2008):1-4.

220. Matsui K, Beasley MB, Nelson WK, et al. Prognostic significance of pulmonary lymphangioleiomyomatosis histologic score. Am J Surg Pathol 2001;25:479-484.

221. Taveira-DaSilva AM, Hedin C, Stylianou MP, et al. Reversible airflow obstruction, proliferation of abnormal smooth muscle cells, and impairment of gas exchange as predictors of outcome in lymphangioleiomyomatosis. Am J Respir Crit Care Med 2001;164:1072-1076.

222. Taveira-DaSilva AM, Steagall WK, Rabel A, et al. Reversible airflow obstruction in lymphangioleiomyomatosis. Chest 2009;136:1596-1603.

223. McCormack FX, Inoue Y, Moss J, et al. Efficacy and safety of sirolimus in lymphangioleiomyomatosis. N Engl J Med 2011;364:1595-1606.

224. Sundar KM, Gosselin MV, Chung HL, Cahill BC. Pulmonary Langerhans cell histiocytosis: Emerging concepts in pathobiology, radiology, and clinical evolution of disease. Chest 2003;123:1673-1683.

225. Dauriat G, Mal H, Thabut G, et al. Lung transplantation for pulmonary Langerhans' cell histiocytosis: A multicenter analysis. Transplantation 2006;81:746-750.

226. Delobbe A, Durieu J, Duhamel A, Wallaert B. Determinants of survival in pulmonary Langerhans' cell granulomatosis (histiocytosis X). Groupe d'Etude en Pathologie Interstitielle de la Societe de Pathologie Thoracique du Nord. Eur Respir J 1996;9:2002-2006.

227. Vassallo R, Ryu JH, Schroeder DR, et al. Clinical outcomes of pulmonary Langerhans'-cell histiocytosis in adults. N Engl J Med 2002;346:484-490.

228. Fartoukh M, Humbert M, Capron F, et al. Severe pulmonary hypertension in histiocytosis X. Am J Respir Crit Care Med 2000;161:216-223.

229. Harari S, Brenot F, Barberis M, Simmoneau G. Advanced pulmonary histiocytosis X is associated with severe pulmonary hypertension. Chest 1997;111:1142-1144.

230. Kiakouama L, Cottin V, Etienne-Mastroianni B, et al. Severe pulmonary hypertension in histiocytosis X: Long-term improvement with bosentan. Eur Respir J 2010;36:202-204.

231. Hosenpud JD, Bennett LE, Keck BM,. Effect of diagnosis on survival benefit of lung transplantation for end-stage lung disease. Lancet 1998;351:24-27.

232. Titman A, Rogers CA, Bonser RS, et al. Disease-specific survival benefit of lung transplantation in adults: A national cohort study. Am J Transplant 2009;9:1640-1649.

233. De Meester J, Smits JM, Persijn GG, Haverich A. Listing for lung transplantation: Life expectancy and transplant effect, stratified by type of end-stage lung disease, the Eurotransplant experience. J Heart Lung Transplant 2001;20:518-524.

234. Goeminne P, Dupont L. Non–cystic fibrosis bronchiectasis: Diagnosis and management in 21st century. Postgrad Med J 2010;86:493-501.

235. Nick JA, Chacon CS, Brayshaw SJ, et al. Effects of gender and age at diagnosis on disease progression in long-term survivors of cystic fibrosis. Am J Respir Crit Care Med 2010;182:614-626.

236. Vizza CD, Yusen RD, Lynch JP, et al. Outcome of patients with cystic fibrosis awaiting lung transplantation. Am J Respir Crit Care Med 2000;162:819-825.

237. Liou TG, Adler FR, Fitzsimmons SC, et al. Predictive 5-year survivorship model of cystic fibrosis. Am J Epidemiol 2001;153:345-352.

238. Sharma R, Florea VG, Bolger AP, et al. Wasting as an independent predictor of mortality in patients with cystic fibrosis. Thorax 2001;56:746-750.

239. Weiss ES, Allen JG, Modi MN, et al. Lung transplantation in older patients with cystic fibrosis: Analysis of UNOS data. J Heart Lung Transplant 2009;28:135-140.

240. Kerem E, Reisman J, Corey M, et al. Prediction of mortality in patients with cystic fibrosis. N Engl J Med 1992;326:1187-1191.

241. Ciriaco P, Egan TM, Cairns EL, et al. Analysis of cystic fibrosis referrals for lung transplantation. Chest 1995;107:1323-1327.

242. Hayllar KM, Williams SG, Wise AE, et al. A prognostic model for the prediction of survival in cystic fibrosis. Thorax 1997;52:313-317.

243. Buzzetti R, Alicandro G, Minicucci L, et al. Validation of a predictive survival model in Italian patients with cystic fibrosis. J Cyst Fibros 2012;11:24-29.

244. Augarten A, Akons H, Aviram M, et al. Prediction of mortality and timing of referral for lung transplantation in cystic fibrosis patients. Pediatr Transplant 2001;5:339-342.

245. Milla CE, Warwick WJ. Risk of death in cystic fibrosis patients with severely compromised lung function. Chest 1998;113:1230-1234.

246. Doershuk CF, Stern RC. Timing of referral for lung transplantation for cystic fibrosis: Overemphasis on FEV$_1$ may adversely affect overall survival. Chest 1999;115:782-787.

247. George PM, Banya W, Pareek N, et al. Improved survival at low lung function in cystic fibrosis: Cohort study from 1990 to 2007. BMJ 2011;342:d1008.

248. Rosenbluth DB, Wilson K, Ferkol T, Schuster DP. Lung function decline in cystic fibrosis patients and timing for lung transplantation referral. Chest 2004;126:412-419.

249. Rosenstein BJ, Zeitlin PL. Prognosis in cystic fibrosis. Curr Opin Pulm Med 1995;1:444-449.

250. Rosenfeld M, Davis R, Fitzsimmons S, et al. Gender gap in cystic fibrosis mortality. Am J Epidemiol 1997;145:794-803.

251. Konstan MW, Morgan WJ, Butler SM, et al. Risk factors for rate of decline in forced expiratory volume in one second in children and adolescents with cystic fibrosis. J Pediatr 2007;151:134-139, 9 e1.

252. Verma N, Bush A, Buchdahl R. Is there still a gender gap in cystic fibrosis? Chest 2005;128:2824-2834.

253. Baghaie N, Kalilzadeh S, Hassanzad M, et al. Determination of mortality from cystic fibrosis. Pneumologia 2010;59:170-173.

254. Ellaffi M, Vinsonneau C, Coste J, et al. One-year outcome after severe pulmonary exacerbation in adults with cystic fibrosis. Am J Respir Crit Care Med 2005;171:158-164.

255. de Boer K, Vandemheen KL, Tullis E, et al. Exacerbation frequency and clinical outcomes in adult patients with cystic fibrosis. Thorax 2011;66:680-685.

256. Venuta F, Rendina EA, Rocca GD, et al. Pulmonary hemodynamics contribute to indicate priority for lung transplantation in patients with cystic fibrosis. J Thorac Cardiovasc Surg 2000;119:682-689.

257. Liou TG, Adler FR, Cahill BC, et al. Survival effect of lung transplantation among patients with cystic fibrosis. JAMA. 2001;286:2683-2689.

258. Chaparro C, Maurer J, Gutierrez C, et al. Infection with *Burkholderia cepacia* in cystic fibrosis: Outcome following lung transplantation. Am J Respir Crit Care Med 2001;163:43-48.

259. Aris RM, Routh JC, LiPuma JJ, et al. Lung transplantation for cystic fibrosis patients with *Burkholderia cepacia* complex. Survival linked to genomovar type. Am J Respir Crit Care Med 2001;164:2102-2106.

260. Alexander BD, Petzold EW, Reller LB, et al. Survival after lung transplantation of cystic fibrosis patients infected with *Burkholderia cepacia* complex. Am J Transplant 2008;8:1025-1030.

261. De Soyza A, Meachery G, Hester KL, et al. Lung transplantation for patients with cystic fibrosis and *Burkholderia cepacia* complex infection: A single-center experience. J Heart Lung Transplant 2010;29:1395-1404.

262. Hadjiliadis D, Steele MP, Chaparro C, et al. Survival of lung transplant patients with cystic fibrosis harboring panresistant bacteria other than *Burkholderia cepacia*, compared with patients harboring sensitive bacteria. J Heart Lung Transplant 2007;26:834-838.

263. Debray D, Kelly D, Houwen R, et al. Best practice guidance for the diagnosis and management of cystic fibrosis–associated liver disease. J Cyst Fibros 2011;10(Suppl 2):S29-S36.

264. Chryssostalis A, Hubert D, Coste J, et al. Liver disease in adult patients with cystic fibrosis: A frequent and independent prognostic factor associated with death or lung transplantation. J Hepatol 2011;55:1377-1382.

265. Klima LD, Kowdley KV, Lewis SL, et al. Successful lung transplantation in spite of cystic fibrosis–associated liver disease: A case series. J Heart Lung Transplant 1997;16:934-938.

266. Nash EF, Volling C, Gutierrez CA, et al. Outcomes of patients with cystic fibrosis undergoing lung transplantation with and without cystic fibrosis–associated liver cirrhosis. Clinical Transplant 2012;26:34-41.

267. Orens JB, Shearon TH, Freudenberger RS, et al. Thoracic organ transplantation in the United States, 1995-2004. Am J Transplant 2006;6:1188-1197.

268. Simonneau G, Robbins IM, Beghetti M, et al. Updated clinical classification of pulmonary hypertension. J Am Coll Cardiol 2009;54(Suppl 1):S43-S54.

269. Hopkins WE, Ochoa LL, Richardson GW, Trulock EP. Comparison of the hemodynamics and survival of adults with severe primary pulmonary hypertension or Eisenmenger syndrome. J Heart Lung Transplant 1996;15:100-105.

270. D'Alonzo GE, Barst RJ, Ayres SM, et al. Survival in patients with primary pulmonary hypertension. Results from a national prospective registry. Ann Intern Med 1991;115:343-349.

271. Sitbon O, Humbert M, Nunes H, et al. Long-term intravenous epoprostenol infusion in primary pulmonary hypertension: Prognostic factors and survival. J Am Coll Cardiol 2002;40:780-788.

272. van de Veerdonk MC, Kind T, Marcus JT, et al. Progressive right ventricular dysfunction in patients with pulmonary arterial hypertension responding to therapy. J Am Coll Cardiol 2011;58:2511-2519.

273. Barst RJ, Rubin LJ, Long WA, et al. A comparison of continuous intravenous epoprostenol (prostacyclin) with conventional therapy for primary pulmonary hypertension. N Engl J Med 1996;334:296-302.

274. McLaughlin VV, Shillington A, Rich S. Survival in primary pulmonary hypertension: The impact of epoprostenol therapy. Circulation 2002;106:1477-1482.

275. Miyamoto S, Nagaya N, Satoh T, et al. Clinical correlates and prognostic significance of six-minute walk test in patients with primary pulmonary hypertension. Comparison with cardiopulmonary exercise testing. Am J Respir Crit Care Med 2000;161:487-492.

276. Raymond RJ, Hinderliter AL, Willis PW, et al. Echocardiographic predictors of adverse outcomes in primary pulmonary hypertension. J Am Coll Cardiol 2002;39:1214-1219.

277. Dandel M, Lehmkuhl HB, Mulahasanovic S, et al. Survival of patients with idiopathic pulmonary arterial hypertension after listing for transplantation: Impact of iloprost and bosentan treatment. J Heart Lung Transplant 2007;26:898-906.

278. Chen H, Shiboski SC, Golden JA, et al. Impact of the lung allocation score on lung transplantation for pulmonary arterial hypertension. Am J Respir Crit Care Med 2009;180:468-474.

279. Nickel N, Golpon H, Greer M, et al. The prognostic impact of follow-up assessments in patients with idiopathic pulmonary arterial hypertension. Eur Respir J 2012;39:589-596.

5

Recipient management before transplantation

GUNDEEP S. DHILLON AND DAVID WEILL

INTRODUCTION

Lung transplantation is an accepted treatment for patients with advanced lung disease in whom all other therapeutic options have been exhausted. Implementation of the lung allocation score (LAS) to prioritize distribution of donor lungs based on medical urgency and posttransplant survival resulted in a decrease in the number of patients awaiting lung transplantation and waiting list time and initially improved waiting list mortality.[1–3] However, the number of patients added to the waiting list has continued to increase, and approximately 1300 patients are active on the lung transplant list at any given time.[4]

Median time on the waiting list in 2012 was 4 months, although it ranged from 3 months for patients with interstitial lung disease to 10 months for those with pulmonary vascular disease. Currently, one third of the patients on the waiting list have been listed for longer than a year. Patients on the waiting list are getting older, 25% of listed patients being older than 65 years. Before implementation of the LAS only 4% of patients were older than 65 years. Also, half of the candidates are listed for interstitial lung disease. After implementation of the LAS, waiting list mortality rates declined, although the rates have reversed course since 2007. From 2010 to 2012 the waiting list mortality rate was 15.4 per 100 waiting list years, which is higher than the rates preceding implementation of the LAS.[4] These data suggest that patients being placed on the waiting list are sicker and require active management to maintain them on the waiting list as suitable candidates for lung transplantation.

This chapter summarizes the transplant-specific monitoring and management of adult patients listed for lung transplantation. In addition, waiting list management is discussed. Disease-specific management is not reviewed; however, close communication between patients, referring physicians, and lung transplant programs is extremely important. Responsibility for management of wait-listed patients' underlying disease should be clearly delineated between referring and transplant providers.

CLINICAL MONITORING AND MANAGEMENT

The clinical status of patients with advanced lung disease can change rapidly within a short time. Patients on the waiting list for a lung transplant need to be closely monitored for the following reasons: to optimize their medical therapy to maintain clinical stability, to update the LAS to reflect patients' current clinical condition and meet the United Network for Organ Sharing (UNOS) reporting requirements, to assess continued suitability of the planned procedure (e.g., single- versus double-lung transplant), and to ascertain ongoing eligibility for maintenance on the waiting list for lung transplantation.

Although monitoring protocols vary significantly between different lung transplant programs, listed outpatients are generally evaluated every 8 to 12 weeks. The focus of the history and physical examination includes any change in symptoms, significant weight gain or loss, exposure to infection, any significant illnesses, and overall debility. The patients are also evaluated for any sensitizing events, such as blood transfusions, since the last evaluation. The usual testing at these clinic visits includes chest radiography, arterial blood gas measurement, pulmonary function tests (PFTs), the 6-minute walk test (6MWT), complete blood counts, and a comprehensive metabolic panel. The variables used in calculation of the LAS should be updated at every evaluation and anytime that the patient's clinical status changes significantly. A change in these variables, especially patients' oxygen requirements and assisted ventilation status, can have a significant impact on their LAS. Additionally, UNOS mandates that most of the clinical variables be updated every 6 months. Moreover, for lung transplant candidates with a LAS greater than 50, UNOS requires that supplemental oxygen use, assisted ventilation status, and Pco_2 be updated every 2 weeks. The clinical variables required for calculation of the LAS and the schedules for updates are summarized in Table 5.1. A transplant program's failure to maintain and update its patients' listing with UNOS can significantly affect their LASs and their access to donor lungs.

In addition, patients with significant preexisting antibodies to human leukocyte antigens (HLAs) or a recent history of a sensitizing event should be monitored for development of new anti-HLA antibodies. Preexisting anti-HLA antibodies have been associated with worse clinical outcomes after lung transplantation.[5-7] The presence of anti-HLA antibodies can restrict the size of the potential donor pool for patients and may lead to prolonged times on the waiting list. Management of highly sensitized lung transplant candidates is discussed later in this chapter. Patients with suppurative lung disease such as cystic fibrosis (CF) should undergo screening at every visit for the development of new infections and to maintain updated information

regarding various antimicrobial susceptibility patterns. Isolation of organisms such as *Burkholderia cenocepacia*[8] and *Mycobacterium abscessus*[9] in lung transplant candidates may, in certain programs, lead to their removal from the lung transplant waiting list. The availability of updated information on antimicrobial susceptibility may allow selection of appropriate antimicrobial therapy and prophylaxis in the preoperative and perioperative periods.

Lung transplant candidates at risk for the development or worsening of pulmonary hypertension should be considered for annual transthoracic echocardiography and, if needed, right-heart catheterization to assess pulmonary artery pressure, the presence or absence of a patent foramen ovale, and right ventricular (RV) function. The development of significant pulmonary hypertension or RV dysfunction may lead to a change in the planned procedure. For example, patients with significant secondary pulmonary hypertension may require double- rather than single-lung transplantation. Similarly, the presence of RV dysfunction could lead to consideration of heart-lung transplantation, intraoperative use of cardiopulmonary bypass, or preemptive use of extracorporeal membrane oxygenation in the postoperative period.

Immunizations

Ideally, potential transplant recipients should undergo a complete evaluation of their immunization status, and all recommended vaccinations should be provided before listing.[10] Pretransplant patients receiving immunosuppressive therapies or patients expected to be listed within 2 weeks should avoid live attenuated vaccinations. Common live attenuated vaccinations include intranasal influenza, measles, mumps, rubella, varicella, and herpes zoster. Household contacts of these patients should also avoid live vaccinations.

Patients on the waiting list for a lung transplant remain at high risk for severe morbidity and mortality secondary to influenza infections.[11-15] These patients should receive seasonal influenza vaccinations at the earliest opportunity. Overall, these vaccinations are deemed safe and efficacious in transplant recipients. However, concerns that administration of seasonal influenza vaccinations might lead to the development of de novo anti-HLA antibodies have been raised.[16] A recent study of kidney transplant recipients from Switzerland demonstrated that anti-HLA antibodies developed in approximately 15% of the recipients. However, the titers of these antibodies were low and short lived, and the vaccination was not associated with an increased incidence of rejection.[17] In our opinion, the risk of influenza infection in patients with advanced lung disease is greater than the risk of development of anti-HLA antibodies in a potential transplant candidate.

Nutritional management

The outcomes of obese as well as underweight patients after lung transplantation are worse than those of recipients with

Table 5.1 Lung allocation score data update requirements

Variables at listing	Update every 6 months	Update every 14 days (if LAS > 50)
Diagnosis		
Date of birth		
Height and weight (BMI)	X	
Diabetes	X	
Supplemental oxygen	X	X
6MWD	X	
PA systolic pressure		
PA mean pressure		
PA occlusion pressure (mean)		
FVC	X	
Serum creatinine	X	
Functional status*	X	
Assisted ventilation*	X	X
Pco_2	X	X

Note: BMI, body mass index; FVC, forced vital capacity; LAS, lung allocation score; 6MWD, 6-minute walk distance; PA, pulmonary artery.

* Zero score is assigned if data are missing or expired.

normal weight. Obesity and underweight are independent risk factors for death after lung transplantation.[18,19] Obesity has also been associated with increased risk for primary graft dysfunction.[20] Underweight patients, with a body mass index (BMI) less than 18.5 kg/m², have a 35% increased risk for death after lung transplantation, and a BMI greater than 34.9 kg/m² is associated with a twofold increase in mortality.[21] Similarly, greater adiposity, as suggested by levels of serum leptin (a hormone produced by adipose tissue), is associated with increased mortality after lung transplantation. In contrast, a recent study did not find moderate obesity (BMI <35 kg/m²) to be a risk factor for worse outcomes after transplantation.[21] Also, markers of malnutrition, such as low serum albumin and total protein levels, have been associated with increased risk for infections and worse survival after lung transplantation.[22]

Lung transplant candidates should be encouraged to achieve and maintain optimal weight. Patients with advanced lung disease can lose significant amounts of weight with progression of their underlying disease. The overall increased energy expenditure to maintain adequate ventilation, coupled with decreased caloric intake related to dyspnea and gastric distention, can lead to rapid weight loss and malnutrition. Patients with CF are at further risk for malnutrition secondary to CF-related pancreatic insufficiency and increased metabolic demands as a result of worsening pulmonary infection burden.[23]

Patients awaiting lung transplantation should undergo comprehensive nutritional assessment and monitoring, preferably at their lung transplant center, by nutritionists trained in the evaluation and management of patients with advanced lung disease. The goals of nutritional evaluation and management include weight gain or loss, as appropriate, and promotion of adequate muscle and energy reserves. Underweight patients awaiting lung transplantation should receive oral high-calorie nutritional supplements. In cases in which patients continue to lose or fail to gain weight, they may benefit from placement of a gastrostomy feeding tube to ensure adequate caloric intake. Usually, experienced interventional radiologists or gastroenterologists can place these feeding tubes in awake patients, thus obviating the need for general anesthesia in patients with advanced pulmonary disease.

It is important to recognize that although underweight patients benefit from preoperative weight gain, they are at high risk for increased mortality before transplantation. Listing for lung transplantation should not be unduly delayed while waiting for weight gain. Similarly, obese patients should be encouraged to lose weight in the pretransplant period. However, in patients with advanced lung disease, rapid weight loss by severe calorie intake restriction could lead to loss of muscle mass and debilitation. The risks of overweight or moderate obesity (BMI = 25 to 35 kg/m²) adversely affecting posttransplant outcomes should be weighed against the risks of poor nutrition related to severe caloric restriction. Patients listed for lung transplantation should be closely monitored for significant changes in their weight, and they may benefit from close collaboration with transplant programs' nutritionists.

Pulmonary rehabilitation

Patients with advanced lung disease can develop decreased exercise tolerance secondary to their ventilatory limitations, skeletal muscle dysfunction, and symptoms associated with their underlying lung disease, such as cough, dyspnea, and fatigue.[24] Patients awaiting a lung transplant can be markedly inactive, with major parts of their waking hours devoted to sitting (54%) and lying (15%).[25,26] Studies of patients with idiopathic pulmonary fibrosis (IPF) and CF have documented that the 6-minute walk distance (6MWD) predicts survival in patients awaiting a lung transplant.[27,28] Candidates' functional status and exercise capacity as measured by 6MWD are associated with waiting list and posttransplant survival. This effect has been described in all lung disease groups.[29] An improvement in exercise tolerance achieved by pulmonary rehabilitation may result in improved clinical outcomes before and after lung transplantation.[30] Both interval and continuous training are effective in improving exercise capacity in patients listed for lung transplantation.[31,32] Similarly, Nordic walking has been shown to be safe, feasible, and effective in patients awaiting lung transplantation.[33] Transplant candidates' access to formal pulmonary rehabilitation programs may be limited by financial or geographic constraints. If feasible, patients should be strongly encouraged to participate in formal exercise programs. Alternatively, they should be encouraged to remain physically active and be provided with educational resources to develop their own home-based exercise regimen. Additionally, their overall exercise tolerance and level of debility should be closely monitored.

Psychosocial support

The pretransplant evaluation and waiting period for lung transplantation can be extremely stressful for patients and their caregivers. Deterioration in health status, uncertainty regarding donor organ availability, financial burden, and ongoing health-related issues can add to their psychosocial stress.[34] Psychiatric disorders during this period are common. A study of 100 lung transplant candidates demonstrated that up to 25% met the criteria for at least one mood disorder, and of these patients, 28% met the criteria for two or more psychiatric disorders, with panic and anxiety disorders being the two most common diagnoses.[35] Another study of 70 lung transplant candidates found that major depression, anxiety disorders, or adjustment disorders were diagnosed in half of the patients.[36] The burden of psychiatric disorders appears to vary depending on patients' underlying disease, and patients with CF seem to report less anxiety than do other patients with advanced lung disease. This might be related to the fact that patients with CF have had to cope with their disease for longer periods.[37]

Psychological distress is also common in transplant recipients' caregivers.[38] The caregiver's coping mechanisms and quality of life (QOL) can significantly affect the transplant recipient's QOL.[39]

Psychosocial problems have been linked to poor outcomes after transplantation. In lung and heart-lung transplant recipients, pretransplant anxiety and depression are associated with physical impairment after transplantation.[40] Similarly, psychosocial difficulties have been associated with increased risk for rejection and longer lengths of hospital stay after heart transplantation.[41,42] In lung transplant patients, nonadherence has been associated with the development of chronic rejection.[43] Alternatively, another study of lung transplant patients found anxiety and depression to be common before transplantation, but psychiatric diagnoses did not affect 1-year survival.[36]

In view of the scarcity of donor organs and concern for less than optimal outcomes after transplantation secondary to nonadherence or other psychosocial disorders, the candidate selection guidelines list these disorders as an absolute contraindication to listing for lung transplantation.[44] However, psychosocial listing criteria are not well established, and the UNOS and various other guidelines provide minimal guidance.

Transplant programs use different techniques, evaluators (social workers, psychologists, or psychiatrists), and psychosocial eligibility criteria to evaluate patients from a psychosocial perspective. At our center we use a recently validated assessment tool: the Stanford Integrated Psychosocial Assessment for Transplantation (SIPAT).[45] In addition to assisting with decisions regarding patients' psychosocial suitability for listing for lung transplantation, this tool has allowed us to identify listed transplant candidates in need of ongoing monitoring and support for nonadherence, substance abuse recidivism, and other psychosocial stressors. Multiple studies have demonstrated that structured interventions involving cognitive behavior therapies can improve lung transplant candidates' QOL, stress level, optimism, relationships with their caregivers, depression, and anxiety.[46–49] We recommend that all patients listed for a lung transplant be monitored for evidence of psychological stressors, nonadherence, and active substance abuse. Candidates at risk for substance abuse may require frequent random drug testing. The patients at risk should be offered access to appropriate behavioral therapies and support groups.

Palliative care

The World Health Organization (WHO) defines palliative care as "an approach that improves the quality of life of patients and their families facing the problem associated with life-threatening illness, through the prevention and relief of suffering by means of early identification and impeccable assessment and treatment of pain and other problems, physical, psychosocial and spiritual." In addition, the WHO reiterates that palliative care should be provided early in the course of illness, in conjunction with other therapies that are intended to prolong life.[50] Similarly, a position statement by the American Thoracic Society states that palliative care should be available at any point during the course of a progressive respiratory disease. An important concept underlined in this position is that in general, palliative care is not in conflict with curative therapies.[51] In practice, however, the goals of palliative care are often in conflict with those of curative care. In the case of lung transplant candidates, the desire to maintain them as acceptable surgical candidates may expose them to greater invasive medical therapies and limit their access to medications such as narcotics and anxiolytics.[52] Additionally, it has been demonstrated that patients with CF listed for lung transplantation are more likely to be admitted to intensive care units and receive mechanical ventilation.[53,54] Patients listed for lung transplantation should be provided with curative and palliative care in parallel rather than sequentially.[49]

BRIDGES TO LUNG TRANSPLANTATION

Implementation of the LAS system in 2005 has resulted in a significant change in the baseline characteristics of patients undergoing lung transplantation. Use of the LAS has allowed listing and transplantation of patients who are sicker and older and in whom IPF is the most common diagnosis.[55] These sicker patients remain at high risk for respiratory decompensation and for needing mechanical support to bridge them to transplantation. In addition, implementation of the LAS prioritizes candidates with high waiting list mortality to receive organs, which has given patients maintained on mechanical support a realistic chance of receiving suitable donor organs. In fact, since implementation of the LAS in 2005, the percentages of transplant candidates receiving transplants while also receiving mechanical ventilation (2.6% versus 6%) or extracorporeal life support (ECLS) (0.6% versus 1.1%) have increased significantly.[55]

Mechanical bridges to lung transplantation can be used to increase candidates' survival on the waiting list and, consequently, their chances of being able to receive suitable organs, as well as to improve their clinical status by allowing a period for aggressive nutrition and physical rehabilitation.[56,57]

Mechanical ventilation

Mechanical ventilation remains the most commonly used bridge to transplantation. The posttransplant outcomes of patients receiving a transplant while on mechanical ventilation are worse than those of other patients.[58–60] Lung transplant candidates on mechanical ventilation remain at risk for the development of ventilator-associated lung injury and heath care–associated pneumonias. Patients with advanced lung disease who are undergoing mechanical ventilation often require sedation to ensure adequate ventilation and oxygenation. Such sedation places them at risk for further deconditioning, malnutrition, and nosocomial infections. In general, it is preferable that potential transplant candidates be fully evaluated before they require mechanical ventilation. Mechanical ventilation and the associated therapies can cause logistic and emotional barriers to thorough pretransplant medical and psychosocial evaluation. Additionally, it may prevent patients from fully understanding transplantation as a therapeutic option and prevent the transplant team from obtaining realistic informed consent.

Extracorporeal life support

The limitations related to bridging patients to lung transplantation have led to renewed interest in ECLS. The earlier experiences with ECLS as a bridge to transplantation or recovery were uniformly disappointing.[61,62] However, the last decade has seen a revival of interest in using extracorporeal membrane oxygenation as a bridge to transplantation. A review of the U.S. experience before 2008 showed that the 1-year survival rate after transplantation was 50% for patients in whom ECLS was used as a bridge as opposed to 79% for unsupported patients. Since then, multiple single-center studies from different countries have reported 1-year posttransplant survival rates of ECLS patients that ranged from 75% to 80% and were statistically similar to those of lung transplant recipients not supported with ECLS.[63–65] The development of new methods of ECLS can provide support with minimal morbidity. The development of smaller oxygenators, heparin-coated circuits, centrifugal pumps, and percutaneously placed dual-lumen catheters has allowed the use of ECLS in awake and ambulatory patients. Patients can be maintained on ECLS for extended periods while awaiting lung transplantation. They can actively participate in nutritional and exercise programs to maintain their transplant candidacy and reduce posttransplant complications.[66] Despite promising reports, the use of ECLS as a bridge to lung transplantation remains controversial. It is associated with significant resource use and medical complications, and the clinical expertise required to provide ECLS is not uniformly available at all lung transplant centers.

ORGAN ALLOCATION AND WAITING LIST MANAGEMENT

In the United States, donor lungs are allocated on the basis of a LAS that is calculated to provide maximal transplant survival benefit to the transplant recipients. One of the goals of the LAS was to reduce waiting list mortality by prioritizing candidates on the basis of urgency rather than time on the waiting list. Since its implementation in 2005, lung transplant recipients have been older, sicker, and more likely to have interstitial lung disease, and transplant rates are highest in individuals 65 years or older and those with diagnoses of interstitial lung disease. Initially, in connection with the ability to perform transplants on sicker patients on an urgent basis, waiting list mortality declined. Since 2010, however, waiting list mortality has increased and is currently 15.4 per 100 waiting list years. Waiting list mortality is highest in patients with a LAS of 50 or greater and

candidates aged 12 to 17 years, followed by those aged 18 to 34 years. Asian, Hispanic, and black candidates have higher waiting list mortality than do whites.[4] A rapid change in the LAS has been associated with worse posttransplant mortality, as well as with increased waiting list mortality over the short term.[67] The median time to transplantation is currently 4 months, although this number varies widely by the geographic location of the transplant center.[4] It is imperative that transplant physicians be aware of the donor supply in their donor service area and of specific barriers to transplantation at their centers. Candidates on the waiting list who are at an increased risk for death should be prospectively identified and closely monitored. The clinical variables included in the LAS, especially oxygen requirement and the use of assisted ventilation, can have a significant impact on candidates' allocation score and thus on the likelihood of their receiving appropriate donor lungs. At our center, patients with a LAS greater than 50 are seen every 4 to 6 weeks, and their clinical status is reviewed at the weekly multidisciplinary candidate selection meeting. The clinical variables that UNOS requires be updated periodically for optimal calculation of the LAS are summarized in Table 5.1.

Sensitized lung transplant candidates

Lung transplant candidates can develop antibodies to HLA if they are ever exposed to a sensitizing event such as pregnancy, blood transfusion, sharing of intravenous needles, or previous organ transplants. The presence of anti-HLA and, especially, donor-specific anti-HLA antibodies is associated with worse graft and patient survival after lung transplantation.[5–7,68,69] The tests used for detection of anti-HLA antibodies have significantly evolved over the last 2 decades. The newer solid-phase assays, especially single-antigen HLA beads, are extremely sensitive in detecting IgG anti-HLA antibodies.[7,70] The clinical significance of these IgG antibodies remains unclear. To ascertain their significance, new assays designed to determine the complement-binding capability of these antibodies have been developed. The presence of complement-binding anti-HLA donor-specific antibodies has been associated with worse outcomes in kidney and heart transplantation.[71,72] It is likely that the presence of complement-binding anti-HLA antibodies rather than IgG antibodies is clinically significant. The presence of anti-HLA antibodies in lung transplant candidates has been associated with lower transplant rates because of the reduced size of the donor pool for sensitized candidates.[68]

Multiple strategies have been used to facilitate transplantation in candidates with preformed anti-HLA antibodies. One approach is to lower the titers of anti-HLA antibodies before transplantation. The results of these "desensitization protocols" in lowering antibody titers in thoracic transplant candidates have been disappointing.[73–75] Despite using an aggressive desensitization protocol consisting of plasmapheresis, methylprednisolone, bortezomib, rituximab, and intravenous immunoglobulin, the investigators were unable to significantly lower the anti-HLA antibodies.[74] At our

Table 5.2 Stanford pre–lung transplant HLA antibody management protocol

HLA antibodies by IgG assay (cPRA%)	HLA antibodies by C1q assay (cPRA%)	Intervention
<50%	Negative	Immediate retrospective crossmatch
≥50%	Negative	Plasmapheresis in the operating room, immediate retrospective crossmatch
Negative or positive	<50%	Virtual crossmatch, followed by immediate retrospective crossmatch
Negative or positive	≥50%	Prospective crossmatch

Note: cPRA, calculated panel-reactive antibodies; HLA, human leukocyte antigen.

center we do not use desensitization protocols; our pre–lung transplant anti-HLA antibody protocol is summarized in Table 5.2. In the United States, the Organ Procurement and Transplantation Network (OPTN) allows an allocation exception for sensitized patients. Lungs can be allocated to sensitized candidates within a donor service area if their physicians deem them to be sensitized against certain HLA antigens, if all lung transplant programs and the organ procurement organization (OPO) in the donor service area agree to allocation of lungs to the candidates in question because the crossmatch between donor and recipient sera is negative, and if all local lung transplant programs and the OPO agree on the level of sensitization at which candidates would qualify for this exception.[76]

Small recipients

With implementation of the LAS, the number of patients with restrictive lung disease who are on the waiting list and undergoing transplantation has increased. Patients with restrictive lung disease are likely to have small thoracic cavities related to their underlying disease. Lung transplant candidates less than 160 cm in height wait 54 days longer for suitable organs than do candidates with an average height of 168 cm.[77] Patients with a high LAS and restrictive lung disease are at higher risk for waiting list mortality. In the case of recipients with small stature, a high LAS, and restrictive lung disease, it is imperative that alternative strategies for transplantation be explored. Possible strategies include living lobar transplantation, cadaveric donor lobar transplantation, and nonanatomic downsizing of the donor lungs to facilitate transplantation of organs from larger donors into smaller recipients. Clinical outcomes of patients undergoing bilateral lobar lung transplantation are similar to those of standard bilateral lung transplant recipients.[78,79]

Lung review board

The OPTN allows a lung transplant program to appeal its patient's LAS if it believes that the candidate's LAS does not reflect appropriate medical urgency for transplantation. The program can request a certain LAS for its patient. All such appeals are reviewed by a lung review board consisting of practicing lung transplant physicians and surgeons.[76]

Multiple listing

Under the current LAS system, donor organs are offered to all the ABO-identical and ABO-compatible candidates within the UNOS donor service area determined by the donor location before being offered outside the area. Median times to transplantation vary significantly between different geographic and donor service areas. All listed patients should be given information regarding listing at multiple centers. Lung transplant candidates at high risk for death, such as those with a LAS higher than 50 or interstitial lung disease with rapid deterioration, should be encouraged to pursue dual listing at transplant centers outside their own OPO's service area. Similarly, sensitized patients and candidates with small stature may benefit from listing at multiple transplant centers, thereby allowing them access to a larger donor pool.

Removal from the waiting list

The clinical status of patients on the lung transplant waiting list can change rapidly. It is essential that all lung transplant candidates be assessed for continued suitability for lung transplantation at all clinic visits, as well as at the time of any significant change in their clinical status. Common reasons for removal from the waiting list before transplantation include the following: progression of illness to the point at which the patient becomes too sick to undergo transplantation; development of another organ failure; uncontrolled sepsis; nonadherence to medical therapy; substance abuse recidivism; change in social support structure; a new absolute or relative contraindication; and rarely, improvement in clinical status. Candidates on mechanical ventilation or ECLS are at high risk for becoming "too ill for transplantation," and their candidacy should be reviewed at least daily or more frequently. If the contraindication to continued candidacy is deemed temporary, patients can be placed on inactive status pending resolution. Positive developments that should lead to consideration of removal from the waiting list include response to medical therapy (most common in the pulmonary hypertension population) and/or improvement in QOL status that would alter the risk-benefit equation away from transplantation at the current time.[44]

REFERENCES

1. Iribarne A, Russo MJ, Davies RR, et al. Despite decreased wait-list times for lung transplantation, lung allocation scores continue to increase. Chest 2009;135:923-928.
2. Kozower BD, Meyers BF, Smith MA, et al. The impact of the lung allocation score on short-term transplantation outcomes: A multicenter study. J Thorac Cardiovasc Surg 2008;135:166-171.
3. Osaki S, Maloney JD, Meyer KC, et al. The impact of the lung allocation scoring system at the single national Veterans Affairs hospital lung transplantation program. Eur J Cardiothorac Surg 2009;36:497-501.
4. Valapour M, Skeans MA, Heubner BM, et al. OPTN/SRTR 2012 annual data report: Lung. Am J Transplant 2014;14(Suppl 1):139-165.
5. Hadjiliadis D, Chaparro C, Reinsmoen NL, et al. Pretransplant panel reactive antibody in lung transplant recipients is associated with significantly worse posttransplant survival in a multicenter study. J Heart Lung Transplant 2005;24(Suppl 7):S249-S254.
6. Shah AS, Nwakanma L, Simpkins C, et al. Pretransplant panel reactive antibodies in human lung transplantation: An analysis of over 10,000 patients. Ann Thoracic Surg 2008;85:1919-1924.
7. Smith JD, Ibrahim MW, Newell H, et al. Pretransplant donor HLA-specific antibodies: Characteristics causing detrimental effects on survival after lung transplantation. J Heart Lung Transplant 2014;33:1074-1082.
8. De Soyza A, Meachery G, Hester KL, et al. Lung transplantation for patients with cystic fibrosis and Burkholderia cepacia complex infection: A single-center experience. J Heart Lung Transplant 2010;29:1395-1404.
9. Taylor JL, Palmer SM. Mycobacterium abscessus chest wall and pulmonary infection in a cystic fibrosis lung transplant recipient. J Heart Lung Transplant 2006;25:985-988.
10. National Center for Immunization and Respiratory Diseases. General recommendations on immunization—recommendations of the Advisory Committee on Immunization Practices (ACIP). MMWR Recomm Rep 2011;60(2):1-64
11. Conway SP, Simmonds EJ, Littlewood JM. Acute severe deterioration in cystic fibrosis associated with influenza A virus infection. Thorax 1992;47:112-114.
12. Flight WG, Bright-Thomas RJ, Tilston P, et al. Incidence and clinical impact of respiratory viruses in adults with cystic fibrosis. Thorax 2014;69:247-253.
13. Poole PJ, Chacko E, Wood-Baker RW, Cates CJ. Influenza vaccine for patients with chronic obstructive pulmonary disease. Cochrane Database Syst Rev 2006;1:CD002733.
14. Umeda Y, Morikawa M, Anzai M, et al. Acute exacerbation of idiopathic pulmonary fibrosis after pandemic influenza A (H1N1) vaccination. Intern Med 2010;49:2333-2336.
15. Whitaker P, Etherington C, Denton M, et al. A/H1N1 flu pandemic. A/H1N1 and other viruses affecting cystic fibrosis. BMJ 2009;339:b3958.
16. Blumberg EA, Fitzpatrick J, Stutman PC, et al. Safety of influenza vaccine in heart transplant recipients. J Heart Lung Transplant 1998;17:1075-1080.
17. Katerinis I, Hadaya K, Duquesnoy R, et al. De novo anti-HLA antibody after pandemic H1N1 and seasonal influenza immunization in kidney transplant recipients. Am J Transplant 2011;11:1727-1733.
18. Lederer DJ, Wilt JS, D'Ovidio F, et al. Obesity and underweight are associated with an increased risk of death after lung transplantation. Am J Respir Crit Care Med 2009;180:887-895.
19. Allen JG, Arnaoutakis GJ, Weiss ES, et al. The impact of recipient body mass index on survival after lung transplantation. J Heart Lung Transplant 2010;29:1026-1033.
20. Lederer DJ, Kawut SM, Wickersham N, et al. Obesity and primary graft dysfunction after lung transplantation: The Lung Transplant Outcomes Group obesity study. Am J Respir Crit Care Med 2011;184:1055-1061.
21. Singer JP, Peterson ER, Snyder ME, et al. Body composition and mortality after adult lung transplantation in the United States. Am J Respir Crit Care Med 2014;190:1012-21.
22. Chamogeorgakis T, Mason DP, Murthy SC, et al. Impact of nutritional state on lung transplant outcomes. J Heart Lung Transplant 2013;32:693-700.
23. Hirche TO, Knoop C, Hebestreit H, et al. Practical guidelines: Lung transplantation in patients with cystic fibrosis. Pulm Med 2014;2014:621342.
24. Rochester CL, Fairburn C, Crouch RH. Pulmonary rehabilitation for respiratory disorders other than chronic obstructive pulmonary disease. Clin Chest Med 2014;35:369-389.
25. Bossenbroek L, ten Hacken NH, van der Bij W, et al. Cross-sectional assessment of daily physical activity in chronic obstructive pulmonary disease lung transplant patients. J Heart Lung Transplant 2009;28:149-155.
26. Langer D, Cebria i Iranzo MA, et al. Determinants of physical activity in daily life in candidates for lung transplantation. Respir Med 2012;106:747-754.
27. Lederer DJ, Arcasoy SM, Wilt JS, et al. Six-minute-walk distance predicts waiting list survival in idiopathic pulmonary fibrosis. Am J Respir Crit Care Med 2006;174:659-664.
28. Sharples L, Hathaway T, Dennis C, et al. Prognosis of patients with cystic fibrosis awaiting heart and lung transplantation. J Heart Lung Transplant 1993;12:669-674.

29. Martinu T, Babyak MA, O'Connell CF, et al. Baseline 6-min walk distance predicts survival in lung transplant candidates. Am J Transplant 2008;8:1498-1505.

30. Rochester CL. Pulmonary rehabilitation for patients who undergo lung-volume-reduction surgery or lung transplantation. Respir Care 2008;53:1196-1202.

31. Gloeckl R, Halle M, Kenn K. Interval versus continuous training in lung transplant candidates: A randomized trial. J Heart Lung Transplant 2012;31:934-941.

32. Spruit MA, Singh SJ, Garvey C, et al. An official American Thoracic Society/European Respiratory Society statement: Key concepts and advances in pulmonary rehabilitation. Am J Respir Crit Care Med 2013;188:e13-e64.

33. Jastrzebski D, Ochman M, Ziora D, et al. Pulmonary rehabilitation in patients referred for lung transplantation. Adv Exp Med Biol 2013;755:19-25.

34. Barbour KA, Blumenthal JA, Palmer SM. Psychosocial issues in the assessment and management of patients undergoing lung transplantation. Chest 2006;129:1367-1374.

35. Parekh PI, Blumenthal JA, Babyak MA, et al. Psychiatric disorder and quality of life in patients awaiting lung transplantation. Chest 2003;124:1682-1688.

36. Woodman CL, Geist LJ, Vance S, et al. Psychiatric disorders and survival after lung transplantation. Psychosomatics 1999;40:293-297.

37. Burker EJ, Carels RA, Thompson LF, et al. Quality of life in patients awaiting lung transplant: Cystic fibrosis versus other end-stage lung diseases. Pediatr Pulmonol 2000;30:453-460.

38. Stukas AA Jr, Dew MA, Switzer GE, et al. PTSD in heart transplant recipients and their primary family caregivers. Psychosomatics 1999;40:212-221.

39. Myaskovsky L, Dew MA, Switzer GE, et al. Quality of life and coping strategies among lung transplant candidates and their family caregivers. Soc Sci Med 2005;60:2321-2332.

40. De Vito Dabbs A, Dew MA, Stilley CS, et al. Psychosocial vulnerability, physical symptoms and physical impairment after lung and heart-lung transplantation. J Heart Lung Transplant 2003;22:1268-1275.

41. Chacko RC, Harper RG, Gotto J, Young J. Psychiatric interview and psychometric predictors of cardiac transplant survival. Am J Psychiatry 1996;153:1607-1612.

42. Shapiro PA, Williams DL, Foray AT, et al. Psychosocial evaluation and prediction of compliance problems and morbidity after heart transplantation. Transplantation 1995;60:1462-1466.

43. Husain AN, Siddiqui MT, Holmes EW, et al. Analysis of risk factors for the development of bronchiolitis obliterans syndrome. Am J Respir Crit Care Med 1999;159:829-833.

44. Weill D, Benden C, Corris PA, et al. A consensus document for the selection of lung transplant candidates: 2014—an update from the Pulmonary Transplantation Council of the International Society for Heart and Lung Transplantation. J Heart Lung Transplant 2015;34:1-15.

45. Maldonado JR, Dubois HC, David EE, et al. The Stanford Integrated Psychosocial Assessment for Transplantation (SIPAT): A new tool for the psychosocial evaluation of pre-transplant candidates. Psychosomatics 2012;53:123-132.

46. Blumenthal JA, Babyak MA, Keefe FJ, et al. Telephone-based coping skills training for patients awaiting lung transplantation. J Consult Clin Psychol 2006;74:535-544.

47. Napolitano MA, Babyak MA, Palmer S, et al. Effects of a telephone-based psychosocial intervention for patients awaiting lung transplantation. Chest 2002;122:1176-1184.

48. Rodrigue JR, Baz MA, Widows MR, Ehlers SL. A randomized evaluation of quality-of-life therapy with patients awaiting lung transplantation. Am J Transplant 2005;5:2425-2432.

49. Rosenberger EM, Dew MA, DiMartini AF, et al. Psychosocial issues facing lung transplant candidates, recipients and family caregivers. Thorac Surg Clin 2012;22:517-529.

50. World Health Organization. WHO definition of palliative care. http://www.who.int/cancer/palliative/definition/en/. Accessed October 14, 2014.

51. Lanken PN, Terry PB, Delisser HM, et al. An official American Thoracic Society clinical policy statement: Palliative care for patients with respiratory diseases and critical illnesses. Am J Respir Crit Care Med 2008;177:912-927.

52. Janssen DJ, Spruit MA, Does JD, et al. End-of-life care in a COPD patient awaiting lung transplantation: A case report. BMC Palliat Care 2010;9:6.

53. Dellon EP, Leigh MW, Yankaskas JR, Noah TL. Effects of lung transplantation on inpatient end of life care in cystic fibrosis. J Cyst Fibros 2007;6:396-402.

54. Ford D, Flume PA. Impact of lung transplantation on site of death in cystic fibrosis. J Cyst Fibros 2007;6:391-395.

55. Maxwell BG, Levitt JE, Goldstein BA, et al. Impact of the lung allocation score on survival beyond 1 year. Am J Transplant 2014;14:2288-2294.

56. Cypel M, Keshavjee S. Extracorporeal life support as a bridge to lung transplantation. Clin Chest Med 2011;32:245-251.

57. Strueber M. Bridges to lung transplantation. Curr Opin Organ Transplant 2011;16:458-461.

58. Gottlieb J, Warnecke G, Hadem J, et al. Outcome of critically ill lung transplant candidates on invasive respiratory support. Intensive Care Med 2012;38:968-975.

59. Mason DP, Thuita L, Nowicki ER, et al. Should lung transplantation be performed for patients on mechanical respiratory support? The US experience. J Thorac Cardiovasc Surg 2010;139:765-773 e761.

60. Singer JP, Blanc PD, Hoopes C, et al. The impact of pretransplant mechanical ventilation on short- and long-term survival after lung transplantation. Am J Transplant 2011;11:2197-2204.

61. Veith FJ. Lung transplantation. Transplant Proc 1977;9:203-208.

62. Zapol WM, Snider MT, Hill JD, et al. Extracorporeal membrane oxygenation in severe acute respiratory failure. A randomized prospective study. JAMA 1979;242:2193-2196.

63. Bermudez CA, Rocha RV, Zaldonis D, et al. Extracorporeal membrane oxygenation as a bridge to lung transplant: Term outcomes. Ann Thoracic Surg 2011;92:1226-1231; discussion 1231-1232.

64. Fuehner T, Kuehn C, Hadem J, et al. Extracorporeal membrane oxygenation in awake patients as bridge to lung transplantation. Am J Respir Crit Care Med 2012;185:763-768.

65. Lang G, Taghavi S, Aigner C, et al. Primary lung transplantation after bridge with extracorporeal membrane oxygenation: A plea for a shift in our paradigms for indications. Transplantation 2012;93:729-736.

66. Diaz-Guzman E, Hoopes CW, Zwischenberger JB. The evolution of extracorporeal life support as a bridge to lung transplantation. ASAIO J 2013;59:3-10.

67. Tsuang WM, Vock DM, Finlen Copeland CA, et al. An acute change in lung allocation score and survival after lung transplantation: A cohort study. Ann Intern Med 2013;158:650-657.

68. Kim M, Townsend KR, Wood IG, et al. Impact of pretransplant anti-HLA antibodies on outcomes in lung transplant candidates. Am J Respir Crit Care Med 2014;189:1234-1239.

69. Lau CL, Palmer SM, Posther KE, et al. Influence of panel-reactive antibodies on posttransplant outcomes in lung transplant recipients. Ann Thoracic Surg 2000;69:1520-1524.

70. Tyan DB. New approaches for detecting complement-fixing antibodies. Curr Opin Organ Transplant 2012;17:409-415.

71. Chin C, Chen G, Sequeria F, et al. Clinical usefulness of a novel C1q assay to detect immunoglobulin G antibodies capable of fixing complement in sensitized pediatric heart transplant patients. J Heart Lung Transplant 2011;30:158-163.

72. Yabu JM, Higgins JP, Chen G, et al. C1q-fixing human leukocyte antigen antibodies are specific for predicting transplant glomerulopathy and late graft failure after kidney transplantation. Transplantation 2011;91:342-347.

73. Patel J, Everly M, Chang D, et al. Reduction of alloantibodies via proteasome inhibition in cardiac transplantation. J Heart Lung Transplant 2011;30:1320-1326.

74. Snyder LD, Gray AL, Reynolds JM, et al. Antibody desensitization therapy in highly sensitized lung transplant candidates. Am J Transplant 2014;14:849-856.

75. Weston M, Rolfe M, Haddad T. Desensitization protocol using bortezomib for highly sensitized patients awaiting heart or lung transplants. Clin Transplant 2009:393-399.

76. Organ Procurement and Transplantation Network (OPTN) policies. http://optn.transplant.hrsa.gov/governance/policies/. Accessed 2014 Oct 14, 2014.

77. Shigemura N, Bhama J, Bermudez C, D'Cunha J. Lobar lung transplantation: Emerging evidence for a viable option. Semin Thorac Cardiovasc Surg 2013;25:95-96.

78. Keating DT, Marasco SF, Negri J, et al. Long-term outcomes of cadaveric lobar lung transplantation: Helping to maximize resources. J Heart Lung Transplant 2010;29:439-444.

79. Marasco SF, Than S, Keating D, et al. Cadaveric lobar lung transplantation: Technical aspects. Ann Thoracic Surg 2012;93:1836-1842.

Donor Management

Allocation of donor lungs

MARK J. RUSSO

In May 2005, the lung allocation score (LAS) was implemented in the United States to allocate organs on the basis of medical urgency (and not strictly waiting time). Since then, waiting list times and mortality have improved, and sicker patients are receiving transplants with no effect on posttransplant survival. However, evidence that the locally based allocation system is impeding the full beneficial potential of the LAS is increasing. Geography continues to play a significant role in lung allocation in the United States, causing lungs to be regularly allocated to low-priority candidates while appropriately matched high-priority regional candidates are being bypassed.

INTRODUCTION

Ideally, a suitable donor organ would be available for every transplant candidate who could benefit from a new organ. Unfortunately, donor organs suitable for transplantation remain in critically short supply.[1] Annually, hundreds of lung transplant candidates die while on the waiting list.[2] The disparity between potential recipients and available donors demands efficient methods of organ allocation to ensure optimal use of a scarce resource.

In prior years, lung allocation in the United States was based on accrued time on the waiting list.[3-5] That is, when organs became available, the candidates with the most days on the list had the highest priority. The system was intended to favor patients who were sick for the longest amount of time, which was considered to be a surrogate for disease severity. However, the system probably led to practices with the opposite effect. Patients were listed earlier in the course of their disease to accrue more time on the waiting list, which resulted in up to 44% of listed patients having an inactive status.[6] The patients who made it to the top of the list were those who were healthy enough to wait the longest. In fact, even when at the top of the list, such patients may have been facing a higher risk by undergoing transplantation than by remaining on the waiting list.[5,7,8] Conversely, the sickest patients, the most urgent cases clinically, may have not been listed at all because of the belief that they would have little chance of surviving the long wait for an available organ.[9] Thus, a revamping of the lung allocation process was necessary.

CURRENT ERA

The lung allocation score

In May 2005, the lung allocation score (LAS) was implemented to allocate organs on the basis of medical urgency (and not strictly waiting time). The LAS, which is a normalized numerical score ranging from 0 to 100, is based on a multivariate model that is a weighted combination of the predicted risk of waiting list death and the predicted likelihood of survival during the first year after transplantation.[10] Specifically, the LAS is calculated as perceived transplant benefit minus waiting list urgency. Transplant benefit is calculated by subtracting waiting list urgency from a posttransplant survival measure.[3,7]

Transplant benefit measure = Posttransplant survival measure - Waiting list urgency measure

Raw LAS = Transplant benefit measure - Waiting list urgency measure

= Posttransplant survival measure - 2 × (Waiting list urgency measure)

Waiting list urgency is measured by taking the area under the waiting list survival curve at 1 year, as estimated by a multivariate regression model. Posttransplant survival is estimated similarly.

The area under the curve corresponds to the number of days alive in the 1-year period.[8] Many factors are used to generate survival curves at 1 year, including functional status, forced vital capacity (percentage of predicted value), age, and diagnosis. The score is then normalized to a 100-point scale.[8] Finally, if the patient deteriorates while on the waiting list, the score can be updated at any time.

Only patients who are at least 12 years old are given a LAS. Dependable models could not be generated for younger patients because of lack of data. Therefore, in those patients, time accrued on the waiting list is the principal determining factor for lung allocation.[8]

Because the LAS assigns greater weight to expected survival on the waiting list than to expected posttransplant survival and therefore preferentially allocates organs to critically ill candidates, it was feared that initiation of the LAS would result in increased posttransplant morbidity and mortality.

Outcomes following implementation of the lung allocation score

The initial studies released after implementation of the new allocation system demonstrated that both the mean LAS of transplant recipients and the mean LAS of listed candidates had increased.[8,10–13] These studies also established that waiting list times had decreased despite an increase in the number of patients listed for a transplant.[9,11]

Because sicker patients were receiving transplants, the post-LAS era was also found to be characterized by higher rates of primary graft dysfunction,[9] longer lengths of stay in the intensive care unit,[9] and greater resource use.[15] Despite these findings, studies have found no evidence of decreased posttransplant survival.[9,12–14]

These beneficial changes notwithstanding, our group has demonstrated that the net benefit of transplantation is not being maximized. We have shown the following: (1) high-priority lung transplant candidates (LAS higher than 75) are continuing to die on the waiting list at high rates, (2) four fifths of lungs are being allocated to low-priority candidates (LAS lower than 50), and (3) low-priority candidates (LAS lower than 50) appear to be receiving little or no benefit survival from transplantation.[2] We postulate that many of these inefficiencies are caused by the local allocation of lungs.

GEOGRAPHY IN LUNG ALLOCATION

The significant impact of geography on organ allocation in the United States has long been recognized. In April 1998, the U.S. Department of Health and Human Services (DHHS) issued the "Final Rule," which states that "allocation of scarce organs will be based on common medical criteria, not accidents of geography."[16] In October 1998, the DHHS and the Institute of Medicine (IOM) assembled an expert panel to assess the impact of the Final Rule on liver allocation and transplantation. The panel's analysis, which was completed in July 1999, had two major conclusions. The first was that broader sharing of organs had many beneficial effects on allocation outcomes, including (1) an overall increase in the rate at which the most severely ill patients were receiving transplants, (2) a concomitant decrease in the excess transplantation of the least severely ill patients, and (3) no increase in pretransplantation mortality. The panel's second major conclusion was that a new allocation system should be designed on the basis of "medical characteristics and disease prognoses rather than waiting times."[17]

The effect of geography on lung transplantation has also long been recognized. When the LAS was implemented in 2005, the Lung Allocation Subcommittee recommended that in addition to allocating organs on the basis of medical urgency, the effects of geography on waiting list outcome be minimized.[3] Despite the introduction of the Final Rule, the findings of the IOM expert panel, and the recommendations of the Lung Allocation Subcommittee, no significant policy changes have been adopted to minimize the impact of geography on the allocation of donor lungs.

Although all candidates are initially prioritized by LAS, organs are first allocated geographically, regardless of LAS. The primary unit of organ allocation is the *local* geographic unit, known as the donor service area (DSA). The next largest unit is the *region*. In the United States and Puerto Rico a total of 58 DSAs form 11 regions. Initially, organs are offered only to the subset of appropriately matched lung transplant candidates (on the basis of blood type and size) within the donor's DSA. If an available organ is accepted for a candidate within the local DSA, it is never offered to potentially more severely ill candidates at the broader *regional* or *national* level, even if those nonlocal candidates have a higher LAS.

Unfortunately, bypassing sicker regional or national candidates for local candidates is a frequent occurrence. In our analysis of all 580 locally allocated double lungs in 2009, 480 (83%) were allocated locally despite the existence of a well-matched candidate with a higher LAS at the regional level.[18] Troublingly, the differences between the LASs of the local candidates and those of the regional candidates in such cases were not trivial. Twenty-four percent of the 480 bypassed regional candidates had LASs more than 10 points higher than the local recipient did. Seven percent had a LAS more than 25 points higher than that of the local recipient. Overall, 185 of these bypassed regional candidates ultimately died while on the waiting list.[18]

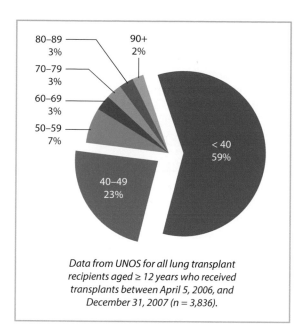

Figure 6.1 Proportion of candidates who received a transplant by LAS at transplant.

Differences in LAS between patients are clinically meaningful. Patients with a LAS lower than 50 are likely to live on the order of years without a transplant, whereas patients with a LAS higher than 75 are likely to live only on the order of days. Those added years of expected survival without a transplant provide time for low-risk patients to wait for available organs—time the high-priority patients do not have.

The locally based allocation system impedes the transplant community's attempts to allocate organs on the basis of severity of disease and limits the full beneficial potential of the LAS. More than 80% of donor lungs continue to be allocated to low-priority candidates (LAS lower than 50) (Figure 6.1).[19] Nearly half of those low-priority candidates receive locally derived organs (Figure 6.2)[20] that may have

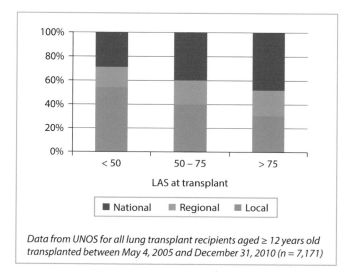

Figure 6.2 Allocation type by LAS.

potentially benefited more severely ill regional candidates. While low-priority recipients are continuing to receive the majority of donor organs, nearly 50% of high-priority candidates (LAS higher than 75) are dying on the waiting list after 1 year of being listed.[2] These observations are even more troublesome because low-priority candidates receive little or no net survival benefit from transplantation (Figure 6.3).[2]

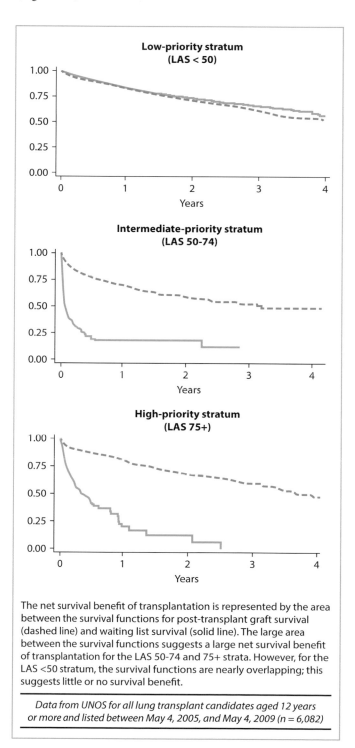

Figure 6.3 Net survival benefit of transplantation by LAS stratum.

POTENTIAL SOLUTION

We advocate for the creation of a priority system for lung transplantation analogous to the allocation system for heart transplantation. In the heart allocation system, organs are first offered to local status 1A candidates (corresponding to the most severely ill candidates). If there are no local 1A candidates, the organ is offered to status 1A candidates in a 500-mile radius. If there are no appropriate 1A candidates in a 500-mile radius, the organ is offered to local 1B candidates. If there are no local 1B candidates, the organ is offered to status 1B candidates in a 500-mile radius. If there are no appropriate 1B candidates in a 500-mile radius, the organ is offered to local status 2 candidates. If there are no local status 2 candidates, the organ is offered to status 2 candidates in a 500-mile radius. If there are no appropriate status 2 candidates in a 500-mile radius, the organ is offered nationally by status level. We argue that lungs could be allocated in a similar manner (Table 6.1), with LAS severity levels lower than 50, from 50 to 75, and higher than 75 and the following geographic strata: local DSA, 500-mile radius, and national.

Our proposed LAS stratifications (LAS less than 50, LAS 50 to 75, and LAS greater than 75) are based on previous studies demonstrating significant differences in pretransplantation survival with each change in LAS stratum.[2,19] However, these thresholds would have to be validated in future studies and may potentially need to be modified. The 500-mile cutoff for regional sharing increases the sharing area enough to increase the donor pool, but not so much as to significantly increase ischemic times and procurement costs. Furthermore, because organ procurement organizations (OPOs), the independent organizations that manage organ allocation within a DSA, are already familiar with the 500-mile cutoff for heart transplantation, it would not be difficult for them to adopt a similar system for lungs.

Other systems, such as the current system used for liver allocation, are conceivable. Liver transplant candidates who are status 1A (i.e., the most severely ill) benefit from regional sharing of organs. The regions correspond to groups of DSAs and are the same regions used for lung allocation. Furthermore, liver transplant candidates with status 1A receive organs in the same way as lung candidates: organs are first distributed locally. If a liver is not accepted locally, it is then offered at the regional and national levels. This model has improved waiting list mortality and post-transplantation outcomes in liver transplant candidates and recipients.[21]

CRITICISMS OF BROADER ORGAN SHARING

The announcement of the Final Rule by the DHHS was followed by many bitter economic and scientific debates within the transplant community.[13,14] Concerns were expressed that implementation of the Final Rule would

- Increase the cost of transplantation.
- Increase ischemic times and worsen outcomes.
- Force the closure of small transplant centers.
- Adversely affect access to transplantation for minorities and low-income patients.
- Discourage organ donation.

As a result of these concerns, in October 1998 the U.S. Congress suspended implementation of the Final Rule for 1 year to allow further study of its impact. It was during this time that Congress asked the IOM to create an expert panel to assess the impact of the Final Rule on liver allocation and transplantation specifically. The panel found no evidence that broader organ sharing would cause any of the aforementioned outcomes.[17,22,23]

Cost of transplantation

One study established that broader sharing of livers at the regional level was not associated with an increase in cost of transplantation.[24] Perhaps more importantly, however, under the current system for lungs, many individuals undergoing transplantation are not receiving a measurable survival benefit (Figure 6.3). This fact suggests that the current approach may not be very cost-effective (as measured by survival benefit divided by cost of transplantation) in comparison to a system that promotes transplantation for high-priority candidates (i.e., those with the greatest survival benefit), as we propose. If, as a result of broader organ sharing, recipients receive a greater net survival benefit from transplantation, the one-time increased cost of procurement may prove to be a worthwhile investment and may actually increase the cost-effectiveness of transplantation.

Prolonged ischemic time

Models created for simulating the increased sharing of livers across regions suggest that broader sharing of organs at the regional level does not significantly increase cold ischemic time.[25] Furthermore, current evidence suggests that an ischemic time of up to 8 hours is not associated with diminished lung graft survival at 1 year.[26] In our proposed system,

Table 6.1 Proposed lung allocation system

Priority level	Geographic requirements	LAS requirements
Highest	Local candidates	LAS >75
	Candidates within a 500-mile radius	LAS >75
	Local candidates	LAS 50-75
	Candidates within a 500-mile radius	LAS 50-75
	Local candidates	LAS <50
	Candidates within a 500-mile radius	LAS <50
Lowest	National candidates	By LAS

Note: LAS, lung allocation score.

which limits the regional sharing radius to 500 miles, most procurement travel times would be less than 2.5 hours.

Smaller programs

The state of New York is currently participating in a state-wide organ-sharing program for liver transplantation that includes several DSAs. One year after implementation, the smaller centers reported an increase in the volume of liver transplants.[27] Additionally, statewide sharing of organs may be associated with improved OPO outcomes. Studies analyzing kidney transplantation and comparing statewide sharing programs (multiple DSAs) with single DSAs showed that statewide sharing is associated with an improvement in transplant rates, waiting time, dialysis time, and graft survival.[28]

Minorities and low-income patients

The most important driver of health care disparities, access to health insurance and high-quality health care services, lies outside the transplantation system. In fact, the IOM panel discovered that once patients are listed for a transplant, no racial disparities in waiting list times exist. Also, the panel found no evidence suggesting that broader geographic sharing of organs would adversely affect minority and low-income patients' access to organ transplants.[17,24] In fact, one study of allocation in liver transplantation suggests that local allocation of livers may increase disparities between whites and Hispanics in local DSAs with a small Hispanic population.[29]

Organ donation

The IOM committee found that most of the factors affecting donation rates have little to do with local allocation policies. Thus, knowledge that donated organs are more likely to stay within the community does not seem to be a significant factor in the decision to donate. The committee found little or no evidence suggesting either that people would decline to donate or that health professionals engaged in organ procurement would be less diligent in their efforts if they knew that a donated organ would be used outside the donor's immediate geographic area.[30] Another study by Egan supports this finding: it reported that more than 60% of the general public declare that they would be more strongly influenced to sign a donor card by a policy that favored national distribution rather than local distribution.[31]

LUNG TRANSPLANTATION IN OTHER COUNTRIES

Lungs can be allocated on the basis of urgency, wait time, or both,[32] with the latter being the most common. One example of a system using both medical urgency and time accrued on the waiting list is Eurotransplant.[33] Until recently, all countries in the Eurotransplant system used a four-step ranking process.[34] The first step is to place the candidate in a rank tier on the basis of location (distance from the donor) and urgency status. A two-leveled urgency system of "high urgency" and "elective" is used. The second step is to rank candidates within a tier on the basis of special situations such as being a pediatric candidate or a heart-lung candidate. The third step is to rank candidates on the basis of time accrued on the waiting list. The fourth, and final, step occurs only if candidates are still tied in rank, at which time a detailed breakdown of time on the waiting list and days with "high urgency" status[34] is considered. Recently, two Eurotransplant countries, Germany (in 2011[35,36]) and the Netherlands (in 2014[37]), adopted the LAS system for their national allocation system, thereby eliminating waiting time from their allocation algorithm.

Organ distribution is also dependent on the type of governing body overseeing allocation. Organ networks can be centralized to govern all transplants throughout an entire country or decentralized to govern all transplantations within a region. Additionally, different systems grant more or less decision-making capacity to transplant centers. For example, in Australia and the United Kingdom, lungs are first made available to the transplant center nearest the donor. If that transplant center is unable to find an appropriate match, the organs are made available to other centers on a rotating basis.[38] This type of system grants greater discretion to the transplant centers, which are able to assess appropriateness of the organ and potential matches on a case-by-case basis. Other countries, such as France and Spain, have strong national networks that are run by governing bodies and similar to the United Network for Organ Sharing (UNOS) in the United States.

Irrespective of the specifics of each organ allocation system, all are influenced by geography. Because of the constraints of ischemic time, prioritizing local allocation of organs is a universal practice.[39] Indeed, even in our proposed model, the arbitrary geographic cutoff point of a 500-mile radius would still influence waiting list outcomes. Accordingly, more studies with country-specific data are required to determine the extent of geographic impact on waiting list outcomes, with the ultimate goal of developing new policies to minimize that impact.

CONCLUSION

Since implementation of the LAS, favorable trends in transplantation outcomes have been observed. Waiting list times and mortality have improved, and transplantation is being performed on sicker patients without affecting post-transplant survival. However, there is increasing evidence that the locally based allocation system is impeding the full beneficial potential of the LAS. Lungs are frequently being allocated to low-priority candidates while appropriately matched, high-priority regional candidates are being bypassed. To maximize the societal benefit of organ donation, we support the implementation of a lung allocation strategy that minimizes the effects of geography similarly to the strategy used for heart transplant patients.

REFERENCES

1. Committee on Organ Procurement and Transplantation Policy, Division of Health Sciences Policy, Institute of Medicine. Organ Procurement and Transplantation: Assessing Current Policies and the Potential Impact of the DHHS Final Rule. Washington, DC: National Academy Press; 1999.
2. Russo MJ, Worku B, Iribarne A, et al. Does lung allocation score maximize survival benefit from lung transplantation? J Thorac Cardiovasc Surg 2011;141:1270-1277.
3. Egan TM, Murray S, Bustami RT, et al. Development of the new lung allocation system in the United States. Am J Transplant 2006;6:1212-1227.
4. Pierson RN, Barr ML, McCullough KP, et al. Thoracic organ transplantation. Am J Transplant 2004;4(Suppl 9):93-105.
5. Travaline JM, Cordova FC, Furukawa S, Criner GJ. Discrepancy between severity of lung impairment and seniority on the lung transplantation list. Transplant Proc 2004;36:3156-3160.
6. Orens JB, Shearon TH, Freudenberger RS, et al. Thoracic organ transplantation in the United States, 1995-2004. Am J Transplant 2006;6:1188-1197.
7. Egan TM, Kotloff RM. Pro/Con debate: Lung allocation should be based on medical urgency and transplant survival and not on waiting time. Chest 2005;128:407-415.
8. Davis SQ, Garrity ER Jr. Organ allocation in lung transplant. Chest 2007;132:1646-1651.
9. Kozower BD, Meyers BF, Smith MA, et al. The impact of the lung allocation score on short-term transplantation outcomes: A multicenter study. J Thorac Cardiovasc Surg 2008;135:166-171.
10. United Network for Organ Sharing. A Guide to Calculating the Lung Allocation Score. http://www.unos.org/docs/lung_allocation_score.pdf. Accessed June 12, 2014.
11. Iribarne A, Russo MJ, Davies RR, et al. Despite decreased wait-list times for lung transplantation, lung allocation scores continue to increase. Chest 2009;135:923-928.
12. Osaki S, Maloney JD, Meyer KC, et al. The impact of the lung allocation scoring system at the single national Veterans Affairs hospital lung transplantation program. Eur J Cardiothorac Surg 2009;36:497-501.
13. Merlo CA, Weiss ES, Orens JB, et al. Impact of U.S. lung allocation score on survival after lung transplantation. J Heart Lung Transplant 2009;28:769-775.
14. Gries CJ, Mulligan MS, Edelman JD, et al. Lung allocation score for lung transplantation: Impact on disease severity and survival. Chest 2007;132:1954-1961.
15. Arnaoutakis GJ, Allen JG, Merlo CA, et al. Impact of the lung allocation score on resource utilization after lung transplantation in the United States. J Heart Lung Transplant 2011;30:14-21.
16. Department of Health and Human Services. Organ Procurement and Transplantation Network: Final Rule. Federal Register 1999. http://www.gpo.gov/fdsys/pkg/FR-1999-10-20/html/99-27456.htm. Accessed June 12, 2014.
17. Gibbons RD, Meltzer D, Duan N. Waiting for organ transplantation. Institute of Medicine Committee on Organ Transplantation. Science 2000;287:237-238.
18. Russo MJ, Meltzer D, Merlo A, et al. Local allocation of lung donors results in transplanting lungs in lower priority transplant recipients. Ann Thorac Surg 2013;95:1231-1234; discussion 1234-1235.
19. Russo MJ, Iribarne A, Hong KN, et al. High lung allocation score is associated with increased morbidity and mortality following transplantation. Chest 20101;137:651-657.
20. Iribarne A, Sonett JR, Easterwood R, et al. Distribution of donor lungs in the United States: A case for broader geographic sharing. Paper presented at the 2011 Annual Meeting of the Western Thoracic Surgical Association, April 1, 2011. Boulder, CO. http://www.westernthoracic.org/Abstracts/2011/CF16.cgi.
21. Washburn K, Harper A, Klintmalm G, et al. Regional sharing for adult status 1 candidates: Reduction in waitlist mortality. Liver Transpl 2006;12:470-474.
22. Kolata G. Acrimony at hearing on revising rules for liver transplants. *The New York Times*. December 11, 1996. http://www.nytimes.com/1996/12/11/us/acrimony-at-hearing-on-revising-rules-for-liver-transplants.html. Accessed June 23, 2014.
23. Stolberg SG. US urges new rule on sharing donated organs. *The New York Times*. June 3, 1998http://www.nytimes.com/1998/06/03/us/us-urges-new-rule-on-sharing-donated-organs.html. Accessed June 23, 2014.
24. Axelrod DA, Gheorghian A, Schnitzler MA, et al. The economic implications of broader sharing of liver allografts. Am J Transplant 2011;11:798-807.
25. Gentry SE, Chow EK, Wickliffe CE, et al. Impact of broader sharing on transport time for deceased donor livers. Liver Transpl 2014;20:1237-1243.
26. Hicks M, Hing A, Gao L, et al. Organ preservation. Methods Mol Biol 2006;333:331-374.
27. Organ procurement and transplantation: Assessing current policies and the potential impact of the DHHS final rule. http://www.nap.edu/openbook.php?isbn=030906578X. Accessed June 12, 2014.
28. Davis AE, Mehrotra S, Kilambi V, et al. The effect of the statewide sharing variance on geographic disparity in kidney transplantation in the United States. Clin J Am Soc Nephrol 2014;9:1449-1460.

29. Volk ML, Choi H, Warren GJW, et al. Geographic variation in organ availability is responsible for disparities in liver transplantation between Hispanics and Caucasians. Am J Transplant 2009;9:2113-2118.

30. Gibbons RD, Duan N, Meltzer D, et al. Waiting for organ transplantation: Results of an analysis by an Institute of Medicine committee. Biostatistics 2003;4:207-222.

31. Egan TM. Ethical issues in thoracic organ distribution for transplant. Am J Transplant 2003;3:366-372.

32. Kirk AD, Knechtle SJ, Larsen CP, et al. Textbook of Organ Transplantation. New York: John Wiley & Sons; 2014.

33. Smits JMA, Vanhaecke J, Haverich A, et al. Waiting for a thoracic transplant in Eurotransplant. Transpl Int 2006;19:54-66.

34. Verleden GM, Massard G, Fisher AJ. European Respiratory Monograph 45: Lung Transplantation. Sheffields, UK: European Respiratory Society Journals, 2009.

35. Kneidinger N, Winter H, Sisic A, et al. Munich Lung Transplant Group: Waiting list during the first 9 months of the lung allocation score era. Thorac Cardiovasc Surg 2014;62:422-426.

36. Gottlieb J, Greer M, Sommerwerck U, et al. Introduction of the lung allocation score in Germany. Am J Transplant 2014;14:1318-1327.

37. Eurotransplant International Foundation. Lung Allocation Score (LAS). 2014. https://www.eurotransplant.org/cms/index.php?page=las.

38. Kotsimbos T, Williams TJ, Anderson GP. Update on lung transplantation: Programmes, patients and prospects. Eur Respir Rev 2012;21:271-305.

39. Berrabah NG. Création d'un service national d'attribution d'organes: Une contribution au débat du point de vue médical sur l'article 18 du projet de loi sur la transplantation d'organes. Laussane, Switzerland: IEMS Institut d'économie et management de la santé UNIL; 2003.

7

Donor selection and management

JOSEPH COSTA, FRANK D'OVIDIO, AND JOSHUA R. SONETT

INTRODUCTION

Lung transplantation has continued to evolve at a rapid pace since Dr. James Hardy performed the first human lung transplant in Jackson, Mississippi, in 1963. In the subsequent 10 years, 36 lung transplants were performed worldwide with catastrophic failures that usually occurred within a few days following transplantation. In 1981, Dr. Norman Shumway and colleagues successfully performed three heart-lung transplants at Stanford University Hospital; two of the three recipients were alive and well 1 year after transplantation. In 1983, the Toronto group performed the first successful single-lung transplant, and in 1986 they reported their experience and stated that the recipient was leading a normal lifestyle with no limitations.

The number of lung transplants has continued to grow at a steady pace; nevertheless, the disparity between the number of patients waiting for transplants and the number of suitable lung allografts available has continued. According to the Organ Procurement and Transplantation Network (OPTN) Web site (www.OPTN.org), of the 78,929 candidates on the active waiting list for some type of transplant as of August 2014, 1653 were wait-listed for a lung transplant in the United States. Over the past 6 years 9223 lung transplants were performed (Table 7.1); however, 1172 (12.7%) candidates died while waiting for suitable allografts.[1] Advances in donor selection, donor management, and surgical techniques have contributed to improving the 1-year survival rate, which currently exceeds 81% worldwide[2] as opposed to approximately 45% in the 1980s.[3] Continued development of organ donor management strategies may increase the number of suitable lung allografts available for transplantation, which is key to the future of helping patients with end-stage lung failure.[4-9]

After the donor's family has given formal consent for organ donation, appropriate management of the donor is critical to keeping organs viable until the explantation operation takes place. Standardization of donor management practices has been introduced to help bridge inconsistencies in care and potentially optimize the number of suitable organ donors.

The United Network for Organ Sharing (UNOS) developed a critical pathway for the organ donor (Figure 7.1) as a clinical management "blueprint" for systematic care of potential donors. The critical pathway promotes uniform collaboration in interaction between organ procurement coordinators and critical care staff at the donor hospital and delineates specific roles and responsibilities to prevent duplication of effort and confusion.

As soon as a patient has been identified as a potential organ donor, a referral should be initiated by contacting the local organ procurement organization (OPO) and the critical pathway implemented. This initial event is critical and often dictates whether the opportunity for donation goes forth or is lost entirely. Most referrals of patients who may be potential organ donors to OPOs are from critical care or intensive care units.[10] Several studies have shown the importance of emergency departments (EDs) as an underused source of potential donors. These studies have found that patients coming to EDs are commonly not identified as potential organ donors. Miller and colleagues reported that patients referred from EDs have donated a greater number

Table 7.1 Lung transplants versus deaths of candidates awaiting transplantation

Year	2009	2010	2011	2012	2013	2014
Deaths	267	234	240	225	173	33
Transplants	1660	1769	1822	1754	1923	295
Percentage	16.1	13.2	13.2	12.8	9.0	11.2

Source: Based on data from UNOS Scientific Registry. http://www.OPTN.org. Accessed May 19, 2014.

Critical pathway for the organ donor

Patient name: _____

ID number: _____

Collaborative practice	Phase I Referral	Phase II Declaration of brain death and consent	Phase III Donor evaluation	Phase IV Donor management	Phase V Recovery phase

The following professionals may be involved to enhance the donation process.
 	
Check all that apply.
○ Physician
○ Critical care RN
○ Organ Procurement Organization (OPO)
○ OPO Coordinator (OPC)
○ Medical Examiner (ME)/ Coroner
○ Respiratory
○ Laboratory
○ Pharmacy
○ Radiology
○ Anesthesiology
○ OR/Surgery staff
○ Clergy
○ Social worker
	○ Notify physician regarding OPO referral
	○ Contact OPO ref: Potential donor with severe brain insult
	○ OPC on site and begins evaluation Time ____ Date ____
	○ Ht ____ Wt ____ as documented
	○ ABO as documented ____
	○ Notify house supervisor/ charge nurse of presence of OPC on unit
		○ Brain death documented Time ____ Date ____
		○ Pt accepted as potential donor
		○ MD notifies family of death
		○ Plan family approach with OPC
		○ Offer support services to family (clergy, etc)
		○ OPC/Hospital staff talks to family about donation
		○ Family accepts donation
		○ OPC obtains signed consent & medical/social history Time ____ Date ____
		○ ME/Coroner notified
		○ ME/Coroner releases body for donation
		○ *Family/ME/Coroner denies donation—stop pathway— initiate post-mortem protocol—support family.*
			○ Obtain pre/post transfusion blood for serology testing (HIV, hepatitis, VDRL, CMV)
			○ Obtain lymph nodes and/ or blood for tissue typing
			○ Notify OR & anesthesiology of pending donation
			○ Notify house supervisor of pending donation
			○ Chest & abdominal circumference
			○ Lung measurements per CXR by OPC
			○ *Cardiology consult as requested by OPC (see reverse side)*
			○ *Donor organs unsuitable for transplant—stop path- way—initiate post-mortem protocol—support family.*
				○ OPC writes new orders
				○ Organ placement
				○ OPC sets tentative OR time
				○ Insert arterial line/2 large- bore IVs
				○ Possibly insert CVP/Pulmonary artery catheter
				○ See reverse side
					○ Checklist for OR
					○ Supplies given to OR
					○ Prepare patient for transport to OR
					  ○ IVs ○ Pumps
					  ○ O₂ ○ Ambu
					  ○ Peep valve
					○ Transport to OR Date ____ Time ____
					○ OR nurse
					  ○ reviews consent form
					  ○ reviews brain death documentation
					  ○ checks patient's ID band

Labs/Diagnostics		○ Review previous lab results ○ Review previous hemody- namics	○ Blood chemistry ○ CBC + diff ○ UA ○ C & S ○ PT, PTT ○ ABO ○ A Subtype ○ Liver function tests ○ Blood culture X 2 / 15 minutes to 1 hour apart ○ Sputum Gram stain & C & S ○ Type & Cross Match ____ # units PRBCs ○ CXR ○ ABGs ○ EKG ○ Echo ○ Consider cardiac cath ○ Consider bronchoscopy	○ Determine need for additional lab testing ○ CXR after line placement (if done) ○ Serum electrolytes ○ H & H after PRBC Rx ○ PT, PTT ○ BUN, serum creatinine after correcting fluid deficit ○ Notify OPC for ____ PT > 14 ____ PTT < 28 ____ Urine output ____ < 1 mL/Kg/hr ____ > 3 mL/Kg/hr ____ Hct < 30 / Hgb > 10 ____ Na > 150 mEq/L	○ Labs drawn in OR as per surgeon or OPC request ○ Communicate with pathology: Bx liver and/ or kidneys as indicated
Respiratory	○ Pt on ventilator ○ Suction q 2 hr ○ Reposition q 2 hr	○ Prep for apnea testing: set FiO₂ @ 100% and anticipate need to decrease rate if PCO₂ < 45 mm Hg	○ Maximize ventilator settings to achieve SaO₂ 98 – 99% ○ PEEP = 5 cm O₂ challenge for lung placement FiO₂ @ 100%, PEEP @ 5 X 10 min ○ ABGs as ordered ○ VS q 1°	○ Notify OPC for ____ BP < 90 systolic ____ HR < 70 or > 120 ____ CVP < 4 or > 11 ____ PaO₂ < 90 or ____ SaO₂ < 95%	○ Portable O₂ @ 100% FiO₂ for transport to OR ○ Ambu bag and PEEP valve ○ Move to OR
Treatments/ Ongoing care		○ Use warming/cooling blanket to maintain temperature at 36.5° C - 37.5 °C ○ NG to low intermittent suction	○ Check NG placement & output ○ Obtain actual Ht ____ & Wt ____ if not previ- ously obtained		○ Set OR temp as directed by OPC ○ Post-mortem care at conclusion of case
Medications			○ Medication as requested by OPC	○ Fluid resuscitation— consider crystolloids, colloids, blood products ○ DC meds except pressors & antibiotics ○ Broad-spectrum antibiotic if not previously ordered ○ Vasopressor support to maintain BP > 90 mm Hg systolic ○ Electrolyte imbalance: consider K, Ca, PO₄, Mg replacement ○ Hyperglycemia: consider insulin drip ○ Oliguria: consider diuretics ○ Diabetes insipidus: consider antidiuretics ○ Paralytic as indicated for spinal reflexes	○ DC antidiuretics ○ Diuretics as needed ○ 350 U heparin/kg or as directed by surgeon
Optimal outcomes	The potential donor is identified & a referral is made to the OPO.	The family is offered the option of donation & their decision is supported.	The donor is evaluated & found to be a suitable candidate for donation.	Optimal organ function is maintained.	All potentially suitable, consented organs are recovered for transplant.

Shaded areas indicate Organ Procurement Coordinator (OPC) activities.

This Critical Pathway was developed under contract with the U.S. Department of Health and Human Services, Health Resources and Services Administration, Division of Transplantation.

Figure 7.1 Critical pathway.

of organs for transplantation per donor than did patients who had been referred from intensive care units, thus highlighting the need to educate ED staff on the importance of organ donor referral.[11]

DONOR SELECTION

Size and sex

Donor-recipient size matching remains an important factor when considering suitable lung allografts and transplantation outcomes. In the United States, potential recipients are listed for a transplant on the basis of acceptable donor height ranges. As a general rule, a donor can be considered without undue worry for a recipient who is 4 inches taller or shorter that the donor. If using this crude rule, one must then make allowance for sex differences, disease-specific modifications of the chest wall, and finally age and quality of the donor lung. Oversizing a donor lung is eminently safer with particularly compliant lungs. Finally, the use of donor lung volume reduction—even selective lobar donation—makes the use of larger donor lungs very possible in many circumstances. With regard to undersized lungs, it is clear that even without taking modified chest walls into account, one can safely use a lung with a volume 20% less than that of the recipient's native lung.

Concerns related to size mismatching have included transplantation of a small donor lung allograft into a large recipient, thus leading to ongoing space management, persistent pneumothorax, hyperexpansion of the lung, and hemodynamic compromise with limited exercise tolerance.[12] Transplantation of large donor lung allografts into smaller recipients may lead to persistent atelectasis and lobar infections. Commonly, the general preference is toward undersizing in recipients with fibrotic lung disease and oversizing in recipients with chronic obstructive pulmonary disease (COPD). In recipients with pulmonary fibrosis, the chest wall shrinks as a result of significant contraction of the intercostal muscles, thereby causing rib crowding. In contrast, patients with COPD who are awaiting transplantation have an increase in the size of their chest cavity along with widening of the intercostal spaces and flattening of the diaphragm.

The literature includes descriptions of excellent results obtained by using oversized lung allografts and performing size reduction by peripheral segmental resection or lobectomy because of a donor-recipient size mismatch.[13,14] Typically, small size discrepancies can be overcome by stapler resection of peripheral lung segments. When size discrepancies are more pronounced, the right middle lobe is often preferentially resected, whereas on the left side, the lingua is the primary target for downsizing. This technique allows a size reduction of approximately 10% to 15%, thereby reducing the graft's size not only in height but also in its anterior-posterior diameter because the upper lobe rotates toward the lower lobe.[13,14]

Donor age

It is well known that lung function generally deteriorates with advancing age. The specific age-related functional changes that occur in the respiratory system are the result of three physiologic events: progressive decreases in compliance of the thorax, static elastic recoil of the lung, and strength of the respiratory muscles.[15] As reductions in chest wall compliance occur with advancing age, compliance of the respiratory system is 20% less in a 60-year-old than in a 20-year-old.[16] With advancing age, notable homogeneous enlargement of the alveolar duct occurs, with the alveolar ducts increasing in diameter and consequently becoming wider and shallower. The elastic fibers of the lung are reduced, thereby resulting in relaxed recoil pressure, which in turn causes distention of the alveolar spaces and increased lung volume.[16] As described by Turner and colleagues, in subjects 20 to 60 years of age, static elastic recoil pressure of the lung decreases as a part of normal aging (0.1 to 0.2 cm H_2O/yr), and the static pressure-volume curve for the lung is shifted to the left and has a steeper slope.[17] Expiratory flow rates show characteristic changes in the flow-volume curves, thus suggesting increased collapsibility of the peripheral airways; however, gas exchange is remarkably well preserved despite the reduced alveolar surface area and increased ventilation-perfusion heterogeneity.[18] These normal changes should not by themselves rule out the use of older lungs, but understanding such changes is still critical when assessing lungs.

Although current lung donor criteria place the age cutoff for suitable lung allografts at younger than 55 years, liberalization of the current donor criteria has resulted in the use of lung allografts from donors as old as 70 with outcomes comparable to those when lung allografts from younger donors are used. Some transplant centers have not reported any association between donor age and outcomes, whereas others have reported decreased long term survival and an increased incidence of bronchiolitis obliterans syndrome (BOS) when lungs from donors older than 55 years are used. De Perrot and associates reported the outcomes of 467 lung transplant recipients, 60 (13%) of whom received lung allografts from donors between the ages of 60 and 77 years, with a median follow-up of 25 months (range = 0 to 136 months); survival rates at 5 and 10 years were significantly decreased in the recipients who received these older lung allografts, and their rates of BOS, which was the most common cause of death in the group younger than 60, were nearly twice as high as those of the reference population, representing the most common cause of death in the group age older than 60.[18]

A retrospective study of the UNOS database conducted by Bittle and colleagues reviewed 10,666 lung transplants performed in the period from 2000 to 2010; they concluded that the use of donors aged 55 to 64 years resulted in outcomes similar to those observed with the use of donors meeting the conventional criterion of age younger than 55 years. Moreover, donor age was not associated with any differences in cause of death, rate of BOS, or time to the development of BOS. The authors did however conclude that the use of donors older than 65 years was associated with decreased immediate-term survival, although no risk for BOS in this group was discovered.[19]

Tobacco history

Given the well-documented adverse effects of smoking on lung allografts, including postoperative pulmonary complications, occult malignancies, decreased pulmonary function, permeability changes, airflow obstruction, parenchymal loss, and increased infection as a result of decreased mucociliary clearance, the threshold value of donor smoking history at which the risk to the recipient is such that it compromises benefit remains unclear. Current International Society for Heart and Lung Transplantation (ISHLT) guidelines recommend using donors with a smoking history of less than 20 pack-years.[20] However, the scarcity of lung allografts suitable for transplantation and the associated high waiting list mortality[21,22] have led to increased efforts to expand the current criteria for donor acceptability and use lung allografts from marginal donors whose lungs were once considered unsuitable for transplantation.

Bonser and colleagues examined the United Kingdom Transplant Registry. The study, which is the largest study examining the use of lung allografts from donors with a smoking history, was limited by their analysis given the inability to quantify donor pack-year smoking history, which is commonly used to evaluate smoking risk. They demonstrated that the use of lung allografts from donors with a smoking history resulted in worse outcomes than when allografts from nonsmoking donors were used; however, survival of patients with allografts from smoking donors remained better than that of patients who remained on the waiting list.[20] The increased mortality seen in recipients of lung allografts from donors with a greater than 20-pack-year smoking history may be due to an increased incidence of primary graft dysfunction.[23-25] Shigemura and colleagues conducted a retrospective review of 532 consecutive lung transplants; 293 (55%) of the donors had a history of smoking and 239 were nonsmokers. The authors' principal findings showed that lungs from donors with no smoking history did not yield better long-term outcomes after transplantation than did lungs from donors who smoked. Lung allografts from donors with a greater than 20-pack-year smoking history had a higher incidence of grade 3 primary graft dysfunction requiring extracorporeal membrane oxygenation support, earlier mortality, and decreased survival at 5 years after transplantation.[23]

Other studies, such as those of Berman and colleagues[26] and Taghavi and associates,[27] have suggested that double-lung transplantation using lung allografts from donors with a greater than 20-pack-year smoking history results in survival similar to that when lung allografts from nonsmokers or those with a less than 20-pack-year smoking history are used. Taghavi and colleagues examined the UNOS database for adult single-lung transplants performed from 2005 to 2011. The authors concluded that single-lung transplant recipients with lung allografts from donors having a greater than 20-year-pack history of smoking had longer intensive care unit and hospital lengths of stay, which is consistent with other studies.[26,27] Interestingly, Taghavi and colleagues noted that lungs received from donors who had a smoking history of greater than 20 pack-years but were not actively smoking at the time of donation did not convey an increased mortality risk.[27] In contrast, the results of a multivariate analysis by Shigemura and colleagues revealed different risk factors for death that contributed to the differences in mortality after lung transplantation between the donor cohorts of smokers and nonsmokers.[23]

Smokers are three to five times more likely than nonsmokers for lung cancer to develop in their lifetime.[28] Transplanted lung allografts explanted from donors with a history of smoking pose the risk of development of cancer in recipients or transplantation of occult lung cancer. The literature includes case reports describing the development of donor-acquired small cell cancer in transplant recipients.[29] Previous studies have failed to demonstrate a link between lung donors with a history of smoking and the development of lung malignancy in transplant recipients.[30,31] Given the limited studies looking at the association between donor smoking history and development of lung malignancy in transplant recipients, caution should be exercised when using lung allografts procured from donors with a smoking history, given the well-established relationship between smoking, malignancy, and immunosuppression.

In view of the similar short-term and midterm survival of recipients who have undergone transplantation with lungs from donors with a smoking history of greater than 20 pack-years, these allografts should be considered on a case-by-case basis, thus allowing increased organ availability and a decrease in waiting list mortality. It is advised that a computed tomography (CT) scan of the chest be performed to screen donors with a history of smoking to rule out occult cancer. Finally and importantly, the data presented to date have quantitated only never-smokers and those with a less than or greater than 20-pack-year smoking history; because of the dangers of transplanting lungs from donors with an accumulation of significantly more than 20 pack-years, such lungs should be used with caution and recipient consent.

It has been our center's experience that donors with a history of smoking illegal chemicals, particularly crack cocaine, have lungs characterized by accelerated parenchymal destruction with resultant emphysema and bullous disease, thus making them unsuitable donors.

Cause of death

The influence of donor cause of death on allograft survival has been described in the literature. The pathophysiologic changes that occur in allografts, directly impairing their function and survival of the transplanted organs, are well known.[32,33] Although one might expect the cause of brain death to impose lung injuries of various types and acuity, studies have found no effect of donor cause of death on survival. Brain death in itself leads to a multitude of pathophysiologic changes that have been demonstrated both in animal models and in clinical investigations to greatly impair the function and survival of transplanted organs.[33]

A retrospective review of 500 consecutive lung transplants performed between July 1988 and December 1999 that was conducted by Ciccone and colleagues[34] showed equivalent early outcomes and no significant difference in long-term survival between lung allografts from donors who suffered traumatic brain injuries and those from donors with non-traumatic brain injuries. However, they noticed that lung allografts from donors with traumatic brain injury were associated with the severity of acute rejection and development of BOS in the recipients who received these allografts. Donors with traumatic brain injury have a much higher incidence of aspiration at time of injury, which increases the possibility of infection, especially when coupled with field intubation in an uncontrolled dirty environment. Wauters and associates[28] had contrasting results in their study that analyzed more than 400 consecutive donors and classified their cause of death as vascular, traumatic, or other. Their study failed to show any association between cause of donor death and outcome, survival, and freedom from BOS. Ganesh and colleagues analyzed transplant outcomes in 580 first-time lung transplant recipients who underwent single- or double-lung transplantation from July 1995 to June 2001.[32] The authors categorized mechanism of death as being due to vascular and tumor, traumatic, or hypoxic brain damage or infective causes, and 5-year mortality was studied. All traumatic donor deaths were the result of blunt trauma only. This study showed no effect of donor cause of death on survival and did not demonstrate any significant difference in early rejection episodes or incidence of BOS in the different recipient groups. Overall 5-year survival was similar to that found in a previous study by Ciccone and colleagues.[34]

In the United States, the yearly estimate of occurrences of drowning and asphyxiation is 6000 to 8000.[35,36] Many transplant centers do not routinely use lungs from donors who have drowned or been asphyxiated. Asphyxiation and drowning are thought to result in changes in lung surfactant with the potential to contribute to pulmonary graft dysfunction.[37] A retrospective analysis of the UNOS/OPTN Standard Transplant Analysis and Research (STAR) database by Whitson and colleagues evaluated the suitability of organ donors whose cause of death was asphyxiation or drowning as a potential option to enlarge the donor pool. The authors concluded that asphyxiation or drowning had no impact on survival and was not associated with poor long-term survival or rejection in the first year after transplantation.[38] With regard to other forms of lung trauma, our experience at Columbia has found no difficulties in using patients with chest tubes or tracheostomies. Concern for

significant contusions in cases of blunt trauma should be addressed by performing CT scans. Donors with large centrally located contusions are likely not to be used; however, smaller peripheral contusions should not contraindicate donation.

Brain-dead donors are at risk for the development of acute lung injury as a result of the hemodynamic, hormonal, and inflammatory changes commonly experienced during the early stages of brain death; as yet, however, no general consensus on specific cause of death influencing lung allograft function and posttransplant outcomes exists.

EVALUATION OF THE POTENTIAL DONOR

Initially, the on-site organ procurement coordinator will conduct a comprehensive medical and social history interview with the appropriate family members or next of kin. As part of the standard review process, deceased donors are screened for any history of treatment of cancer, diabetes, heart disease, and hypertension; use of drugs, alcohol, and tobacco; and high-risk behavior. During this interview the family history of the donor is also evaluated.

Events leading to the patient's admission are evaluated by reviewing emergency medical services' pre–hospital care reports and ED admission notes. Information such as mechanism of injury, chest, or abdominal trauma, and cardiopulmonary arrest and resuscitation time, along with administered and ongoing medications, is noted. Completing the required serologic and general hematologic laboratory analysis is extremely important to expedite the overall process and decrease the interval between donor management and the operative recovery phase.

Infectious agents

Given the expansion of donor criteria for lungs, increasing age in particular may present challenges given the greater potential for infection and malignancies. All potential organ donors undergo a comprehensive screening evaluation for infections that could be transmitted to recipients via transplanted allografts. This evaluation process not only includes an in-depth interview about deceased donors' medical and social history with the donors' next of kin but may also include interviews with other individuals, such as friends, who may have information regarding any risky behavior in which the deceased donors may have engaged, thereby exposing them to certain diseases.

The few absolute medical contraindications to organ donation to date are as follows:

- Infections.
  - Viral: Human immunodeficiency virus (HIV), reactive hepatitis B surface antigen, active herpes simplex, varicella zoster or cytomegalovirus (CMV) viremia, West Nile virus (WNV) encephalitis.
  - Bacterial: Tuberculosis, meningitis, gangrenous bowel or intra-abdominal sepsis.

- Fungal infections: cryptococcosis, aspergillosis, histoplasmosis, coccidiosis, active candidemia.
- Prion: Creutzfeldt-Jakob disease.
- Parasitic infections: Chagas disease, rabies, leishmaniasis, strongyloidiasis, or malaria.
- Cancer.
  - History of cancer, except nonmelanoma skin cancer (basal cell and squamous cell), within the past 5 years.
  - Primary central nervous system (CNS) tumors without evidence of metastatic disease.
  - Any previous malignant neoplasms with current evident metastatic disease.
- History of melanoma, hematologic malignancy (leukemia, Hodgkin disease, lymphoma, multiple myeloma).

Standard serologic testing for hepatitis B virus (HBV), hepatitis C virus (HCV), HIV, human T-lymphotrophic virus (HTLV), and CMV, along with screening for treponemal antigen (syphilis), is routinely ordered during the workup of any potential donor. Unfortunately, in some cases unexpected transmission of HIV, HCV, lymphocytic choriomeningitis virus (LCVM), *Mycobacterium tuberculosis*, rabies, and WNV may potentially occur irrespective of the current screening guidelines.

Viral infections persist mainly in hepatic cells, but also in other locations such as endothelial cells,[39,40] as in the case of HBV and HCV. HBV is characterized by resolution through immune containment in 90% of cases and persistent viral replication with variable symptoms in 10%. The current population includes individuals who have asymptomatic, undiagnosed, ongoing HBV infection but die of unrelated causes and become organ donors, thus making donor serology testing an absolutely essential part of testing. A donor who is positive for an isolated hepatitis B surface antibody usually implies vaccination (Table 7.2), whereas a donor who has serology positive for hepatitis B surface antigen reflects active hepatitis B infection or a remote infection that has not cleared. The incidence of hepatitis B core antibody positivity in organ donors naturally parallels the prevalence of HBV in the general population. Therefore, the incidence of core antibody positivity in organ donors is much higher in Asia (50%) than in Europe (7% to 12%) or the United States (3%)[41]; it is becoming more of a concern given the influx of immigrants from other countries.

Table 7.3 Hepatitis C serology interpretation

Anti-HCV IgM	Anti-HCV IgG	HCV-RNA	Interpretation
+	–	+	Active acute infection
–	+	–	Remote controlled infection
–	+	+	Remote infection, chronic active
–	–	+	Remote infection, patient or donor unable to make antibody

Note: Anti-HCV IgG, IgM antibodies against hepatitis C virus antigens; Anti-HCV IgM, IgM antibodies against hepatitis C virus antigens.

HCV is a much more persistent virus, with a higher rate of transmission than that of HBV. Any potential organ donor with a positive serologic test for hepatitis C antibody should be considered infectious and unsuitable for lung donation in view of the virus's high rate of transmission. The literature suggests the rate of transmission of HCV to be between 25% and 100%.[42,43] HCV serology testing is traditionally based on antibody testing (Table 7.3); however, false-negative antibody results do occur, and HCV RNA nucleic acid amplification testing is more reliable.

A donor with a positive screening result does not necessarily rule out organ donation. In cases in which the recipient is HCV positive, reserving organs from donors who are also HCV positive makes it possible for organs from HCV-positive donors to be used. When HCV-positive donor livers are transplanted into HCV-positive recipients, no increased morbidity or mortality is evident. Comparatively speaking, an HCV-positive lung allograft may be considered for transplantation into a recipient who is not HCV positive if no alternative exists, death is imminent, and the recipient or next of kin has given appropriate informed consent to accept a high-risk donor.[44,45] Table 7.4 shows the risk for viral transmission of HBV and HCV viruses.

Cancer

The potential for cancer being transmitted from an organ donor to a recipient is a well-recognized complication of transplantation. Cancer may be transmitted to a recipient from a donor with a history of cancer but no active disease.

Table 7.2 Interpretation of hepatitis B testing

HBsAg/IgG	Anti-HBc IgM	Anti-HBc IgG	Anti-HBsAb	Interpretation
+	–	–	–	Recent or active viral replication
+	+	–	–	Recent or active viral replication
–	+	–	–	"Window" phase, recent infection
–	–	+	+/–	Natural infection resolved
–	–	–	+	Vaccine immune response

Note: Anti-HBc IgG, IgG antibody against hepatitis B core antigen; Anti-HBc IgM, IgM antibody against hepatitis B core antigen; Anti-HBsAb, hepatitis B surface antibody; HBsAg/IgG, IgG antibody against hepatitis B surface antigen.

Table 7.4 Risk for viral transmission

Donor serology	HBsAb⁺ recipient	HBsAb⁻ recipient
HBsAg⁺	Liver: Insufficient data	Liver: High
	Nonliver: Insufficient data	Nonliver: High
HBcAb⁺	Liver: Low to moderate	Liver: Moderate to high
	Nonliver: Very low	Nonliver: Low
HCVAb⁺	Liver: High	Liver: High
	Nonliver: Insufficient data	Nonliver: High

Source: From Rosengard BR. Feng S, Alfrey EJ, et al. Report of the Crystal City meeting to maximize the use of organs recovered from the cadaver donor. Am J Transplant 2002;2:701-711.

Note: Data indicate that the risk for viral infection may be lower in recipients who are immune from previous HBV infection (HBsAB⁺/HBcAb⁺) than in recipients who are immune from vaccination (HBsAb⁺/ABcAb⁻); HBsAb, hepatitis B surface antibody; HBsAg, hepatitis B surface antigen; HBcAb, hepatitis B core antibody; HCVAb, hepatitis C virus antibody; HBV, hepatitis B virus.

The literature overwhelmingly supports the use of kidneys with small, solitary, well-differentiated renal cell carcinoma for transplantation, provided that the lesion has been completely resected. A search for extrarenal tumors should be conducted because approximately 7% of small tumors may demonstrate metastatic activity.[46] The literature does not currently include any high-level evidence establishing the true transmission rate of donor-related malignancies to the recipient after transplantation. Currently, the OPTN collects and maintains the most robust published data on donor-derived disease transmission via organ transplantation globally.[47] Data collection began in 2005, and since then the data have shown an increase in the number of cases of disease from 7 reports in 2005 to 152 reports in 2009. This increase probably reflects not a true increase in the number of cases but rather an underreporting of cases.[48] A summary by Ison and Nalesnik[48] of potential donor-derived malignancy transmission reported between 2005 and 2009 (Table 7.5) showed that of 146 submitted reports, 20 involved confirmed cases of donor-derived malignancy transmission with 9 deaths attributed to the following: lung cancer (3), lymphoma (2), neuroendocrine carcinoma (2), melanoma (1), and glioblastoma multiforme (1). The cause of brain death must be considered when it comes to potential occult malignancy, especially in donors with unclear causes of intracranial hemorrhage. There is always the possibility of malignant transmission resulting from misdiagnosis of the cause of the donor's brain death.

In some instances donors with a medical history of certain types of cancer may still donate their organs for transplantation; this includes certain types of primary CNS tumors. Donors with high-grade CNS tumors such as

Table 7.5 Potential donor-derived malignancy transmissions reported to the OPTN, 2005-2009

Malignancy	No. donor reports[a]	No. recipients with confirmed transmission[b]	No. recipient deaths attributable to donor-derived malignancy[c]
Renal cell carcinoma	64	7	1[d]
Lung cancer	12	4	3
Lymphoma	8	6	2
Thyroid carcinoma	7	0	0
Glioblastoma multiforme	7	1	1
Prostate	5	0	0
Liver cancer	3	1	0
Melanoma	5	2	1
Pancreatic cancer	2	3	0
Neuroendocrine cancer	4	2	2
Ovarian carcinoma	2	2	0
Other[e]	26	0	0
Total malignancies	145	28	10

Source: From Ison MG, Nalesnik MA. An update on donor-derived disease transmission in organ transplantation. Am J Transplant 2011;11:1123-1130.

[a] Each report reflects a single donor but may involve multiple recipients.

[b] Number of recipients with a confirmed malignancy transmission; transmission classified by the disease transmission advisory committee (DTAC) as either proven, probable, or possible.

[c] Number of recipients with a confirmed malignancy transmission who died directly as the result of the transmitted malignancy.

[d] One patient with probable or proven disease expired; final tumor assessment pending.

[e] Other reported malignancies without confirmed transmission: astrocytoma, breast (3), colon cancer (2), dermatofibrosarcoma protuberans, Kaposi sarcoma, leukemia (chronic lymphocytic leukemia), medulloblastoma, myeloid sarcoma, pineoblastoma, liposarcoma, gastrointestinal stromal tumor, spindle cell carcinoma, carcinoma not otherwise specified (4), and urothelial carcinoma.

astrocytoma or medulloblastoma or previous craniotomy with ventriculoperitoneal or ventriculoatrial shunts have a very high rate of transmission and should not be considered for organ donation.[49] Lung allografts from donors with a history of nonmelanoma skin cancer, as well as certain CNS tumors, may still be used if the cancers are low grade and no biopsy or shunt operation has been performed.

A history of cancer does not automatically exclude an individual from organ donation. A low incidence of transmission of malignant disease from organ donors to patients awaiting a transplant is still feasible provided that a thorough assessment is performed, a detailed history of the donor is available, and informed consent is obtained from the recipient after he or she has been made aware of the donor's history and the potential for transmission if the transplant is performed.

DONOR MANAGEMENT

Donor management begins by using strategies aimed at limiting the amount of damage that lung allografts may sustain as a result of the physiologic disarray common during brain death. Such limitation is possible only when physicians are well versed in the pathophysiology of brain death and, accordingly, perform rational maneuvers to minimize lung injury. Successful organ transplantation is directly dependent on donor management strategies. The period during and shortly after brain death is critical, and potential donors will manifest profound metabolic and hemodynamic instability that often results in the loss of already scarce organs for transplantation. Even with aggressive donor management strategies, only approximately 15% to 20% of lung allografts are suitable for transplantation.[50]

Brain death

The vast majority of organs for transplantation come from patients who have progressed to brain death. Brain death is well known for its significant and detrimental effects on organ systems—in particular, for causing lung injury. Implementing early aggressive donor management once brain death has been determined is important for maximizing the yield of lungs from multiorgan donors and improving recipient outcomes. Specifically, the aim of implementing early aggressive donor management is to minimize the incidence of donor lung injury and prevent its escalation.

Establishing brain death is often a daunting task for physicians; it requires not only speed but also accuracy in patient assessment to provide clear-cut evidence of brain death to family members and to determine what the care plan will include. The diagnosis of brain death involves three distinct findings: apnea, absence of brainstem reflexes, and irreversible and unresponsive coma. The two main tests required to conclusively declare a patient brain-dead are an assessment of brainstem reflexes and an apnea test.

Evidence indicates that during the brain death cascade, the lung is the first organ to incur injury.[51] Clinical

Table 7.6 Physiologic changes associated with brain death

Hematologic
  Coagulopathy
    Disseminated intravascular coagulopathy
    Factor and platelet dilution
Endocrine and metabolic
  Decreased aerobic metabolism (early phase)
  Increased anaerobic metabolism (late phase)
  Decreased circulating pituitary hormones
    Diabetes insipidus ($\downarrow$ ADH)
  Electrolyte disturbances
    Hypernatremia ($\downarrow$ ADH)
    Hyperglycemia ($\downarrow$ insulin levels)
    Hypocalcemia
    Hypophosphatemia
    Hypomagnesemia
    Hypokalemia
Cardiopulmonary
  Pulmonary edema (neurogenic)
  Increased pulmonary artery pressure (secondary to systemic vasoconstriction)
  Myocardial ischemia
  Reduced myocardial contractility ($\downarrow$ T_3 and cortisol)
  Cardiac arrest
  Arrhythmias
  Tachycardia (early phase)
  Bradycardia (late phase)
  Hypertension (early phase)
  Hypotension (late phase)

Source: From Faropoulos K, Apostolakis E. Brain death and its influence on the lungs of the donor: How is it prevented? Transplant Proc 2009;41:4114-4119.
Note: ADH, antidiuretic hormone; T_3, triiodothyronine.

and experimental studies have demonstrated the cataclysmic sympathetic discharge commonly associated with brain death.[52] This "autonomic storm" releases enormous amounts of catecholamines such as dopamine, epinephrine, and norepinephrine into the circulation. Table 7.6 illustrates many of the physiologic changes that occur during brain death. Having a clear understanding of the brain death cascade and how it affects lung allografts allows better appreciation of the importance of developing rapid and effective donor management strategies aimed at inhibiting these detrimental physiologic effects of brain death and increasing the number of usable lung allografts while also attempting to decrease the incidence of pulmonary graft dysfunction in recipients.

Hemodynamic management

Hemodynamic management of an organ donor is the foundation and most crucial intervention that can be delivered. It is estimated that 80% of organ donors will require vasoactive support and approximately 25% of organ donors are lost during this phase.[53] Hypovolemia is a common event, especially because of the osmotic agents administered to treat rising intracranial pressure, poorly treated diabetes insipidus, and blood loss in the case of trauma, all of which are contributing factors to hypotension. Traditional trauma and donor management includes significant fluid loading to improve hemodynamic instability, especially in trauma-related cases; however, this strategy may not be ideal for optimal organ recovery.

Restrictive fluid balance has been associated with higher rates of lung procurement[54-56] despite the controversial theory of fluid restriction affecting donor kidney function after transplantation. Minambres and colleagues demonstrated for the first time that an aggressive management strategy in potential lung donors, which includes ventilator recruitment maneuvers, positive end-expiratory pressure (PEEP) greater than 8 cm H_2O, use of hormonal replacement therapy, and restrictive fluid balanced to keep the central venous pressure (CVP) lower than 8 mmHg, results in higher lung utilization while not affecting kidney recovery and post-transplant renal function.[57] The authors' recommendation for restrictive fluid balance to keep the CVP lower than 8 mm Hg was at the higher limit recommended by the Crystal City conference[45] and the Spanish consensus document on donor lung management,[58] which recommended keeping the CVP between 6 and 8 mm Hg. When it comes to fluid resuscitation, the goal is to establish euvolemia rather than hypervolemia, which coupled with neurogenic pulmonary edema, can have grave effects on lung allografts, thereby directly affecting oxygenation. The goal of hemodynamic management should be to maintain an adequate volume, proper cardiac output, and suitable perfusion, hence ensuring optimal oxygen delivery to organs being evaluated for transplantation.

The use of hormone replacement therapy (HRT) has become accepted as the standard of care and has resulted in increased use of both cardiac and lung grafts, although not all centers are convinced of its absolute benefit.[56, 59-62] Arginine vasopressin has been shown to impart several favorable hemodynamic effects.[60,63,64] Vasopressin stabilizes systemic blood pressure, corrects serum hyperosmolarity, improves maintenance of energy metabolism in solid organs, and decreases or eliminates the need for catecholamines.[65,66] Commonly, vasopressin is administered initially as a bolus of 5 units, followed by a maintenance infusion of 0.5 to 4 U/hr, thus keeping systemic vascular resistance between 800 and 1200 dynes/sec/cm[5]. Vasopressin supplementation commonly begins with dopamine, low doses of which will result in increased renal perfusion and subsequent increased urine output, thereby reducing lung edema in brain-dead donors.

Hemodynamic instability has been suggested because of the significantly decreased levels of circulating thyroxine, which in turn leads to reduced myocardial energy stores and a shift from aerobic to less efficient anaerobic metabolism, thus resulting in increased lactate levels. Triiodothyronine (T_3), which is commonly used in brain-dead donors, has

been shown to improve donor heart function.[65,66] T_3 is generally administered as an initial bolus of 4 µg, followed by an infusion at a rate of 3 µg/hr. Reduced left atrial pressure and improved overall cardiac function may limit lung edema; in addition, T_3 increases alveolar fluid clearance. The use of thyroid hormone therapy is not without debate. Several studies have shown no correlation between hemodynamic instability and decreased levels of thyroid hormones.

Given the ongoing shortage of suitable donor organs, routine use of HRT is important and should be initiated without delay in any potential organ donor. Withholding HRT in an unstable potential organ donor with a catastrophic brain injury will allow hemodynamic instability to take its toll, as a result of which potentially suitable organs may no longer be adequate for transplantation.

Pulmonary management

Brain-dead donors should have their heads raised between 35 and 45 degrees and a nasogastric tube placed to prevent any possibility of silent aspiration. All potential lung donors should have a baseline chest radiograph, although it has been shown to be somewhat unreliable in the definitive diagnosis of pneumonia. Chest radiograph findings show a predictive accuracy of only 50% to 60% for pneumonia and 60% to 80% for pulmonary edema.[67] CT of the chest, though not routinely performed on donors, is a more precise technique for imaging the chest in that it offers greater accuracy and consistency when it comes to findings of pneumonia, contusions, and lesions that are often missed on routine chest radiography. Donors with a history of greater than 20 pack-years of smoking should have a baseline CT of the chest done as part of the process of evaluating lung allografts for transplantation.

Smoking history, along with the results of sputum Gram stains and ongoing arterial blood gas (ABG) tests, should be made available to all transplant centers considering lungs for transplantation. A bronchoscopic examination is performed to assess the quality of the airways (hyperemia) and look for evidence of aspiration, foreign bodies, and blood and secretions (mucoid, purulent, bloody); it also allows direct collection of secretions for Gram stain and culture. Noting whether secretions reaccumulate is important because this may indicate an ongoing process such as pneumonia. Thoracic teams should emphasize to the OPO on site that pediatric bronchoscopy is not suitable for the management of copious, thick, tenacious secretions. A bronchoscopic examination should be performed as close as possible to the time when organs are being allocated. Procuring teams should always perform their own bronchoscopic evaluation.

The approach to ventilator management in brain-dead donors is variable, with some centers using volume control and others pressure control ventilation with or without the use of PEEP. A protective ventilator strategy consists of low tidal volumes (6 to 8 mL/kg) and a PEEP value less than 8 cm H_2O. High tidal volumes should be avoided or limited as much as possible because of the potential for barotrauma to the lung. High levels of PEEP are discouraged and potentially harmful because they exacerbate the donor lung injury already triggered by the systemic inflammatory response to brain death. Ideally, PEEP should be maintained at less than 8 with a peak inspiratory pressure of less than 30 cm H_2O.

Blood gases should be measured approximately every 3 hours to permit ongoing pulmonary interventions and determine trends. Minute ventilation should be adjusted to keep CO_2 and pH levels within the range for mild respiratory alkalosis. Overall, reducing ventilation frequency rather than tidal volume is better for preventing atelectatic changes in the lung. Recruitment maneuvers without barotrauma are an extremely important component of optimizing lung allografts for possible transplantation, although the optimal method is still debated.[68]

Traditionally, volume-controlled modes of mechanical ventilation have entailed using assist/control mode (A/C) or synchronized intermittent mandatory ventilation (SIMV), limiting flow during inspiration, and requiring the inspiratory flow rate and pattern to be set to complement patient demand. Aside from the detrimental effects of the cascade of events associated with brain death on lungs, alveolar injury secondary to mechanical ventilation results from shearing forces, which in turn produce alveolar stress. Epithelial and endothelial damage and augmentation of the cytokine response also occur. These effects are exacerbated by the preservation solution and by ischemia-reperfusion injury.

The use of pressure-regulated volume control (PRVC) allows automatic adjustments in inspiratory pressure in response to dynamic changes in the lung donor's mechanics. Because respiratory mechanics will change on a breath-by-breath basis in any mechanically ventilated patient, using PRVC in lung donors makes it possible to adjust target pressures to achieve the required tidal volume. Although the use of PRVC in patients has not been shown in the literature to improve clinical outcomes, achieving lower airway pressures will help offset alveolar injury in potential donors.

The arterial partial pressure of oxygen (Pao_2) remains a critical element in the assessment of donor lung function. The standard lung donor criteria in the literature recommends that the donor Pao_2 set point be 300 mm Hg or greater with a fraction of inspired oxygen (Fio_2) of 1.0 when a lung is being considered for transplantation. Although many centers would most likely no longer consider a donor with a Pao_2 less than 300 mm Hg, Zafar and colleagues questioned this standard. The authors' retrospective study examined UNOS data on 12,545 lung transplants performed between 2000 to 2009 to assess the effect of donor Pao_2 on graft survival. At the time, their study revealed that 20% of lung transplants performed in the United States over the previous decade had a Pao_2 lower than 300 mm Hg at the time of procurement. The authors concluded that using lung allografts from donors with a Pao_2 lower than 300 mm Hg did not affect early or midterm graft survival in double-lung transplants. Although the authors suggested that donor Pao_2 does not appear to affect pulmonary graft survival, this result may provide another avenue to decrease the disparities between suitable lung allografts and patients awaiting a transplant.[68]

Although the standard donor criteria suggest a Pao_2 higher than 300 mm Hg as a suitable criterion, "challenge gases" with an Fio_2 of 100% following pulmonary recruitment may not accurately represent the true quality of the lungs. Often, when other values, such as those from radiographic studies and bronchoscopy, and trends in Pao_2 values are favorable, a donor team is sent and further evaluation can be performed by the donor surgeon, as in the case of evaluation of selective pulmonary vein gases after intraoperative recruitment procedures. Intraoperative selective pulmonary vein gas values provide corroborative support to the intraoperative findings during palpation and visual assessment of the lungs and the support bronchoscopic examination performed by the donor surgeon. Large differences in Po_2 (>100) are indicative of selective lobar injury, such as pneumonia or contusion, that may have significant postoperative consequences.

Recruitment maneuvers are sustained increases in airway pressure with the goal of opening collapsed alveolar units in the lung, after which sufficient PEEP is applied to prevent recollapse (derecruitment). Pulmonary recruitment strategies consist of different ventilator modes, such as pressure control and airway pressure release ventilation (APRV). Actual recruitment strategies vary from center to center. Typically, the preferred ventilation mode is pressure control ventilation with an inspiratory pressure of 25 cm H_2O, a PEEP value of 10 cm H_2O, and an inspiratory-to-expiratory time ratio (I/E ratio) of 1:1 delivered for 2 hours. Following this 2-hour interval, ventilation is returned to the previous settings, with the Fio_2 kept at 1.0 and the ABGs remeasured. Fio_2 may be decreased to its previous setting after the ABG measurement. A successful pulmonary recruitment strategy is defined as an improvement in the Pao_2/Fio_2 ratio (P/F ratio) to at least 300 mm Hg and improvement in the follow-up chest radiograph. APRV is a mode of ventilation that was originally developed as a lung-protective mode that allows alveolar recruitment while minimizing ventilator-induced injury. The use of APRV in potential donors may be of benefit because the release time in this mode is much shorter than the equilibrium time, thereby resulting in a residual volume of air remaining in the lungs, creating an intentional auto-PEEP, and avoiding derecruitment. Unfortunately, in patients with no respiratory drive, such as brain-dead donors or heavily sedated patients, the lack of spontaneous breathing efforts result in loss of this mode's physiologic advantages.

In the APRV mode, auto-PEEP is controlled by adjusting the vent settings that restrict expiratory flow. This procedure will provide relatively high mean airway pressure, which will prevent the derecruitment of alveoli while over time continuing recruitment of additional alveolar units in the lung. With other modes of ventilation, recruitment maneuvers require changes in ventilator parameters, such as PEEP, rate, and tidal volume; once set, however, the APRV mode can serve as an ongoing recruitment strategy that allows serial oxygen challenge gas samples to be drawn and evaluated at a F_{IO_2} of 100%. The auto-PEEP encountered with APRV may suggest that lung allografts are suitable if the P/F ratio is greater than 300. Although the APRV mode is useful because of its ability to recruit collapsed alveoli and prevent derecruitment, physiologically, it is important to assess oxygen challenge gases while donors are on pressure control ventilation with a F_{IO_2} of 100%. When APRV is used in potential organ donors, expiratory time should be short enough to prevent any derecruitment of the lung and long enough to deliver a suitable tidal volume. Expiratory time should be set between 0.4 to 0.6 second with a tidal volume of 6 to 8 mL/kg.

Plateau pressure (P high) should be kept between 20 and 25 cm H_2O and not exceed 35 cm H_2O. The respiratory rate is initiated at 10 to 12 breaths per minute, and the inspiratory time (T high) is set between 4 and 6 seconds and progressively increased over time to a maximum of 10 to 15 seconds and adjusted on the basis of oxygenation. Mean airway pressure is maintained by setting high PEEP at 5 to 10 cm H_2O and low PEEP at 0 cm H_2O.

Often the auto-PEEP associated with APRV may mask the true physiologic assessment of the lung, thereby resulting in a false sense of an acceptable P/F ratio. This situation has often been the case when dramatic changes in chest radiographs and measurements of O_2 challenge gases have occurred after the APRV mode was changed to pressure control ventilation, thus resulting in the deterioration of what would have been a suitable allograft had the decision to accept a lung been made while the donor was on APRV.

Recruitment maneuvers may be repeated multiple times during the course of managing a donor, and they are typically repeated by the thoracic procurement team intraoperatively while central and selective pulmonary vein gases are evaluated. Pulmonary recruitment maneuvers should always be accompanied by aggressive pulmonary toileting, such as regular suctioning, chest physiotherapy, position changes, and elevation of the head between 30 and 45 degrees at all times.

In cases in which sputum cultures are positive, these lung allografts should not be immediately declined unless the cultures are positive for significant hospital-acquired pathogens. In cases with radiographic evidence of lobar or multilobar infiltrates along with poor challenge gas measurements and reaccumulating purulent secretions on bronchoscopy, the lung allografts may be declined outright. Bonde and colleagues did a retrospective review of 80 consecutive single- and double-lung transplants performed between 1998 and 2001 and found that of 61 donor lungs, 57 (93%) grew organisms, 46 (81%) of which were polymicrobial. The most common donor organisms were *Staphylococcus* species (61.4%), *Streptococcus* species (57.9%), *Haemophilus* species (28.1%), *Candida* (24.6%), and *Pseudomonas* species. (7%). Posttransplant pneumonia developed in 24 of the 71 recipients, with *Pseudomonas* being the most common causative agent (54.2%). Nineteen of these 24 recipients (79.2%) had received lung allografts

from a donor with positive cultures; however, the causative organism was identified in the donor cultures in only 5 of 19 cases (26.3%).[69] In the vast majority of cases, donors should receive prophylactic broad-spectrum antibiotic coverage early as part of their management protocol.

Maintaining adequate perfusion to ensure optimal organ viability is important; however, cautious repeated fluid challenges should be closely monitored to avoid volume overloading the lungs. Crystalloid and blood products may be infused to maintain a systolic blood pressure higher than 90 mm Hg; however, fluid administration should be used judiciously with the aim of maintaining the lowest central venous pressure and thereby allowing adequate urine output and perfusion pressure. Common findings of neurogenic pulmonary edema and general pulmonary edema from volume resuscitation should be treated with intermittent doses of intravenous furosemide (Lasix). Given the newest technology, ex vivo lung perfusion is an alternative assessment pathway in many cases and has been successfully used with lungs that are characterized by volume overload, thereby greatly reducing edema as a result of its hyperosmotic perfusate.

CONCLUSION

The incidence of end-stage lung disease continues to grow at a rapid pace all over the world,[70] and lung transplantation has been accepted as the only treatment option for many patients listed for a transplant. Despite the increased incidence of end-stage lung disease, the availability of suitable lungs for transplantation has not increased to meet the growing demands but has instead remained steady. In view of the fact that a large number of donors are not meeting the standard criteria for lung donation (Table 7.7), many centers are continuing to expand current donor criteria in the hope of yielding more lung allografts for transplantation.

Donor optimization increases the number of organs suitable for transplantation and improves organ function in the allografts. Initiating early and attentive management of a brain-dead donor may help optimize the potential for increased organ recovery given the growing list of patients

Table 7.7 Standard lung donor criteria

Age <55 years
Clear chest radiograph
Pao_2 >300 mm Hg (F_{IO_2} 1.0, PEEP 5 mm Hg)
History of smoking <20 pack-years
Absence of chest trauma
Absence of microbiologic endobronchial organisms
Absence of malignancy
Absence of purulent secretions or signs of endobronchial aspiration
Inconspicuous virology

Source: From Frost AE. Donor criteria and evaluation. Clin Chest Med 1997;18:231-237.

Note: PEEP, positive end-expiratory pressure.

awaiting a transplant. Organ treatment plans and protocols are designed to help direct critical care staff and OPOs in the required critical and ongoing management of potential organ donors in the hope of avoiding any sacrifice in the quality of these organs. Having an in-depth appreciation of the physiologic manifestations of brain death is imperative to formulating and adopting donor organ management strategies for optimal preservation of the quality and function of organs.

REFERENCES

1. UNOS Scientific Registry. http://www.OPTN.org. Accessed May 19, 2014.

2. Christie JD, Edwards LB, Kucheryavaya AY, et al. The Registry of the International Society of Heart and Lung Transplantation: Twenty-seventh official adult lung and heart-lung transplant report—2010. J Heart Lung Transplant 2010;29:1104-1118.

3. Grossman RF, Frost A, Zamel N, et al. Results of single-lung transplantation for bilateral pulmonary fibrosis. The Toronto Lung Transplant Group. New Engl J Med 1990;322:727-733.

4. Van Raemdonck D, Neyrinck A, Verleden GM, et al. Lung donor selection and management. Proc Am Thorac Soc 2009;6:28-38.

5. Dahlman S, Jeppsson A, Scherstén H, Nilsson F. Expanding the donor pool: Lung transplantation with donors 55 years and older. Transplant Proc 2006;38:2691-2693.

6. Pizanis N, Heckman J, Tsagakis K, et al. Lung transplantation using donors 55 years and older: Is it safe or just a way out of organ shortage? Eur J Cardiothorac Surg 2010;38:192-197.

7. Botha P, Trivedi D, Weir C, et al. Extended donor criteria in lung transplantation: Impact on organ allocation. J Thorac Cardiovasc Surg 2006;131:1154-60.

8. Sommer W, Kühn C, Tudorache I, et al. Extended criteria donor lungs and clinical outcome: Results of an allocation algorithm. J Heart Lung Transplant 2013;32:1065-1072.

9. Pierre AF, Sekine Y, Hutcheon MA, et al. Marginal donor lungs: A reassessment. J Thorac Cardiovasc Surg 2002;123:421-428.

10. Michael GE, O'Connor RE. The importance of emergency medicine in organ donation: Successful donation is more likely when potential donors are referred from the emergency department. Acad Emerg Med 2009;16:850-858.

11. Miller LD, Gardiner ST, Gubler KD. Emergency department referral for organ donation: More organ donors and more organs per donor. Am J Surg 2013;207;728-734.

12. Shigemura N, Bermudez C, Hattler BG, et al. Impact of graft volume reduction for oversized grafts after lung transplantation on outcome in recipients with end-stage restrictive pulmonary diseases. J Heart Lung Transplant 2009;28:130-134.

13. Santos F, Lama R, Alvarez A, et al. Pulmonary tailoring and lobar transplantation to overcome size disparities in lung transplantation. Transplant Proc 2005;37:1526-1529.

14. Aigner C, Winkler G, Jaksch P, et al. Size-reduced lung transplantation: An advanced operative strategy to alleviate donor organ shortage. Transplant Proc 2004;36:2801-2805.

15. Janssens JP, Aging of the respiratory system: Impact on pulmonary function tests and adaptation to exertion. Clin Chest Medicine 2005;26:496-484.

16. Sharma G, Goodwin J, Effect on aging on respiratory system physiology and immunology. Clin Interv Aging 2006;1:253-260.

17. Turner J, Mead J, Wohl M. Elasticity of human lungs in relation to age. J Appl Physiol 1968;25:664-671.

18. De Perrot M, Waddell TK, Shargall Y, et al. Impact of donors aged 60 years or more on outcome after lung transplantation: Results of an 11-year single-center experience. J Thorac Cardiovasc Surg 2006;133:525-531.

19. Bittle GJ, Sanchez PG, Kon ZN, et al. The use of lung donors older than 55 years: A review of the United Network of Organ Sharing database. J Heart Lung Transplant 2013;32:760-768.

20. Bonser RS, Taylor R, Collett D, et al. Effect of donor smoking on survival after lung transplantation: A cohort study of a prospective registry. Lancet 2012;380:747-755.

21. Gabbay E, Williams TJ, Griffiths AP, et al. Maximizing the utilization of donor organs offered for lung transplantation. Am J Respir Crit Care Med 1999;160:265-271.

22. Bhorade SM, Vigneswaran W, McCabe MA, Garrity ER. Liberalization of donor criteria may expand the donor pool without adverse consequences in lung transplantation. J Heart Lung Transplant 2000;19:1199-1204.

23. Shigemura N, Toyoda Y, Bhama JK, et al. Donor smoking history and age in lung transplantation: A revisit. Transplantation 2013;95:513-518.

24. Christie JD, Kotloff RM, Pochettino A, et al. Clinical risk factors for primary graft failure following lung transplantation. Chest 2003;124:1232-1241.

25. Diamond JM, Lee JC, Kawut SM, et al. Clinical risk factors for primary graft dysfunction after lung transplantation. Am J Respir Crit Care Med 2013;187:527-534.

26. Berman M, Goldsmith K, Jenkins D, et al. Comparison of outcomes from smoking and non-smoking donors: Thirteen year experience. Ann Thorac Surg 2010;90:1786-1792.

27. Taghavi S, Jayarajan S, Komaroff E, et al. Double-lung transplantation can be safely performed using donors with heavy smoking history. Ann Thorac Surg 2013;95:1912-1917.

28. Wauters S, Verleden GM, Belmans A, et al. Donor cause of brain death and related time intervals: Does it affect outcome after lung transplantation? Eur J Cardiothorac Surg 2011;39:68-76.

29. De Soyza AG, Dark JH, Parums DV, et al. Donor-acquired small cell cancer following pulmonary transplantation. Chest 2001;120: 1030-1031.

30. Oto T, Griffiths A, Levvey B, et al. A donor history of smoking affects early but not late outcome in lung transplantation. Transplantation 2004;78:599-606.

31. Lam T, Ho S, Hedley A, et al. Mortality and smoking in Hong Kong: Case-control study of all adult deaths in 1998. BMJ 2001;323:361.

32. Ganesh SJ, Rogers CA, Banner NR, Bonser RS. Donor cause of death and mid-term survival in lung transplantation. J Heart Lung Transplant 2005;24:1544-1549.

33. Faropoulos K, Apostolakis E. Brain death and its influence on the lungs of the donor: How is it prevented? Transplant Proc 2009;41:4114-4119.

34. Ciccone AM, Stewart KC, Meyers BF, et al. Does donor cause of death affect the outcome of lung transplantation? J Thorac Cardiovasc Surg 2002;123:429-435.

35. Falk JL, Escowitz HE. Submersion injuries in children and adults. Semin Respir Crit Care Med 2002;23:47-55.

36. McNamee CJ, Modry DL, Lien D, Conlan AA. Drowned donor lung for bilateral lung transplantation. J Thorac Cardiovasc Surg 2003;126:910-912.

37. Miyoshi K, Oto T, Otani S, et al. Effect of donor pre-mortem hypoxia and hypotension on graft function and start of warm ischemia in donation after cardiac death lung transplantation. J Heart Lung Transplant 2011;30:445-451.

38. Whitson BA, Hertz MI, Kelly RF, et al. Use of donor lung after asphyxiation or drowning: Effect on lung transplant recipients. Ann Thorac Surg 2014;98:1145-1151.

39. Xu DZ, Yan YP, Choi BC, et al. Risk factors and mechanism of transplacental transmission of hepatitis B virus: A case-control study. J Med Virol 2002;67:20-26.

40. Agnello V, Abel G. Localization of hepatitis C in cutaneous vasculitic lesions in patients with type II cryoglobulinemia. Arthritis Rheum 1997;40:2007-2015.

41. Salvadori M, Rosso G, Carta P, et al. Donors positive for hepatitis B core antibodies in nonliver transplantations. Transplant Proc 2011;43:277-279.

42. Fagiuoli S, Minniti F, Pevere S, HBV and HVC infections in heart transplant recipients. J Heart Lung Transplant 2001;20:718-724.

43. Marelli D, Bresson J, Laks H. Hepatitis C–positive donors in heart transplantation. Am J Transplant 2002;2:443-444.

44. Delmonico FL. Cadaver donor screening for infectious agents in solid organ transplantation. Clin Infect Dis 2000;31:781-786.

45. Rosengard BR, Feng S, Alfrey EJ, et al. Report of the Crystal City meeting to maximize the use of organs recovered from the cadaver donor. Am J Transplant 2002;2:701-711.

46. Klatte T, Patard JJ, deMartino M, et al. Tumor size does not predict risk of metastatic disease or prognosis of small renal cell carcinomas. J Urol 2008;179:1719-1726.

47. Ison MG, Hager J, Blumberg E, et al. Donor-derived disease transmission events in the United States: Data reviewed by the OPTN/UNOS Disease Transmission Advisory Committee. Am J Transplant 2009;9:1929-1935.

48. Ison MG, Nalesnik MA. An update on donor-derived disease transmission in organ transplantation. Am J Transplant 2011;11:1123-1130.

49. Buell, JF, Trofe J, Sethuraman G, et al. Donors with central nervous system malignancies: Are they truly safe? Transplantation 2003;76:340-343.

50. Trulock EP. Lung transplantation. Am J Respir Crit Care Med 1997;155:789-818.

51. Fisher AJ, Donelly SC, Hirani N, et al. Enhanced pulmonary inflammation in organ donors following fatal non-traumatic brain injury. Lancet 1999;24:353:1412-1413.

52. de Perrot M, Weder W, Patterson GA, Keshavjee S. Strategies to increase limited donor resources. Eur Respir J 2004;23:477-82.

53. Wood KE, Coursin DB. Intensivists and organ donor management. Curr Opin Anesthesiol 2007;20:97.

54. Angel LF, Levine DJ, Restrepo MI, et al. Impact of a lung transplantation donor-management protocol on lung donation and recipient outcomes. Am J Respir Crit Care Med 2006;174:710-716.

55. Roche AM, James FM. Fluid therapy in organ transplantation. Curr Opin Organ Transplant 2007;12:281-286.

56. Abdelnour T, Rieke S. Relationship of hormonal resuscitation therapy and central venous pressure on increasing organs for transplant. J Heart Lung Transplant 2009;28:480-485.

57. Minambres E, Ballesteros MA, Rodriqo E, et al. Aggressive lung donor management increases graft procurement without increasing renal graft loss after transplantation. Clin Transplant 2013;27:52-59.

58. Protocolo de manejo del donante toracico: estrategias para mejorar el approvechamiento de organos. http://www.ont.es/infesp/Paginas/Documentosde Consenso.aspx. Accessed 9 Oct 2014.

59. Taniguchi S, Kitamura S, Kawachi K, et al. Effects of hormonal supplements on the maintenance of cardiac function in potential donor patients after cerebral death. Eur J Cardiothorac Surg 1992;6:96-101; discussion 102.

60. Rosendale JD, Kauffman HN, Mc Bride MA, et al. Hormonal resuscitation yields more transplanted hearts, with improved early function. Transplantation 2003;75:1336-1341.

61. Shah VR. Aggressive management of multiorgan donor. Transplant Proc 2008;40:1087-1090.
62. Venkateswaran RV, Patchell VB, Wilson IC, et al. Early donor management increases the retrieval of lungs for transplantation. Ann Thorac Surg 2008;85:278-286.
63. Rosendale JD, Kauffman HM, McBride MA, et al. Aggressive pharmacologic donor management results in more transplanted organs. Transplantation 2003;75:482-487.
64. Pennefather SH, Bullock RE, Mantle D, Dark JH. Use of low dose arginine vasopressin to support brain-dead organ donors. Transplantation 1995;59:58-62.
65. Rosendale JD, Kauffman HM, McBride MA, et al. Hormonal resuscitation yields more transplanted hearts, with improved early function. Transplantation 2003;75:1336-1341.
66. Hing AJ, Hicks M, Garlick SR, et al. The effects of hormone resuscitation on cardiac function and hemodynamics in a porcine brain-dead organ donor. Am J Transplant 2007;7:809-817.
67. Powner DJ, Biebuyck JC. Introduction to the interpretation of chest radiographs during donor care. Prog Transplant 2005;15:240-248.
68. Zafar F, Khan MS, Heinle JS, et al. Does donor arterial partial pressure of oxygen affect outcomes after lung transplantation? A review of more than 12,000 lung transplants. J Thorac Cardiovasc Surg 143:912-925.
69. Bonde PN, Patel ND, Borja MC, et al. Impact of donor lung organisms on post-lung transplant pneumonia. J Heart Lung Transplant 2007;25:99-105.
70. Yusen RD, Christie JD, Edwards LB, et al. The Registry of the International Heart and Lung Society for Heart and Lung Transplantation: Thirtieth adult lung and heart-lung transplant report—2013; focus theme: Age. J Heart Lung Transplant 2013;32:965-978.

8

Non–heart-beating donors

DAVID GÓMEZ DE ANTONIO, JOSE LUIS CAMPO CAÑAVERAL DE LA CRUZ, LUCAS HOYOS MEGÍA, DANIEL VALDIVIA CONCHA, AND ANDRÉS VARELA DE UGARTE

INTRODUCTION

The scarcity of grafts for lung transplantation is a major problem that is due mainly to the low yield of viable lungs from potential multiorgan donors and the increasing number of patients who are being referred to lung transplant units and seeking a last chance to alleviate their suffering.

James Hardy is credited as being the first surgeon to perform lung transplantation and, at the same time, the first to use a donation after cardiac death (DCD) donor for that purpose.[1]

During the 1990s, Thomas Egan and colleagues revisited the possibility of using lungs from DCD donors, thus reopening the door for others to investigate the viability of these grafts in relation to warm ischemia and best preservation.[2] During the late 1990s and early 2000s, experimental evidence came to light suggesting that a warm ischemic time (WIT) longer than 90 minutes might be extreme and also confirming topical cooling as the best way to preserve lungs in situ for DCD, the importance of retrograde perfusion in DCD donors, and the potential of ex vivo evaluation as a tool to improve graft quality.[3-8]

After the first international workshop focused on DCD donors, which was held in Maastricht (the Netherlands) in 1995, such donors were classified into two main categories: (1) uncontrolled donation after cardiac death (uDCD) donors (dead on arrival [category I] or unsuccessful resuscitation [category II]) and (2) controlled (cDCD) donors (awaiting cardiac arrest [category III] and cardiac arrest in a brain-dead donor [category IV]).[9]

Recently, another controlled category (V) has been added for patients suffering an unexpected sudden death in an intensive care unit (ICU) or critical care facility.

In this chapter we summarize the criteria for, methods of preservation used in, and results of transplantation of lungs obtained via DCD.

UNCONTROLLED NON–HEART-BEATING DONORS

Steen and coworkers in 2001 successfully transplanted a single lung from a donor after failed cardiac resuscitation,[10] thus inspiring others to focus on this source of grafts. The uncontrolled scenario is a logistic challenge because it depends on a wide network of hospital emergency services, as well as on transplant coordinators' skills and motivation to request consent for organ donation in a delicate situation. For this reason, 14 years after Steen's report, only our group in Madrid is reporting a consistent number of lung transplants from uDCD donors.[11]

Donor management and preservation

The uDCD program includes a multidisciplinary medical and surgical team that is on site upon arrival of a potential donor. This team includes surgeons, anesthesiologists, perfusionists, and nurses. Also essential are out-of-hospital emergency teams trained to provide high-quality basic and advanced life support.

The "code" starts after a witnessed cardiac arrest, with emergency units initiating basic and advanced resuscitation maneuvers within 15 minutes of the code. If no recovery of spontaneous circulation has occurred after 30 minutes of advanced cardiopulmonary resuscitation (CPR), the patient is transported to the emergency department while still receiving advanced CPR.

When the patient arrives, death is declared by the ICU staff independently of the transplant team. Declaration of death is based on cardiopulmonary criteria and defined as irreversible or permanent cessation of respiration and circulation after a certain period.[12,13] Signs of death are absence of heart sounds and pulse, as well as lack of spontaneous respiration during a no-touch period of 5 minutes in accordance with the Institute of Medicine recommendations, provided that hypothermia, drowning, penetrating trauma, or suspected intoxication has not occurred.[14]

After the declaration of death, legal permission for organ preservation is requested from the judge on duty, after which serologic samples, blood samples, anthropometric measurements, and chest radiographs are obtained.

Spain follows an opting-in principle, but the in case of uDCD, legislation usually allows preservation of organs while the family's consent is obtained or the deceased's advanced directives are consulted.

This situation may raise controversy related to patient autonomy. If the deceased wished to donate, but a delay in obtaining consent leads to organ loss, the deceased's wishes may be disregarded. Alternatively, if the individual did not wish to donate or CPR would be futile, the patient's dignity and self-respect would be at risk should CPR continue. Given the uncontrolled scenario, where an appropriate opportunity to request consent is lacking, Spanish law allows emergency service personnel to proceed with CPR until arrival at the hospital.[15]

Once legal permission for preservation is obtained, heparin (3 to 5 mg/kg) is given to the potential donor to reduce the risk for pulmonary thromboembolism,[16-19] cold (at 4° C) Perfadex (Medisan, Uppsala, Sweden) is instilled into both pleural cavities through chest drains to bring the lung temperature to below 21° C,[11,20,21] and venoarterial extracorporeal membrane oxygenation is implemented for preservation of the abdominal organs, with insertion of a Fogarty catheter supradiaphragmatically to prevent abdominal solutions from entering the chest.[22,23]

At this point, the same criteria for potential donation apply as for brain-dead donors, with the accepted maximum WIT (from absence of circulation until effective topical cooling) being 90 minutes (Table 8.1). Once topical cooling is achieved, consent can be obtained. In the interim, the grafts are cooled to below 21° C, after which a maximum of 240 minutes may pass while the graft remains viable (preservation time).[10,11,16]

Table 8.1 Standard criteria for lung donation from an uncontrolled non–heart-beating donor

Age younger than 65 years
Less than a 20-pack-year smoking history
Appropriate size matching with the prospective recipient
Blood type compatibility
Absence of previous cardiopulmonary surgery
Absence of bronchoscopic or chest radiographic evidence of pulmonary edema, infection, or aspiration Po_2/Fio_2 ratio >400
Topical cooling with a target pleural temperature <21° C
Time sequence
• No-touch period after cardiac arrest ≤15 min
• Warm ischemic time ≤100 min
• Topical cooling total time ≤240 min

Once consents have been obtained, organ retrieval and in situ graft evaluation begin. The topical cooling preservation solution is drained from both pleural cavities, and 100% oxygen (Fio_2 = 1.0) with 5 cm H_2O of positive endexpiratory pressure lung ventilation is started with a low tidal volume and slowly increased to 5 to 7 mL/kg.[24,25] Bronchoscopic exploration is performed to rule out gastric aspiration, pulmonary edema, or other endobronchial lesions.

Following surgical exposure of the cadaveric lung, a macroscopic evaluation is performed the same way as for braindead donors. Flush perfusion through the pulmonary artery is implemented until the effluent through the left atrium is clear. Next, 300 mL of donor blood is passed through the system and an analysis of gas from the left atrium and each pulmonary vein is conducted with temperature correction, with the goal being a partial pressure of oxygen greater than 400 mm Hg[11,26] (Figure 8.1). The procedure is completed with retrograde perfusion[8] of 200 mL of Perfadex through each pulmonary vein to wash the bronchial vasculature and improve graft preservation.

The decision whether to use the donor graft is based on a stringent evaluation during which donor characteristics, WIT, macroscopic appearance, the collapse test results, perfect flush perfusion, and gas exchange are assessed.

Ex vivo lung perfusion in uncontrolled donation after cardiac death

Normothermic ex vivo lung perfusion (EVLP) makes it possible to assess organ viability before transplantation. Its first clinical application was described by Steen and coworkers at University Hospital of Lund in 2001.[10] EVLP as a platform to deliver different medications has also been tested and proven beneficial in most reports. It is fully described in Chapter 11 of this book.[24,25,27,28]

In general terms, the foundations of EVLP include gradual rewarming, an increase in vascular flow up to

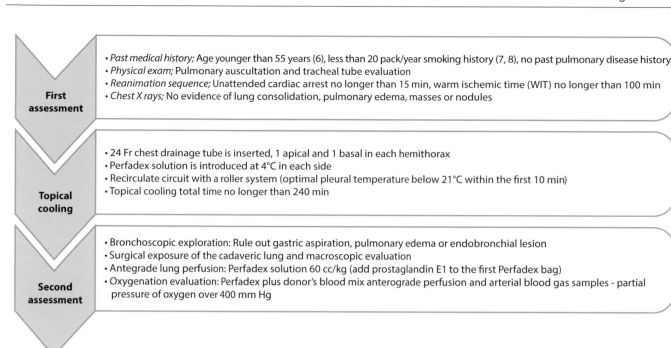

First assessment
- *Past medical history;* Age younger than 55 years (6), less than 20 pack/year smoking history (7, 8), no past pulmonary disease history
- *Physical exam;* Pulmonary auscultation and tracheal tube evaluation
- *Reanimation sequence;* Unattended cardiac arrest no longer than 15 min, warm ischemic time (WIT) no longer than 100 min
- *Chest X rays;* No evidence of lung consolidation, pulmonary edema, masses or nodules

Topical cooling
- 24 Fr chest drainage tube is inserted, 1 apical and 1 basal in each hemithorax
- Perfadex solution is introduced at 4°C in each side
- Recirculate circuit with a roller system (optimal pleural temperature below 21°C within the first 10 min)
- Topical cooling total time no longer than 240 min

Second assessment
- Bronchoscopic exploration: Rule out gastric aspiration, pulmonary edema or endobronchial lesion
- Surgical exposure of the cadaveric lung and macroscopic evaluation
- Antegrade lung perfusion: Perfadex solution 60 cc/kg (add prostaglandin E1 to the first Perfadex bag)
- Oxygenation evaluation: Perfadex plus donor's blood mix anterograde perfusion and arterial blood gas samples - partial pressure of oxygen over 400 mm Hg

Figure 8.1 Assessments.

normothermia to a predetermined percentage of the predicted cardiac output, protective lung ventilation, and perfusion with a solution with high colloid osmotic pressure to remove water from the lung parenchyma.[29]

A variety of techniques, solutions, and devices exist to perform EVLP. The Lund technique, for example, differs from the Toronto technique in terms of the open left atrium, use of Steen solution mixed with red blood cells, and perfusion at flows corresponding to 100% of the donor predicted cardiac output instead of 40%.[30]

Furthermore, a growing body of evidence has focused on the application of EVLP to assess and repair lungs obtained via DCD. The low clinical utilization rate of these lungs is probably due to the fact that the injuries (such as warm ischemia, hypoxia, hypotension, and aspiration) are different from those associated with brain-dead donors.[29]

The initial clinical experience with transplantation of lungs obtained via uDCD showed a high incidence of severe (grade 3) primary graft dysfunction (PGD),[31] thus leading to focused efforts to reassess and repair grafts with some form of EVLP. A detailed discussion of our experience is available in the "Results" section of this chapter.

From this experience we have adopted EVLP as part of uDCD evaluation in the following situations:

- Best Pao$_2$ less than 400 mm Hg.
- Signs of pulmonary edema on the chest radiograph or macroscopic examination during procurement.
- Poor lung compliance at the procurement assessment.
- Donors with more than one risk factor, including age older than 65 years, questionable history of aspiration, history of heavy smoking, and expected long ischemic time.

CONTROLLED NON–HEART-BEATING DONORS

The controlled scenario offers several advantages over the uncontrolled scenario, including the ability to schedule, assess graft viability, conduct more controlled recipient selection, and engage in careful communication with the donor's relatives.

Limitation of therapeutic efforts

Withdrawal of life-sustaining therapy (WLST) must be proposed by the ICU staff in an irreversible clinical situation characterized by no response to therapy and little likelihood of progression to brain death. The most common cases result from catastrophic and irreversible neurologic injuries, terminal neuromuscular disorders, severe and irreversible spinal cord injuries, and terminal pulmonary diseases (the latter are obviously not considered for lung donation). Recently, some countries (Belgium and Holland) have started to consider donation after euthanasia. Such donors are included in Maastricht category III.

At a separate time and completely independently of the decision in favor of WLST, the patient is considered for lung donation and a transplant coordinator contacts the potential donor's relatives for consent.

Selection criteria for potential donation after cardiac death

The selection criteria for potential donors are similar to those for brain-dead donors[32-34]:

- Age younger than 55 years, although some groups include 65-year-old donors.
- Po_2/Fio_2 ratio of 300 or higher.
- Less than 20-pack-year smoking history.
- Absence of significant abnormalities on the chest radiograph.
- Absence of purulent secretions or signs of aspiration through the orotracheal tube or during bronchoscopy.
- Absence of malignant diseases, except for brain tumors other than glioblastoma multiforme or astrocytoma and skin tumors in the last 2 years.
- Absence of previous cardiac or pulmonary surgery.

Some algorithms have been proposed to help predict the likelihood of death within 2 hours after the withdrawal of life support.[35,36]

Potential donor management and monitoring

Once the decision to donate has been made, WLST is carried out by the ICU personnel in the operating room or in the ICU. Until cardiac arrest, regular analgesia and sedative drugs are administered for patient comfort. The following variables are closely monitored:

- Invasive arterial pressure (systolic, diastolic, and mean).
- Heart rate and rhythm.
- Respiratory rate.
- Saturation of O_2.
- Diuresis.

A time limit of 2 hours until cardiac arrest is accepted, after which the patient is returned to the ICU.

Some controversy surrounds the criteria for declaration of death. Most protocols require not only confirmation of permanent or irreversible cessation of circulation and respiration by indirect findings but also implementation of specific diagnostic measures such as invasive arterial monitoring or Doppler interrogation.[37] Electrocardiography (ECG) is advisable but not essential; however, it should be consistent with the clinical observation of circulatory cessation.

Another concern is duration of the no-touch observation period. Depending on the local protocol, the period lasts from 2 to 20 minutes.[38,39] The aim of this period is to detect signs of autoresuscitation (arterial pulse, respiration effort, or spontaneous muscular activity). Most units have adopted a 5-minute no-touch period to confirm death. Transplant coordination team members must be absent during the whole process.

Ischemic time and agonal phase

As has already been mentioned, extensive experimental work has helped establish that the maximum tolerable WIT ensuring viability of the organs ranges from 60 to 90 minutes.[2,5,6,40,41]

Different definitions for WIT have been proposed; they vary depending on the local protocol. The American Society of Transplant Surgeons (ASTS) guidelines define WIT as the period between WLST and cold perfusion of the graft. However, these guidelines also define a "true WIT," which is the interval between a significant ischemic insult and initiation of cold perfusion in view of the fact that real ischemic damage starts when mean arterial pressure drops below 60 mm Hg.[38]

Some authors also take oxygenation into account when considering the initiation of ischemia. Oto and colleagues found that organ injury starts when systolic arterial pressure drops below 50 mm Hg and oxygen saturation below 85%.[42] Other groups consider WIT to be the time between circulatory arrest and cold perfusion.[43,44] This lack of consensus makes the data extremely difficult to compare. However, most groups agree on the critical time points from WLST, which include the time when WLST is initiated, mean arterial pressure falls below 60 mm Hg, systolic arterial pressure drops below 50 mm Hg, cardiac arrest occurs, and cold flush perfusion is initiated. Therefore, recording and publication of these variables can help make outcomes comparable. An international effort to form a multicenter registry was started within the International Society for Heart and Lung Transplantation (ISHLT). In April 2013, this registry reported outcomes comparable to those for brain-dead donors in terms of early and intermediate survival.[45]

Agonal phase is another applicable concept; it is defined as the period between WLST and declaration of death. The agonal phase is essentially a period of cardiopulmonary instability, and its length appears to be crucial for graft viability. Some experimental and clinical studies have suggested an inverse correlation between the length of the agonal phase and graft viability and function. In a porcine model, Van de Wauwer and colleagues showed that the mode of death in non–heart-beating donors is also important; they addressed the inferior quality of grafts after hypoxic cardiac arrest when compared with exsanguination.[46] Interestingly, in a different animal model, Miyoshi and colleagues showed that oxygenation and ventilation management may be even more critical than circulatory instability itself.[47] In the clinical setting in 2008, Snell and colleagues showed a trend of correlation of longer WITs with both lower Pao_2/Fio_2 ratio and longer ICU stay after transplantation.[48] Conversely in 2012, in 72 lung transplants they found a weak correlation between these parameters when WIT was always below 60 minutes.[49]

In conclusion, most protocols accept between 60 and 90 minutes of WIT, depending on the definitions. Our institution considers 60 minutes acceptable for "true WIT" (between the occurrence of mean arterial pressure below 60 mm Hg and cold preservation).

Donor evaluation and preservation

As stated previously, donor evaluation includes obtaining a medical history; measuring arterial gases; and performing chest radiography, bronchoscopy, and a macroscopic examination after death has been declared.

Before WLST, most protocols include the administration of a bolus of heparin. Although this is the only intervention before declaration of death, some ethical concerns may exist depending on local policy. The major ethical conflict is in balancing the risk of the perception that heparin is hastening death against the risk of decreasing the likelihood of donation by avoiding adequate graft preservation.[50] In our protocol the patient receives heparin at a rate of 1000 IU/kg, but again the dosage and moment of administration vary between groups.[51]

After cardiac arrest plus a 5-minute no-touch period, an ICU staff member involved in the WLST process usually determines death. Reintubation is then performed quickly, ventilation is restarted, and the donor is transferred to the operating room. The airway is checked by bronchoscopy to rule out aspiration during the agonal phase. Simultaneous rapid opening of the chest and flush perfusion through the pulmonary artery are performed. Although several flush solutions are available, our preference is a low-potassium dextran product (Perfadex).

If the donor fulfills the acceptance criteria, recipient anesthesia is started and graft procurement is carried out in the standard fashion. Retrograde perfusion through the pulmonary veins is advisable at any time and is usually performed at the back table.[8,52]

In the event of concerns about the grafts' suitability (extended criteria, marginal donors), ex vivo lung perfusion (EVLP) assessment could be carried out if feasible to ensure graft viability.

Ex vivo lung perfusion in controlled donation after cardiac death

EVLP has become a potentially useful tool to reassess, preserve, or recover grafts, thus expanding the donor pool. In 2012 the Toronto group reported 50 lung transplants after EVLP, 22 of which were from cDCD donors and had outcomes similar to those of the control group (no EVLP perfusion).[53] It advocates the use of EVLP in cDCD grafts because of concerns regarding the incidence of PGD. With this strategy the group has increased the acceptable time between WLST and cardiac arrest to 2 hours.

Other groups have reported successful outcomes without EVLP in situations involving cDCD.[20,49] In fact, only 13% of all reported transplants from cDCD donors in the ISHLT DCD registry in April 2013 were performed after EVLP assessment.[45] EVLP may well prove to be a valuable tool to improve utilization of these donor lungs, especially when extended donor criteria are used.

RESULTS

Uncontrolled donation after cardiac death

In our experience, approximately 5% of all potential uDCD donors become effective lung donors. The primary reasons for

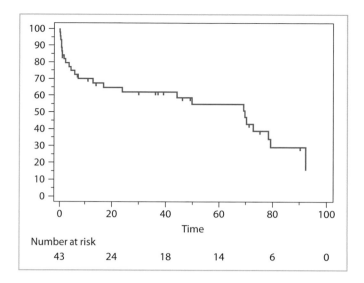

Figure 8.2 Kaplan-Meier survival curve, uncontrolled donation after cardiac death.

rejection of a donor include lack of family consent, prolonged ischemic times, and a history of malignancy. After preservation of potentially suitable organs, the main reasons for not implanting lungs from uDCD donors are gastric aspiration, pulmonary contusion, extrathoracic tumor, and suspected pulmonary embolism. Through May 2014, we performed 46 lung transplants from uDCD donors, including 11 with EVLP (4 with the OCS portable system) (unpublished data).

The rate of grade 3 PGD was 37%, and 30-day mortality was 16%. The 1-, 3-, and 5-year survival rates were 70%, 62%, and 54%, respectively (Figure 8.2).[54] Multivariate analysis revealed severe secondary pulmonary hypertension and extracorporeal support as clinically relevant factors associated with mortality. The risks associated with recipient diagnosis, demographics, acute rejection, method of preservation, or PGD did not reach statistical significance.

Although the hope is that EVLP will improve graft function and reduce PGD, it appears that PGD is still a major concern with uDCD. The current EVLP systems focus on preservation solutions specifically designed to dry the lungs, which is a crucial factor after brain death and, in some cases, in cDCD. In uDCD, the principal foe is warm ischemia, which leads to immediate cell death and architectural damage culminating in pulmonary edema. We speculate that the mode of vascular injury increases the risk for PGD despite extravascular water extraction and excellent performance ex vivo. The chronic allograft rejection rates at 3 and 5 years are 23% and 54%, respectively, which are comparable to those reported in the international registry.[55]

Controlled donation after cardiac death

Currently, more than 10 centers are reporting lung transplants from cDCD donors,[20,21,42-44,48,49,51,53,56-65] with such transplants representing about 10% of their average transplant volume. Without a doubt, such donors are the most promising additional source of grafts to increase the donor pool. The results in terms of graft function and early and midterm survival are uniformly excellent.

In 2011, Erasmus's group reported their experience with 35 cases that were compared with a group of cases involving transplants from brain-dead donors. They showed comparable results in terms of PGD and survival.[43] The group from Australia reported on 72 cases in 2012, with impressive survival rates (97% the first year and 90% at 5 years) and no difference in the incidence of PGD within the first 72 hours as compared with in their cases involving brain-dead donors.[49]

The group from Cleveland[21] reported on 32 cases, with survival rates of 97%, 91%, 91%, and 71% at 3 and 4 years. Similar results were reported by the group from Leuven.[44]

Zych and colleagues[65] reported on 26 transplants from cDCD donors; the results with regard to graft function, survival, and chronic rejection were similar to those for their cohort of recipients of transplants from brain-dead donors in the same period. Cypel and associates[45] published the results of a collaborative initiative focused on cDCD, with nine reporting centers showing 97% and 89% survival rates at 30 days and 1 year, respectively.

A recent meta-analysis[66] looking for differences between DCD and brain-dead donors in terms of early mortality, PGD, and chronic rejection did not show any disparities, thus supporting the concept of DCD as an effective method to increase the donor pool.

CONCLUSIONS

When lungs from uDCD donors are being considered, the pivotal factor besides complexity of the logistics is cell damage secondary to warm ischemia, and solution of this problem should be the target toward which to strive. EVLP systems are the most valuable tool for investigating both measurable parameters to detect grafts at risk for the development of PGD and also for finding specific therapeutic strategies to repair ongoing damage.

Evidence showing the viability of cDCD programs is mounting, with excellent clinical outcomes and great potential to overcome the scarcity of lungs for transplantation.

REFERENCES

1. Hardy JD, Webb WR, Dalton ML, Walker GR. Homotransplantation in man. JAMA 1963;186:1065-1074.
2. Egan TM, Lambert CJ, Reddick R, et al. A strategy to increase the donor pool: Use of cadaver lungs for transplantation. Ann Thorac Surg 1991;52:1113-1121.
3. Homatas J, Bryant L, Eiseman B. Time limits of cadaver lung viability. J Thorac Cardiovasc Surg 1968;56:132-140.
4. Loehe F, Mueller C, Annecke T, et al. Pulmonary graft function after long-term preservation of non–heart-beating donor lungs. Ann Thorac Surg 2000;69:1556-1562.
5. Greco R, Cordovilla G, Sanz E, et al. Warm ischemic time tolerance after ventilated non–heart-beating lung donation in piglets. Eur J Cardiothorac Surg 1998;14:319-325.
6. Van Raemdonck DE, Jannis NC, De Leyn PR, et al. Warm ischemic tolerance in collapsed pulmonary grafts is limited to 1 hour. Ann Surg 1998;228:788-796.
7. Rega FR, Jannis NC, Verleden GM, et al. Should we ventilate or cool the pulmonary graft inside the non–heart-beating donor? J Heart Lung Transplant 2003;22:1226-1233.
8. Van De Wauwer C, Neyrinck AP, Geudens N, et al. Retrograde flush following topical cooling is superior to preserve the non–heart-beating donor lung. Eur J Cardiothorac Surg 2007;31:1125-1132.
9. Kootstra G, Daemen JH, Oomen AP. Categories of non–heart-beating donors. Transplant Proc 1995;27:2893-2894.
10. Steen S, Sjöberg T, Pierre L, et al. Transplantation of lungs from a non–heart-beating donor. Lancet 2001;357:825-829.
11. Gomez-de-Antonio D, Campo-Canaveral JL, Crowley S, et al. Clinical lung transplantation from uncontrolled non–heart-beating donors revisited. J Heart Lung Transplant 2012;31:349-353.
12. Bernat JL, D'Alessandro AM, Port FK, et al. Report of a National Conference on Donation after cardiac death. Am J Transplant 2006;6:281-291.
13. Elgharably H, Shafii A, Mason D. Expanding the donor pool donation after cardiac death. Thorac Surg Clin 2015;25:35-46.
14. Ethics Committee, American College of Critical Care Medicine, Society of Critical Care Medicine. Recommendations for non–heart-beating organ donation. A position paper by the Ethics Committee, American College of Critical Care Medicine, Society of Critical Care Medicine. Crit Care Med 2001;29:1826-1831.
15. Real Decreto 2070/1999 del 30 de Diciembre. B.O.E. 4 de Enero de 2000. http://www.boe.es/g/es/bases_datos/webBOE.php.
16. Okazaki M, Date H, Inokawa H, et al. Optimal time for post-mortem heparinization in canine lung transplantation with non–heart-beating donors. J Heart Lung Transplant 2006;25:454-460.
17. Akasaka S, Nishi H, Aoe M, et al. The effects of recombinant tissue-type plasminogen activator (rt-PA) on canine cadaver lung transplantation. Surg Today 1999;29:747-754.
18. Sugimoto R, Date H, Sugimoto S, et al. Post-mortem administration of urokinase in canine lung transplantation from non–heart-beating donors. J Heart Lung Transplant 2006;25:1148-1153.
19. Hayama M, Date H, Oto T, et al. Improved lung function by means of retrograde flush in

canine lung transplantation with non–heart-beating donors. J Thorac Cardiovasc Surg 2003;125: 901-906.

20. De Oliveira NC, Osaki S, Maloney JD, et al. Lung transplantation with donation after cardiac death donors: Long-term follow-up in a single center. J Thorac Cardiovasc Surg 2010;139:1306-1315.

21. Mason DP, Brown CR, Murthy SC, et al. Growing single-center experience with lung transplantation using donation after cardiac death. Ann Thorac Surg 2012;94:406-411; discussion: 411-412.

22. Brook NR, Waller JR, Nicholson ML. Non–heart-beating donation: Current practice and future developments. Kidney Int 2003;63:1516-1529.

23. Mateos Rodríguez AA, Navalpotro Pascual JM, del Río Gallegos F. Lung transplant of extrahospitalary donor after cardiac death. Am J Emerg Med 2013;31:710-711.

24. Cypel M, Yeung JC, Hirayama S, et al. Technique for prolonged normothermic ex vivo lung perfusion. J Heart Lung Transplant 2008;27:1319-1325.

25. Cypel M, Rubacha M, Yeung J, et al. Normothermic ex vivo perfusion prevents lung injury compared to extended cold preservation for transplantation. Am J Transplant 2009;9:2262-2269.

26. Meneses JC, Gámez AP, Mariscal MA, et al. Comparative experimental study of pulmonary function evaluation in outpatient NHBLD among exsanguinating donors and sudden death donors. Paper presented at the 31st Annual Meeting and Scientific Sessions of the ISHLT, April 14, 2011, San Diego, California.

27. Nakajima D, Chen F, Yamada T, et al. Reconditioning of lungs donated after circulatory death with normothermic ex vivo lung perfusion. J Heart Lung Transplant 2012;31:187-193.

28. Mulloy DP, Stone ML, Crosby IK, et al. Ex vivo rehabilitation of non–heart-beating donor lungs in preclinical porcine model: Delayed perfusion results in superior lung function. J Thorac Cardiovasc Surg 2012;144:1208-1215.

29. Machuca TN, Cypel M. Ex vivo lung perfusion. J Thorac Dis 2014;6:1054-1062.

30. Machuca TN, Cypel M, Keshavjee S. Advances in lung preservation. Surg Clin North Am 2013;93:1373-1394.

31. Gomez-de-Antonio D, Campo-Cañaveral JL, Crowley S, et al. Clinical lung transplantation from uncontrolled non–heart-beating donors revisited. J Heart Lung Transplant 2012;31:349-53.

32. De Perrot M, Waddell TK, Shargall Y, et al. Impact of donors aged 60 years or more on outcome after lung transplantation: Results of an 11 year single-center experience. J Thorac Cardiovasc Surg 2006;133:525-531.

33. Oto T, Griffiths AP, Levvey B, et al. A donor history of smoking affects early but not late outcomes in lung transplantation. Transplantation 2004;78:599-606.

34. Bonser RS, Taylor R, Collett D, et al. Effect of donor smoking on survival after lung transplantation: A cohort study of a prospective registry. Lancet 2012;380:747-755.

35. Lewis J, Peltier J, Nelson H, et al. Development of the University of Wisconsin donation after cardiac death evaluation tool. Prog Transplant 2003;13:265-273.

36. DeVita MA, Mori Brooks M, Zawistowski C, et al. Donors alter cardiac death: Validation of identification criteria (DVIC) study for predictors of rapid death. Am J Transplant 2008;8:432-444.

37. The Organ and Tissue Authority. National Protocol for Donation after Cardiac Death. Canberra, Australia: The Organ and Tissue Authority; July 2010.

37a. Steinbrook R. Organ donation after cardiac death. N Engl J Med 2007;357:209-213.

38. Reich DJ, Mulligan DC, Abt PL, et al. ASTS recommended practice guidelines for controlled donation after cardiac death organ procurement and transplantation. Am J Transplant 2009;9:2004-2011.

39. Detry O, Le Dinh H, Noterdaeme T, et al. Categories of donation after cardiocirculatory death. Transplant Proc 2012;44:1189-1195.

40. Van Raemdonck DE, Jannis NC, Rega FR, et al. Extended preservation of ischemic pulmonary graft by postmortem alveolar expansion. Ann Thorac Surg 1997;64:801-808.

41. Kuang JQ, Raemdonck DE, Jannis NC, et al. Pulmonary cell death in warm ischemic rabbit lung is related to the alveolar oxygen reserve. J Heart Lung Transplant 1998;17:406-414.

42. Oto T, Levvey B, McEgan R, et al. A practical approach to clinical lung transplantation from a Maastricht Category III donor with cardiac death. J Heart Lung Transplant 2007;26:196-299.

43. Van De Wauwer C, Verschuuren EA, van der Bij W, et al. The use of non–heart-beating lung donors category III can increase the donor pool. Eur J Cardiothorac Surg. 2011 Jun;39:e175-e280.

44. De Vleeschauwer SI, Wauters S, Dupont LJ, et al. Medium-term outcome after lung transplantation is comparable between brain-dead and cardiac-dead donors. J Heart Lung Transplant 2011;30:975-981.

45. Cypel M, Levvey B, Van Raemdonck D, et al. Favorable outcomes of donation after cardiac death in lung transplantation: A multicenter study. J Heart Lung Transplant 2013;32:S15.

46. Van de Wauwer C, Neyrinck AP, Geudens N, et al. The mode of death in the non–heart-beating donor has an impact on lung graft quality. Eur J Cardiothorac Surg 2009;36:919-926.

47. Miyoshi K, Oto T, Otani S, et al. Effect of donor premortem hypoxia and hypotension on graft function and start of warm ischemia in donation after cardiac death lung transplantation. J Heart Lung Transplant 2011;30:445-451.

48. Snell GI, Levvey BJ, Oto T, et al. Early lung transplantation success utilizing controlled donation after cardiac death donors. Am J Transplant 2008;8:1282-1289.

49. Levvey BJ, Harkess M, Hopkins P, et al. Excellent clinical outcomes from a national donation-after-determination-of-cardiac-death lung transplant collaborative. Am J Transplant 2012;12:2406-2413.

50. Oto T, Rabinov M, Griffiths AP, et al. Unexpected donor pulmonary embolism affects early outcomes after lung transplantation: A major mechanism of primary graft failure? J Thorac Cardiovasc Surg 2005;130:1446.

51. Erasmus ME, Verschuuren EA, Nijkamp DM, et al. Lung transplantation from nonheparinized category III non–heart-beating donors. A single-centre report. Transplantation 2010;89:452-457.

52. Varela A, Cordoba M, Serrano-Fiz S, et al. Early lung allograft function after retrograde and antegrade preservation. J Thorac Cardiovasc Surg 1997;114:1119-1120.

53. Cypel M, Yeung JC, Machuca T, et al. Experience with the first 50 ex vivo lung perfusions in clinical transplantation. J Thorac Cardiovasc Surg 2012;144:1200-1206.

54. Gómez de Antonio D. Non–heart-beating donors Maastricht II. Spanish experience. Presented at the Fifth Annual Marie Lannelongue Alumni Day Meeting, May 2014, Paris, France.

55. Yusen RD, Edwards LB, Kucheryavaya AY, et al. The Registry of the International Society for Heart and Lung Transplantation: Thirty-first adult lung and heart-lung transplant report—2014; focus theme: Retransplantation. J Heart Lung Transplant 2014;33:1009-1024.

56. D'Alessandro AM, Fernandez LA, Chin LT, et al. Donation after cardiac death: The University of Wisconsin experience. Ann Transplant 2004;9:68-71.

57. Mason DP, Murthy SC, Gonzalez-Stawinski GV, et al. Early experience with lung transplantation using donors after cardiac death. J Heart Lung Transplant 2008;27:561-563.

58. Levvey BJ, Westall GP, Kotsimbos T, et al. Definitions of warm ischemic time when using controlled donation after cardiac death lung donors. Transplantation 2008;86:1702-1706.

59. De Vleeschauwer S, Van Raemdonck D, Vanaudenaerde B, et al. Early outcome after lung transplantation from non–heart-beating donors is comparable to heart-beating donors. J Heart Lung Transplant 2009;28:380-387.

60. Cypel M, Sato M, Yildirim E, et al. Initial experience with lung donation after cardiocirculatory death in Canada. J Heart Lung Transplant 2009;28:753-758.

61. Puri V, Scavuzzo M, Guthrie T, et al. Lung transplantation and donation after cardiac death: A single center experience. Ann Thorac Surg 2009;88:1609-1614; discussion 1614-1615.

62. McKellar SH, Durham LA 3rd, Scott JP. Successful lung transplant from donor after cardiac death: A potential solution to shortage of thoracic organs. Mayo Clin Proc 2010;85:150-152.

63. Wigfield CH, Love RB. Donation after cardiac death lung transplantation outcomes. Curr Opin Organ Transplant 2011;16:462-468.

64. Zych B, Popov AF, Simon AR, et al. Ex vivo evaluation of lungs from donation after cardiac death after recent cardiac surgery with cardiopulmonary bypass. Transplant Proc 2011;43:4029-4031.

65. Zych B, Popov AF, Amrani M, et al. Lungs from donation after circulatory death donors: An alternative source to brain-dead donors? Midterm results at a single institution. Eur J Cardiothorac Surg 2012;42:542-549.

66. Krutsinger D, Reed RM, Blevins A, et al. Lung transplantation from donation after cardiocirculatory death: A systematic review and meta-analysis. J Heart Lung Transplant 2015;34:675-684.

9

Donor lung preservation

WIEBKE SOMMER AND GREGOR WARNECKE

The quality of preservation of donor lungs between explantation and implantation in the recipient is of utmost importance for early and midterm outcomes. Surgical technique, choice of perfusion solution, and duration of ischemic time may all contribute to the quality of organ preservation. Excitingly, with ex vivo lung perfusion (EVLP), a new modality for lung preservation that potentially raises the bar for graft preservation in the future has been introduced. Faulty donor lung preservation may result in ischemia-reperfusion injury, which in lung transplantation is called *primary graft dysfunction* (PGD). Because the occurrence of PGD is associated with later onset of chronic rejection, lung graft preservation influences not only short-term but also long-term outcomes in lung transplantation.

PATHOGENESIS OF PRIMARY GRAFT DYSFUNCTION

PGD is defined as a malfunction of lung grafts occurring within the first 72 hours after transplantation, and it is significantly associated with poor long-term outcomes. The underlying disease has historically been termed *ischemia-reperfusion injury* and is characterized by noncardiogenic pulmonary edema, radiographic consolidation, and hypoxia. Severe PGD consistently occurs in 10% to 20% of all lung transplants according to most reports.[1]

Ischemia-reperfusion injury develops from alveolar cell damage, release of reactive oxygen species, and activation of proinflammatory cytokines.[2] For many years, the lack of a consistent and widely accepted definition of ischemia-reperfusion injury after lung transplantation has hindered systematic correlations with risk factors in multicenter studies and registry analyses. In 2005, a standardized definition of PGD was introduced; it is based on oxygenation and radiologic appearance of the allograft.[3] Once this simple but effective definition was established, various risk factors for the development of PGD were detected. In a multicenter effort, Diamond and associates discovered six independent risk factors for grade 3 PGD: donor smoking history, overweight recipient, sarcoidosis and pulmonary arterial hypertension as underlying diseases, single-lung transplantation, and transplantation after extracorporeal circulation.[1] In a study by Liu and colleagues, female sex, Afro-American race, and underlying diseases such as idiopathic pulmonary fibrosis, sarcoidosis, and idiopathic pulmonary hypertension were identified as risk factors for PGD.[4] With regard to retrieval methods, prolonged cold ischemic time and use of intracellular preservation solution have been recognized as independent risk factors for the development of PGD.[5,6] Because many of these risk factors, and especially most recipient risk factors, simply must be accepted if we wish to perform transplants in such patients, strategies to decrease the overall risk for PGD need to be focused on optimizing retrieval and preservation strategies.

LUNG ASSESSMENT BEFORE RETRIEVAL

During the donor lung retrieval procedure, accurate assessment of the lungs is important. Generally, bronchoscopy is performed to evaluate endobronchial abnormalities and secretions, hemorrhage, or the aspirated foreign material that is occasionally present. In our experience, purulent secretions are frequently found in brain-dead donors even after only short mechanical ventilation times. Purulent endobronchial secretions rarely represent serious pulmonary infection. In the vast majority of donors, endobronchial mucus can be removed by bronchoscopy. In the case of reappearance of purulent secretions after the initial bronchoscopy, macroscopic assessment of the lung parenchyma is necessary for further evaluation. Bronchoalveolar lavage (BAL) fluid should be preserved for microbiologic analysis. However, positive cultures from lung donor BAL fluid do not translate into postoperative infections in lung recipients.[7]

After median sternotomy, the pleural cavities are opened and macroscopic assessment of the lungs is performed. Frequently, lengthy mechanical ventilation, hypoventilation, and supine position of the donor cause atelectasis of dorsal lung areas; in particular, both lower lobes often require active recruitment. While lung recruitment maneuvers are being performing, hemodynamic instability might occur as a result of increased ventilation pressure and concomitant reduced backflow of blood to the heart. Therefore, opening the pericardium and thereby allowing estimation of cardiac function before recruitment is advisable.

Typically, extensive recruitment maneuvers with the thorax opened improve gas exchange, thus leading to considerably increased Pao_2/Fio_2 ratios.

Further inspection and palpation of the lungs are performed to exclude potentially malignant tumors. With regard to the lung parenchyma, it is checked for structural defects such as beginning or established emphysematous tissue alterations or severe inflammatory changes. If impaired oxygenation persists after the recruitment maneuvers, separate analyses of blood gases from each lung vein can further contribute to evaluation of the organ and may be especially useful in cases in which a lobar transplant is being considered.

SURGICAL TECHNIQUE

Flushing the lung with perfusion solution and thereby instituting cold ischemia can be performed from either an antegrade or retrograde direction. Antegrade flushing is performed by cannulating the pulmonary artery, whereas for retrograde flushing, the cannula is inserted into the left atrial appendage. Theoretically, retrograde perfusion leads to a more homogeneous distribution, thus effectively reaching both the perfusion area of the pulmonary artery tree and the area perfused by bronchial arteries. Additionally, retrograde perfusion may clear the pulmonary vasculature bed of the blood clots and occult emboli that are present rather frequently.[8] Experiments examining the use of low-potassium dextran (LPD) solution in pigs suggest that it results in better early postoperative oxygenation, lower airway pressures for mechanical ventilation, and improved lung compliance with retrograde perfusion.[9-11] Also, retrograde perfusion leads to improved postoperative surfactant function in a porcine model.[12]

Thus far, however, no clinical trials prospectively comparing retrograde and antegrade perfusion have been published. Partly because of concern regarding potential damage to the heart during procurement if perfusion pressure in the left atrium is too high, several lung transplant programs have adopted a combined perfusion technique, first performing antegrade flushing through the pulmonary

artery and then retrograde perfusion through each lung vein after retrieval of the heart.[13]

Pulmonary artery vasoconstriction when a hypothermic solution is flushed through the lung is a concern because it potentially causes inhomogeneous distribution of the lung preservation fluid. Porcine experiments in which the preservation solution was supplemented with phosphodiesterase-5 inhibitor found improved pulmonary microcirculation following transplantation.[14] Also in a pig lung transplantation model, primary graft dysfunction and surfactant dysfunction proved to be less severe when prostaglandin E_2 was added to the perfusion solution.[15] Consequently, application of nitroglycerin, prostaglandins, or comparative agents, either directly into the pulmonary artery before flushing or as an additive to the preservation fluid, has become an accepted routine.[13]

In preparation for antegrade lung flushing, the superior vena cava is encircled and the pulmonary artery is cannulated after full heparinization of the donor. Importantly, cannulation of the pulmonary artery should take place at a sufficient distance from the pulmonary valve to ensure competence of the valve while the lung is being flushed as well as antegrade direction of the perfusate flow. However, the cannulation site must also allow for equal distribution of the preservation solution in the left and right lungs to avoid unilateral and therefore heterogeneous perfusion. Before initiation of the lung flushing, the superior vena cava is ligated and the inferior vena cava is incised. For left atrial drainage, the left atrial appendage is opened. In the case of simultaneous heart retrieval, clamping of the ascending aorta is necessary before initiating cardioplegia and then pulmoplegia. During perfusion and the subsequent surgical dissection for retrieval of the lungs, ventilation is continued until clamping of the trachea. A collapse test, which is performed by briefly opening the tracheal clamp, provides information regarding possible airway obstruction of the donor lung. The optimum degree of inflation during cold ischemia is unknown; however, fully collapsed lungs show higher pulmonary vascular resistance and impaired distribution of preservation fluid.[16] In contrast, overinflated lungs may suffer from barotrauma, which could lead to severe ischemia-reperfusion injury.[17] Also, transportation by air might lead to further expansion of the lung parenchyma as a result of barometric pressure differences at great altitudes. Animal models find the optimum inflation status to be 50% of total lung capacity[18] and inflation to be 30 cm H_2O[19] or 75% to 100% of vital capacity[20]; however, the comparability of these different experimental setups is limited owing to their varying perfusion solutions and treatment protocols. Most transplant centers prefer a medium level of inflation because exact volume measurements are difficult to obtain in practice.

STORAGE ON ICE

After retrieval, the lungs are stored in three sterile bags with perfusion solution in the first bag and cold saline in the

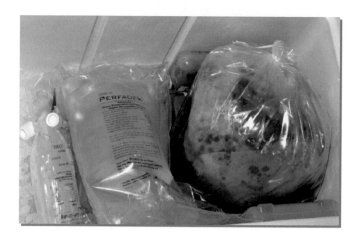

Figure 9.1 Donor lungs in a coolbox ready for transportation.

second bag. The lungs are then placed in a coolbox and typically kept on ice at 4° C during transportation (Figure 9.1). In a rat lung transplantation model, the optimum temperature for lung storage was found to be 10° C; however, other research groups could not confirm these findings and favor storage at 4° C.[21] In clinical practice, aiming for an exact temperature requires extensive technical equipment; consequently, a regular refrigerator with an assumed average temperature of 4° C is used.

PRESERVATION SOLUTION

The ideal choice of lung preservation solution has been a focus of research for decades. Preservation solutions are used to maintain the hypothermic organ in optimal condition from the time of retrieval until reperfusion and rewarming upon implantation. Organ preservation solutions must fulfill several requirements, some of which are very likely organ specific. First, the donor organ has to undergo homogeneous exsanguination to reduce intravascular thrombosis. Second, cell membrane integrity must be maintained to avoid the development of edema. Additionally, hypothermia needs to be established to reduce cellular metabolism.

In the early days of clinical lung transplantation, intracellular lung perfusion solutions such as Euro-Collins (which was originally developed for kidney preservation) or University of Wisconsin solution were routinely used for the preservation of lungs. However, the introduction of extracellular perfusion solutions such as LPD solution (Perfadex) or Celsior solution into lung transplantation led to a marked improvement in lung preservation, which in turn resulted in a significant decrease in ischemia-reperfusion injury and ensuing PGD (Table 9.1). When extracellular preservation solutions were used in animal experiments, more homogeneous lung flushing possibly resulting from less vasoconstriction was observed. Additionally, distinctly

Table 9.1 Composition of the most important lung preservation solutions

	Intracellular perfusion solution	Extracellular perfusion solutions		
	Euro-Collins	LPD	Celsior	HTK
Na^+ (mmol/L)	10	138	100	15
K^+ (mmol/L)	108	6	15	9
Cl^- (mmol/L)	14	142	41.5	
Mg^{2+} (mmol/L)		0.8	13	4
Ca^{2+} (mmol/L)		0.3	0.25	0.015
Glucose (g/L)	35	5		
Ketoglutarate/ glutamic acid (mmol/L)				1
Lactobionate (mmol/L)			80	
Dextran 40 (g/L)		50		
Mannitol (mmol/L)			60	30
Hydroxyethyl starch (g/L)				
SO_4^{2-} (mmol/L)	8	0.8		
HCO_3^- (mmol/L)	8	1		
PO_4^{3-} (mmol/L)	93	0.8		
Histidine (mmol/L)			30	198
Tryptophan (mmol/L)				2
Trometamol (mmol/L)		1		
Glutamic acid (mmol/L)			20	
Glutathione (mmol/L)			3	
pH	7.4	7.4	7.4	7.4
Osmolarity (mOsm/L)	452	335	320	310

less pulmonary edema was present in grafts preserved with LPD solution. This effect is supposedly based on the solutions' low potassium content and on the addition of dextran and glucose.[22] Yamazaki and colleagues proved the superiority of LPD over Euro-Collins solution in a lung reperfusion model involving the use of rabbit lungs; they found better oxygenation and a more favorable wet/dry ratio in the LPD-preserved grafts.[23] Also, in a rat model of flushing and reperfusion in an artificial lung perfusion system, airway resistance and lung compliance were superior in the grafts that were preserved with an extracellular lung perfusion solution such as LPD solution as opposed to several intracellular solutions (namely, Euro-Collins solution and similar substrates).[24] Low-potassium preservation solution was also shown to have a protective effect on lung epithelial cells in a cell culture model in which adult rat alveolar type II cells were exposed to Euro-Collins solution as well as to LPD solution. After exposure to LPD solution, the type II alveolar cells showed intracellular metabolic activity superior to that when exposed to Euro-Collins solution.[25]

In a rabbit lung transplantation model, oxygenation was significantly better for up to 3 days after lung transplantation in the grafts preserved with LPD solution than in those preserved with Euro-Collins solution.[26]

Several retrospective analyses comparing intracellular and extracellular perfusion solution in clinical lung transplantation have been published; thus far, however, no prospective randomized trials have been conducted to our knowledge. The great majority of studies have found improved lung protection when an extracellular-type perfusion solution is used.

Starting in the 1990s, LPD solution (Perfadex) was introduced into clinical lung transplantation. According to a retrospective study by Mueller and colleagues, early postoperative oxygenation was considerably better when LPD solution was used for preservation than when Euro-Collins solution was used; moreover, survival rates at 30 days and 1 year after lung transplantation were also improved.[27] In addition to finding lower overall mortality in the case of LPD-preserved grafts, a retrospective analysis by Strueber and associates also discovered that the recipients of such grafts had significantly shorter mechanical ventilation times and shorter intensive care unit stays. Furthermore, significantly improved early postoperative lung function parameters were found for the LPD-preserved grafts.[28] Similar findings were demonstrated by Fischer and colleagues, who demonstrated significantly better Pao_2/Fio_2 ratios in LPD-preserved lungs, although total ischemic time was significantly longer in the LPD group than in the Euro-Collins group.[29] In another single-center study comparing Euro-Collins ($n = 79$), Papworth ($n = 38$), and LPD ($n = 40$) solutions, no clear advantage of one preservation solution could be detected, but LPD solution tended toward preventing moderate to severe primary graft dysfunction.[30]

As a result of these studies, LPD solution is the worldwide "gold standard" today and has been adopted by most lung transplantation programs.

Celsior solution is another extracellular organ preservation solution; it was first introduced into clinical practice in 1994. Containing mannitol and lactobionate, Celsior solution contains strong osmotic carriers that prevent swelling of cells and therefore the development of pulmonary edema. Additionally, Celsior solution contains glutathione, which is an antioxidant that potentially inhibits injury from oxygen free radicals. Glutathione may be an important component contributing to amelioration of ischemia-reperfusion injury in a porcine model using LPD solution and LPD solution plus glutathione.[31] In animal studies, Celsior solution was superior to LPD solution from the standpoint of postpreservation graft function. In studies involving different models of isolated rat lung perfusion, several groups found that Celsior solution results in significantly better oxygenation capability and less pulmonary microvascular permeability contributing to ischemia-reperfusion injury than do other preservation solutions. Additionally, lung compliance was superior in the Celsior-preserved grafts.[32-34] Experiments in a comparable model then showed that Celsior preservation of rat lungs is superior to preservation with LPD solution when cold ischemic time is prolonged up to 4 hours.[35] In a minipig model of lung ischemia-reperfusion injury comparing Euro-Collins, histidine-tryptophan-ketoglutarate (HTK), and Celsior solutions for preservation, Celsior demonstrated improved oxygenation and reduced pulmonary vascular resistance after reperfusion.[36] In a Landrace pig lung transplantation model, cold preservation of the donor lungs for 24 hours with Celsior solution led to a significantly lower pulmonary vascular resistance index and less sequestration of neutrophils than did preservation with LPD solution.[37] Celsior solution has recently been introduced into clinical practice at several centers; yet no prospective clinical trial comparing Celsior with other lung preservation solutions exist. In addition, in Germany, for example, the manufacturer of Celsior solution had an approved indication for lung transplantation earlier than the manufacturer of LPD solution did, which led to most German centers switching to Celsior solution. A similar development occurred in France earlier.

The volume used for flushing the lungs with cold preservation fluid has not been the subject of clinical trials, but most centers use a perfusion volume of approximately 60 mL/kg, as Haverich and colleagues proposed a long time ago after confirming in a dog model that higher volumes and higher flow rates lead to homogeneous perfusion of the lungs, thereby achieving balanced cooling of all lung lobes.[38]

COLD ISCHEMIC TIME

Reports have described experiments on several animal models in which cold ischemic times exceeding 24 hours have been used.[39-41] In clinical practice, however, cold ischemic times exceeding 10 to 12 hours are rare, with many centers accepting ischemic times no longer than 6 hours. An older analysis of United Network for Organ Sharing (UNOS) data for the period from 1987 to 1997 found no impact on early recipient mortality when the total ischemic time was longer than 7 hours. Nevertheless, in the case of advanced donor age (older than 55 years) and prolonged cold ischemic time, an increased risk for death in recipients was found.[42] An analysis in which donor and recipient factors were examined in 27 pairs of single-lung recipients in which both members of each pair received a single-lung donation from the same donor and underwent transplantation in the same center found no influence of graft ischemic time on post-transplant outcome.[43] Several older reports from the 1990s that evaluated ischemic times longer than 4 or 5 hours did not find any negative effects of prolonged cold ischemic time on postoperative oxygenation, mechanical ventilation time, or survival.[44-46] More importantly, ischemic time is a variable monitored in the International Society for Heart and Lung Transplantation (ISHLT) database. As of 2014, close to 40,000 lung transplants had been entered into the database, and no statistically significant association between ischemic time and important clinical end points, including survival, existed.[47] The only limitation of this database analysis is the fact that very long ischemic times beyond 8 hours are not represented in high numbers, as a result of which the upper cutoff of acceptable ischemic time remains ill defined.

NORMOTHERMIC EX VIVO LUNG PERFUSION

Over the past 10 years EVLP has been developed to tackle the need for methods to evaluate extended criteria donor lungs and lungs obtained via donation after cardiac death. The technology in this field has been exceedingly successful[48] and, as a side note, has suggested that with normothermic perfusion, preservation overall could be similar to or better than that with cold static storage, which is currently the standard of care. Preservation and storage at 4° C remains unphysiologic and detrimental to integrity of the organ, as a result of which avoiding it by performing ex vivo perfusion and ventilation in a normothermic milieu might provide better preservation. Several devices have been developed recently and are currently in clinical use: the OCS Lung (TransMedics, Andover, Massachusetts), the Vivoline LS1 (VivoLine Medical, Lund, Sweden), the Lung Assist (Organ Assist, Groningen, the Netherlands), and the XPS (XVIVO Perfusion AB, Göteborg, Sweden).[49] All share a common principle: donor lungs undergo normothermic perfusion and ventilation. Only one of these commercially available devices, the OCS Lung, is actually portable and thus designed especially for preservation of grafts.[50] When this device is used, cold ischemic time is reduced to only the time immediately following cold flushing in the donor, after which the graft is connected to the device via the pulmonary artery for perfusion and via the trachea for ventilation. The left atrium drains passively into the reservoir. The perfusion solution usually consists of either Steen solution or OCS lung solution enriched with erythrocytes and several additives, including antibiotic agents. After the graft is connected to the device, slow rewarming of the graft is initiated by slowly increasing the temperature of the perfusion solution. Ventilation is started at 34° C and perfusion flow is kept at approximately 1.5 L/min. Continuous monitoring of pulmonary artery pressure and pulmonary vascular resistance allows close surveillance of the graft. For cessation, the perfusion solution can be cooled by using a heat exchanger; alternatively, a second cold flush with LPD solution can be performed. As of 2014, preservation of donor lungs meeting the standard criteria was the subject of an ongoing large prospective, multicenter, randomized trial (INSPIRE Trial NCT01630434), which compared normothermic EVLP with the standard of care, static cold storage, with the primary end point being a composite of PGD at any time in the first 72 hours and hospital mortality. Interim reports of this trial have shown that normothermic perfusion is at the very least not inferior and is showing a trend toward improved outcomes in comparison to those with static cold storage.[51]

REFERENCES

1. Diamond JM, Lee JC, Kawut SM, et al. Clinical risk factors for primary graft dysfunction after lung transplantation. Am J Respir Crit Care Med 2013;187:527-534.
2. Suzuki Y, Cantu E, Christie JD. Primary graft dysfunction. Semin Respir Crit Care Med 2013;34:305-319.
3. Christie JD, Carby M, Bag R, Corris P. ISHLT Working Group on Primary Lung Graft Dysfunction. Report of the ISHLT Working Group on Primary Lung Graft Dysfunction. Part II: Definition. A consensus statement of the International Society for Heart and Lung Transplantation. J Heart Lung Transplant 2005;24:1454-1459.
4. Liu Y, Su L, Jiang SJ. Recipient-related clinical risk factors for primary graft dysfunction after lung transplantation: A systematic review and meta-analysis. PLoS One 2014;9:e92773.
5. Kuntz CL, Hadjiliadis D, Ahya VN, et al. Risk factors for early primary graft dysfunction after lung transplantation: A registry study. Clin Transplant 2009;23:819-830.
6. de Perrot M, Bonser RS, Dark J, et al. Report of the ISHLT Working Group on Primary Lung Graft Dysfunction. Part III: Donor-related risk factors and markers. J Heart Lung Transplant 2005;24:1460-1467.
7. Mattner F, Kola A, Fischer S, et al. Impact of bacterial and fungal donor organ contamination in lung, heart-lung, heart, and liver transplantation. Infection 2008;36:207-212.
8. Ware LB, Fang X, Wang Y, et al. High prevalence of pulmonary arterial thrombi in donor lungs rejected for transplantation. J Heart Lung Transplant 2005;24:1650-1656.
9. Kofidis T, Strüber M, Warnecke G, et al. Antegrade versus retrograde perfusion of the donor lung: Impact on the early reperfusion phase. Transplant 2003;16:801-805.

10. Wittwer T, Franke U, Fehrenbach A, et al. Impact of retrograde graft preservation in Perfadex-based experimental lung transplantation. J Surg Res 2004;117:239-248.

11. Wittwer T, Franke UF, Fehrenbach A, et al. Experimental lung transplantation: Impact of preservation solution and route of delivery. J Heart Lung Transplant 2005;24:1081-1090.

12. Strüber M, Hohlfeld JM, Kofidis T, et al. Surfactant function in lung transplantation after 24 hours of ischemia: Advantage of retrograde flush perfusion for preservation. J Thorac Cardiovasc Surg 2002;123:98-103.

13. Van Raemdonck D, Neyrinck A, Verleden GM, et al. Lung donor selection and management. Proc Am Thorac Soc 2009;6:28-38.

14. Pizanis N, Heckmann J, Wendt D, et al. Improvement of pulmonary microcirculation after lung transplantation using phosphodiesterase-5 inhibitor modified preservation solution. Eur J Cardiothorac Surg 2009;35:801-806.

15. Gohrbandt B, Sommer SP, Fischer S, et al. Iloprost to improve surfactant function in porcine pulmonary grafts stored for twenty-four hours in low-potassium dextran solution. J Thorac Cardiovasc Surg 2005;129:80-86.

16. Baretti R, Bitu-Moreno J, Beyersdorf F, et al. Distribution of lung preservation solutions in parenchyma and airways: Influence of atelectasis and route of delivery. J Heart Lung Transplant 1995;14:80-91.

17. Patel MR, Laubach VE, Tribble CG, Kron IL. Hyperinflation during lung preservation and increased reperfusion injury. J Surg Res 2005;123:134-138.

18. DeCampos KN, Keshavjee S, Liu M, Slutsky AS. Optimal inflation volume for hypothermic preservation of rat lungs. J Heart Lung Transplant 1998;17:599-607.

19. Puskas JD, Hirai T, Christie N, et al. Reliable thirty-hour lung preservation by donor lung hyperinflation. J Thorac Cardiovasc Surg 1992;104:1075-1083.

20. Tanaka Y, Shigemura N, Noda K, et al. Optimal lung inflation techniques in a rat lung transplantation model: A revisit. Thorac Cardiovasc Surg 2014;62:427-433.

21. Munneke AJ, Rakhorst G, Petersen AH, et al. Flush at room temperature followed by storage on ice creates the best lung graft preservation in rats. Transpl Int 2013;26:751-760.

22. Munshi L, Keshavjee S, Cypel M. Donor management and lung preservation for lung transplantation. Lancet Respir Med 2013;1:318-328.

23. Yamazaki F, Yokomise H, Keshavjee SH, et al. The superiority of an extracellular fluid solution over Euro-Collins solution for pulmonary preservation. Transplantation 1990;49:690-694.

24. Sasaki S, McCully JD, Alessandrini F, LoCicero J. Impact of initial flush potassium concentration on the adequacy of lung preservation. J Thorac Cardiovasc Surg 1995;109:1090-1095; discussion 1095-1096.

25. Maccherini M, Keshavjee SH, Slutsky AS, et al. The effect of low-potassium-dextran versus Euro-Collins solution for preservation of isolated type II pneumocytes. Transplantation 1991;52:621-626.

26. Keshavjee SH, Yamazaki F, Cardoso PF, et al. A method for safe twelve-hour pulmonary preservation. J Thorac Cardiovasc Surg 1989;98:529-534.

27. Müller C, Fürst H, Reichenspurner H, et al. Lung procurement by low-potassium dextran and the effect on preservation injury. Munich Lung Transplant Group. Transplantation 1999;68:1139-1143.

28. Strüber M, Wilhelmi M, Harringer W, et al. Flush perfusion with low potassium dextran solution improves early graft function in clinical lung transplantation. Eur J Cardiothorac Surg 2001;19:190-194.

29. Fischer S, Matte-Martyn A, De Perrot M, et al. Low-potassium dextran preservation solution improves lung function after human lung transplantation. J Thorac Cardiovasc Surg 2001;121:594-596.

30. Oto T, Griffiths AP, Rosenfeldt F, et al. Early outcomes comparing Perfadex, Euro-Collins, and Papworth solutions in lung transplantation. Ann Thorac Surg 2006;82:1842-1848.

31. Sommer SP, Gohrbandt B, Fischer S, et al. Glutathione improves the function of porcine pulmonary grafts stored for twenty-four hours in low-potassium dextran solution. J Thorac Cardiovasc Surg 2005;130:864-869.

32. Reignier J, Mazmanian M, Chapelier A, et al. Evaluation of a new preservation solution: Celsior in the isolated rat lung. Paris-Sud University Lung Transplantation Group. J Heart Lung Transplant 1995;14:601-604.

33. Roberts RF, Nishanian GP, Carey JN, et al. A comparison of the new preservation solution Celsior to Euro-Collins and University of Wisconsin solutions in lung reperfusion injury. Transplantation 1999;67:152-155.

34. Xiong L, Legagneux J, Wassef M, et al. Protective effects of Celsior in lung transplantation. J Heart Lung Transplant 1999;18:320-327.

35. Wittwer T, Wahlers T, Fehrenbach A, et al. Improvement of pulmonary preservation with Celsior and Perfadex: Impact of storage time on early post-ischemic lung function. J Heart Lung Transplant 1999;18:1198-1201.

36. Warnecke G, Strüber M, Hohlfeld JM, et al. Pulmonary preservation with Bretscheider's HTK and Celsior solution in minipigs. Eur J Cardiothorac Surg 2002;21:1073-1079.

37. Sommer SP, Warnecke G, Hohlfeld JM, et al. Pulmonary preservation with LPD and Celsior solution in porcine lung transplantation after 24 h of cold ischemia. Eur J Cardiothorac Surg 2004;26:151-157.

38. Haverich A, Aziz S, Scott WC, et al. Improved lung preservation using Euro-Collins solution for flush-perfusion. Thorac Cardiovasc Surg 1986;34:368-376.

39. Yoshida O, Yamane M, Yamamoto S, et al. Impact of prolonged cold preservation on the graft function and gene expression levels in an experimental lung transplantation model. Surg Today 2013;43:81-87.

40. Dedeilias P, Koletsis E, Apostolakis E, et al. The effectiveness of an extracellular low-potassium solution in 24-hour lung graft preservation. Med Sci Monit 2006;12:BR355-BR361.

41. Gohrbandt B, Fischer S, Warnecke G, et al. Glycine intravenous donor preconditioning is superior to glycine supplementation to low-potassium dextran flush preservation and improves graft function in a large animal lung transplantation model after 24 hours of cold ischemia. J Thorac Cardiovasc Surg 2006;131:724-729.

42. Novick RJ, Bennett LE, Meyer DM, Hosenpud JD. Influence of graft ischemic time and donor age on survival after lung transplantation. J Heart Lung Transplant 1999;18:425-431.

43. Sommers KE, Griffith BP, Hardesty RL, Keenan RJ. Early lung allograft function in twin recipients from the same donor: Risk factor analysis. Ann Thorac Surg 1996;62:784-790.

44. Kshettry VR, Kroshus TJ, Burdine J, Savik K. Does donor organ ischemia over four hours affect long-term survival after lung transplantation? J Heart Lung Transplant 1996;15:169-174.

45. Winton TL, Miller JD, deHoyos A, et al. Graft function, airway healing, rejection, and survival in pulmonary transplantation are not affected by graft ischemia in excess of 5 hours. Transplant Proc 1993;25:1649-1650.

46. Glanville AR, Marshman D, Keogh A, et al. Outcome in paired recipients of single lung transplants from the same donor. J Heart Lung Transplant 1995;14:878-882.

47. Yusen RD, Christie JD, Edwards LB, et al. The Registry of the International Society for Heart and Lung Transplantation: Thirtieth adult lung and heart-lung transplant report—2013. J Heart Lung Transplant 2013;32:965-978.

48. Cypel M, Yeung JC, Liu M, et al. Normothermic ex vivo lung perfusion in clinical lung transplantation. N Engl J Med 2011;364:1431-1440.

49. Van Raemdonck D, Neyrinck A, Cypel M, Keshavjee S. Ex-vivo lung perfusion. Transpl Int 2015;28:643-656.

50. Warnecke G, Moradiellos J, Tudorache I, et al. Normothermic perfusion of donor lungs for preservation and assessment with the Organ Care System Lung before bilateral transplantation: A pilot study of 12 patients. Lancet 2012;380:1851-1858.

51. Warnecke G, Van Raemdonck D, Massard G, et al. The INSPIRE Lung International Trial Evaluating the Impact of Portable Ex-Vivo Perfusion Using the Organ Care System (OCS) Lung Technology on Routine Lung Transplant Outcome. Presented at the 34th Annual Meeting of the International Society of Heart and Lung Transplantation, San Diego, CA, April 10-13, 2014.

10

Donor procurement

HASSAN MICHAEL NEMEH AND NATALIE MADOUN

The process of donor procurement includes the final—and possibly most critical—step in evaluation of a lung's suitability for transplantation. A methodical approach should be followed. Clear communication with the teams on site and with the implanting team regarding their needs is crucial. Sharing the estimated time for cross-clamping the donor's aorta and the organ's estimated time of arrival at the recipient hospital helps in timing the procedure on the recipient to minimize the ischemic burden.

INITIAL EVALUATION OF THE DONOR

The evaluation starts with an examination of the medical records to verify the medical history, course of hospitalization, blood test results, brain death note, and consent form for organ donation. Attention is then directed toward confirming blood group compatibility between the donor and recipient. Next is a review of the available chest imaging studies, including a chest radiograph within the last 24 hours to ensure the absence of any significant abnormalities. At this stage a discussion is held with the anesthesia staff to develop a plan for minimizing fluid administration to protect the lungs[1] by keeping central venous pressure at 6 to 8 mm Hg and to also maintain normal ventilation until the end of the procedure.

Flexible bronchoscopy is performed to assess the anatomy for normalcy. Some accumulation of secretions is commonly encountered. Complete clearance of the mucus is performed, and a sample is collected for microbiologic testing. The mucosa is then examined to exclude signs of infection, such as erythema and purulent secretions, which continue to reaccumulate despite proper removal with the bronchoscope. Secretions that clear easily with the bronchoscope, thus revealing normal underlying mucosa, are not significant.[2]

The ventilator is set at a tidal volume between 6 and 8 mL/kg with a positive end-expiratory pressure of 5 cm H_2O and F_{IO_2} of 1.0 to protect the lungs from the barotrauma of the higher tidal volumes that are traditionally recommended.[3-5] An arterial blood sample for blood gas assessment is obtained within 15 to 20 minutes after the bronchoscopy procedure. Peak and mean airway pressures are monitored to ensure normal lung compliance.

The chest is accessed through a standard median sternotomy incision, and the pleural spaces are opened wide to complete the initial evaluation of the lungs. After a visual inspection to exclude emphysema, consolidation, or trauma, the endotracheal tube is quickly disconnected from the ventilator at the end of inspiration; instantaneous deflation of the lungs is observed to confirm normal compliance.[6] While the lungs are being deflated, they are palpated to check for nodules or masses. The lungs are inflated manually to an airway pressure of approximately 20 cm H_2O until atelectasis is completely eliminated, after which the donor is placed back on the ventilator. At the end of this assessment, the recipient team is informed of the adequacy of the lungs and the estimated time of arrival so that the recipient operation can be scheduled to keep ischemia time at 8 hours or less.[7]

The basic principles of the technique detailed in this chapter were well described in the early days of successful lung transplantation[8,9]; however, some modifications have been made to reflect developments in the field over time and our preferences.

At this stage of the procedure we work with the cardiac procurement team on circumferential dissection of the aorta from the pulmonary artery. The superior vena cava is freed at a level just above the azygos vein and encircled with a 0 silk tie. The inferior vena cava is freed circumferentially within the pericardium. The spot at which the cannula will be inserted into pulmonary artery, lines of incision, and the site of left atrial venting are agreed upon with the cardiac team.

CANNULATION AND LUNG PRESERVATION

When the donor and recipient teams are ready to proceed, 300 U/kg heparin is given to the donor as an intravenous bolus.[6] A cannula is inserted into the pulmonary artery with a purse-string suture of 4-0 monofilament that is placed just proximal to the origin of the right pulmonary artery. We prefer to use a 6-mm Sarns Soft-Flow aortic cannula (Terumo, Ann Arbor, Michigan) or an equivalent cannula with a flow-diffusing tip to ensure even distribution of the flush solution to both lungs.

After the cannulas have been inserted, de-aired, and connected, 500 μg prostaglandin E_1 (alprostadil) in a 10-mL syringe is infused into the main pulmonary artery next to the cannula. It serves to dilate the pulmonary vascular bed to improve flushing and has a protective effect against graft dysfunction.[10] An additional 500 μg prostaglandin E_1 is added to the first liter of lung perfusion fluid.

Low-potassium dextran (Perfadex) is used for lung preservation because of its association with a superior outcome.[11-13] The effective dose is 60 mL/kg at a pressure of 10 to 15 mm Hg (high-volume, low-pressure infusion). This pressure can be reached by hanging the Perfadex bag 30 cm above the level of the donor and allowing the solution to flow by gravity. The ideal temperature of the solution is 10° C, but most programs use temperatures between 4° C and 8° C to retain some margin of clinical safety.[14]

The right heart is unloaded by ligation of the superior vena cava and incision of the inferior vena cava anteriorly. High-power suction is applied inside the inferior vena cava opening, the aorta is cross-clamped, and cardioplegia infusion is started. The left heart is vented by resection of the tip of the left atrial appendage and the pulmonary flush is initiated. Alternatively, the left atrium can be vented by opening the level of Sondergaard (Figure 10.1). Cold saline slush is placed in the pleural spaces and around the heart, and ventilation is continued throughout the process until the trachea is stapled shut. The lungs are uniformly cooled mainly by infusing a cold Perfadex flush and maintaining ventilation. The topical cold fluid in the pleural space is usually insulated from the deeper layers of the lung by the air in the lung.

During infusion, the heart is not manipulated but is monitored closely to prevent ventricular distention, which can have a negative impact on the quality of cardiopulmonary flush delivery. The fluid exiting the left atrium is monitored; it should become clear during the course of effective perfusion.

After removal of the lungs from the field, a retrograde flush is performed on the back table with a 14 French self-inflating, balloon-tipped retrograde cardioplegia catheter (Edwards Lifesciences, Irvine, California). A quantity of 250 mL of Perfadex is infused into the orifice of each pulmonary

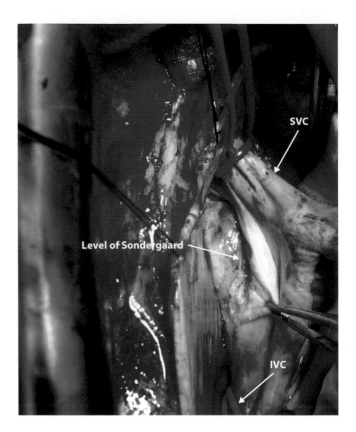

Figure 10.1 The interatrial groove (the level of Sondergaard) dissected before entry into the left atrium. IVC, inferior vena cava; SVC, superior vena cava.

vein, and the effluent is monitored as it exits the pulmonary artery. The infusion is continued until the return is clear (Figure 10.2). Small to medium pulmonary emboli exiting the pulmonary artery during retrograde infusion are very common.[15] The retrograde infusion should be accomplished by gravity to keep the infusion pressure low. The positive effect of retrograde infusion on outcome is evident in both the experimental and the clinical literature.[16-18]

RESECTION

After infusion of the cardiopulmonary flush solution, the field is cleared. The inferior edge of the right inferior pulmonary vein is freed from the soft tissue attachment to the inferior vena cava to prevent injury. The inferior vena cava resection line is completed circumferentially within the pericardium. The apex of the heart is elevated toward the right shoulder to expose the confluence of the left-sided pulmonary veins. The left atrium is entered by using a No. 11 blade at the point halfway between the coronary sinus and the left-sided pulmonary vein confluence (Figure 10.3). This approach leaves enough of a rim of left atrial tissue for both the heart and the lung grafts. Scissors are used to extend the left atrial incision superiorly toward the base of the left atrial appendage, leaving the appendage remaining with the cardiac side of the graft. The incision is then extended inferiorly and across the midline toward the right-sided pulmonary veins. Clear visualization of the right-sided pulmonary vein

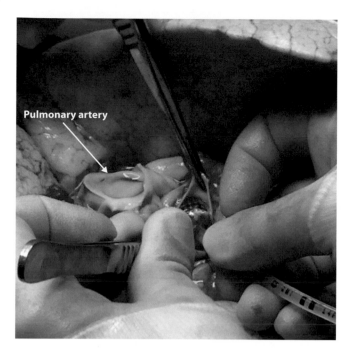

Figure 10.2 Retrograde flush in the orifice of the pulmonary veins. Clear return is noted in the pulmonary artery.

orifices from the inside is critical to guiding the resection so that ample tissue margins are left on both the heart and lung grafts. A rim of 4 to 5 mm on the left atrial cuff is sufficient for the recipient anastomosis. Previous dissection of the level of Sondergaard greatly facilitates this portion of the procurement (see Figure 10.1). Next, the superior aspect

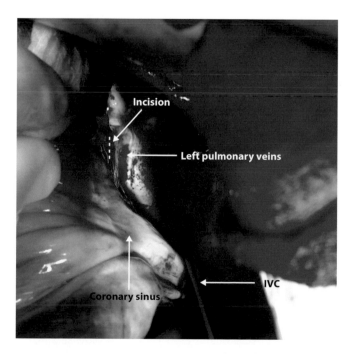

Figure 10.3 The left-sided pulmonary venous confluence as seen with the apex of the donor heart elevated toward the donor's right shoulder. The dotted line depicts the incision line in the left atrium halfway between the veins and the coronary sinus. IVC, inferior vena cava.

of the left atrium (the roof) is incised to complete the left atrial incision.

The pulmonary artery is incised anteriorly at the point of cannulation (just below the bifurcation); the incision is extended circumferentially with clear visualization of the artery from inside to avoid injury to the posterior wall of the bifurcation or unnecessary shortening of the pulmonary artery on the cardiac or pulmonary side. The ascending aorta is transected at the base of the origin of the innominate artery, and the superior vena cava is transected proximal to the tie that was applied at the beginning of the harvest. With the heart removed from the field, the pericardium is incised at the level of the diaphragm down to the level of the inferior pulmonary ligaments on both sides. Care is taken to avoid injury to the opening of the inferior vena cava at the level of the diaphragm. The inferior pulmonary ligaments are taken down to the inferior edges of the inferior pulmonary veins. At this point, each lung is in turn delivered outside the pleural space by medial rotation to expose the posterior aspect of the hilum, and the mediastinal pleura is incised posterior to the hilum (at the level of the aorta on the left and the esophagus on the right) all the way up to the lung apices. On the right side, the dissection is continued very carefully to separate the esophagus from the trachea while avoiding injury to the membranous portion of the trachea.

The innominate vein is transected, and the trachea is exposed anteriorly at the level of the base of the neck. The trachea is mobilized circumferentially and surrounded by umbilical tape. The endotracheal tube is palpated through the trachea to ensure a clear area for application of the stapler. If necessary, the anesthesia staff is asked to pull the tube back slightly. We use a TA 30 stapler with 4.8-mm staples to surround the trachea. The lungs are hand-inflated with 50% F_{IO_2} to eliminate any atelectasis. The lungs are allowed to deflate slightly to near half the volume of total lung capacity to avoid hyperinflation and barotrauma during transport.[14] At this point the stapler is closed and deployed twice. The trachea is transected between the staple lines and mobilized posteriorly all the way down to the carina via blunt and sharp dissection. The pericardium is transected across the midline inferiorly. The remaining soft tissue attachments superior to the pulmonary arteries are incised sharply. When the superior aspect of the left pulmonary artery is being freed, care is taken to avoid injury to the artery at the level of the ligamentum arteriosum. The lung block is carefully removed from the chest and taken to the back table for a retrograde flush as described earlier. To minimize warm ischemia time, we prefer to separate the two lungs and package them separately. The pulmonary artery is transected at the level of the bifurcation ridge, and the left atrium is transected in the center between the left- and right-sided pulmonary venous confluences. The origin of the left main bronchus is exposed and transected at the level of the carina by using a GIA 60 stapler with 4.8-mm staples.

Each lung is placed in a sterile bowel bag with 1 L of cold Perfadex. The bag is tied securely after the air is evacuated (Figure 10.4). The first bag is then placed successively into

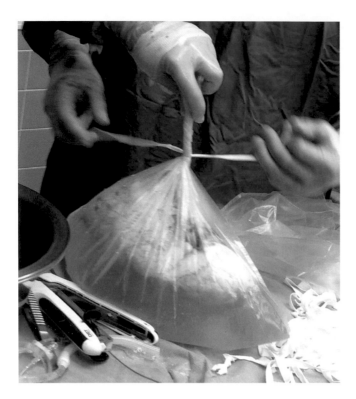

Figure 10.4 The lung bagging process in a Perfadex-filled bowel bag.

two more bowel bags, each of which is filled with cold saline and evacuated of air. The last bag is clearly labeled for laterality and placed inside the ice-filled cooler to keep the temperature of the organ at 4° C to 6° C during transportation.

PITFALL

Occasionally the membranous portion of the trachea can be injured during harvest, which results in deflation of the lungs. To correct this problem, a sterile endotracheal tube is inserted into the trachea below the tear and secured in place by inflation of the balloon, after which the lungs are inflated by an assistant using an Ambu bag connected to 50% FIO_2. Once the desired inflation level is reached, the trachea is clamped below the tube and stapled to keep the lungs inflated.

DONATION AFTER CARDIAC DEATH DONORS

Donation after cardiac death donors are covered in detail elsewhere; however, a few points pertaining to the harvest procedure are worth mentioning here.

The gastric contents of the donor should be thoroughly aspirated via an orogastric or nasogastric tube before removal of the endotracheal tube to reduce the risk for aspiration.

Heparin is usually administered to the donor before extubation. However, in certain institutions this step may not be permitted because it is viewed as an intervention that could hasten the donor's death. If heparin is not given before cardiac death, it can be injected directly into the pulmonary artery at the time of harvest and the heart massaged a few times. Animal experiments suggest that not administering heparin before death does not lead to clotting or have a negative effect on the graft.[18-20] In all other respects, the harvest procedure can follow the technique already described.

REFERENCES

1. Tuttle-Newhall JE, Collins BH, Kuo PC, Schoeder R. Organ donation and treatment of the multi-organ donor. Curr Probl Surg 2003;40:266-310.
2. Botha P, Rostron AJ, Fisher AJ, Dark JH. Current strategies in donor selection and management. Semin Thorac Cardiovasc Surg 2008;20:143-151.
3. Ventilation with lower tidal volumes as compared with traditional tidal volumes for acute lung injury and the acute respiratory distress syndrome. The Acute Respiratory Distress Syndrome Network. N Engl J Med 2000;342:1301-1308.
4. Determann RM, Royakkers A, Wolthuis EK, et al. Ventilation with lower tidal volumes as compared with conventional tidal volumes for patients without acute lung injury: A preventive randomized controlled trial. Crit Care 2010;14:R1.
5. Mascia L, Pasero D, Slutsky AS, et al. Effect of a lung protective strategy for organ donors on eligibility and availability of lungs for transplantation: A randomized controlled trial. JAMA 2010;304:2620-2627.
6. Puri V, Patterson GA. Adult lung transplantation: Technical considerations. Semin Thorac Cardiovasc Surg 2008;20:152-164.
7. Hartwig MG, Davis RD. Surgical considerations in lung transplantation: Transplant operation and early postoperative management. Respir Care Clin N Am 2004;10:473-504.
8. Sundaresan S, Trachiotis GD, Aoe M, et al. Donor lung procurement: Assessment and operative technique. Ann Thorac Surg 1993;56:1409-1413.
9. Todd TR, Goldberg M, Koshal A, et al. Separate extraction of cardiac and pulmonary grafts from a single organ donor. Ann Thorac Surg 1988;46:356-359.
10. de Perrot M, Fischer S, Liu M, et al. Prostaglandin E_1 protects lung transplants from ischemia-reperfusion injury: A shift from pro- to anti-inflammatory cytokines. Transplantation 2001;72:1505-1512.
11. Ganesh JS, Rogers CA, Banner NR, et al. Does the method of lung preservation influence outcome after transplantation? An analysis of 681 consecutive procedures. J Thorac Cardiovasc Surg 2007;134:1313-1321.
12. Muller C, Furst H, Reichenspurner H, et al. Lung procurement by low-potassium dextran and the effect on preservation injury. Munich Lung Transplant Group. Transplantation 1999;68:1139-1143.

13. Wu M, Yang Q, Yim AP, et al. Cellular electrophysiologic and mechanical evidence of superior vascular protection in pulmonary microcirculation by Perfadex compared with Celsior. J Thorac Cardiovasc Surg 2009;137:492-498.

14. Munshi L, Keshavjee S, Cypel M. Donor management and lung preservation for lung transplantation. Lancet Respir Med 2013;1:318-328.

15. Oto T, Rabinov M, Griffiths AP, et al. Unexpected donor pulmonary embolism affects early outcomes after lung transplantation: A major mechanism of primary graft failure? J Thorac Cardiovasc Surg 2005;130:1446.

16. Novick RJ. Innovative techniques to enhance lung preservation. J Thorac Cardiovasc Surg 2002;123:3-5.

17. Sarsam MA, Yonan NA, Deiraniya AK, et al. Retrograde pulmonaryplegia for lung preservation in clinical transplantation: A new technique. J Heart Lung Transplant 1993;12:494-498.

18. Van De Wauwer C, Neyrinck AP, Rega FR, et al. Retrograde flush is more protective than heparin in the uncontrolled donation after circulatory death lung donor. J Surg Res 2014;187:316-323.

19. Erasmus ME, Fernhout MH, Elstrodt JM, Rakhorst G. Normothermic ex vivo lung perfusion of non–heart-beating donor lungs in pigs: From pretransplant function analysis towards a 6-h machine preservation. Transpl Int 2006;19:589-593.

20. Keshava HB, Farver CF, Brown CR, et al. Timing of heparin and thrombus formation in donor lungs after cardiac death. Thorac Cardiovasc Surg 2013;61:246-250.

11

Ex vivo lung perfusion

THORSTEN KRUEGER, MARCELO CYPEL, AND SHAF KESHAVJEE

INTRODUCTION

The shortage of lungs available for lung transplantation is to a great extent a result of the low acceptance rate of potential donor lungs; it is known to be one of the limiting factors of the surgical treatment of end-stage lung disease. In the past, donor lung injury resulting from neurogenic pulmonary edema following brain death, pneumonia, aspiration of gastric contents, or trauma made up to 80% of lungs from multiorgan donors unusable.[1] Different strategies have been developed to expand the number of suitable donor lungs used for transplantation. Whereas approaches such as donation after cardiac death or living donor lobar donation[2-5] allow an increase in the pool of potential donors, ex vivo lung perfusion (EVLP) aims for more efficient use of lungs from the existing pool, thereby offering a chance to expand the pool through the use of lungs that had been turned down in the past.

Normothermic EVLP maintains the donor lung in physiologic condition after procurement. As a result, cell metabolism in the graft is preserved, which allows assessing and regenerating the lung before transplantation. The technique requires an EVLP system and a ventilator.

From a historical perspective, successful ex vivo perfusion of isolated organs at body temperature was first reported in the third decade of the last century.[6] This pioneering work was followed by the development of experimental isolated organ perfusion systems that later became key tools for research in physiology.[7] The use of ex vivo perfusion to assess the function of lungs[8] was described in 1970, and its first application for organ preservation after procurement was reported in 1987.[9] In 2001 Steen revisited the technique of clinical EVLP as a tool for pretransplant assessment of lungs obtained via donation after cardiac death (DCD).[10]

This chapter focuses on the technical aspects, current clinical applications, and results of EVLP.

CLINICAL USE OF EX VIVO LUNG PERFUSION

Functional assessment of the lung

EVLP has significant potential to improve the assessment of donor lungs. Without EVLP, evaluation of the lung is limited to the period from the donor's brain death to procurement; it can be greatly influenced by the experience and clinical judgment of the retrieval team, the therapeutic management of the donor at the remote hospital, and the ongoing inflammatory processes and hemodynamic instability induced by brain death in the donor. The difficulty of determining a lung's suitability for transplantation on the basis of donor clinical parameters is well demonstrated by the fact that significant primary graft dysfunction (PGD) will develop in up to 20% of grafts even when established, relatively conservative donor lung selection criteria have been applied.[11,12] On the other hand, lungs that are frequently considered unusable would probably be appropriate for transplantation.

Evaluation of donor lungs in the EVLP system appears to be more reliable for the following reasons: lung function can be assessed repeatedly over several hours, the preset perfusion and ventilation parameters during the assessment are well defined and constant, brain death–related effects are not present ex vivo, and a more detailed lung assessment can be performed by the transplant surgeon together with the team.

Once the donor lung has arrived at the transplant center, cold ischemic preservation is interrupted and the lung is mounted in the EVLP circuit, after which an initial phase of progressive reperfusion, warming, and reventilation of the graft is begun (Figure 11.1). Next, with steady-state conditions, suitability for transplantation can be determined by assessing various parameters, such as lung compliance and airway pressure, oxygenation, pulmonary artery and left atrial pressure, and pulmonary vascular resistance. After lung mechanics and hemodynamics have been evaluated, the lung's oxygenation capacity is determined by measuring the difference between Pao_2 in the effluent (pulmonary veins or left atrium) and in the inflow perfusion solution (pulmonary artery). These measurements need to be performed repeatedly with the pulmonary perfusion, flow, and ventilatory parameters set according to the EVLP protocol being applied. After these measurements have been completed, the graft is palpated to identify parenchymal abnormalities, endobronchial status is assessed by bronchoscopy, and radiographs are obtained.

The decision whether a lung can be accepted or needs to be declined is based on the trend of the aforementioned parameters over 4 to 6 hours of EVLP. So far, no single individual parameter to indicate suitability for transplantation has been identified. According to the Toronto EVLP protocol, a lung will be declined if the Pao_2/Fio_2 ratio is less than 400 mm Hg after 4 to 6 hours of perfusion or if pulmonary artery pressure, compliance, or peak airway pressure worsen more than 15% during EVLP; conversely, lungs are accepted with a Pao_2/Fio_2 ratio higher than 400 mm Hg, stable or decreasing pulmonary artery and peak airway pressure, and stable or improving compliance.[13] Importantly, some deviation from the aforementioned criteria can occur when one of the two lungs has a significantly different appearance during EVLP. In this case, careful assessment of the lung radiograph, bronchoscopy findings, and results of the selective pulmonary vein gas analyses and the deflation test should be performed to determine the suitability of a single lung for transplantation. Obviously, the use of EVLP for assessment of donor lungs is of particular interest in cases in which the risk for unidentified graft damage is high, such as in the case of lungs not fulfilling standard International Society for Heart and Lung Transplantation (ISHLT) criteria for transplant suitability or lungs obtained as a result of DCD. A more reliable graft evaluation is performed to help decrease the incidence of PGD and early and late mortality in such situations.[14] Whether EVLP should be used routinely with controlled DCD donors is currently being debated. Experimental studies have shown that EVLP has at least the potential to determine the quality and suitability of DCD lungs before transplantation.[15-18] However, most centers still practice selective use of EVLP for DCD donors.

Regeneration, repair, and preparation for transplantation

The preserved cell metabolism in donor lungs during normothermic EVLP allows more than functional tests. More importantly, EVLP presents the opportunity to treat or repair common donor lung injuries.

Thus far, EVLP has been shown to assist in treating typical donor lung injuries in the clinical setting, such as neurogenic edema related to brain death, atelectasis, and pulmonary embolism.[19,20] In the future, pneumonitis secondary to aspiration of gastric contents and bacterial infection may become targets of such treatment. Experimental data also indicate that EVLP may be useful in preparing a graft for the events following transplantation, for example, to prime the graft for ischemia and blood reperfusion or to modulate the recipient's immune response to the graft.[21-23]

EVLP can be used as a therapeutic platform for administering drugs into the airways and pulmonary vessels. The perfusate itself has therapeutic properties permitting treatment of lung edema: because of the optimized oncotic pressure of the perfusate fluid, interstitial fluid is eliminated from the donor lung during EVLP. Adequate perfusion and ventilation also stimulate clearance of alveolar fluid.

Multiple pharmacologic interventions involving adding drugs to the perfusate have been evaluated in clinical and experimental settings; such drugs include anti-infective drugs,[24] anti-inflammatory drugs such as steroids or cytokine scavengers,[25] gene therapy agents,[19] antioxidant drugs,[26] vasodilators, bronchodilators,[27] surfactants,[28,29] and fibrinolytics.[30] Because these agents are applied to an isolated organ rather than to the whole organism, the drug doses used are

Toronto Ex Vivo Lung Perfusion (EVLP) system

Gas for deoxygenation
86% N_2, 8% CO_2, 6% O_2

Red: Venous (oxygenated) perfusate
Blue: Arterial (deoxygenated) perfusate
Perfusate: Acellular Steen solution

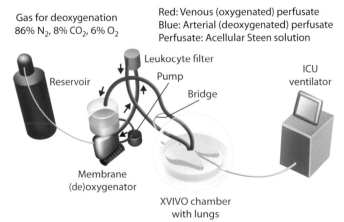

Reservoir
Leukocyte filter
Pump
Bridge
ICU ventilator
Membrane (de)oxygenator
XVIVO chamber with lungs

Ventilator Perfusion: 40% CO
Ventilation: 7cc/kg, 7 BPM, PEEP 5, FiO_2 = 21%

Figure 11.1 Essential components of the Toronto ex vivo lung perfusion system.

limited only by direct tissue toxicities and not by systemic adverse effects. Drugs can be administered repeatedly. However, potential therapies and treatment targets are limited by the maximal duration of EVLP. For instance, resolution of an established bacterial pneumonia will probably require prolonged ex vivo anti-infective therapy.

In addition to allowing these drug-mediated therapeutic interventions, EVLP provides the ability to perform pulmonary endoscopy to clear bronchial secretions and facilitate proper recruitment maneuvers in the case of atelectasis, thereby improving function and ventilation-perfusion matching of the potential grafts.

Finally, the EVLP procedure may be modified to have a dialysis function: integrating a filter into the system could serve to remove mediators of inflammation.

As already mentioned, EVLP may also prepare the graft for adverse events following lung transplantation, such as ischemia-reperfusion injury or rejection. Limited clinical data support this hypothesis.[31] It is expected that in the future EVLP will be able to decrease the incidence of PGD and chronic allograft dysfunction. This decrease may occur by several mechanisms, including by "washing" the graft free of donor white blood cells and cytokines. Alternatively, preconditioning could be promoted by an active approach through therapeutic intervention. The ex vivo administration of mesenchymal stem cells to lung allografts to exploit their therapeutic properties in the context of lung injury has attracted major interest.[32-34] Similarly, ex vivo gene therapy for immunologic preparation of grafts would be another promising strategy.[19]

Lung preservation

Normothermic EVLP can be applied to allow longer total graft preservation times. With conventional cold static preservation, cell metabolism is reduced, the lung's substrate need is diminished, and total preservation times are limited to 12 hours[35]; however, most clinical programs limit the preservation time to less than 6 to 10 hours.[13,36,37] Pig studies have shown that EVLP can be performed safely for up to 12 hours and that doing so prevents lung injury (as occurs with extended cold preservation).[38] When EVLP is used, the total preservation time is fractioned into a first cold ischemic preservation time (CIT_1), the normothermic preservation time (EVLP), and a second cold ischemic preservation time (CIT_2). Total preservation times up to 25 hours, including 5 hours of normothermic preservation, have been reported as being safe in patients. Interestingly, a total cold ischemic time (CIT_1 plus CIT_2) of up to 20 hours was shown to have no influence on graft function and posttransplant outcome in the clinical application of EVLP.[39] Thus, whether prolonged preservation is best carried out with continuous normothermic EVLP or whether the cold ischemic preservation simply can be interrupted by rejuvenating periods of EVLP is open to debate.

In the future, EVLP may help overcome the current restrictions related to graft preservation times (such as the maximal acceptable travel time from harvest to transplant center or the need to perform the transplantation within a very limited time frame after procurement), thereby facilitating the logistics of lung transplantation.

TECHNICAL ASPECTS

General considerations

Maintenance of lung tissue metabolism is the main principle of normothermic EVLP. This requires ventilation and perfusion of the organ. After the donor lung has been retrieved in the standard manner, it is stored at 4° C, transported to the transplant center, and then mounted in the EVLP circuit. Alternatively, the lung can be mounted in a mobile EVLP device immediately after the cold flush and before transport.

EVLP requires a perfusion circuit with the following elements: an organ chamber to create a protective environment for the graft during perfusion, a pump to drive the perfusate, a reservoir and tubing containing the perfusion solution, a gas exchange membrane to supply the circuit with a gas mixture to remove oxygen and add carbon dioxide, a heat exchanger for temperature control, and a filter to continuously remove white blood cells. To mount the lung in the perfusion circuit the system is primed with the perfusion solution, a straight cannula is inserted in the pulmonary artery, and a funnel-shaped cannula is sutured to the left atrium. The resultant closed circuit of lung and perfusion system allows control of pulmonary artery and left atrial pressure during perfusion. Alternatively, some systems use an "open" circuit,[40] in which the influent enters the graft through a cannula placed in the pulmonary artery and the effluent runs out from the open left atrium and is then collected from the surface below the organ. With both systems the perfusate flows from the lung to a reservoir and then to the gas and heat exchange system and the leukocyte filter before reentering the lung. To ventilate the lung, a standard single-lumen tube is inserted into the trachea and connected to a standard intensive care unit (ICU) ventilator.

Instead of the component setup of the EVLP circuit with equipment from extracorporeal life support systems, a number of EVLP devices have been developed and are commercially available (see later). Their potential advantages are their simplified setup, the fact that they provide a ready-to-use solution, and reduced personnel requirements. Their disadvantages are their cost, which is particularly relevant for smaller transplant centers, and their rigid technology, which does not allow adoption of anticipated refinements of EVLP.

Since the report on the clinical results of the Toronto EVLP technique,[41] investigations of two other EVLP protocols have been undertaken. Common aspects of and differences in these approaches are discussed in the following section.

The Toronto technique of ex vivo lung perfusion

Most cases from series in the literature describe the outcome of EVLP based on the Toronto technique, which can be considered the best-evaluated approach to date.[42-45] Once the pulmonary artery and left atrial cannulas and an endotracheal tube have been inserted into the lung, it is connected to the primed perfusion circuit and its vascular system is de-aired. The lung is then connected to the ventilator in a semi-inflated state. The perfusion is performed with an extracellular solution complemented with dextran and albumin to achieve optimal rheologic properties and high colloid pressure (Steen Solution, XVIVO, Denver, Colorado). Antibiotics and steroids are added. The inflow Pco_2 is corrected by controlling the CO_2 supply through the gas exchange membrane. Perfusion is initiated slowly, the graft is warmed progressively, the flow is increased gradually, and ventilation is started when the circuit reaches a temperature of 32° C. The respiratory rate is 7 breaths per minute, tidal volume is 7 mL/kg, positive end-expiratory pressure (PEEP) is 5 cm H_2O, and Fio_2 is 21%. When lung temperature reaches 37° C, the perfusion flow is increased to a maximum of 40% of the cardiac output calculated on the basis of the donor's ideal body weight. Left atrial pressure is set at 3 to 5 mm Hg; pulmonary artery pressure is monitored and depends on the vascular resistance of the lung and the preset flow. In general, clinical EVLP is performed for a period of 4 to 6 hours and the graft is cooled down and preserved at 4° C until implantation.

The Toronto technique of EVLP requires assembly of the components of the perfusion system as described earlier. It can also be approximated by using the commercially available XPS device (XVIVO Perfusion, Göteborg, Sweden), which includes all the components of the aforementioned perfusion circuit, a ventilator, a reservoir for gas supply, and a pressure and flow control unit.

The Lund technique of ex vivo lung perfusion

Steen was the first to use EVLP for the assessment of DCD donor lungs in clinical lung transplantation. The lungs of a Maastricht Category II donor were assessed during 1 hour of EVLP, and a single lung was transplanted successfully.[46] In contrast to the Toronto technique, the Lund protocol uses a cellular perfusate consisting of Steen solution with red blood cells added to obtain a hematocrit of 15%. The underlying intent was to come closer to the properties of blood and improve assessment of gas exchange capacity during EVLP (because oxygen will bind to the hemoglobin). An important difference is that with the Lund procedure, the lung is not entirely connected to the circuit and the effluent perfusate runs out from the left atrium into a plastic dish before being recirculated. Thus, sewing a cannula to the left atrium is not necessary. This so-called open circuit does not permit control and maintenance of a physiologic left atrial pressure. The flow is set higher, at 100% of cardiac output. Fio_2 is 50%, the respiratory rate is 20 breaths per minute, tidal volume is 7 mL/kg body weight, and the PEEP value is 5 cm H_2O.

The principles of the Lund protocol were used to construct the commercially available Vivoline LS1 device (Vivoline Medical, Lund, Sweden). It is a stationary device with an integrated perfusion circuit but no ventilator, and it allows the operator to set and measure perfusion flow and temperature, as well as to monitor pulmonary artery pressure.

The Organ Care System

The third EVLP technique is based on the presumption that EVLP must be started as early as possible after lung retrieval to avoid exposure to cold. For this reason, a transportable EVLP device called the OCS lung (Organ Care System lung, TransMedics, Andover, Massachusetts) was developed. It allows EVLP during transport of an organ from the procurement center to the transplant center. The system's batteries give it energy autonomy; another of its unique features is that the integrated roller pump is able to create a pulsatile-like flow of perfusate.

The perfusion procedure and ventilatory settings are quite similar to those of the Lund protocol. The OCS lung uses an "open" circuit. The cellular perfusate recommended for use with the system contains red blood cells with a hematocrit up to 25%, but in contrast to Steen solution, the OCS solution (TransMedics, Andover, Massachusetts) does not contain human albumin. The perfusion flow rate is 2.5 L/min, with pulmonary artery pressure set below 20 mm Hg. Tidal volume is 6 mL/kg body weight, the respiratory rate is 10 breaths per minute, and the PEEP value is 5 cm H_2O.

The potential advantages of this system are that it allows early recruitment of the graft after cold flushing and continuous monitoring of the graft's function during transport. Its drawbacks are the complexity of the system during transport, in particular during air travel, and its cost in comparison to that of other marketed solutions. In contrast to the underlying hypothesis about the beneficial effect of immediate normothermic EVLP, studies have shown that cold ischemic preservation before EVLP may actually have a beneficial effect on posttransplant lung function[47] and that varying the length of cold static preservation from 6 to 20 hours, if followed by 4 to 5 hours of EVLP according to the Toronto protocol, has no influence on short-term outcome after clinical lung transplantation.[39]

All the aforementioned techniques and concepts have the common intent of keeping the potential graft in a protective environment that allows preservation, assessment, and reconditioning of the lung without harming it. No comparative studies of the different approaches have been performed.

RESULTS OF CLINICAL EX VIVO LUNG PERFUSION

The Toronto protocol

To date, 15 single-center and multicenter case series examining clinical EVLP have been published since the first report of the Lund group in 2001, with 8 groups reporting their results of using the Toronto technique (Toronto,[42] Vienna,[43] Paris,[48] Newcastle,[49] Harefield,[45,50] Madrid,[51] Turin[44]) or a modified Toronto technique (Milan[52]), 3 groups describing their results with the Lund protocol (Lund,[40] Göteborg,[53] Brisbane[54]), and 1 report from Hannover and Madrid on use of the OCS approach.[55]

After extensive preclinical work to establish the technique of prolonged normothermic EVLP involving a closed circuit and an acellular perfusate, the Toronto group published (in 2011 and 2012) the results of a prospective nonrandomized trial of clinical EVLP.[41,42] Fifty-eight EVLP procedures were performed to assess and recondition high-risk donor lungs and resulted in 50 lung transplants (86% utilization rate). Lungs were selected for transplantation on the basis of improved physiologic function, including compliance and airway pressure, as well as improved oxygenation capacity and pulmonary vascular resistance. The incidence of grade 3 PGD was 2% in the EVLP group as opposed to 9% in a control group of 253 conventional transplants ($P < .14$). No adverse effects related to EVLP were found, outcomes (ICU stay, mechanical ventilation, or hospital stay) did not differ, 30-day mortality rates were 3.5% and 4% (EVLP), and 1-year survival rates were 86% and 87% (EVLP), respectively.

Aigner and colleagues from Vienna reported 13 EVLP procedures in which the Toronto protocol was used with donor lungs that were initially unacceptable.[43] Four lungs with traumatic injury did not improve in the circuit; all the other nine lungs were transplanted after EVLP (100% use of high-risk lungs without trauma, 69% use of all lungs) with no grade 3 PGD and no 30-day mortality. All the secondary study end points were similar to those of the 119 conventional transplants performed during the same period.

The Harefield experience with the Toronto EVLP-based protocol was reported in 2012, at which time it consisted of 13 EVLP procedures. Of 13 marginal donor lungs, 6 were used for transplantation after a mean of 140 minutes of EVLP (46%). Short-term survival was excellent (a rate of 100% at 3 months). The rate of PGD from this study is not known.[45]

The Turin group perfused 11 lungs that were initially considered unsuitable according to the Toronto protocol, with 8 of the lungs subsequently being transplanted (73%). Grade 3 PGD was not present in any of the reconditioned grafts at 72 hours, but it was present in 25% of the 28 conventional grafts transplanted during the same period (not significant).[44]

Dark and colleagues reported on a series of 18 donor lungs (4 single and 14 bilateral) that had been deemed unusable for immediate transplantation. In this study only 39% of the lungs (7) were used for transplantation after the group's modified EVLP technique, with one case of grade 3 PGD at 72 hours. The 90-day survival rate was 100%.[49]

Further results with the Toronto technique were presented by Sage from Paris (32 EVLPs) and by the group in Madrid (8 EVLPs).[48,51] The rate of conversion to transplantable lungs was 95% in the first center and 50% in the second; rates of PGD 72 hours after transplantation were 10 % and 0%, and survival rates at 30 days were 95% and 100%, respectively.

From these different series that include more than 150 EVLP procedures, it can be concluded that the Toronto approach is safe for assessment and reconditioning of extended criteria donor lungs with a rate of conversion to transplantable lungs of up to 90%, a similar or even lower incidence of severe PGD, and early outcomes in terms of survival and morbidity similar to those with conventional transplanted lungs.

The Lund protocol

Steen is to be recognized for pioneering the introduction of EVLP into clinical lung transplantation in the modern era. He performed the first clinical transplant of a lung that was obtained by DCD and deemed transplantable after short-term EVLP with an open circuit and a cellular perfusate.[10] He was also the first to report assessment by EVLP and subsequent transplantation of an initially unacceptable donor lung.[16] These case reports were preceded by the development of Steen solution (XVIVO Perfusion, Sweden) in experimental studies.

In 2009 and 2011 the Lund group published its experience with six lung transplants involving reconditioned grafts that were initially considered unusable for transplantation.[40,56] The rate of their conversion to transplantable lungs after EVLP was 66%. The rate of PGD is not specified; however, the survival rate was 100% at 3 months and 66% at 2 years. Postoperative outcomes did not differ from those of the 15 patients who received a conventional transplant during the same period.

The Lund approach of short-term open-circuit EVLP with cellular perfusate was also assessed by the Göteborg group and reported in publications in 2012 and 2014.[53] Eleven pairs of lungs were subjected to EVLP, and all but two single lungs were subsequently considered transplantable. After transplantation, the rate of grade 3 PGD at 72 hours was 9%; the median time to extubation and length of ICU stay were actually significantly longer in the EVLP group than in the group of patients undergoing transplantation with conventional grafts at the same institution during the same time. The 30-day survival rate was 100%.

Additional information on the Lund approach is available from Hopkins and colleagues in Brisbane. They transplanted four of five lungs subjected to EVLP according to the Lund protocol (80% utilization rate). No PGD was observed at 72 hours, and the 30-day survival rate was 100%.[54]

The Organ Care System approach

The transportable OCS has been reported to be a safe and feasible preservation approach for donor lungs fulfilling the standard criteria for transplantation. One clinical study of the system has been published so far: Instead of being transported under conditions of cold static preservation, 12 standard criteria lungs were transported from the procurement site to the transplant center under normothermic conditions.[55] Short-term outcomes were similar to those of the controls. The device's capacity to recondition damaged grafts has not been proven thus far but is under investigation in the EXPAND trial.[57]

Several randomized and nonrandomized trials are currently examining the role of EVLP; in particular, various commercially available EVLP devices are being tested. The primary end points are 30-day mortality, PGD, and 1-year survival rate. The results are pending. The NOVEL trial is a prospective nonrandomized multicenter trial in which standard criteria lungs are being compared with extended criteria lungs that have been reconditioned according to the Toronto protocol by using the XPS EVLP device.[58] The DEVELOP-UK trial is a prospective nonrandomized multicenter trial that is assessing the Lund protocol and the Vivoline device.[59] The aim of both the INSPIRE and EXPAND trials is to evaluate the OCS device; the first trial is comparing static preservation with normothermic preservation in standard criteria lungs, and the second is examining the value of this device for reconditioning of extended criteria grafts.[57,60]

CONCLUSION

EVLP is an important tool for overcoming the shortage of grafts available for lung transplantation. It has been shown to increase the utilization rate of donor lungs by different means: normothermic EVLP permits more detailed and accurate donor lung assessment, as well as reconditioning or preservation of potential grafts. In the future it may serve as a unique treatment platform for advanced ex vivo therapies, either to repair common donor lung injuries or to prepare the graft for posttransplantation events, such as ischemia-reperfusion injury or rejection.

REFERENCES

1. Yeung JC, Cypel M, Waddell TK, et al. Update on donor assessment, resuscitation, and acceptance criteria, including novel techniques—non–heart-beating donor lung retrieval and ex vivo donor lung perfusion. Thorac Surg Clin 2009;19:261-274.
2. Date H. Update on living-donor lobar lung transplantation. Curr Opin Organ Transplant 2011;16:453-457.
3. Cypel M, Keshavjee S. Expanding lung donation: The use of uncontrolled non–heart beating donors. Eur J Cardiothorac Surg 2013;43:419-420.
4. Cypel M, Keshavjee S. Strategies for safe donor expansion: Donor management, donations after cardiac death, ex-vivo lung perfusion. Curr Opin Organ Transplant 2013;18(5):513-517.
5. Cypel M, Sato M, Yildirim E, et al. Initial experience with lung donation after cardiocirculatory death in Canada. J Heart Lung Transplant 2009;28:753-758.
6. Carrel A, Lindbergh CA. The culture of whole organs. Science 1935;81:621-623.
7. Lochner W, Bartels H, Beer R, et al. [Research on gas exchange in an isolated dog's lung lobe during blood perfusion.] Pflugers Arch 1957;264:294-305.
8. Jirsch DW, Fisk RL, Couves CM. Ex vivo evaluation of stored lungs. Ann Thorac Surg 1970;10:163-168.
9. Hardesty RL, Griffith BP. Autoperfusion of the heart and lungs for preservation during distant procurement. J Thorac Cardiovasc Surg 1987;93:11-18.
10. Steen S, Sjoberg T, Pierre L, et al. Transplantation of lungs from a non–heart-beating donor. Lancet 2001;357:825-829.
11. Angel LF, Levine DJ, Restrepo MI, et al. Impact of a lung transplantation donor-management protocol on lung donation and recipient outcomes. Am J Respir Crit Care Med 2006;174:710-716.
12. Naik PM, Angel LF. Special issues in the management and selection of the donor for lung transplantation. Semin Immunopathol 2011;33:201-210.
13. Machuca TN, Cypel M, Keshavjee S. Advances in lung preservation. Surg Clin North Am 2013;93:1373-1394.
14. Gomez-de-Antonio D, Campo-Canaveral JL, Crowley S, et al. Clinical lung transplantation from uncontrolled non–heart-beating donors revisited. J Heart Lung Transplant 2012;31:349-353.
15. Snell GI, Oto T, Levvey B, et al. Evaluation of techniques for lung transplantation following donation after cardiac death. Ann Thorac Surg 2006;81:2014-2019.
16. Steen S, Liao Q, Wierup PN, et al. Transplantation of lungs from non–heart-beating donors after functional assessment ex vivo. Ann Thorac Surg 2003;76:244-252; discussion 252.
17. Neyrinck AP, Van De Wauwer C, Geudens N, et al. Comparative study of donor lung injury in heart-beating versus non–heart-beating donors. Eur J Cardiothorac Surg 2006;30:628-636.
18. Egan TM, Haithcock JA, Nicotra WA, et al. Ex vivo evaluation of human lungs for transplant suitability. Ann Thorac Surg 2006;81:1205-1213.
19. Cypel M, Liu M, Rubacha M, et al. Functional repair of human donor lungs by IL-10 gene therapy. Sci Transl Med 2009;1:4ra9.
20. Machuca TN, Hsin MK, Ott HC, et al. Injury-specific ex vivo treatment of the donor lung: Pulmonary thrombolysis followed by successful lung transplantation. Am J Respir Crit Care Med 2013;188:878-880.

21. Ott HC, Clippinger B, Conrad C, et al. Regeneration and orthotopic transplantation of a bioartificial lung. Nat Med 2010;16:927-933.

22. Song JJ, Kim SS, Liu Z, et al. Enhanced in vivo function of bioartificial lungs in rats. Ann Thorac Surg 2011;92:998-1005; discussion 1006.

23. Yeung JC, Wagnetz D, Cypel M, et al. Ex vivo adenoviral vector gene delivery results in decreased vector-associated inflammation pre– and post–lung transplantation in the pig. Mol Ther 2012;20:1204-1211.

24. Andreasson A, Karamanou DM, Perry JD, et al. The effect of ex vivo lung perfusion on microbial load in human donor lungs. J Heart Lung Transplant 2014;33:910-916.

25. Meers CM, Wauters S, Verbeken E, et al. Preemptive therapy with steroids but not macrolides improves gas exchange in caustic-injured donor lungs. J Surg Res 2011;170:e141–e148.

26. Rega FR, Wuyts WA, Vanaudenaerde BM, et al. Nebulized N-acetyl cysteine protects the pulmonary graft inside the non–heart-beating donor. J Heart Lung Transplant 2005;24:1369-1377.

27. Valenza F, Rosso L, Coppola S, et al. Beta-adrenergic agonist infusion during extracorporeal lung perfusion: Effects on glucose concentration in the perfusion fluid and on lung function. J Heart Lung Transplant 2012;31:524-530.

28. Inci I, Hillinger S, Arni S, et al. Reconditioning of an injured lung graft with intrabronchial surfactant instillation in an ex vivo lung perfusion system followed by transplantation. J Surg Res 2013;184:1143-1149.

29. Khalife-Hocquemiller T, Sage E, Dorfmuller P, et al. Exogenous surfactant attenuates lung injury from gastric-acid aspiration during ex vivo reconditioning in pigs. Transplantation 2014;97:413-418.

30. Inci I, Zhai W, Arni S, et al. Fibrinolytic treatment improves the quality of lungs retrieved from non–heart-beating donors. J Heart Lung Transplant 2007;26:1054-1060.

31. Fildes J, Regan S, Al-Aloul M, et al. Improved clinical outcome of patients transplanted with reconditioned donor lungs via EVLP compared to standard lung transplantation. Transpl Int 2011;2:77.

32. Gotts JE, Matthay MA. Mesenchymal stem cells and acute lung injury. Crit Care Clin 2011;27:719-733.

33. Lee JW, Fang X, Gupta N, et al. Allogeneic human mesenchymal stem cells for treatment of E. coli endotoxin–induced acute lung injury in the ex vivo perfused human lung. Proc Natl Acad Sci U S A 2009;106:16357-16362.

34. Van Raemdonck D, Neyrinck A, Rega F, et al. Machine perfusion in organ transplantation: A tool for ex-vivo graft conditioning with mesenchymal stem cells? Curr Opin Organ Transplant 2013;18:24-33.

35. Keshavjee SH, Yamazaki F, Cardoso PF, et al. A method for safe twelve-hour pulmonary preservation. J Thorac Cardiovasc Surg 1989;98:529-534.

36. Munshi L, Keshavjee S, Cypel M. Donor management and lung preservation for lung transplantation. Lancet Respir Med 2013;1:318-328.

37. Van Raemdonck D. Thoracic organs: Current preservation technology and future prospects; part 1: Lung. Curr Opin Organ Transplant 2010;15:150-155.

38. Cypel M, Rubacha M, Yeung J, et al. Normothermic ex vivo perfusion prevents lung injury compared to extended cold preservation for transplantation. Am J Transplant 2009;9:2262-2269.

39. Krueger T, Machuca T, Linacre V, et al. Impact of extended cold ischemic times on the outcome of clinical lung transplantation using ex vivo lung perfusion. J Heart Lung Transplant 2014;33(Suppl):S94.

40. Ingemansson R, Eyjolfsson A, Mared L, et al. Clinical transplantation of initially rejected donor lungs after reconditioning ex vivo. Ann Thorac Surg 2009;87:255-260.

41. Cypel M, Yeung JC, Liu M, et al. Normothermic ex vivo lung perfusion in clinical lung transplantation. N Engl J Med 2011;364:1431-1440.

42. Cypel M, Yeung JC, Machuca T, et al. Experience with the first 50 ex vivo lung perfusions in clinical transplantation. J Thorac Cardiovasc Surg 2012;144:1200-1206.

43. Aigner C, Slama A, Hotzenecker K, et al. Clinical ex vivo lung perfusion—pushing the limits. Am J Transplant 2012;12:1839-1847.

44. Boffini M, Ricci D, Barbero C, et al. Ex vivo lung perfusion increases the pool of lung grafts: Analysis of its potential and real impact on a lung transplant program. Transplant Proc 2013;45:2624-2626.

45. Zych B, Popov AF, Stavri G, et al. Early outcomes of bilateral sequential single lung transplantation after ex-vivo lung evaluation and reconditioning. J Heart Lung Transplant 2012;31:274-281.

46. Steen S, Ingemansson R, Eriksson L, et al. First human transplantation of a nonacceptable donor lung after reconditioning ex vivo. Ann Thorac Surg 2007;83:2191-2194.

47. Mulloy DP, Stone ML, Crosby IK, et al. Ex vivo rehabilitation of non–heart-beating donor lungs in preclinical porcine model: Delayed perfusion results in superior lung function. J Thorac Cardiovasc Surg 2012;144:1208-1215.

48. Sage E, Mussot S, Trebbia G, et al. Lung transplantation from initially rejected donors after ex vivo lung reconditioning: The French experience. Eur J Cardiothorac Surg 2014;46:794-799.

49. Dark J, Karamanou DM, Clark SC, et al. Successful transplantation of unusable donor lungs using ex-vivo lung perfusion: The Newcastle experience. J Heart Lung Transplant 2012;31:115.

50. Garcia Saez D, Zych B, Mohite PN, Simon AR. Transplantation of lungs after ex vivo reconditioning in a patient on semi-elective long-term veno-arterial extracorporeal life support. Eur J Cardiothorac Surg 2014;45:389-390.

51. Moradiellos F, Naranjo J, Córdoba M, et al. Clinical lung transplantation after ex vivo evaluation of uncontrolled non heart-beating donors lungs: Initial experience. J Heart Lung Transplant 2011;30:S38.

52. Valenza F, Rosso L, Gatti S, et al. Extracorporeal lung perfusion and ventilation to improve donor lung function and increase the number of organs available for transplantation. Transplant Proc 2012;44:1826-1829.

53. Wallinder A, Ricksten SE, Silverborn M, et al. Early results in transplantation of initially rejected donor lungs after ex vivo lung perfusion: A case-control study. Eur J Cardiothorac Surg 2014;45:40-44; discussion 45.

54. Hopkins P, Chambers D, Naidoo R, et al. Australia's experience with ex-vivo lung perfusion of highly marginal donors. J Heart Lung Transplant 2013;32:S154.

55. Warnecke G, Moradiellos J, Tudorache I, et al. Normothermic perfusion of donor lungs for preservation and assessment with the Organ Care System lung before bilateral transplantation: A pilot study of 12 patients. Lancet 2012;380:1851-1858.

56. Lindstedt S, Hlebowicz J, Koul B, et al. Comparative outcome of double lung transplantation using conventional donor lungs and non-acceptable donor lungs reconditioned ex vivo. Interact Cardiovasc Thorac Surg 2011;12:162-165.

57. TransMedics. International EXPAND Lung Pivotal Trial (EXPANDLung). http://www.clinicaltrials.gov/ct2/show/NCT01963780. 2013.

58. XVIVO Perfusion, Novel Lung Trial: Normothermic ex vivo lung perfusion (EVLP) as an assessment of extended/marginal donor lungs. http://www.clinicaltrials.gov/ct2/show/NCT01365429. 2011.

59. Newcastle upon Tyne Hospitals NHS Foundation Trust, DEVELOP-UK: A study of donor ex-vivo lung perfusion in United Kingdom lung transplantation. UKCRN Portfolio Database. http://www.nets.nihr.ac.uk/projects/hta/108201. 2012. Accessed:

60. TransMedics. International Randomized Study of the TransMedics Organ Care System (OCS Lung) for Lung Preservation and Transplantation (INSPIRE). http://www.clinicaltrials.gov/ct2/show/NCT01630434. 2011.

Recipient Management and Outcome

12

The humoral response to lung transplantation

GLEN P. WESTALL, MIRANDA A. PARASKEVA, AND GREG I. SNELL

MANAGING SENSITIZED PATIENTS BEFORE LUNG TRANSPLANTATION

Detection of antibodies against the human leukocyte antigen (HLA) present on the donor lung allograft is central to determining the pathophysiology and diagnosis of antibody-mediated rejection (AMR). The influence of donor-recipient HLA mismatches on subsequent clinical outcomes was demonstrated in a number of early studies in lung transplantation.[1-4] Additionally, the ability to define the presence or absence of circulating anti-HLA antibodies in patients awaiting lung transplantation facilitates the identification of a suitable donor against whom that recipient is not sensitized.

Detecting anti-HLA antibodies

Methods to detect anti-HLA antibodies have evolved from cell-based assays such as the complement-dependent cytotoxicity (CDC) assay and flow cytometry to solid-phase assays such as the Luminex platform. Consensus guidelines on the different methodologies to identify HLA and non-HLA antibodies and their relevance to transplantation have recently been published.[5]

CELLULAR ASSAYS

Both the CDC and flow cytometric assays rely on cellular targets. The CDC assay determines whether recipient serum can lyse non-self T or B lymphocytes. The lymphocytes are collected from a local representative population, as in the case of the panel-reactive antibody (PRA) assay or from the potential lung donor in the crossmatch test. The presence of autoantibodies may provide a false-positive crossmatch result, which is a scenario that can be avoided by the addition of dithiothreitol. The CDC does not differentiate between HLA class I and class II antibodies, nor between HLA and non-HLA antibodies.

The readout of the PRA is a percentage (%PRA) and refers to the proportion of cells that are lysed following addition of the patient's serum. A high %PRA suggests that the patient is highly sensitized; it has generally been associated with a longer time waiting for a transplant,[6] acute rejection episodes following transplantation,[7] and reduced allograft survival,[8-10] although the latter has not been confirmed in all studies.[11,12] The PRA readout may vary between laboratories because the local reference population from which the donor cells are sourced may differ with regard to relative frequencies of the different HLA alleles. Given the potential for between-center variability, the term *calculated PRA* (cPRA) is preferred; it represents the percentage of donors in a given area against whom the recipient has anti-HLA antibodies. In the United States, this figure can be obtained by the cPRA calculator provided at the Organ Procurement and Transplantation Network (OPTN) Web site (http://optn.transplant.hrsa.gov).

The flow cytometry assay offers improved sensitivity and can distinguish between class I and class II anti-HLA antibodies. Flow cytometric results may vary between centers and are difficult to standardize. The addition of Pronase (Roche Diagnostics, Indianapolis, Indiana) reduces background nonspecific reactivity.

Cellular assays are useful screening tools for the presence of anti-HLA antibodies but are limited in that they do not determine the specificity of or quantify anti-HLA antibodies.

SOLID-PHASE ASSAYS

Solid-phase assays such as the Luminex assay are widely used in lung transplantation to assess for the presence of anti-HLA antibodies. The Luminex platform consists of solubilized HLA molecules fixed to a solid microbead matrix. The microbeads are coated with two fluorescent dyes that when excited by laser energy, allow detection of the resultant emitted light by a dedicated Luminex flow cytometer. The patterns of discharged light permit identification of up to 100 distinct beads, each of which represents a specific HLA molecule. The readout from the Luminex assay, mean fluorescence intensity (MFI), is semiquantitative in that the recorded MFI is not completely representative of the true titer of the circulating anti-HLA antibody.

Different Luminex panels provide increasing specificity with regard to allosensitization. The pooled antigen panel consists of beads coated with either HLA class I (HLA-A, -B, and -C) or HLA class II (HLA-DR, -DQ, and -DP) antigens collected from many individuals; it provides a qualitative assessment of the presence or absence of antibodies against either HLA class I or class II antigens. The pooled antigen panel is relatively inexpensive but does not provide specificity. Quantification of a specific antibody is provided by the single-antigen bead (SAB) assay in which each bead is coated by a single HLA class I or class II allele. The SAB assay is more expensive and is typically performed only if the pooled antigen panel assay is positive to precisely identify which circulating recipient anti-HLA antibodies may be cytotoxic in a potential organ donor.

The Luminex assay is more sensitive than the CDC assay and flow cytometry and can detect low levels of anti-HLA antibodies. Although absolute cutoffs may vary between laboratories, levels of anti-HLA antibodies, as defined by the MFI, are typically graded as low (MFI <2000), moderate (MFI 2000 to 5000), or high (MFI >8000). Luminex results are semiquantitative; however, studies in lung transplantation have demonstrated a correlation between the MFI value and both positive crossmatch results and subsequent clinical outcomes.[6]

INTERPRETATION OF THE LUMINEX ASSAY

MFI levels represent the percentage of antigens on any given bead that are bound by antibody. However, antigenic density varies between beads, which means that MFI does not truly represent antibody titer. HLA-cW, HLA-DQ, and HLA-DP have antigenic density on each bead within the SAB assay. Additionally, once antigens are fully saturated with antibody, a maximal MFI is achieved for that given bead, which means that increasing amounts of antibody

will not be reflected in a further increase in antibody. To better determine the titer of antibody present, dilutions of the serum are required. Interference from IgM or C1 may also affect antigen-antibody binding, and further treatment with hypotonic dialysis is required to remove these confounders.[13] Determining the efficacy of desensitization in reducing antibody levels, particularly in cases of a maximal MFI reading, requires dilution and titration of the antibody. It should, however, be noted that therapeutic drugs, such as intravenous immunoglobulin (IVIG), antithymocyte globulin, bortezomib, and the complement C5 inhibitor eculizumab, may interfere with the sensitivity of the Luminex assay. Solid-phase assays such as Luminex have provided a major advance in how we interpret HLA sensitization. One challenge for the future is to ensure standardization of reagents, assays, and data analysis to allow between-center comparisons of HLA sensitization in patients awaiting lung transplantation.

C1Q ASSAY

Binding of an anti-HLA donor-specific antibody (DSA) with its cognate HLA ligand on the lung allograft triggers a potentially deleterious immune response that results in allograft injury and dysfunction. Amplification of the immune response is dependent on activation of the complement system via the classical pathway. It is now understood that not all DSAs are complement-fixing antibodies; specifically, not all anti-HLA antibodies activate the complement system after binding with HLA molecules. The role of non–complement-fixing antibodies in AMR remains controversial, but an evolving consensus suggests that they are less likely to be alloreactive. The C1q assay aims to distinguish complement-fixing from non–complement-fixing antibodies by identifying only antibodies that can bind to C1q, the first step of the classical complement pathway. C1q-positive anti-HLA DSAs have been shown to be associated with poor outcomes in heart transplantation.[14,15] A landmark paper by Loupy and colleagues[16] demonstrated that following kidney transplantation, patients with C1q-positive DSAs experienced greater graft loss than did patients with DSAs that were C1q negative. Of note, stratification of patients before transplantation according to C1q positivity did not predict subsequent poor outcomes. Equivalent studies in lung transplantation are awaited.

HLA epitopes

Sensitization against donor HLA and the production of anti-HLA DSAs is associated with transplant rejection and reduced graft survival. The HLA antibodies recognize specific fragments or epitopes of the HLA peptides. These distinct structural motifs are defined by their amino acid sequence and are not specific to any one HLA allele; rather, they are shared among different HLA alleles. The existence of shared epitopes was first suggested by the discovery of antibodies specific for serologically cross-reactive epitope groups (CREGs) such as the A2- and B7-CREGs.

The antigenicity (reactivity with antibody) and immuno-genicity (ability to induce an antibody response) of HLA epitopes define their clinical relevance, which are in turn dictated by the structural relationship or bond that exists between the HLA epitope and its corresponding antibody. HLAMatchmaker is a structurally based matching program that interprets each HLA antigen as a sequence of epitopes defined by its amino acid composition at the sites of antibody-antigen binding.[17] HLAMatchmaker assesses areas of surface-exposed non-self amino acids that are referred to as eplets. The 16th International Histocompatibility and Immunogenetics Workshop project has developed a Web-based registry of antibody-defined HLA epitopes (http://epregistry.com.br). To date, epitope maps have been designated for the antibodies HLA-ABC; HLA-DR, -DQ, and -DP; and MICA.[18-20] HLAMatchmaker can be used to define sensitization in patients awaiting transplantation and to identify potential donors with acceptable epitope mismatches.[21]

Non-HLA antibodies

Although HLA antigens are the major transplant antigens, other antigens, either donor or self derived, that may also provoke an antibody response against the transplanted organ also exist. They include autoantigens, such as collagen, vimentin, angiotensin receptor, and α-tubulin, as well as minor histocompatibility antigens (MICA and MICB).[22] The associations with lung allograft dysfunction come largely from single-center studies in which local research tools were used.

Antibodies against the donor lung matrix proteins collagen type V [col(V)] and K-α1-tubulin (KαlT) have been shown to be associated with primary graft dysfunction[23] and bronchiolitis obliterans syndrome (BOS),[24] as well as with the development of anti-HLA DSA. Both col(V) and KαlT are self antigens against which tolerance would be expected. Following lung transplantation, self-tolerance to these antigens is disrupted and autoimmunity develops, particularly in patients with chronic rejection. Recent studies in mouse models have demonstrated that inoculation with antibodies against col(V) and KαlT following orthotopic lung transplantation leads to graft infiltration of col(V)- and KαlT-specific interferon-γ T cells and epitope spreading for other lung-specific self-antigens. The de novo development of autoimmunity to self-antigens precedes and induces the more classical T-cell alloimmune response to transplantation, the resultant pathology being airway inflammation and fibrosis.[25] The authors concluded that future strategies to reduce chronic rejection may need to target these autoreactive antibodies.

Angiotensin II type 1 receptor (AT1R) mediates a number of physiologic pathways of its endogenous ligand, angiotensin II, including arterial blood pressure and salt-water balance.[26] Antibodies against AT1R are associated with vascular remodeling and hypertension. In renal transplantation, AT1R antibodies are associated with AMR in

the absence of anti-HLA DSAs.[27] The combination of both AT1R and HLA antibodies may have a synergistic effect that results in accelerated rejection following renal transplantation.[28] Similar studies in heart transplantation have demonstrated that AT1R is upregulated in the coronary arteries of heart transplant recipients in whom transplant vasculopathy develops.[29] Antibodies against both AT1R and the endothelin-1 type A receptor induce endothelial activation,[30] which is an important precursor of transplant vasculopathy. The studies in lung transplantation are limited to two abstract reports that do not describe an association between elevated AT1R antibodies and lung function and rejection within 12 months of transplantation. Further studies are required to establish whether AT1R antibodies are associated with chronic rejection phenotypes such as BOS or chronic vascular rejection.

A need still exists for broader clinical translation of these novel findings by using commercially developed and validated antibody assays against these putative antigenic targets.

Pretransplant assessment of immune sensitization

Optimal clinical outcomes following lung transplantation require matching the transplant recipient with a suitable donor lung. Central to this pairing is an assessment of immunologic compatibility and, in particular, determination of the presence of DSAs in the recipient. At the time of wait-listing, potential lung transplant recipients can be screened for the presence of anti-HLA antibodies with the Luminex pooled antigen assay. If the result is positive, the Luminex SAB assay is performed to specify and quantify the antibodies. Knowledge of the anti-HLA antibody profile in any given wait-listed patient facilitates identification of a compatible donor (i.e., a donor whose haplotype does not include HLA alleles against which the proposed recipient has anti-HLA DSAs).

Highly sensitized patients with multiple anti-HLA antibodies require a prospective CDC crossmatch to ensure donor-recipient compatibility. Given the typical time and geographic constraints of organ donation, running this assay may not always be possible because recipient serum must be analyzed against donor lymphocytes. An alternative to the CDC crossmatch is "virtual crossmatching," whereby the recipient anti-HLA profile is known. The cytotoxicity of the anti-HLA antibody is inferred, although not confirmed, by the magnitude of MFI as measured by Luminex.[31] Identified antibodies are deemed unacceptable; hence, a prospective CDC crossmatch is not required because the identified donor has already been declared unsuitable for the intended recipient. A number of studies have confirmed that the virtual crossmatch is an adequate, albeit not perfect surrogate for the CDC crossmatch.[32] A virtual crossmatch presupposes that all antibodies are equally alloreactive; however, much of the published literature on renal transplantation focuses on AMR associated with HLA-A, -B, -DR, and -DQ, with less emphasis on the injurious role of antibodies against HLA-Cw and HLA-DP.[5] A weakness of the virtual crossmatch as shown in renal transplantation relates to the identification and clinical interpretation of antibodies with low MFI, many of which will not be associated with a positive CDC crossmatch or with deleterious clinical outcomes following transplantation.[33] Equivalent studies in lung transplantation are awaited.

Recommendations: pretransplant sensitization

No consensus statements on the pretransplant management of sensitized patients awaiting lung transplantation exist. Guidelines that arose from a consensus conference on managing sensitized patients awaiting heart transplantation have been published.[34] Despite recognizing the limitations of extrapolating data from the heart transplant literature to the lung transplant setting, the report does provide useful pointers on how to manage sensitized patients waiting for a lung transplant. The recommended frequency of antibody screening includes the following:

- In nonsensitized patients, antibody screening every 6 months.
- In patients with anti-HLA DSAs, repeated screening every 3 months.
- Repeated screening following potentially sensitizing events such as blood transfusions.
- Repeated screening following any desensitization procedure.

A more recent consensus conference[5] on the testing and clinical management issues associated with HLA and non-HLA antibodies in transplantation that reviewed all forms of solid-organ transplantation made the following additional recommendations:

- Transplantation risk stratification should be based on antibody detection and crossmatch results.
- Interpretation of antibody results should include consideration of previous sensitizing events.
- To minimize risk of sensitization, administration of blood products should be avoided if possible.
- DSAs should be avoided in view of the subsequent risk of AMR and graft loss.

Future direction and areas for research

The members of the Transplantation Society's antibody consensus group also highlighted the following future research directions and research gaps that must be addressed to optimize the care and management of sensitized patients:

- Application of the C1q assay.
- Relevance of antibodies against MICA, endothelial cells, AT1Rs, and other non-HLA targets.

- The role of antibodies against epitopes on HLA-E.
- The long-term clinical sequelae of a low titer of anti-HLA DSAs.
- Randomized controlled studies of different desensitization protocols.
- The differential role of complement-fixing- and non–complement-fixing antibodies.

Pretransplant desensitization

Desensitization refers to therapeutic interventions that are performed on highly sensitized individuals with a view to reducing the "load" of circulating anti-HLA antibodies for the purpose of facilitating lung transplantation with an immunologically compatible donor. Several modalities can be used to reduce levels of DSAs; they can be broadly divided into those that reduce the ongoing production of antibodies by B cells or plasma cells and those that remove preexisting antibodies from the circulation (Table 12.1). Typically, a combination of methods is used; the most common is a regimen based on the use of plasmapheresis with IVIG, rituximab, or both. Experience is based largely in the renal transplantation literature, with only a few emerging reports of efficacy in lung transplantation[35-37]

Whether anti-HLA DSAs are produced primarily by B cells or the more differentiated plasma cells remains unclear, the importance being that rituximab has efficacy only against the former. The proteasome inhibitor bortezomib drives apoptosis in plasma cells and has a more selective action against plasma cells.[38]

IVIG has a number of effects that include reducing B-cell numbers, promoting B-cell apoptosis, inhibiting DSA-HLA binding, and inhibiting complement activation.[39] Typically,

Table 12.1 Desensitization strategies

Desensitization strategy	Comment
Removal of circulating DSAs	
Plasmapheresis	Typically 5 or 6 courses over 2-week period
Immunoadsorption	Does not deplete coagulation factors
Neutralize DSAs	
Intravenous immunoglobulin	Targets multiple immune pathways
Eculizumab	Inhibits complement activation
Prevent DSA production	
Rituximab	Anti-CD20 antibody targeting B cells
Bortezomib	Proteasome inhibitor targeting plasma cells
Splenectomy	Limited experience in lung transplantation

Note: DSA, donor-specific antibody.

the dose of IVIG used in desensitization protocols is higher (1 g/kg) than the usual replacement monthly dose of 0.4 g/kg that is given to patients with hypogammaglobulinemia.

Appel and colleagues[36] described a peritransplant desensitization protocol applied to patients who were sensitized to third-party HLA antigens by using IVIG and extracorporeal immunoadsorption. Of 35 sensitized patients identified before transplantation, 12 were desensitized. Of the 7 patients with class I anti-HLA antibodies, desensitization resulted in elimination of the antibody in 6 patients (85.7%), whereas elimination was observed in only 1 of 3 patients with class II anti-HLA antibodies. Acute rejection or BOS was less likely to develop in sensitized patients who underwent desensitization than in sensitized patients who did not undergo desensitization.

Two wait-listed lung transplant patients who underwent combination desensitization with IVIG, plasmapheresis, rituximab, and bortezomib demonstrated only a transient decrease in anti-HLA antibodies with a subsequent rebound to the levels before transplantation.[40]

In a more recent study, the Duke lung transplant group has described a more sobering experience with regard to pretransplant desensitization.[37] Potential lung transplant candidates with anti-HLA antibodies and a cPRA value greater than 80% were considered for desensitization. The protocol was run for 26 days and included intravenous methylprednisolone (50 to 100 mg, four doses), plasmapheresis (seven courses), bortezomib (1.3 mg/m² subcutaneously, four doses), rituximab (375 mg/m² intravenously, two doses), and monthly IVIG (0.5 g/kg). Sensitized patients waited longer for a transplant, and of the 18 patients who started desensitization, only 8 finished the complete protocol. Despite the intensity of the desensitization protocol, no significant change in PRA or cPRA occurred. Nine of the 18 sensitized patients subsequently underwent transplantation and had a 65% 1-year survival rate, a figure similar to that for a comparison group of sensitized patients who did not undergo sensitization. The group concluded that its aggressive multimodal desensitization protocol did not significantly reduce pretransplant levels of anti-HLA antibodies.

Peritransplant management of sensitized patients

A significant proportion of wait-listed patients with anti-HLA antibodies will remain sensitized despite the implementation of pretransplant desensitization protocols. Proceeding to lung transplant surgery in a sensitized patient may result in immediate allograft dysfunction because of the development of hyperacute AMR. However, the Duke experience suggests that transplantation can be performed successfully on sensitized patients, albeit with a reduced 1-year survival rate of 65%. In our own center, we insist on a negative prospective T-cell crossmatch before undertaking transplant surgery in a sensitized patient. Further management of sensitized patients depends on the magnitude of the identified DSAs. Lung transplant recipients with anti-HLA DSA levels graded low (MFI <5000) receive standard triple-therapy immunotherapy consisting of corticosteroids, mycophenolate mofetil, and tacrolimus. In addition to receiving standard immunosuppression, patients with a DSA level graded high (MFI >5000) and a negative crossmatch, undergo plasmapheresis in the hours before transplant surgery and then receive five further courses of plasmapheresis on alternate days during the immediate postoperative period.

Conclusion

Sensitized patients represent a challenge in lung transplantation. Such patients wait longer for a transplant, have higher wait-list mortality, and despite augmented immunosuppression are more likely to experience acute and chronic rejection episodes following transplantation. Pretransplant assessment of sensitized patients has moved beyond cytotoxicity tests to the routine use of solid-phase assays to provide qualitative and quantitative data on the presence of anti-HLA antibodies. Functional assays that determine the ability of DSA to activate the complement system will further enhance assessment of the sensitized patient. Future implementation of molecular tools and predictive software will allow identification of the distinct structural motifs that antibody-producing immune cells recognize. Epitope matching will further optimize donor-recipient compatibility, thereby reducing the incidence of AMR. More than ever, management of sensitized patients requires a multidisciplinary approach that involves both the transplanting team and the local HLA laboratory.

ANTIBODY-MEDIATED REJECTION

In 1990, the first iteration of the grading system for pulmonary allograft rejection was adopted by the International Society of Heart and Lung Transplantation (ISHLT); it focused on histologic interpretation of the cellular rejection pathways first described by Peter Medawar more than 70 years earlier.[41] With further, albeit subtle, revisions in 1996[42] and 2007,[43] we now define classical T-cell alloreactivity as the presence of perivascular and interstitial mononuclear infiltrates.

Humoral alloreactivity has been considerably more difficult to characterize. The histopathologic features of lung AMR were not addressed in the first two ISHLT workshops on lung allograft rejection and were indistinctly defined in the "2007 Revision of the Working Formulation for the Standardization of Nomenclature in the Diagnosis of Lung Rejection." But AMR is not a newly recognized entity. A 1972 descriptive study of the alveolar manifestations of rejection following lung transplantation included histologic features that today would be best attributed to AMR.[44] In contrast, the diagnostic tenets on which AMR following renal transplantation is defined are more established. The Banff classification of renal AMR[45] is based on the following diagnostic features: (1) circulating DSAs, (2) immunologic evidence of complement activation (C4d staining),

(3) characteristic histopathology, and (4) renal allograft dysfunction. In this section we examine the applicability of each of these diagnostic tools in defining AMR following lung transplantation.

The Banff classification and antibody-mediated rejection after lung transplantation

DEFINITION OF DONOR-SPECIFIC ANTIBODIES

Alloreactivity, the immune response to the transplanted lung, is largely directed against non-self HLA present within the donor lung allograft. The humoral immune pathway involves activation of B cells or plasma cells to produce DSAs, which in turn activate the complement system, the end result being histopathologic change and allograft dysfunction. Very few studies have precisely defined the antigenic targets within the lung that promote the alloreactive response. Classical immunology teaching states that whereas class I HLA expression is universal, HLA class II expression is seen only selectively on antigen-presenting cells. Yet, at a clinical level it is common for DSAs against both HLA class I and class II to develop equally in patients, thus suggesting that HLA class II expression is upregulated in the lung allograft, as has been suggested by studies of lung injury[46] or chronic lung allograft dysfunction (CLAD).[47]

The presence of circulating DSAs does not automatically imply allograft damage. Levels of DSAs in the circulation may remain high if they are not being bound to their cognate antigen within the lung allograft. Likewise, a drop in circulating DSAs may imply that the potentially injurious antibody is remaining within the lung allograft, thereby increasing the likelihood of complement activation and amplification of the immune response against the transplanted lung.

DSAs are defined by using solid-phase assays such as the Luminex platform. MFI does not truly represent the titer of the circulating DSAs, but for the clinician by the bedside, MFI has been largely adopted as a surrogate for the "strength" of the alloantibody. To date, most studies of Luminex in lung transplantation have focused on the clinical relevance of antibodies against donor HLA, but the Luminex platform can also detect the presence of other transplant-relevant antibodies, such as those against minor histocompatibility antigens (MICA/MICB) and AT1R.

Finally, DSAs per se are not injurious; rather, allograft damage occurs because of their role in activating other complement-dependent or complement-independent immune pathways. A modification of the standard Luminex platform, the C1q assay, detects complement-fixing antibodies.[14] Further studies are required to see whether the C1q assay can improve risk stratification in lung transplantation, as has been suggested in renal transplantation.[16]

DEFINITION OF COMPLEMENT ACTIVATION

Demonstration of positive C4d (or C3d staining or both), which suggests complement activation, has historically been central to the diagnosis of AMR. C4d deposition can be detected in transbronchial biopsy samples by either immunofluorescence or immunohistochemistry. However, the diagnostic utility of C4d staining in AMR is under scrutiny.[48] A recent study has shown poor reproducibility for immunofluorescence and immunohistochemistry between pathologists, and the correlation between the two methods for detecting C4d is low.[49] C4d staining in the lung is often nonspecific and can be associated with primary graft dysfunction and infection of the lung allograft.[50] Although the complement system can be activated by antibodies (the "classical" pathway), it can also be driven by exposure to bacteria or mannose-binding lectin, both of which have been described in lung transplantation.[51]

We also now recognize that AMR can arise from complement-independent immune pathways which by definition would not result in C4d deposition. DSAs, acting through the low-affinity Fc receptor on natural killer (NK) cells and macrophages, can lyse target cells through a pathway known as antibody-dependent cell-mediated cytotoxicity. The importance of NK cell activation in AMR has recently been shown in a study in renal transplantation. Genomic analysis in patients with DSAs and presumed AMR demonstrated selective expression of NK cell, and not T-cell, transcripts.[52] When all these points are taken into consideration, the presence of positive C4d staining may on the one hand be suggestive of a diagnosis of AMR; on the other hand, its absence does not necessarily rule out the diagnosis. Accordingly, C4d is no longer a pillar on which AMR is built but is instead viewed as a minor secondary diagnostic tool with a supportive rather than confirmatory role.

HISTOLOGIC FEATURES OF ANTIBODY-MEDIATED REJECTION

The histologic features of AMR have been notoriously difficult to define. The 2007 working group revision of the diagnosis of lung rejection concluded that AMR is a controversial entity in the lung, and no consensus on its diagnostic features could be reached. In 2012, the pathology council of the ISHLT reviewed the morphologic and immunologic criteria for pulmonary AMR.[53] The most overt, albeit rare, form of AMR is "hyperacute rejection" manifested as primary graft dysfunction in sensitized patients. This rejection is associated with the histologic features of fibrin thrombi in alveolar septa, fibrinoid necrosis of alveolar septal walls, and hemorrhage. In clinical practice, AMR typically develops at times later after transplantation, when the differential diagnosis includes more commonly encountered causes of allograft rejection such as T-cell–mediated rejection and infection. Confounding the ability to diagnose AMR is the fact that the histopathologic features of AMR are nonspecific and include patterns of injury that can be seen with infection, ischemia-reperfusion injury, drug reactions, and acute cellular rejection. Features suggestive of AMR are focused on the capillary and include neutrophilic capillaritis and neutrophilic septal margination. The pathology council highlighted the limitations of histology in diagnosing AMR by stating that any histologic abnormality in the setting of de novo DSAs may be indicative of antibody-driven damage to the lung allograft. AMR should not necessarily be ruled out by normal transbronchial biopsy findings in view of the limitations of sampling error and also because AMR can be pauci-immune in that activation of the complement system may not be associated with histologic changes.

ALLOGRAFT DYSFUNCTION

As already discussed, unlike renal transplantation,[45] there is no consensus regarding the features that characterize lung transplant allograft dysfunction. In the setting of lung transplantation all the symptoms, signs, and investigations of decreased allograft performance are nonspecific and potentially confounded by other diseases or processes and even by therapy for AMR (e.g., steroid myopathy). Potential symptoms of AMR include dyspnea, exercise limitation, or rarely in severe cases, hemoptysis. Potential signs include lung crepitation. Lung function testing typically shows a new restrictive spirometric picture. Radiologic evidence of new diffuse infiltrates or focal fibrosis may also exist.[54,55]

Sudden-onset (acute) AMR might have all these features of allograft dysfunction. In the presence of other Banff-style DSA and MFI criteria[45] and additional exploration and investigation of the differential diagnosis, it is possible to make a compelling case that AMR is present and that potentially complex and expensive therapies are indicated.[56] Slow-onset chronic AMR may be characterized simply by chronic dyspnea and a relatively subtle restrictive spirometric picture.[54] As already discussed, in this situation the subsequent poor utility of lung histology and DSA assessment makes a firm diagnosis of chronic AMR essentially impossible. Figure 12.1 attempts to schematically demonstrate the different stages of AMR and their relationship to acute lung allograft dysfunction (ALAD) and CLAD "syndromes."[57,58] In a significant number of cases, a firm diagnosis of chronic AMR can be made only in retrospect after a significant response to presumptive AMR therapy or after

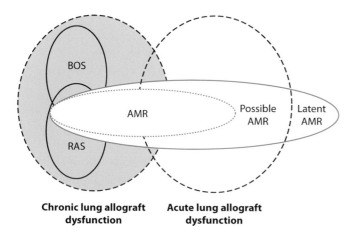

Chronic lung allograft dysfunction   **Acute lung allograft dysfunction**

Figure 12.1 Antibody-mediated rejection (AMR) and its relationship to acute and chronic lung allograft dysfunction. BOS, bronchiolitis obliterans syndrome; RAS, restrictive allograft syndrome.

a postmortem examination or review of explant histology following retransplantation.[55,59]

Evidence for antibody-mediated rejection in lung transplantation

AMR following lung transplantation remains difficult to define. The preceding discussion makes it clear that the diagnostic tenets inherent to the Banff classification of AMR in renal transplantation may not be directly applicable to the lung allograft. Although the evidence for AMR and its negative effects on the lung allograft is not as robust as in cardiac and renal transplantation, the ability of DSAs to mediate lung allograft damage has been acknowledged. The clearest example of this is hyperacute rejection during which preformed DSAs mediate allograft destruction. Numerous case reports and case series have described clinicopathologic findings consistent with acute AMR as well as the various treatment strategies and outcomes.[56,60,61] In addition, an emerging body of evidence has associated the presence of DSAs with acute and chronic allograft dysfunction.[56,60-67]

The association between pretransplant DSAs and poor early graft survival in all solid-organ transplant groups has long been understood. As discussed earlier, higher pretransplant PRA and DSA levels and greater HLA mismatches predict worse outcomes in lung transplant recipients, with rates of graft loss as high as 70% at 5 years after transplantation.[6,9,68]

The detrimental role of de novo HLA antibodies detected after transplantation has also been explored. Whereas acute and chronic AMR are vascular phenomena in renal transplantation, in lung transplantation detection of HLA antibodies has been associated with acute cellular rejection[66] and lymphocytic bronchiolitis.[67] Several early studies had linked the development of DSAs to BOS.[10,67,69,70] A later study by Hachem and colleagues indirectly highlighted this association.[61] In this interventional study patients with de novo DSAs were treated with IVIG and rituximab or IVIG alone. BOS was more likely to develop in those with persistent DSAs despite treatment than in those in whom DSAs were decreased successfully. More recent studies have confirmed de novo DSA development as an independent risk factor for BOS. In addition, such de novo DSA development has been associated with accelerated BOS kinetics and severity and worse survival.[33,64,65]

Unfortunately, despite the increasing evidence implicating the role of DSAs and antibody-mediated allograft dysfunction in BOS, few if any studies have examined the link between AMR and other problematic CLAD syndromes, including restrictive allograft syndrome and acute fibrinous and organizing pneumonia.[71,72]

Therapy for antibody-mediated rejection

Although AMR is clearly a serious complication of lung transplantation requiring treatment, the therapeutic strategies continue to slowly evolve from lung transplant case reports and small series based primarily on emerging renal transplant data. No randomized controlled trials to direct practice are currently available in lung transplantation.

Prevention by avoiding transplanting known DSA donor HLA targets is the primary approach.[37,55] Preemptive perioperative DSA desensitization with a combination of plasmapheresis, antithymocyte globulin, IVIG, and mycophenolate has recently been reported as being reasonably tolerated and appears to be successful in reducing early rejection (including AMR) episodes in lung transplantation.[73] Other earlier lung transplant case series with less intense therapies are less convincing.[37,56,61]

For treatment of established AMR, combinations of corticosteroids, IVIG, plasmapheresis, antithymocyte globulin, and rituximab (a B-cell–depleting monoclonal antibody) are the most commonly described[37,56,60,61,74] and have yielded variable results. Our own approach is to start with mycophenolate, intravenous corticosteroids, and IVIG and escalate to plasmapheresis and rituximab in cases in which improvement is not forthcoming or not sustained.[54,55] The amount of lung transplantation data suggesting additional efficacy with bortezimab (a monoclonal antibody inducer of plasma cell apoptosis)[75,76] and eculizimab (a monoclonal antibody inhibitor of complement activation) is very small.[77,78] A therapeutic response appears to have some relation to a subsequent decrease in the target DSA MFI, but this is not universally true.[55,60] These therapies are complex, associated with significant side effects, and expensive (particularly the monoclonal antibodies), and evidence of clinical success can be hard to produce.

Future directions

The diagnosis and management of AMR of a transplanted lung are immediate challenges to conquer. Studies involving Luminex pretransplant DSA and C1q screening, careful characterization of recipients' risk for sensitization, and development of a protocol for perioperative DSA monitoring and therapy will provide hard data on which to base future multicenter lung transplant trials. Lung physiology and alloresponses are sufficiently different from renal transplantation to suggest that direct lung transplant studies must be performed.[48] Indirect renal transplant data will only hint at the direction to investigate. Epitope matching rather than antigen matching must be explored.[17] Non-HLA autoantibodies against lung structural antigens, including col(V) and anti–α_1-tubulin, should also be considered as potential stimulants of fibroproliferation.[74] The expensive reality of broad DSA testing and AMR therapeutic agents will mandate the need to pair clinicians with industry partners to answer these questions. Robust international collaborations to create definitions are now critical. Determining where chronic AMR fits into the emerging new entities of restrictive allograft syndrome and CLAD is particularly important.[54,57,58]

Conclusion

Pulmonary AMR is probably real and likely contributes significantly to the previously unexplained "noise" affecting allograft performance early and late after transplantation. Presently, AMR manifestations, phenotypes, and therapeutic responsiveness are still only poorly defined. Current definitions and facts are neither consistent nor bulletproof—so an open mind is important. Notwithstanding, potentially significant clinical gains are to be made by exploring these issues and creating new lung transplant rejection paradigms.

REFERENCES

1. Harjula AL, Baldwin JC, Glanville AR, et al. Human leukocyte antigen compatibility in heart-lung transplantation. J Heart Lung Transplant 1987;6:162-166.
2. Schulman LL, Weinberg AD, McGregor CC, et al. Influence of donor and recipient HLA locus mismatching on development of obliterative bronchiolitis after lung transplantation. Am J Respir Crit Care Med 2001;163:437-442.
3. Chalermskulrat W, Neuringer IP, Schmitz JL, et al. Human leukocyte antigen mismatches predispose to the severity of bronchiolitis obliterans syndrome after lung transplantation. Chest 2003;123:1825-1831.
4. Quantz MA, Bennett LE, Meyer DM, Novick RJ. Does human leukocyte antigen matching influence the outcome of lung transplantation? An analysis of 3,549 lung transplantations. J Heart Lung Transplant 2000;19:473-479.
5. Tait BD, Susal C, Gebel HM, et al. Consensus guidelines on the testing and clinical management issues associated with HLA and non-HLA antibodies in transplantation. Transplantation 2013;95:19-47.
6. Kim M, Townsend KR, Wood IG, et al. Impact of pretransplant anti-HLA antibodies on outcomes in lung transplant candidates. Am J Respir Crit Care Med 2014;189:1234-1239.
7. Mangi AA, Mason DP, Nowicki ER, et al. Predictors of acute rejection after lung transplantation. Ann Thorac Surg 2011;91:1754-1762.
8. Lau CL, Palmer SM, Posther KE, et al. Influence of panel-reactive antibodies on posttransplant outcomes in lung transplant recipients. Ann Thorac Surg 2000;69:1520-1524.
9. Hadjiliadis D, Chaparro C, Reinsmoen NL, et al. Pretransplant panel reactive antibody in lung transplant recipients is associated with significantly worse posttransplant survival in a multicenter study. J Heart Lung Transplant 2005;24(Suppl 7):S249-S254.
10. Palmer SM, Davis RD, Hadjiliadis D, et al. Development of an antibody specific to major histocompatibility antigens detectable by flow

cytometry after lung transplant is associated with bronchiolitis obliterans syndrome. Transplantation 2002;74:799-804.

11. Gammie JS, Pham SM, Colson YL, et al. Influence of panel-reactive antibody on survival and rejection after lung transplantation. J Heart Lung Transplant 1997;16:408-415.

12. Shah AS, Nwakanma L, Simpkins C, et al. Pretransplant panel reactive antibodies in human lung transplantation: An analysis of over 10,000 patients. Ann Thorac Surg 2008;85:1919-1924.

13. Zachary AA, Lucas DP, Detrick B, Leffell MS. Naturally occurring interference in Luminex assays for HLA-specific antibodies: Characteristics and resolution. Hum Immunol 2009;70:496-501.

14. Zeevi A, Lunz J, Feingold B, et al. Persistent strong anti-HLA antibody at high titer is complement binding and associated with increased risk of antibody-mediated rejection in heart transplant recipients. J Heart Lung Transplant 2013;32:98-105.

15. Chin C, Chen G, Sequeria F, et al. Clinical usefulness of a novel C1q assay to detect immunoglobulin G antibodies capable of fixing complement in sensitized pediatric heart transplant patients. J Heart Lung Transplant 2011;30:158-163.

16. Loupy A, Lefaucheur C, Vernerey D, et al. Complement-binding anti-HLA antibodies and kidney-allograft survival. N Engl J Med 2013;369:1215-1226.

17. Duquesnoy RJ. Human leukocyte antigen epitope antigenicity and immunogenicity. Curr Opin Organ Transplant 2014;19:428-435.

18. Duquesnoy RJ, Marrari M, Mulder A, et al. First report on the antibody verification of HLA-ABC epitopes recorded in the website-based HLA Epitope Registry. Tissue antigens 2014;83:391-400.

19. Duquesnoy RJ, Marrari M, Tambur AR, et al. First report on the antibody verification of HLA-DR, HLA-DQ and HLA-DP epitopes recorded in the HLA Epitope Registry. Hum Immunol 2014;75:1097-1103.

20. Duquesnoy RJ, Mostecki J, Marrari M, et al. First report on the antibody verification of MICA epitopes recorded in the HLA epitope registry. Int J Immunogenet 2014;41:370-377.

21. Claas FH, Dankers MK, Oudshoorn M, et al. Differential immunogenicity of HLA mismatches in clinical transplantation. Transpl Immunol 2005;14:187-191.

22. Stastny P. Introduction: What we know about antibodies produced by transplant recipients against donor antigens not encoded by HLA genes. Hum Immunol 2013;74:1421-1424.

23. Iwata T, Philipovskiy A, Fisher AJ, et al. Anti-type V collagen humoral immunity in lung transplant primary graft dysfunction. J Immunol 2008;181:5738-5747.

24. Bharat A, Saini D, Steward N, et al. Antibodies to self-antigens predispose to primary lung allograft dysfunction and chronic rejection. Ann Thorac Surg 2010;90:1094-1101.

25. Subramanian V, Ramachandran S, Banan B, et al. Immune response to tissue-restricted self-antigens induces airway inflammation and fibrosis following murine lung transplantation. Am J Transplant 2014;14:2359-2366.

26. Dzau VJ, Bernstein K, Celermajer D, et al. The relevance of tissue angiotensin-converting enzyme: Manifestations in mechanistic and endpoint data. Am J Cardiol 2001;88:1L-20L.

27. Reinsmoen NL, Lai CH, Heidecke H, et al. Anti-angiotensin type 1 receptor antibodies associated with antibody mediated rejection in donor HLA antibody negative patients. Transplantation 2010;90:1473-1477.

28. Kelsch R, Everding AS, Kuwertz-Broking E, et al. Accelerated kidney transplant rejection and hypertensive encephalopathy in a pediatric patient associated with antibodies against angiotensin type 1 receptor and HLA class II. Transplantation 2011;92:e57-e59.

29. Yousufuddin M, Cook DJ, Starling RC, et al. Angiotensin II receptors from peritransplantation through first-year post-transplantation and the risk of transplant coronary artery disease. J Am Coll Cardiol 2004;43:1565-1573.

30. Schneider MP, Boesen EI, Pollock DM. Contrasting actions of endothelin ET(A) and ET(B) receptors in cardiovascular disease. Annu Rev Pharmacol Toxicol 2007;47:731-759.

31. Reinsmoen NL, Lai CH, Vo A, et al. Acceptable donor-specific antibody levels allowing for successful deceased and living donor kidney transplantation after desensitization therapy. Transplantation 2008;86:820-825.

32. Stehlik J, Islam N, Hurst D, et al. Utility of virtual crossmatch in sensitized patients awaiting heart transplantation. J Heart Lung Transplant 2009;28:1129-1134.

33. Morath C, Opelz G, Zeier M, Susal C. Clinical relevance of HLA antibody monitoring after kidney transplantation. J Immunol Res. 2014;2014:845040. doi: 10.1155/2014/845040.

34. Kobashigawa J, Mehra M, West L, et al. Report from a consensus conference on the sensitized patient awaiting heart transplantation. J Heart Lung Transplant 2009;28:213-225.

35. Robinson JA. Apheresis in thoracic organ transplantation. Ther Apher 1999;3:34-39.

36. Appel JZ 3rd, Hartwig MG, Davis RD, Reinsmoen NL. Utility of peritransplant and rescue intravenous immunoglobulin and extracorporeal immunoadsorption in lung transplant recipients sensitized to HLA antigens. Hum Immunol 2005;66:378-386.

37. Snyder LD, Gray AL, Reynolds JM, et al. Antibody desensitization therapy in highly sensitized lung transplant candidates. Am J Transplant 2014;14:849-856.

38. Sadaka B, Alloway RR, Shields AR, et al. Proteasome inhibition for antibody-mediated allograft rejection. Semin Hematol 2012;49:263-269.

39. Jordan SC, Toyoda M, Vo AA. Intravenous immunoglobulin a natural regulator of immunity and inflammation. Transplantation 2009;88:1-6.

40. Weston M, Rolfe M, Haddad T, Lopez-Cepero M. Desensitization protocol using bortezomib for highly sensitized patients awaiting heart or lung transplants. Clin Transplant 2009:393-399.

41. Medawar PB. The behaviour and fate of skin autografts and skin homografts in rabbits: A report to the War Wounds Committee of the Medical Research Council. J Anat 1944;78(Pt 5):176-199.

42. Yousem SA, Berry GJ, Cagle PT, et al. Revision of the 1990 working formulation for the classification of pulmonary allograft rejection: Lung Rejection Study Group. J Heart Lung Transplant 1996;15:1-15.

43. Stewart S, Fishbein MC, Snell GI, et al. Revision of the 1996 working formulation for the standardization of nomenclature in the diagnosis of lung rejection. J Heart Lung Transplant 2007;26:1229-1242.

44. Veith FJ, Hagstrom JW. Alveolar manifestations of rejection: An important cause of the poor results with human lung transplantation. Ann Surg 1972;175:336-348.

45. Takemoto SK, Zeevi A, Feng S, et al. National conference to assess antibody-mediated rejection in solid organ transplantation. Am J Transplant 2004;4:1033-1041.

46. Nakayama A, Nagura H, Yokoi T, et al. Immunocytochemical observation of paraquat-induced alveolitis with special reference to class II MHC antigens. Virchows Arch B Cell Pathol Incl Mol Pathol 1992;61:389-396.

47. Taylor PM, Rose ML, Yacoub M. Expression of class I and class II MHC antigens in normal and transplanted human lung. Transplant Proc 1989;21:451-452.

48. Westall GP, Snell GI. Antibody-mediated rejection in lung transplantation: Fable, spin, or fact? Transplantation 2014;98:927-930.

49. Roden AC, Maleszewski JJ, Yi ES, et al. Reproducibility of complement 4d deposition by immunofluorescence and immunohistochemistry in lung allograft biopsies. J Heart Lung Transplant 2014;33:1223-1232.

50. Westall GP, Snell GI, McLean C, et al. C3d and C4d deposition early after lung transplantation. J Heart Lung Transplant 2008;27:722-728.

51. Carroll KE, Dean MM, Heatley SL, et al. High levels of mannose-binding lectin are associated with poor outcomes after lung transplantation. Transplantation 2011;91:1044-1049.

52. Hidalgo LG, Sellares J, Sis B, et al. Interpreting NK cell transcripts versus T cell transcripts in renal transplant biopsies. Am J Transplant 2012;12:1180-1191.

53. Berry G, Burke M, Andersen C, et al. Pathology of pulmonary antibody-mediated rejection: 2012 update from the pathology council of the ISHLT. J Heart Lung Transplant 2013;32:14-21.

54. Fuller J, Paraskeva M, Thompson B, et al. A spirometric journey following lung transplantation. Respirol Case Rep 2014;2:120-122.

55. Otani S, Davis AK, Cantwell L, et al. Evolving experience of treating antibody-mediated rejection following lung transplantation. Transpl Immunol 2014;31:75-80.

56. Daoud AH, Betensley AD. Diagnosis and treatment of antibody mediated rejection in lung transplantation: A retrospective case series. Transpl Immunol 2013;28:1-5.

57. Snell GI, Paraskeva M, Westall GP. Managing bronchiolitis obliterans syndrome (BOS) and chronic lung allograft dysfunction (CLAD) in children: What does the future hold? Paediatr Drugs 2013;15: 281-289.

58. Verleden GM, Raghu G, Meyer KC, et al. A new classification system for chronic lung allograft dysfunction. J Heart Lung Transplant 2014;33:127-133.

59. Martinu T, Howell DN, Davis RD, et al. Pathologic correlates of bronchiolitis obliterans syndrome in pulmonary retransplant recipients. Chest 2006;129:1016-1023.

60. Witt CA, Gaut JP, Yusen RD, et al. Acute antibody-mediated rejection after lung transplantation. J Heart Lung Transplant 2013;32:1034-1040.

61. Hachem RR, Yusen RD, Meyers BF, et al. Anti-human leukocyte antigen antibodies and preemptive antibody-directed therapy after lung transplantation. J Heart Lung Transplant 2010;29:973-980.

62. Lobo LJ, Aris RM, Schmitz J, Neuringer IP. Donor-specific antibodies are associated with antibody-mediated rejection, acute cellular rejection, bronchiolitis obliterans syndrome, and cystic fibrosis after lung transplantation. J Heart Lung Transplant 2013;32:70-77.

63. Snyder LD, Wang Z, Chen DF, et al. Implications for human leukocyte antigen antibodies after lung transplantation: A 10-year experience in 441 patients. Chest 2013;144:226-233.

64. Safavi S, Robinson DR, Soresi S, et al. De novo donor HLA-specific antibodies predict development of bronchiolitis obliterans syndrome after lung transplantation. J Heart Lung Transplant 2014;33:1273-1281.

65. Morrell MR, Pilewski JM, Gries CJ, et al. De novo donor-specific HLA antibodies are associated with early and high-grade bronchiolitis obliterans syndrome and death after lung transplantation. J Heart Lung Transplant 2014;33:1288-1294.

66. Girnita AL, McCurry KR, Iacono AT, et al. HLA-specific antibodies are associated with high-grade and persistent-recurrent lung allograft acute rejection. J Heart Lung Transplant 2004;23:1135-1141.

67. Girnita AL, Duquesnoy R, Yousem SA, et al. HLA-specific antibodies are risk factors for lymphocytic bronchiolitis and chronic lung allograft dysfunction. Am J Transplant 2005;5:131-138.

68. Smith JD, Ibrahim MW, Newell H, et al. Pre-transplant donor HLA-specific antibodies: Characteristics causing detrimental effects on survival after lung transplantation. J Heart Lung Transplant 2014;33:1074-1082.

69. Jaramillo A, Smith MA, Phelan D, et al. Temporal relationship between the development of anti-HLA antibodies and the development of bronchiolitis obliterans syndrome after lung transplantation. Transplant Proc 1999;31:185-186.

70. Smith MA, Sundaresan S, Mohanakumar T, et al. Effect of development of antibodies to HLA and cytomegalovirus mismatch on lung transplantation survival and development of bronchiolitis obliterans syndrome. J Thorac Cardiovasc Surg. 1998;116:812-820.

71. Paraskeva M, McLean C, Ellis S, et al. Acute fibrinoid organizing pneumonia after lung transplantation. Am J Respir Crit Care Med 2013;187:1360-8.

72. Sato M, Waddell TK, Wagnetz U, et al. Restrictive allograft syndrome (RAS): A novel form of chronic lung allograft dysfunction. J Heart Lung Transplant 2011;30:735-742.

73. Tinckam KJ, Keshavjee S, Chaparro C, et al. Survival in sensitized lung transplant recipients with perioperative desensitization. Am J Transplant 2015;15:417-426.

74. McManigle W, Pavlisko EN, Martinu T. Acute cellular and antibody-mediated allograft rejection. Semin Respir Crit Care Med 2013;34:320-335.

75. Baum C, Reichenspurner H, Deuse T. Bortezomib rescue therapy in a patient with recurrent antibody-mediated rejection after lung transplantation. J Heart Lung Transplant 2013;32:1270-1271.

76. Stuckey LJ, Kamoun M, Chan KM. Lung transplantation across donor-specific anti–human leukocyte antigen antibodies: Utility of bortezomib therapy in early graft dysfunction. Ann Pharmacother 2012;46:e2.

77. Commereuc M, Karras A, Amrein C, et al. Successful treatment of acute thrombotic microangiopathy by eculizumab after combined lung and kidney transplantation. Transplantation 2013;96:e58-e59.

78. Dawson KL, Parulekar A, Seethamraju H. Treatment of hyperacute antibody-mediated lung allograft rejection with eculizumab. J Heart Lung Transplant 2012;31:1325-1326.

79. Snell GI, Westall GP, Paraskeva MA. Immuno-suppression and allograft rejection following lung transplantation: Evidence to date. Drugs 2013;73:1793-1813.

13

Anesthesia for lung transplantation

J. DEVIN ROBERTS, MOHAMMED MINHAJ, AND MARK A. CHANEY

INTRODUCTION

The first human lung transplant was performed in 1963; however, it was not until the 1980s that improvements in surgical technique and improved immunosuppression regimens made lung transplantation the "gold standard" treatment for a variety of end-stage lung diseases. Since that time, the number of reported lung transplants has been increasing steadily, with more than 3800 transplants performed worldwide in 2012 and recorded in the Registry of the International Society for Heart and Lung Transplantation (ISHLT).[1]

Survival rates have also gradually improved over the past 3 decades, and interest in the anesthetic management of patients undergoing lung transplantation and its contribution to patient outcomes has increased in recent years.[2-6] Anesthesiologists taking part in these procedures need to have specific skills in the areas of thoracic and cardiac anesthesia. Such skills include the ability to address both technical and physiologic concerns, such as achieving adequate lung isolation and oxygenation, using and interpreting invasive monitoring (such as transesophageal echocardiography [TEE]), and managing respiratory and myocardial impairments. This chapter provides an overview of these perioperative anesthetic management considerations.

PREOPERATIVE EVALUATION AND INDUCTION

The criteria for patients to be considered for lung transplantation are reviewed elsewhere in this textbook, but it is important for the anesthesiologist to realize that organ allocation in the United States is now based on a priority system that balances the risk for death while on the waiting list with the likelihood of survival after transplantation.[7] The result is that although all patients will have some degree of functional impairment as a result of their underlying disease, the degree of hypoxia and oxygen requirements can vary significantly and thus affect their perioperative management. Older patients now represent an important growing subset of lung recipients, especially in the United States, where 26% of candidates on the lung waiting list in 2012 were 65 years or older in comparison to just 6% in 2004.[8]

Patients will have a variety of underlying pulmonary disorders (Table 13.1). Idiopathic pulmonary fibrosis, chronic obstructive pulmonary disease (COPD), and cystic fibrosis are the leading indications for lung transplantation worldwide, but primary pulmonary hypertension and other diseases may result in patients requiring transplantation.[1] Careful consideration of the underlying pathology is important because it will predict the type of surgical procedure (single-lung versus bilateral lung transplantation) and the intraoperative techniques that are used (e.g., cardiopulmonary bypass [CPB]). These decisions in turn affect anesthetic management with respect to lung isolation and the use of epidural anesthesia. For example, patients with idiopathic pulmonary fibrosis or COPD usually receive a single-lung transplant (SLT), whereas patients with cystic fibrosis will undergo bilateral lung transplantation because the native lung can contaminate the transplanted lung. Most bilateral lung transplants are now bilateral sequential single-lung transplants.

Various studies and practitioners have proposed that epidural anesthesia be considered in all lung transplant patients because the technique has been associated with improved pain control and better pulmonary function after transplantation.[2,9] However, complications of epidural anesthesia include a risk for hematoma resulting in potential

Table 13.1 2012 International Society for Heart and Lung Transplantation diagnosis categories

Diagnosis	Total (n = 3828)
Idiopathic pulmonary fibrosis	26.9%
Emphysema/chronic obstructive pulmonary disease	25%
Cystic fibrosis	15.7%
α_1-Antitrypsin deficiency	3%
Primary pulmonary hypertension	2.8%
Retransplant or graft failure	1.5%
Congenital heart disease	0.2%
Other	21.8%
Not reported	3.2%

Source: Adapted from the International Society for Heart and Lung Transplantation Web site: www.ishlt.org/. Accessed May 24, 2014.

permanent neurologic injury. The likelihood of using CPB (which requires anticoagulation) and whether the patient is receiving other anticoagulants that may preclude preoperative placement of a thoracic epidural should be considered carefully.[10]

Usually, the time between donor identification and the start of surgery is sufficient to review the patient's history, laboratory test results, and other data (including pulmonary function tests and echocardiograms) and establish an optimal time line for the ensuing operation. Communication between the harvesting surgical team and the surgeons, anesthesiologists, and other staff at the recipient site is vital to minimize organ ischemic time and establish appropriate times for induction of anesthesia, surgical incision, and cross-clamping.

When the anesthetic plan is reviewed with the patient and family, they should be counseled regarding the stages of the upcoming surgery. Operating room availability at the donor site and bronchoscopy of the donor lungs to assess viability can result in lengthy wait times or cancellation of the procedure. During that time a decision regarding epidural placement can also be made, taking the aforementioned considerations into account. When intravenous access has been secured, samples for laboratory testing should be obtained if recent results are not available, and typing and crossmatching of the patient's blood for blood products should be performed.

It is our practice to sedate patients in the preoperative holding area with caution if at all—even if they are undergoing epidural placement. Increased oxygen requirements, declining functional status, and depression of their respiratory drive may result in exaggerated responses to intravenous sedation and cause hypoxia or hypercapnia. When placing preinduction arterial lines and thoracic epidurals, the authors use local anesthetic liberally instead of sedation, and they counsel the patients extensively regarding the technical aspects of these procedures to minimize discomfort.

When the patient is brought into the operating room, American Society of Anesthesiologists (ASA) standard monitors are applied, oxygen is administered via face mask (preoxygenation), and the arterial line is connected. Hemodynamic instability leading to cardiac arrest after induction of general anesthesia has been reported in these patients.[11,12] Most patients will have elevated pulmonary artery pressure and Paco$_2$ levels. Potential hypoxia during preinduction or induction can trigger dramatic increases in pulmonary vascular resistance and precipitate right ventricular failure. Adequate preoxygenation and avoidance of apnea and hypercapnia are essential during this period. Particular emphasis should be placed on assessment of the airway because these patients will not generally tolerate the prolonged periods of apnea resulting from a difficult intubation. Contingency plans for potential difficult airway access should be carefully formulated and include a variety of readily available endotracheal tubes.

It is our practice to use a "cardiac"-style induction that relies heavily on narcotics (fentanyl or sufentanil) and benzodiazepines (midazolam). Depending on the patient's underlying disease and baseline hemodynamic profile, etomidate may also be administered. At all times, vasoactive medications should be available for hemodynamic support and resuscitation. Neuromuscular blockade is administered and the airway secured rapidly (the choice of endotracheal tube is discussed later).

A central line is typically not placed until after induction because most patients may not tolerate Trendelenburg or even fully supine positioning while awake. A pulmonary artery catheter and a TEE probe are placed. The use of TEE intraoperatively is well established in lung transplantation; it allows evaluation of ventricular function, volume status, and flow from the pulmonary veins into the left atrium after surgical anastomosis.[4] TEE can also identify potential complications such as the presence of air and thrombus formation.[13,14]

A baseline arterial blood gas analysis is also obtained after the initiation of mechanical ventilation with 100% oxygen because a large alveolar-arterial (A-a) gradient may predict difficulty during a bilateral lung transplant and suggest that use of CPB may be of benefit for the procedure. Antibiotic and immunosuppressant regimens should be initiated.

INTRAOPERATIVE MANAGEMENT

Ventilation strategies

Intraoperative anesthetic management depends largely on the patient's underlying pathology. For example, mechanical ventilation strategies that follow guidelines for patients with adult respiratory distress syndrome have been described for lung transplant patients with obstructive disease.[5] Such strategies include the use of tidal volumes of 6 to 8 mL/kg, careful administration of positive end-expiratory pressure (PEEP), and performance of alveolar recruitment maneuvers.

Patients who have pulmonary fibrosis and low pulmonary compliance are at risk for mechanical ventilation-associated barotrauma. Use of pressure control ventilation rather than volume control modes may be preferable in patients undergoing thoracic surgery to decrease the airway pressure transmitted to the diseased lungs.[15,16] However, despite the reduction in airway pressure associated with pressure control ventilation, the only randomized trial comparing the two modes of ventilation found no improvement in oxygenation when pressure control ventilation was used during one-lung ventilation.[17] A limitation of this study was its relatively small size, and additional work is needed in this area.

Care should be taken when ventilating transplanted lungs; a period of low compliance associated with reinflating the donor lung may occur initially, but as compliance improves, pressure control ventilation may result in higher than desired tidal volumes. In general, the goals of mechanical ventilation should be to maintain normocapnia and avoid hypoxia while exposing the lungs to minimal airway pressure. This status is especially important after transplantation because high airway pressure and tidal volume may be associated with trauma to bronchial anastomoses.

In cases not involving CPB, one-lung ventilation is necessary. The authors typically use left-sided double-lumen endotracheal tubes (ETTs) inasmuch as they have been described as being more favorable for lung transplantation.[18] Right-sided ETTs can interfere with ventilation of the right upper lobe even with proper placement because of the variability of the location of the right upper lobe orifice. Proper tube position is confirmed by fiberoptic bronchoscopy. In comparison to bronchial blockers, double-lumen ETTs also offer the advantages of more effective suctioning and application of continuous positive airway pressure (CPAP). However, double-lumen ETTs usually need to be replaced with a single-lumen ETT at the conclusion of the procedure, which may be less than ideal, especially with a difficult initial intubation. If a single-lumen ETT is used with a bronchial blocker, the blocker can simply be removed, in which case a second laryngoscopy is not required.

The initiation of one-lung ventilation can produce significant hemodynamic instability. Shunting can worsen hypoxia, hypercapnia, and acidosis, all of which can adversely affect right ventricular function by increasing pulmonary vascular resistance. These factors, coupled with the prospect of ventilating lungs with significant underlying pathology, can make maintenance of adequate oxygenation challenging. Treatment strategies for hypoxia during one-lung ventilation include application of CPAP to the nonventilated lung (thereby reducing intrapulmonary shunt) and PEEP to the ventilated lung (thereby potentially improving atelectasis), although both strategies have disadvantages. Surgical exposure can be impaired by lung reinflation with the application of CPAP to the nonventilated lung. Potential disadvantages of PEEP include decreased venous return, impaired hypoxic pulmonary vasoconstriction, and elevated pulmonary vascular resistance resulting in right ventricular strain while increasing unwanted shunt. Its use must be carefully titrated in an attempt to maintain a balance between improving oxygenation and minimizing potential negative effects.

After implantation and anastomoses of the donor lung have been completed, antegrade flow through the graft is permitted and the lung is gently reinflated. Aggressive reexpansion of the lung can result in pulmonary edema or barotrauma.[19] At our institution inhaled nitric oxide (iNO) is routinely administered during this period because it has been demonstrated to reduce pulmonary artery pressure without affecting systemic blood pressure, thereby reducing workload on the right ventricle while maintaining ventricle perfusion and potentially avoiding the need for CPB.[20,21] However, the routine use of iNO is controversial. A randomized controlled trial involving 30 bilateral lung transplant patients did not reveal any reduction in extravascular lung water or improvement in gas exchange associated with the use of iNO.[22] One should note that this was a small trial focusing only on bilateral lung transplant patients. No randomized controlled studies establishing a reduction in morbidity (time to extubation, length of intensive care unit [ICU] or hospital stay) or mortality exist currently.[23] Further work in this area needs to be completed to definitively determine the benefits of iNO in this patient population.

Hemodynamic management

Hemodynamic instability can occur at various points during the procedure. Usually, patients undergoing lung transplantation procedures have preserved left ventricular function, but their right ventricular function may be diminished, especially during periods of increased afterload. Dopamine and dobutamine infusions augment right ventricular contractility and may also increase systemic blood pressure. Hypotension is not well tolerated and may worsen right ventricular function secondary to inadequate perfusion, particularly in patients with elevated right ventricular pressures. Given preserved left ventricular function, infusions of vasoconstrictor agents such as norepinephrine or phenylephrine can increase systemic vascular resistance and blood pressure. Phosphodiesterase inhibitors can also provide some inotropic support while reducing pulmonary vascular resistance, although decreases in systemic vascular resistance may limit their use.

Surgical clamping of the pulmonary artery during removal of the diseased lung can improve the intrapulmonary shunt but also has the effect of increasing right ventricular afterload. The use of TEE can help determine whether the right ventricle will tolerate pulmonary artery clamping. If the patient's cardiac hemodynamics do not appear reassuring during this period, one should consider the possibility of initiation of CPB.

Hypotension can also occur as a result of the plegia solution and metabolites from the ischemic donor lung entering into the circulation and air entering the coronary arteries.

Air is more likely to enter the right coronary artery given its anatomic location, and this can further impair right ventricular function. This period often requires vasoactive support to maintain adequate perfusion pressures.

In addition to protective lung ventilation strategies, fluid restriction is typically described in the literature as being beneficial in reducing pulmonary complications.[24] Increased central venous pressure has been associated with prolonged mechanical ventilation and increased mortality.[25] A recent retrospective review found an inverse relationship between the volume of intraoperative colloid administered and early graft dysfunction and a reduced rate of extubation.[3] However, fluid restriction strategies can precipitate hypotension, thus requiring a carefully administered balance of fluid administration and use of vasoconstrictors or inotropic agents to optimize end-organ perfusion.

If the procedure entails bilateral sequential single-lung transplantation, it is important to assess the first transplanted lung to rule out technical issues that may affect adequate ventilation and perfusion of the transplanted lung during explantation of the remaining diseased organ. This includes evaluating flow through both pulmonary arteries and veins via TEE to ascertain the presence of any immediate stenosis.[5] Bronchoscopy can identify potential kinking of the bronchial anastomoses.

Use of cardiopulmonary bypass

The use of CPB in lung transplantation is a source of considerable debate.[26-32] Proponents of using CPB cite the greater hemodynamic stability that it affords, the avoidance of one-lung ventilation (which can be technically difficult and physiologically poorly tolerated in some patients), and the fact that it provides a safe and controlled reperfusion period.[32] Opponents of the routine use of CPB state that it is associated with longer periods of postoperative ventilation, increased blood transfusions, increased pulmonary edema, and early graft dysfunction.[28,31] More recent studies in patients with COPD have suggested a survival benefit and no adverse outcomes associated with CPB.[29,30] The absence of randomized, controlled trials involving the use of CPB for lung transplantation should be recognized. Most of the literature consists of small retrospective studies. The heterogeneity of patients' underlying pathology and disease severity makes it difficult to broadly apply available study results to current clinical practice. Overall, the role of CPB as an independent risk factor for early graft dysfunction remains controversial.

For the anesthesiologist, cases involving CPB obviously necessitate a different approach. If CPB is planned from the outset, one-lung ventilation will not routinely be necessary. However, we still commonly use a double-lumen ETT for cases involving CPB at our institution. If a complication such as pulmonary hemorrhage occurs, lung isolation will be required, and one-lung ventilation would be more difficult to establish with a single-lumen ETT in a patient whose airway has now been compromised by bleeding. Additionally, probable or planned CPB may affect epidural placement in the preoperative period (see earlier). Even if CPB is not initially planned, perfusion teams should be readily available and the anesthesiologist prepared for initiation of CPB if hemodynamic instability (e.g., right-sided heart failure) is encountered.

Anesthetic maintenance

Several reports on centers' anesthetic maintenance regimens during lung transplantation have been published.[5,24,33] Most of them have described the use of benzodiazepines and narcotics in large doses (so-called cardiac induction and maintenance). Myles and colleagues[4] described the use of intravenous propofol infusions or volatile anesthetics in their series of patients undergoing lung transplantation as part of anesthetic maintenance, whereas Raffin and associates[24] advocated that no volatile anesthetics be administered because of concerns regarding decreased hypoxic pulmonary vasoconstriction during one-lung ventilation and the potential for reperfusion injury associated with their use. Other advantages of administering an anesthetic involving higher doses of narcotics are that it blunts the sympathetic stress response to surgery and avoids depression of myocardial function from volatile anesthetics.

In cases involving CPB the anesthesiologist needs to consider the pharmokinetics of narcotics in relation to the bypass circuit. The initiation of CPB is associated with a decrease in plasma concentration of all the narcotic agents.[34] In addition, the lungs themselves contribute to a "first-pass" effect on narcotics. The combination of these factors suggests that narcotic concentrations decrease when the lung is removed and when the transplanted lung is reperfused, thus making patient awareness a possible concern. This period is also associated with potential hemodynamic instability, and patients may not tolerate increases in volatile anesthetic levels or propofol administration; thus, the anesthesiologist should be prepared to recalculate the doses of and titrate benzodiazepines and narcotics as tolerated.

At our institution we typically administer an anesthetic that relies more heavily on narcotic and benzodiazepine administration, with volatile anesthetic levels titrated to the patient's hemodynamics. Propofol infusions are not typically administered during the procedure, but low-dose infusions (20 to 50 µg/kg/min as tolerated) are used for sedation while the patient is transported to the ICU. If an epidural has been placed preoperatively, its activation and use are dependent on the hemodynamic status of the patient. If hypotension is a concern, it is prudent to delay epidural dosing until hemodynamic stability is achieved. Typically at our institution, epidural infusions are started postoperatively after consultation with the acute pain service. Epidural anesthesia has been associated with earlier extubation and improved pain control, and catheters are typically left in place until after the chest tubes are removed.[5]

POSTOPERATIVE CARE

Management of these patients in the ICU is addressed elsewhere in this book; the immediate postprocedural care of these patients begins in the operating room. At the conclusion of the procedure, the anesthesiologist needs to be prepared for several facets of the patient's care:

1. Changing the double-lumen ETT (if one has been placed) to a single-lumen one.
2. Maintaining anesthesia for bronchoscopic evaluation of the transplanted lung or lungs.
3. Preparing the patient for transport to the ICU.
4. Signing out care to the ICU team.

When changing a double-lumen ETT to a single-lumen one, the anesthesiologist should consider the initial intubation conditions and difficulty, administration of fluid intraoperatively, and anticoagulation status of the patient. If the initial intubation conditions were ideal, fluid restriction was used (reducing the risk for oropharyngeal edema), and the patient is not currently receiving anticoagulants, direct laryngoscopy is often the technique of choice. However, if any of these factors are less than ideal, use of an airway exchange catheter may be prudent. Care should be taken when using such catheters because they can be associated with trauma and the bronchial anastomoses may be susceptible to traumatic injury.[35] A final option may be to leave the double-lumen tube in place until edema, anticoagulation, and so forth have been corrected. Because ICU care teams may not be as familiar with double-lumen tubes, they should be carefully educated regarding their differences from single-lumen ETTs.

At the end of the surgery patients remain intubated for bronchoscopy and immediate postoperative care in the ICU. The authors typically maintain the patient's anesthetic, including neuromuscular blockade, for the bronchoscopy, and they initiate low-dose propofol infusions for transport. Reversal of neuromuscular blockade before extubation is vital and can be initiated either in the operating room or in the ICU before sedation is discontinued.

Transport of critical care patients to and from the ICU is associated with potential complications; recommendations include providing patients with the same care and monitoring as they would have in the ICU or operating room.[36] Essential monitoring during transport includes an electrocardiogram, measurement of arterial line pressure, and pulse oximetry. In addition, the anesthesiologist should be prepared with emergency airway equipment and resuscitative drugs. Finally, coordination with various members of the transport team is vital to ensure safe transport. This includes communicating with the surgical team members and respiratory therapists, especially if nitric oxide is being used.

Finally, transfer of care to the ICU team (including the nurses, physician assistants, and intensivists) involves detailed reporting of intraoperative events and the patient's current hemodynamic state. Unfortunately, incomplete postoperative handoffs are described in the literature as occurring commonly, and they may contribute to adverse outcomes.[37] A handoff checklist or protocol can reduce the risks associated with incomplete handoffs between providers and care teams. Intraoperative fluid administration should be noted, any vasoactive infusions verified, and the status of antibiotics, immunosuppressant regimens, and neuromuscular blockade status relayed to the ICU team. Ventilator settings should reflect the goals of using a protective lung strategy and minimizing airway pressure while maintaining oxygenation. If an epidural catheter is in place or postoperative placement of one is planned, the acute pain service should be included in this discussion. The hemodynamic status of the patient at the time of transfer of care to the ICU team should be documented before the anesthesiologist signs off.

CONCLUSION

In the future, a continually greater number of patients will benefit from lung transplantation procedures thanks to advances in technology and pharmacology combined with liberalization of donor and recipient criteria. From helping to coordinate the optimal timing of anesthetic induction and minimizing organ ischemia time to safely guiding patients through an operation that is psychologically, physiologically, and hemodynamically challenging, the anesthesiologist plays a role in perioperative care that is vital to favorable outcomes for such patients.

REFERENCES

1. International Society for Heart and Lung Transplantation. Organization Web site. http://www.ishlt.org. Accessed May 24, 2014.
2. Baez B, Castillo M. Anesthetic considerations for lung transplantation. Semin Cardiothorac Vasc Anesth 2008;12:22-127.
3. McIlroy DR, Pilcer DV, Snell GI. Does anaesthetic management affect early outcomes after lung transplant? An exploratory analysis. Br J Anaesth 2009;102:506-514.
4. Myles PS, Snell GI, Westall GP. Lung transplantation. Curr Opin Anaesthesiol 2007;20:21-26.
5. Miranda A, Zink R, McSweeney M. Anesthesia for lung transplantation. Semin Cardiothorac Vasc Anesth 2005;9:205-212.
6. Singh H, Bossard RF. Perioperative anaesthetic considerations for patients undergoing lung transplantation. Can J Anaesth 1997;44:284-299.
7. Egan TM, Murray S, Bustami RT, et al. Development of the new lung allocation system in the United States. Am J Transplant 2006;6:1212-1227.
8. Valapour M, Paulson K, Smith JM, et al. OPTN/SRTR 2011 annual data report: Lung. Am J Transplant 2013;13:149-177.
9. Ballantyne JC, Carr DB, deFerranti S, et al. The comparative effects of postoperative analgesic therapies

on pulmonary outcome: Cumulative meta-analyses of randomized, controlled trials. Anesth Analg 1998;86:598-612.

10. Chaney MA. Intrathecal and epidural anesthesia and analgesia for cardiac surgery. Anesth Analg 2006;102:45-64.

11. Horan BF, Cutfield GR, Davies IM. Problems in the management of the airway during anesthesia for bilateral sequential lung transplantation performed without cardiopulmonary bypass. J Cardiothorac Vasc Anesth 1996;10:387-390.

12. Myles PS, Hall JL, Berry CB, Esmore DS. Primary pulmonary hypertension: Prolonged cardiac arrest and successful resuscitation following induction of anesthesia for heart lung transplantation. J Cardiothorac Vasc Anesth 1994;8:678-681.

13. Huang YC, Cheng YJ, Lin YH, et al. Graft failure caused by pulmonary venous obstruction diagnosed by intraoperative transesophageal echocardiography during lung transplantation. Anesth Analg 2000;91:558-560.

14. Cywinski JB, Wallace L, Parker BM. Pulmonary vein thrombosis after sequential double-lung transplantation. J Cardiothorac Vasc Anesth 2005;19:225-227.

15. Schilling T, Kozian A, Huth C, et al. The pulmonary immune effects of mechanical ventilation in patients undergoing thoracic surgery. Anesth Analg 2005;101:957-965.

16. Michelet P, D'Journo XB, Roch A, et al. Protective ventilation influences systemic inflammation after esophagectomy: A randomized controlled study. Anesthesiology 2006;105:911-919.

17. Unzueta MC, Casas JI, Moral VM. Pressure-controlled versus volume-controlled ventilation during one-lung ventilation for thoracic surgery. Anesth Analg 2007;104:1029-1033.

18. Gelzinis T, Firestone L. Anesthesia for lung transplantation. In Thys DM, Hillel Z, Schwartz AJ, eds. Cardiothoracic Anesthesiology. New York: McGraw-Hill; 2001:817-823.

19. Trachiotis GD, Vricella LA, Aaron BL, Hix WR. As originally published in 1988: Reexpansion pulmonary edema. Updated in 1997. Ann Thorac Surg 1997;63:1206-1207.

20. Rocca GD, Coccia C, Pugliese F, et al. Intraoperative inhaled nitric oxide during anesthesia for lung transplant. Transplant Proc 1997;29:3362-3366.

21. Ardehali A, Laks H, Levine M, et al. A prospective trial of inhaled nitric oxide in clinical lung transplantation. Transplantation 2001;72:112-115.

22. Perrin G, Roch A, Michelet P, et al. Inhaled nitric oxide does not prevent pulmonary edema after lung transplantation measured by lung water content: A randomized clinical study. Chest 2006;29:1024-1030.

23. Tavare AN, Tsakok T. Does prophylactic inhaled nitric oxide reduce morbidity and mortality after lung transplantation? Interact Cardiovasc Thorac Surg 2011;13:516-520.

24. Raffin L, Michel-Cherqui M, Sperandio M, et al. Anesthesia for bilateral lung transplantation without cardiopulmonary bypass: Initial experience and review of intraoperative problems. J Cardiothorac Vasc Anesth 1992;6:409-417.

25. Pilcher DV, Snell GI, Scheinkestel CD, et al. A high central venous pressure is associated with prolonged mechanical ventilation and increased mortality following lung transplantation. J Thoracic Cardiovasc Surg 2005;129:912-918.

26. Myles PS. Pulmonary transplantation. In Kaplan JA, Slinger P, eds. Thoracic Anesthesia. Philadelphia, PA: Elsevier Science; 2003:295-314.

27. Guillén RV, Briones FR, Marín PM, et al. Lung graft dysfunction in the early postoperative period after lung and heart lung transplantation. Transplant Proc 2005;37:3994-3995.

28. Dalibon N, Geffroy A, Moutafis M, et al. Use of cardiopulmonary bypass for lung transplantation: A 10-year experience. J Cardiothorac Vasc Anesth 2006;20:668-672.

29. De Boer WJ, Hepkema BG, Loef BG, et al. Survival benefit of cardiopulmonary bypass support in bilateral lung transplantation for emphysema patients. Transplantation 2002;73:1621-1627.

30. Szeto WY, Kreisel D, Karakousis GC, et al. Cardiopulmonary bypass for bilateral sequential lung transplantation in patients with chronic obstructive pulmonary disease without adverse effect on lung function or clinical outcome. J Thorac Cardiovasc Surg 2002;124:241-249.

31. McRae K. Con: Lung transplantation should not be routinely performed with cardiopulmonary bypass. J Cardiothorac Vasc Anesth 2000;14:746-750.

32. Marczin N, Royston D, Yacoub M. Pro: Lung transplantation should be routinely performed with cardiopulmonary bypass. J Cardiothorac Vasc Anesth 2000;14:739-745.

33. Myles PS, Weeks AM, Buckland MR, et al. Anesthesia for bilateral sequential lung transplantation: Experience of 64 cases. J Cardiothorac Vasc Anesth 1997;11:177-183.

34. Stoelting RK. Pharmacology and Physiology in Anesthetic Practice, 3rd ed. Philadelphia: Lippincott-Raven; 1999.

35. Thomas V, Neustein SM. Tracheal laceration after the use of an airway exchange catheter for double-lumen tube placement. J Cardiothorac Vasc Anesth 2007;21:718-719.

36. Braxton CC, Reilly PM, Schwab CW. The traveling intensive care unit patient: Road trips. Surg Clin North Am 2000;80:949-956.

37. Nagpal K, Arora S, Abboudi M, et al. Postoperative handover: Problems, pitfalls and prevention of error. Ann Surg 2010;252:171-176.

Mechanical ventilation and extracorporeal membrane oxygenation (ECMO): Bridges to lung transplantation

JAMES J. YUN AND DAVID P. MASON

INTRODUCTION

Lung transplantation is an established therapy for end-stage lung disease. Following implementation of the lung allocation score in 2005, the use of mechanical ventilation, extracorporeal membrane oxygenation (ECMO), or both as a bridge to transplantation increased. Mechanical ventilation and ECMO have successfully bridged selected patients to transplantation but are associated with higher resource use and mortality. Refinements in patient selection, ECMO circuits, and perioperative care now permit ECMO support in awake and sometimes ambulatory patients before transplantation. Bridging patients to transplantation with mechanical ventilation or ECMO is increasingly common, and in properly selected patients, it may be the only lifesaving option for critically ill patients awaiting a donor lung.

MECHANICAL VENTILATION (NONINVASIVE AND INVASIVE): A BRIDGE TO LUNG TRANSPLANTATION

Before lung transplantation for mechanically ventilated patients gained wider acceptance, noninvasive positive pressure ventilation (NPPV) was a more commonly used, temporizing "bridge" therapy for transplant candidates with acute respiratory decompensation despite maximal medical therapy.[1] NPPV was successful for acute control of hypercapnia and aversion of endotracheal intubation in both adult patients with chronic obstructive pulmonary disease and young patients with cystic fibrosis (CF) who were awaiting a transplant.[1,2] Although still used today, NPPV is not always well tolerated, particularly in anxious or uncooperative patients. Furthermore, NPPV remains contraindicated in patients who are unable to maintain a patent airway, those with excessive secretions, and those with hemodynamic compromise.

In the early experience with lung transplantation, invasive mechanical ventilation (endotracheal intubation) was considered an absolute or strong contraindication to transplantation.[2] Through the early 1990s, pretransplant mechanical ventilation was believed to be associated with insurmountable morbidity and mortality related mainly to respiratory muscle weakness and nosocomial infection.[3,4] Delisting lung transplant candidates who required invasive mechanical ventilation while awaiting donor lungs was common practice in that era.[1]

Nevertheless, multiple centers have reported some success with performing transplants on mechanically ventilated candidates. In 1994, Flume and associates reported a series of seven double-lung recipients (six for CF and one for acute lung injury) who were between the ages of 15 and 30 years and had been bridged to transplantation with pretransplant mechanical ventilation for 7 to 115 days. The authors found no early infections or deaths attributable to the ventilatory support. Only the patient supported for 115 days before transplantation required prolonged post-transplant ventilation (27 days).[4] Bartz and colleagues from the University of Wisconsin compared 8 patients with CF who received a double-lung transplant following pretransplant mechanical ventilation with a group of 24 control patients with CF who did not receive ventilatory support. Although the patients requiring ventilation before transplantation needed significantly longer support postoperatively (11 versus 4 days), no significant difference was observed between the groups in terms of time to discharge, 1-year survival, or forced expiratory volume at 1 year.[5] More recently, Elizur and colleagues reported the results for 18 pediatric patients with CF who had been supported with pretransplant mechanical ventilation through 2007. The authors cautioned that patients who were intubated before transplantation had longer post-transplant intubation periods and lengths of intensive care unit stay and lower short-term (1-year) survival than did age-matched controls who had not been mechanically ventilated before transplantation.[6] It is difficult to draw definitive conclusions from these and other single-center reports in the literature, all of which are limited by small sample size and some selection bias. Consequently, although growing evidence suggests that lung transplantation after mechanical ventilation is feasible and not absolutely contraindicated, it still is not universally practiced because of its higher-risk nature.

The risks associated with mechanical ventilation before lung transplantation in the U.S. experience were further assessed by analyzing the United Network for Organ Sharing (UNOS) lung transplantation database. Mason and associates reviewed the U.S. outcomes of lung transplantation after pretransplant mechanical ventilation from 1987 to 2008 and found that of 15,934 primary lung transplants (586 patients were mechanically ventilated before transplantation), the unadjusted survival rate for mechanically ventilated patients was inferior to that for nonsupported patients (83% versus 93% at 1 month, 62% versus 79% at 12 months, and 57% versus 70% at 24 months).[7] The trend of decreased survival persisted after transplant year and propensity for mechanical support were taken into account. Nevertheless, patients who survived the early postoperative period had longer-term survival rates that were comparable to those of patients not requiring pretransplant mechanical ventilation. Because the survival rate of those requiring pretransplant support was far from "dismal" and, in many cases, a transplant was their only option for survival, the authors noted that the inherent question when deciding whether to perform a transplant on a mechanically ventilated patient is as follows: is the therapeutic goal of lung transplantation to maximize the survival of an individual who is more likely to have early complications, or is it instead to provide the highest likelihood of benefit to the maximum number of patients?[7]

Given the controversy in this area, pretransplant mechanical ventilation remains a relative, not absolute contraindication to transplantation in current practice.

ECMO: A BRIDGE TO LUNG TRANSPLANTATION

History and background

The first reported use of ECMO as a bridge to lung transplantation in humans dates back to the 1970s, when Veith performed a double-lung transplant on a patient with respiratory failure following trauma who was being supported with ECMO.[8] Although the patient died on the 10th postoperative day, this case established the feasibility of ECMO support as a bridge to transplantation. In the 1980s, the Toronto group notably used ECMO as a salvage bridge to transplantation twice in the same patient, a 31-year-old man with Paraquat poisoning who was originally supported with ECMO for refractory respiratory failure despite mechanical ventilation and then bridged successfully to a right single-lung transplant.[9] ECMO was then reinstituted less than a week later for respiratory failure (which was believed to have resulted from Paraquat reentering the circulation from muscle stores) until a successful left lung transplant 19 days later. The patient died of a cerebral vascular accident related to a tracheobrachiocephalic artery fistula 3 months postoperatively, but the case demonstrated the feasibility of ECMO as a rescue bridge to transplant therapy.[9]

In the early 1990s, the Hannover (Federal Republic of Germany) group reported several cases of a successful bridge to lung transplantation with ECMO. Jurmann and colleagues reported two cases in which ECMO was used as rescue therapy for recent lung transplant recipients with early graft dysfunction refractory to mechanical ventilation.[10] In the first case refractory graft dysfunction developed in a 46-year-old woman who had received a right single-lung transplant for pulmonary fibrosis 11 days earlier. She was supported with venoarterial (VA) ECMO for 8 hours; it was subsequently discontinued in the operating room following successful emergency right lung retransplantation. She was discharged after 3 months and was alive and well 1 year after retransplantation. The second patient was a 32-year-old woman with pulmonary fibrosis in whom refractory graft dysfunction with hemodynamic compromise developed immediately following implantation of a right single lung. VA ECMO was instituted intraoperatively and continued for 232 hours until urgent right lung retransplantation. The patient had multiple postoperative complications but lived for approximately 5 months. Despite their small number of cases, these reports demonstrated that ECMO was possible as a bridge to emergency retransplantation under adverse circumstances and offered the chance of a positive outcome.

Shortly thereafter, Jurmann and the Hannover group reported three additional cases of ECMO used as a bridge to primary lung transplantation (not retransplantation).[11] The first involved a 19-year-old man with refractory pulmonary hemorrhage and respiratory failure following blunt trauma; a bilateral lung transplant after 5 days of ECMO support was successful, and the patient returned to work after discharge. The second case involved a 43-year-old woman who had undergone a combined liver and kidney transplant; she had pulmonary endarteritis obliterans, was bridged to a left single-lung transplant within 2 weeks of ECMO, and also did well (she survived for at least 1 year after transplantation). The third patient was a 32-year-old man with multiorgan failure following trauma and suspected sepsis; he was successfully bridged to a transplant with ECMO for 6 days but died during an attempted salvage via a left single-lung transplant. This series, although also small, provided further evidence that ECMO as a bridge to transplantation was feasible, with good results for urgent (versus salvage) primary lung transplantation.

Other early experiences with ECMO as a bridge to lung transplantation have also recently been well summarized by Diaz-Guzman and colleagues.[12]

Evolution of ECMO therapy

In the 1990s, ECMO was used primarily for graft failure after lung transplantation and only rarely as a bridge to transplantation. According to UNOS data, from 1990 to 2000 only 22 patients were listed for a lung transplant while on ECMO.[12] Factors hindering the clinical utility of ECMO included (1) limited membrane performance and durability, (2) membrane plasma leakage, (3) limited performance of the older roller head pumps, and (4) bleeding related to systemic anticoagulation.[12,13] More recently, ECMO oxygenators with polymethylpentene (PMP) membranes (Maquet Quadrox) have replaced the older silicone or polypropylene membrane oxygenators. PMP based membranes not only have superior gas exchange characteristics but can also support ECMO for several weeks without plasma leakage or need for exchange. In addition, newer centrifugal pumps cause less hemolysis than the older roller designs did. Furthermore, increased use of heparin-bonded circuits has decreased the need for aggressive anticoagulation.[12-14]

In the 2000s, the results of the CESAR trial also further validated contemporary ECMO as a clinically effective therapy.[15] Briefly, the CESAR trial demonstrated that intention-to-treat acute respiratory distress syndrome (ARDS) with ECMO in a centralized fashion conferred a greater survival advantage at 6 months than did conventional ventilator therapy alone. Although this trial did not involve transplant patients, it established the efficacy of modern adult ECMO therapy for respiratory failure, and it has changed the perception of ECMO, which is now seen not as a salvage therapy tool with an inevitably negative outcome but rather as a useful tool for cases of severe respiratory illness. Not surprisingly, the increased interest in adult ECMO as a bridge to lung transplantation has paralleled the increased use of ECMO for ARDS.

ECMO as a bridge to transplantation: patient selection

Because of the limited clinical experience with ECMO as a bridge to lung transplantation, no registry or randomized clinical trials exist to define the ideal characteristics of ECMO candidates. However, the consensus of opinion suggests that among transplant candidates, favorable characteristics for ECMO bridge-to-transplant therapy include (1) younger age, (2) absence of multiorgan failure, (3) absence of systemic infection or sepsis, and (4) adequate nutritional status before and during ECMO support.[12-14] Controversial areas include (1) the upper chronologic age limits for ECMO candidacy before transplantation, (2) the "acceptable" duration of continued ECMO support before transplantation, and (3) the ideal timing of initiation of ECMO support.[12-14] ECMO was used for 107 days as a bridge to successful transplantation in a 24-year-old man with severe ARDS; he lived for 351 days after transplantation before dying of pneumonia.[16]

In practice, the decision to use ECMO before lung transplantation, patient selection and age criteria for ECMO support before transplantation, and timing of initiation of ECMO support vary significantly between transplant centers. In a 2013 survey of 33 U.S. lung transplant programs, 18 reported having used ECMO as a bridge to transplantation.[17] Fifteen programs reported age older than 65 years as a contraindication to pretransplant ECMO, whereas 12 (including the 5 highest-volume centers) had no age contraindication. The majority of programs (17 of 33) instituted ECMO only in cases of failure or impending failure of mechanical ventilation.[17]

Modes of ECMO bridge-to-transplantation therapy

ECMO can be delivered in two modes depending on patient needs: venovenous (VV) or VA. In the VV mode, deoxygenated venous blood removed from the patient is pumped through the ECMO circuit and oxygenated blood is returned to a vein. For VA ECMO, a central or peripheral artery is the return site. For simple relief of hypercapnia and hypoxia before lung transplantation, VV ECMO may be adequate, particularly when native cardiac function is preserved. However, in cases of end-stage lung disease with significant pulmonary hypertension, particularly with associated severe right ventricular dysfunction, VA ECMO may be required for adequate peripheral oxygen delivery.[13,18]

Most commonly, VV ECMO with peripheral cannulation involves femoral venous cannulation with return to the contralateral femoral vein, an internal jugular vein, or one of the subclavian veins. For VA ECMO with peripheral cannulation, circuit inflow occurs most commonly from a femoral or jugular vein with arterial return to a femoral or subclavian artery.[18] Central cannulation options for pretransplant ECMO include VV ECMO with right atrial-to–pulmonary artery cannulation and VA ECMO with pulmonary artery–to–left atrial cannulation, in addition to simple right atrial–to–aortic cannulation. For hypoxia associated with significant pulmonary hypertension, VV ECMO with atrial septostomy is also an alternative to VA ECMO.[19]

Ambulatory ECMO

A recent major paradigm shift in ECMO therapy is the concept that ECMO is no longer exclusively for use in sedated immobile patients but should be applied to avoid intubation, permit extubation, and promote mobility in a patient awaiting lung transplantation.[12-14] Previously, ECMO as a bridge-to-transplant therapy was used only when mechanical ventilation failed or its failure was imminent. Older ECMO cannulation strategies involving only femoral vessel cannulation also precluded ambulation and thus contributed to ongoing continued intubation and sedation.[18] ECMO support in an awake, extubated, and mobile patient circumvents the sequelae of intubation and sedation, including diaphragmatic and skeletal muscle deconditioning, no active participation in physical therapy, and preclusion of oral intake. Beginning in the 2000s, several case reports described upper body cannulation strategies that allowed short-term VV and VA ECMO support in awake, ambulatory patients.[12-14,20-22]

An important advance in VV ECMO cannula design that stimulated interest in ambulatory VV ECMO was U.S. Food and Drug Administration (FDA) approval in 2009 of the Avalon double-lumen cannula (DLC) developed by Drs. Wang and Zwischenberger.[23] The Avalon cannula has two cannula lumina in one catheter, thereby enabling VV ECMO therapy from a single venous access site.[12] The cannula is inserted percutaneously into an upper body vein with fluoroscopic or transesophageal echocardiography guidance. By aligning the oxygenated blood return lumen port with the tricuspid valve, the Avalon DLC cannula facilitates VV ECMO with upper body cannulation only, thereby allowing patient extubation, mobilization, and possibly ambulation.[21,22]

For patients requiring VA ECMO, an upper body cannulation strategy that facilitates ambulation during a bridge to transplantation is right internal jugular vein cannulation for inflow to the ECMO circuit with blood return via the subclavian artery.[18,20] This strategy also offers optimal cerebral oxygen saturation (in contrast to femoral artery return). Possible cannulation complications (in addition to bleeding) include upper extremity ischemia (with direct cannulation) and upper extremity hyperperfusion (which is preventable by beveling and properly angling the graft sewn to the subclavian artery). Transient upper extremity neurapraxia has also been observed with this strategy and may result from manipulation of the brachial plexus during axillary artery access or prolonged ECMO support.

The experience with pediatric ambulatory pretransplant ECMO is even more limited than in adults. However, Hayes and associates reported two cases in which adolescent lung transplant candidates were successfully mobilized while receiving ECMO support with tracheostomy performed in conjunction with VV ECMO.[24] Tracheostomy allowed intermittent mechanical ventilation and physical therapy, with avoidance of sedation and paralytics during a pretransplant ECMO duration of up to 23 days. The only adverse incident associated with tracheostomy during pretransplant ECMO support was a single episode of self-limited bleeding that was corrected surgically.[24]

ECMO as a bridge to lung transplantation: recent clinical results

In a study based on UNOS data, Mason and associates reported outcomes of lung transplantation in patients in the United States who were supported with ECMO before transplantation from 1987 to 2008.[7] Of 15,934 primary lung transplant recipients, 51 (0.3%) had been supported with pretransplant ECMO. The unadjusted survival rates for those who received ECMO support were inferior to those of nonsupported patients (72% versus 93% at 1 month, 50% versus 79% at 12 months, and 45% versus 70% at 24 months), with the trend toward decreased survival persisting after propensity matching. However, following the high-risk early phase, patients supported with ECMO before transplantation had survival rates similar to those of patients not supported with ECMO (and also survival rates similar to those of patients supported with mechanical ventilation before transplantation).

The frequency of ECMO bridge-to-transplant therapy increased significantly in the United States from 2000 to 2010 and after 2010,[12] particularly at higher-volume transplant centers. Accordingly, multiple single-center experiences with encouraging short- and intermediate-term survival rates emerged (mainly after 2008). Shafii and coworkers retrospectively reviewed 19 cases in which pretransplant ECMO was performed by the Cleveland Clinic group from 2008 to 2011.[25] Fourteen patients supported with ECMO (74%) received successful transplants, with survival rates of 75% at 1 year and 63% at 3 years after transplantation. The best results occurred in patients with interstitial lung disease who were bridged to transplantation with VV ECMO. The Columbia (New York) group reported 13 patients supported with ECMO from July 2007 to April 2012 with the intent to transplant.[26] Ten received successful transplants, with a median duration of ECMO support of 6 days (three recovered and were weaned from ECMO); all the transplant recipients were alive at early follow-up (as long as 2 years after transplantation). The Pittsburgh group reported 17 patients who received transplants after being supported with ECMO from 1991 to 2010 (notably, 12 operations occurred after 2005), with a mean duration of ECMO support of only 3.2 days (shorter than in most other reports).[27] The respective 30-day, 1 year, and 3-year survival rates in the ECMO-supported patients were 81%, 74%, and 65% versus 93%, 78%, and 62% in the controls. Hoopes and colleagues reported the results of using ECMO as a bridge to transplantation in 31 patients (19 ambulatory) at two institutions (the University of California at San Francisco and University of Kentucky). Survival rates at 1, 3, and 5 years were 93%, 80%, and 66%, respectively.[28]

Encouraging results from the U.S. centers were reproduced internationally. Cypel and associates from Toronto reported a 70% 1-year survival rate for 10 patients from 2010 who were successfully bridged to a lung transplant with ECMO (including 4 with pumpless membrane support).[29] Fuehner and colleagues reported an 80% survival rate at 1 year in 26 patients who were bridged with ECMO.[30] The Vienna group (Lang and coworkers) noted that the 1- and 3-year survival rates for 34 patients supported with ECMO who received transplants from 1998 to 2011 were 60% and 60%.[31] Notably, for patients who survived 3 months, the survival rates at 1, 3, and 5 years were similar to those of non–ECMO-supported transplant patients during the same period.

Most recently, Dellgren and associates from Sweden reported that of 16 patients supported with ECMO from 2005 to 2013, 12 received successful transplants and 9 of the 12 (75%) were alive at 1 year.[32] Crotti and colleagues from Italy noted that 17 of 25 patients who were supported with ECMO and subsequently received a transplant had a 76% 1-year survival rate and that their mortality risk was correlated with duration of ECMO support (hazard ratio, 1.06 per day of ECMO support).[33] Taken together, these international reports further support the findings of the U.S. groups. Although these single-center reports have small sample sizes, they collectively suggest that contemporary ECMO therapy used as a bridge to lung transplantation can yield acceptable short-term outcomes at selected centers.

Extracorporeal pulmonary support with an interventional lung assist device as a bridge to lung transplantation

The pumpless Novalung interventional lung assist (iLA) device uses a PMP membrane placed in an arteriovenous configuration (without a pump) to assist in gas exchange by simple diffusion.[12] It has been used successfully as an extracorporeal pulmonary support alternative to ECMO in Europe and Canada[29,30] but is not yet FDA approved in the United States. Because the iLA device is pumpless, it is most effective in patients with hypercapnic respiratory failure.[12] Flow through the iLA device is dependent on adequate native cardiac function and the patient's native blood pressure (arteriovenous) gradient; gas exchange occurs via simple diffusion across the low-resistance membrane. When compared with ECMO, the iLA device is pumpless and more compact.

Internationally, the iLA device has been used both as a bridge to lung recovery from ARDS, and as a bridge to lung transplantation.[29,30,34-36] Major adverse effects include bleeding and complications of arterial cannulation.[36] Despite not being ambulatory because of femoral cannulation, many patients in whom the iLA device was used were able to be extubated. The Novalung iLA device holds promise as a low-morbidity bridge to lung transplantation in selected patients with hypercapnic respiratory failure. The process of FDA approval in the United States is currently under way.

CONCLUSIONS

Successful bridge to lung transplantation with mechanical ventilation, ECMO, or both is not only feasible but increasingly common in the current era of donor lung allocation. Although patients bridged to transplantation with mechanical ventilation or ECMO have increased early morbidity and mortality, they typically have few other options for survival and their survival is comparable to that of nonsupported patients after the early postoperative period. The improved early clinical outcomes in mechanically ventilated and ECMO-bridged patients reflect better patient selection and improved pretransplant and post-transplant care, as well as improvements in ECMO therapy, including the recent adoption of ambulatory ECMO systems.

In the current era of limited organ donors and health care resources, further longer-term studies and the development of appropriate registries are needed to identify the lung transplant patients who will reap the greatest benefit from pretransplant mechanical ventilation and ECMO.

REFERENCES

1. O'Brien G, Criner GJ. Mechanical ventilation as a bridge to lung transplantation. J Heart Lung Transplant 1999;18:255-265.
2. Hodson ME, Madden BP, Steven MH, et al. Non-invasive mechanical ventilation for cystic fibrosis patients—a potential bridge to transplantation. Eur Respir J 1991;4:524-527.
3. Vermeijden JW, Zijlstra JG, Erasmus ME, et al. Lung transplantation for ventilation-dependent respiratory failure. J Heart Lung Transplant 2009;28:347-351.
4. Flume PA, Egan TM, Westerman JH, et al. Lung transplantation for mechanically ventilated patients. J Heart Lung Transplant 1994;13:15-21.
5. Bartz RR, Love RB, Leverson GE, et al. Pre-transplant mechanical ventilation and outcome in patients with cystic fibrosis. J Heart Lung Transplant 2003;22:433-438.
6. Elizur A, Sweet SC, Huddleston CB, et al. Pre-transplant mechanical ventilation increases short-term morbidity and mortality in pediatric patients with cystic fibrosis. J Heart Lung Transplant 2007;26:127-131.
7. Mason DP, Thuita L, Nowicki E, et al. Should lung transplantation be performed for patients on mechanical respiratory support? The US experience. J Thorac Cardiovasc Surg 2010;139:765-773.
8. Veith FJ. Lung transplantation. Transplant Proc 1977;9:203-208.
9. Toronto Lung Transplant Group. Sequential bilateral lung transplantation for Paraquat poisoning. A case report. J Thorac Cardiovasc Surg 1985;89:734-742.
10. Jurmann MJ, Haverich A, Demertzis S, et al. Extracorporeal membrane oxygenation as a bridge to lung transplantation. Eur J Cardiothorac Surg 1991;5:94-98.

11. Jurmann MJ, Schaefers HJ, Demertzis S, et al. Emergency lung transplantation after extracorporeal membrane oxygenation. ASAIO J 1993;39:M448-M452.

12. Diaz-Guzman ED, Hoopes CW, Zwischenberger JB. The evolution of extracorporeal life support as a bridge to lung transplantation. ASAIO J 2013;59:3-10.

13. Javidfar J, Bacchetta M. Bridge to lung transplantation with extracorporeal membrane oxygenation support. Curr Opin Organ Transplant 2012;17:496-502.

14. Strueber M. Bridges to lung transplantation. Curr Opin Organ Transplant 2011;16:458-461.

15. Peek GJ, Mugford M, Tiruvoipati R, et al. Efficacy and economic assessment of conventional ventilatory support versus extracorporeal membrane oxygenation for severe adult respiratory failure (CESAR): A multicentre randomised controlled trial. Lancet 2009;374:1351-1363.

16. Iacono A, Groves S, Garcia J, Griffith BA. Lung transplantation following 107 days of extracorporeal membrane oxygenation. Eur J Cardiothorac Surg 2010;37:969-971.

17. Fidul R, McCurry KR, Budev MM, Yun JJ. Extracorporeal membrane oxygenation (ECMO) practices for bridging to lung transplantation in North America: A multi-center survey. J Heart Lung Transplant 2014;33:S246-S247.

18. Stulak JM, Dearani JA, Burkhart HM, et al. ECMO cannulation controversies and complications. Semin Cardiothorac Vasc Anesth 2009;13:176-182.

19. Hoopes CW, Gurley JC, Zwischenberger JB, et al. Mechanical support for pulmonary venoocclusive disease: Combined atrial septostomy and venovenous extracorporeal membrane oxygenation. Semin Thorac Cardiovasc Surg 2012;24:232-234.

20. Mangi A, Mason D, Yun J, et al. Bridge to lung transplantation using short-term ambulatory extracorporeal membrane oxygenation. J Thorac Cardiovasc Surg 2010; 40:713-715.

21. Garcia J, Iacono A, Kon ZN, Griffith BP. Ambulatory ECMO: A new approach for bridge to lung transplantation. J Thorac Cardiovasc Surg 2010;139:e137-e139.

22. Turner DA, Cheifetz IM, Rehder KJ, et al. Active rehabilitation and physical therapy during extracorporeal membrane oxygenation while awaiting lung transplantation: A practical approach. Crit Care Med 2011;39:2593-2598.

23. Wang D, Zhou X, Liu X, et al. Wang-Zwische double lumen cannula—toward a percutaneous and ambulatory paracorporeal artificial lung. ASAIO J 2008:54;606-611.

24. Hayes D, Galantowicz M, Preston JJ, et al. Tracheostomy in adolescent patients bridged to lung transplantation with ambulatory venovenous extracorporeal membrane oxygenation. J Artif Organs 2014;17:103-105.

25. Shafii A, Mason DP, Brown C, et al. Growing experience with extracorporeal membrane oxygenation as a bridge to lung transplantation. ASAIO J 2012;58:526-529.

26. Javidfar J, Brodie D, Iribarne A, et al. Extracorporeal membrane oxygenation as a bridge to lung transplantation and recovery. J Thorac Cardiovasc Surg 2012;144:716-721.

27. Bermudez CA, Rocha RV, Zaldonis D, et al. Extracorporeal membrane oxygenation as a bridge to lung transplant: Midterm outcomes. Ann Thorac Surg 2011;92:1226-1232.

28. Hoopes CW, Kukreja J, Golden J, et al. Extracorporeal membrane oxygenation as a bridge to pulmonary transplantation. J Thorac Cardiovasc Surg 2013;145:862-867.

29. Cypel M, Waddell TK, de Parrot M, Keshavjee S. Safety and efficacy of the Novalung interventional lung assist (iLA) device as a bridge to lung transplantation. J Heart Lung Transplant 2010;29(Suppl 2):588.

30. Fuehner T, Kuehn C, Hadem J, et al. Extracorporeal membrane oxygenation in awake patients as bridge to lung transplantation. Am J Respir Crit Care Med 2012;185:763-768.

31. Lang G, Taghavi S, Aigner C, et al. Primary lung transplantation after bridge with extracorporeal membrane oxygenation: A plea for a shift in our paradigms for indications. Transplantation 2012;93:729-736.

32. Dellgren G, Riise GC, Sward K, et al. Extracorporeal membrane oxygenation as a bridge to lung transplantation: A long-term study. Eur J Cardiothorac Surg 2015;47:95-100.

33. Crotti S, Iotti GA, Lissoni A, et al. Organ allocation waiting time during extracorporeal bridge to lung transplant affects outcomes. Chest 2013;144:1018-1025.

34. Christie JD, Edwards LB, Aurora P, et al. Registry of the International Society for Heart and Lung Transplantation: Twenty-fifth official adult lung and heart/lung transplantation report—2008. J Heart Lung Transplant 2008:27:957-969.

35. Fischer S, Hoeper MM, Tomaszek S, et al. Bridge to lung transplantation with the extracorporeal membrane ventilator Novalung in the veno-venous mode: The initial Hannover experience. ASAIO J 2007;53;168-170.

36. Flörchinger B, Philipp A, Klose A, et al. Pumpless extracorporeal lung assist: A 10 year institutional experience. Ann Thorac Surg 2008:86:410-417.

15

Single-lung transplantation: Technical aspects

CHRISTOPHER WIGFIELD AND WICKII T. VIGNESWARAN

INTRODUCTION

Lung transplantation remains the only hope for survival in most patients with end-stage lung disease (ESLD). The challenges inherent to lung transplantation continue to be a shortage of available donor organs, primary graft dysfunction, rejection, and infection. Excellent progress with perioperative strategies, including technical advances and improvement in critical care, has been made over the last decade. Although both bilateral and single-lung transplants provide valid options for selected patients with ESLD, single-lung transplantation is often a pragmatic means of providing a suitable lung allograft.[1] This chapter describes the history, technique, and outcomes of single-lung transplantation.

HISTORY

The history of thoracic transplantation began in the laboratories of the University of Chicago, where Alexis Carrel pioneered the technique of blood vessel anastomosis and orthotopic heart transplantation in canines.[2] The first human lung transplant was performed by Dr. Hardy at the University of Mississippi in 1963.[3] It was not until the introduction of cyclosporine and cardiopulmonary bypass that lung transplantation became a viable and increasingly safe treatment option for patients with ESLD. The surgical refinement of tracheal to bilateral sequential bronchial anastomoses allowed consideration of single-lung transplantation via thoracotomy. The first single-lung transplant with prolonged postoperative survival is credited to Dr. Joel Cooper at Toronto General Hospital in 1983.[4] Since then, refinements in technique, immunosuppression, and perioperative care have made single-lung transplantation routinely available for many patients with selected types of ESLD.

INDICATIONS FOR SINGLE-LUNG TRANSPLANTATION

Single-lung transplantation is considered primarily for nonsuppurative ESLD. It is a viable option in the absence of idiopathic or secondary pulmonary hypertension. In particular, patients with chronic obstructive pulmonary disease, α_1-antitrypsin deficiency–related lung disease, or idiopathic pulmonary fibrosis (IPF) may be considered candidates provided that detailed assessment of laterality and possible aggravating factors is performed. Disease-specific guidelines must be followed on an individual basis when considering lung transplantation.[5] Single-lung transplants offer several advantages, including procurement of the contralateral donor organ for an additional recipient. Reduced waiting times, shorter operating times, and rapid recovery have been noted and may well reduce the risk for mortality while on the waiting list for individual candidates.

Perioperatively, the contralateral, native lung may provide a recipient with temporary support for gas exchange if significant primary allograft graft dysfunction is encountered. Some advocates of bilateral lung transplantation cite several advantages, including long-term survival benefits in subgroups of lung transplant recipients. Concern for native lung–induced donor compromise and the decreased incidence of bronchiolitis obliterans have been mentioned in the past, but they must be reconciled with the practicalities of a scarce commodity for recipients within a reasonable time frame.[6,7] Single-lung transplantation provides a survival advantage in selected patients, such as those with IPF, particularly in the absence of secondary pulmonary hypertension.[8,9] Such patients have benefited from introduction of the lung allocation score in the United States.[10] In addition, recent data suggest that bilateral lung transplantation offers little benefit over single-lung transplantation in patients 60 years of age and older with a diagnosis of chronic obstructive pulmonary disease.[11,12] Thus, it has become imperative to individualize the transplantation strategy and to consider factors such as underlying lung disease, age, and associated comorbidity for each recipient in this context. Extended criteria donor options may also include procurement from donors whose contralateral lung was not deemed suitable, thereby increasing the donor pool to some extent.

The technical details of preservation of the donor lung and its implantation into a recipient are even more critical in this setting, and success depends totally on having the transplanted single lung functioning at its maximum potential. Strategies for single and bilateral lung transplants will continue to evolve as more evidence emerges and with the advent of ex vivo lung perfusion. Some centers have developed expertise in transplants from living related donors and split lung lobar transplantation. This practice is restricted to relatively few situations and is beyond the scope of this chapter (see Chapter 18). In summary, single-lung transplantation should be considered a viable option for selected recipients with ESLD and has a proven record of good short- and long-term outcomes.

TECHNIQUE

Donor pneumonectomy

Donor selection (see Chapter 7) and procurement (see Chapter 10) are addressed in detail elsewhere in this book. During donor evaluation flexible bronchoscopy is always performed to examine the airways and remove any secretions. Anatomic variations may occasionally be present, and they are evaluated during bronchoscopy. Invariably, lung donor procurement occurs in the setting of multiorgan procurement. Lungs are procured "en bloc" and the surgical approach is via a midline sternotomy. Initially the lung is inspected to evaluate its suitability for transplantation by checking for pathology, including evidence of trauma, infection, tumor, or other parenchymal disease. Static compliance and oxygenation are assessed routinely for each lung, and selective pulmonary venous blood gas measurements can help differentiate a viable single lung.[13]

Procedures performed on the recipient of a single lung

Once a donor has been verified and a lung has been deemed suitable for transplantation, the recipient is brought into the operating room for transplantation. We prefer to place a thoracic epidural before the transplantation procedure unless cardiopulmonary bypass and full systemic anticoagulation are expected. General anesthesia is provided, and the patient is ventilated with a double-lumen endotracheal tube. The tube's position is verified by fiberoptic bronchoscopy. Arterial and venous access lines, including a Swan-Ganz catheter, are placed. At this stage we also insert a transesophageal echocardiography (TEE) probe. The patient is placed in a lateral decubitus position for an anterolateral thoracotomy or in a semilateral position if a limited submammary incision is planned. An axillary roll should be placed under the axilla of the dependent arm to prevent injuries to the brachial plexus. A body-warming device (Bair Hugger) is used for the lower part of the body. The chest, abdomen, and groin are exposed, and the field is prepared with antiseptic solution and draped in sterile fashion (in case cardiopulmonary bypass via femoral access is needed). It is helpful to insert a femoral arterial line for a later Seldinger approach in this position if the need for extracorporeal support appears to be likely.

INCISIONS

A number of incisions may be used in this setting, including a posterolateral incision, anterior submammary incision, or lateral incision that either spares all the large muscles or partially divides the muscle. Our preferred approach is a submammary anterolateral incision that splits the pectoral muscles but preserves the latissimus dorsi muscle. When the chest cavity is normal size or larger, as in patients with obstructive airway disease, we perform a muscle-sparing submammary incision. In patients with small chest cavities, such as those with severe IPF, we perform an anterolateral thoracotomy, occasionally partially dividing the latissimus dorsi muscle but preserving the serratus anterior muscle. The incision is placed in such a way that it is over the hilum of the lung, ideally entering the pleural space through no lower than the fifth intercostal space. Developing a good understanding of unilateral, dependent lung ventilation and the intraoperative shunting mechanisms involved is essential.

RECIPIENT PNEUMONECTOMY

The recipient pneumonectomy is prepared while the donor organ is being procured, but the lung is not excised until the donor organs are received in the recipient operating room. Adhesions between the lung and chest wall are treated by electrocautery. The hilum is dissected with care to preserve the phrenic nerves. Injury to the phrenic nerve may occur during division of the inferior pulmonary ligament, dissection of the hilum, placement of vascular clamps, or excessive retraction. The right phrenic nerve is more vulnerable because of its position adjacent to the hilum. The vagal neurovascular bundles need to be carefully preserved. Particular attention is warranted on the left side where the recurrent laryngeal nerve emerges and encircles the ligamentum arteriosum. The recurrent laryngeal nerve may be injured during dissection of the left main pulmonary artery, and heightened awareness of this possibility will help avoid neurapraxia or more permanent injury.

The pulmonary artery and veins are dissected as distally as possible from the surrounding tissues and isolated with vessel loops. Dissection around the main bronchus is kept to a minimum to preserve its blood supply. This procedure can be particularly demanding in patients with marked lymphadenopathy because the arterial supply may be abundant. Good hemostasis is essential. The pericardium is opened circumferentially along the superior and inferior pulmonary veins to release the left atrium in preparation for later placement of a proximal vascular clamp to allow a "left atrial cuff" anastomosis. It is important to recognize the anterior-posterior distribution of the pulmonary veins and the repositioning that may occur with cardiac rotation as a result of ventricular enlargement; in particular, the left-sided anastomosis can be affected, thus making adequate exposure difficult in this region.

When the donor lung has been received in suitable condition in the operating room, the recipient is given 5000 units of heparin intravenously. The pulmonary artery catheter needs to be withdrawn at this stage if it is palpable in the ipsilateral pulmonary artery. After adequate circulation of the heparin, the pulmonary veins and artery are divided well within the hilum with a linear cutting vascular stapler while providing as much length as possible. The main bronchus is divided at the lobar branch level by electrocautery. Once the lung has been resected, the main bronchus is sharply divided with a knife no further than two to three rings away from the carina. This division is generally achieved shorter on the right side than on the left. Good communication with the anesthesiologist at this stage is clearly required to address any issues related to positioning of the left main bronchus tip of the double-lumen endotracheal tube. Any bronchial vessels are identified and cauterized or closed with a metal clip. Lymph node vascularity may require attention at this stage inasmuch as later hemostasis may be difficult because of the allograft obstructing direct access. Studies have demonstrated the feasibility of bronchial arterial anastomosis. Although this concept is an intriguing one, it is not routinely performed at most institutions because it adds considerable time to the transplantation procedure with no clear benefit.[14]

BACK-BENCH PREPARATION OF THE DONOR LUNG

At the back table, final preparations for implantation are made to the donor lung, including removal of excess mediastinal tissue and mobilization of the main pulmonary artery and the left atrial and venous structures from any bronchial attachments. Any extra pulmonary artery is left untrimmed at this point; the final length is determined in situ at the time of anastomosis. A second retrograde flushing of the pulmonary vascular bed before implantation is optional. The retrograde flush that is performed at the donor hospital during procurement may drain residual blood and intravascular debris and reveal a thrombotic or embolic burden otherwise not discovered. The main bronchus is opened, which allows deflation in the presence of adequate static compliance, and a microbiological specimen is collected. The bronchus is then divided with a knife, leaving no more than two cartilaginous rings from the origin of the upper lobe bronchus.

A recent review describes superior results and low complications associated with bronchial anastomosis by trimming the donor main bronchus to the lobar take-off.[15]

ALLOGRAFT IMPLANTATION

The donor lung is then brought to the operative field in its normal orientation. Because of its most posterior location, the bronchus is anastomosed first; the procedure is performed as an end-to-end anastomosis. This approach "frames" the lung inasmuch as it is the most rigid of the three anastomoses required. We routinely use two separate suturing techniques for the bronchial anastomosis. The membranous portion of the bronchus is anastomosed by using a running 4-0 synthetic absorbable suture (polyglyconate [Maxon, Covidien, Minneapolis, Minnesota] or polydioxanone [PDS, Ethicon, Somerville, New Jersey]), whereas the cartilaginous portion is secured with interrupted figure-of-eight sutures (Figure 15.1). Single running suture techniques have also been described in the literature and appear to be equally efficacious. This technique is most useful when both bronchi are fairly pliable.[16] The "telescoping technique" is a useful alternative technique in cases involving a significant size discrepancy between the donor and the recipient. In this setting especially, it is essential to avoid geometric distortion and ensure adequate alignment and size matching of the membranous aspect. Early intraoperative intraluminal examination can be performed with a pediatric bronchoscope at the time of completion of the bronchial anastomosis.

Bronchoplastic techniques are rarely needed; division and reinforcement of a stump is usually adequate in the unusual case of an aberrant bronchus requiring division. In one report apical segmental branches were found to originate from the donor trachea; the anomalous segmental bronchus was excised from the donor trachea with a cuff, which was then incorporated into the bronchial suture line.[17]

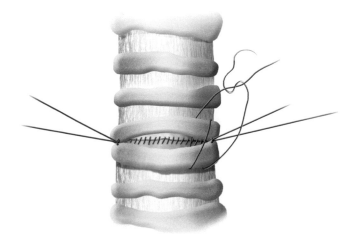

Figure 15.1 We routinely use a monofilament absorbable suture (4-0 Maxon) and figure-of-eight sutures for the cartilaginous portion and continuous suturing for the membranous portion.

Next, attention is turned to the venous anastomosis. After the vascular clamp has been placed to include a sufficient portion of the left atrium without compromising the left atrial cavity for adequate filling, the recipient left pulmonary vein orifices are connected by dividing the bridge of the atrial wall to create an oval "atrial cuff." The donor atrial cuff is then anastomosed to the recipient atrial cuff in an end-to-end fashion by using a single double-armed running 4-0 polypropylene suture (Figure 15.2). When the donor "cuff" is inadequate, various augmentation techniques can be used to overcome this inadequacy.[18,19] Some of these maneuvers are described in Chapter 16.

Finally, the pulmonary artery is prepared for the anastomosis. Frequently, this anastomosis is left for last because it is the most delicate of the three anastomoses. Alternatively, it may follow the bronchial anastomosis if required in cases in which access is limited. Excess length of the pulmonary artery is removed after the vessel has been appropriately sized to prevent any kinking or tension in the anastomosis. This step is particularly important on the right side because extra length is available on the donor artery. The donor pulmonary artery is anastomosed to the recipient in an end-to-end fashion with a single, double-armed running 5-0 polypropylene suture (Figure 15.3). Occasionally, the recipient pulmonary artery is larger than the donor pulmonary artery; in the event of such a size mismatch, the larger inferior pulmonary trunk arising from the main pulmonary artery is anastomosed end to end with the donor main pulmonary artery. Occasionally an arteriotomy may be needed to extend the anastomotic circumference to accommodate end-to-end anastomosis. Size matching requires gradual adjustments to reduce the risk for posterior bleeding points because they are difficult to access without complete forward lift of the implanted lungs, which would create considerable tension at the newly formed hilum. A vascular snugger may be applied for accommodation of the suture line and to allow full reexpansion during reperfusion. Stricture ought to be avoided at all costs because it will adversely affect short- and long-term outcome of the allograft.

Intravenous administration of 500 mg of methylprednisolone sodium succinate (Solu-Medrol) systemically before

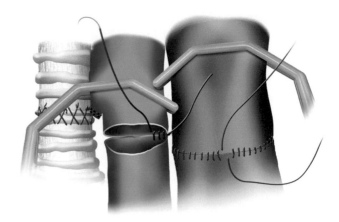

Figure 15.3 Pulmonary arterial anastomosis is performed end to end; however, at times the recipient pulmonary artery is large, and the larger lower trunk is anastomosed end to end to the donor (5-0 polypropylene).

reperfusion of the graft is imperative; it is best done by having the anesthetist infuse the medication while the last anastomosis is being performed. In preparation for reperfusion, a cross-clamp is placed distal to the anastomosis on the donor pulmonary artery to vent clots, air, and debris. The patient is placed in Trendelenburg position. Pulmonary plegia solution is allowed to vent from the left atrial cuff anastomosis by partially releasing the arterial clamp to allow a slow flush. While the left atrium is observed by TEE, the left atrial clamp is removed and the anastomosis is secured. The reperfusion is controlled by slow release of the arterial clamp over several minutes, and any hypotension is treated promptly by judicious volume or vasoactive agents as required. Low-pressure reperfusion of the new graft over several minutes is advocated to mitigate the dreaded adverse effects of acute reperfusion injury.[20] The chest is inspected carefully for hemostasis. The appearance of the lung is observed and the lungs are inflated while the left atrium is monitored by TEE. A "leak test" may be performed at this time by carefully ventilating the new lung with the bronchus submerged in normal saline and observing for bubbles. The irrigation is evacuated and a chest tube is placed posterior to the apex, with a second placed if required. Once stable hemodynamics and good oxygenation have been achieved, the ribs are re-approximated by using interrupted 1-0 Dexon pericostal sutures. The fascia and skin are approximated with running 2-0 and 4-0 Dexon sutures or equivalent. With the patient returned to a supine position, the double-lumen endotracheal tube is replaced by a single-lumen tube, and fiberoptic bronchoscopy is performed to inspect the bronchial anastomosis and remove any clots or secretion present in the bronchial tree.

CARDIOPULMONARY BYPASS FOR SINGLE-LUNG IMPLANTATION

Cardiopulmonary bypass is rarely necessary during single-lung transplantation. Ideally, the ipsilateral groin is prepared to create a sterile field during draping if cannulation of the

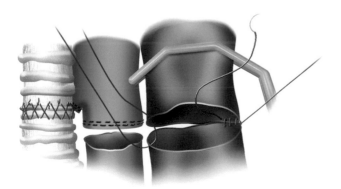

Figure 15.2 Pulmonary venous anastomosis created by using an atrial cuff technique (4-0 polypropylene).

groin becomes necessary. When right-sided lung transplantation is being performed, the aorta and right atrium can be accessed for cannulation from the chest; therefore, groin cannulation is needed less frequently. When left single-lung transplantation is performed, the groin provides the best access for cannulation if cardiopulmonary bypass is required. It is our practice to have a perfusionist available in the hospital in all cases during lung transplants. Most often when cardiopulmonary support is required for single-lung transplantation, a partial flow bypass will suffice and full systemic flow is rarely required.

TROUBLESHOOTING AND PITFALLS DURING SINGLE-LUNG TRANSPLANTATION

During procurement it is critical to preserve an adequate donor left atrial cuff around the confluence of the superior and inferior pulmonary veins. An inadequate donor left atrial cuff may occur as a result of technical error or during cardiac procurement. In this case a "neoatrial cuff" in the form of a gusset may be fashioned from donor pericardium or alternative nonthrombogenic conduit material. This gusset may be created with a running 5-0 polypropylene suture around the divided edges of the two pulmonary veins. The resultant pericardial gusset is trimmed to match the recipient's left atrium (see Chapter 16). More complex donor vein reconstructions with excellent outcomes have been described.[18,19] Interrogating the pulmonary venous return flow with the TEE probe at the end of the reperfusion phase is crucial to identify any venous obstruction that could result in serious graft dysfunction postoperatively.

Occasionally, donor lungs will have congenital venous anomalies. For instance, the donor right upper lobe pulmonary vein may be seen draining into the superior vena cava or the innominate vein. The normal donor inferior veins can be anastomosed to the recipient inferior pulmonary vein. The donor and recipient superior veins may then be anastomosed to each other individually with a conduit of donor iliac vein or autologous pericardium.[17]

Patients with IPF pose a particular surgical challenge because their intrathoracic volumes tend to be restricted and adhesions are abundant. Using donor with smaller lung volumes may be helpful in this setting. Predicted total lung capacity within 20% is a general rule.[21] In addition, strategies to depress the diaphragm by using either a suture placed on the dome retracted through the potential chest tube site or a malleable retractor may be helpful during implantation. Some have advocated keeping this retracting suture at the end of the surgery to avoid postoperative atelectasis in the early period and then slowly releasing it. Graft atelectasis must be diligently avoided, and physiotherapy and early mobilization are essential.

OUTCOMES

Single-lung transplantation offers the advantages of shorter operating times, rare need for cardiopulmonary bypass, and maximal utilization of lungs. The donor shortage is a prime reason for long waiting list times and fewer available lung transplants. It is critical for transplant surgeons to be familiar with the single-lung transplant technique and to offer it to carefully selected patients. Analysis of long-term outcomes in the International Society for Heart and Lung Transplantation (ISHLT) registry data indicates that double-lung transplantation may be associated with a survival advantage in more recent recipient subgroups.[22] The unadjusted median survival for single-lung transplantation is 4.6 years as compared with 6.9 years for double-lung transplantation. Registry data have to be considered in the context of selection bias and other confounders. The indications for and outcomes following single-lung transplantation will evolve with time depending on donor availability, the type of patients on the waiting list, and the process for selecting donors and recipients. In the abscence of a randomized prospective study comparing outcomes after single- and double-lung transplantation the clinical value for individual patients has to be considered. Data from the ISHLT registry and individual center experience as well as improvements in critical care, immunosuppression, and operative strategies have made single-lung transplantation a viable option for selected patients with ESLD.[8,9,23]

CONCLUSION

Single-lung transplantation is an efficient and economical way to treat patients with ESLD who need lung transplantation. The technique may be applied in a minimally traumatic manner through a muscle-sparing thoracotomy in a relatively shorter operating time. Venous anastomotic challenges and other technical difficulties with the donor may be overcome by a variety of reconstructive strategies. In a significant number of patients with ESLD, single-lung transplantation yields a symptomatic or survival benefit comparable to that of double-lung transplantation and is an excellent means of maximizing lung allografts in the prevailing scarcity.

REFERENCES

1. Christie JD, Edwards LB, Aurora P, et al. Registry of the International Society for Heart and Lung Transplantation: Twenty-fifth official adult lung and heart/lung transplantation report—2008. J Heart Lung Transplant 2008;27:957-969.
2. Akerman J. Alexis Carrel: Nobel Prize for physiology and medicine, 1912. By Professor Jules Akerman, member of the Medical Nobel Committee. Transplant Proc 1987;19(4 Suppl 5):9-11.
3. Hardy JD, Eraslan S, Webb WR. Transplantation of the lung. Ann Surg 1964;60:440-448.
4. Unilateral lung transplantation for pulmonary fibrosis. Toronto Lung Transplant Group. N Engl J Med 1986;314:1140-1145.
5. DeMeo DL, Ginns LC. Lung transplantation at the turn of the century. Annu Rev Med 2001;52:185-201.

6. Bavaria JE, Kotloff R, Palevsky H, et al. Bilateral versus single lung transplantation for chronic obstructive pulmonary disease. J Thorac Cardiovasc Surg 1997;113:520-527; discussion 528.

7. Gammie JS, Keenan RJ, Pham SM, et al. Single- versus double-lung transplantation for pulmonary hypertension. J Thorac Cardiovasc Surg 1998;115:397-402; discussion 402-403.

8. Mason DP, Brizzio ME, Alster JM, et al. Lung transplantation for idiopathic pulmonary fibrosis. Ann Thorac Surg 2007;84:1121-1128.

9. Meyers BF, Lynch JP, Trulock EP, et al. Single versus bilateral lung transplantation for idiopathic pulmonary fibrosis: A ten-year institutional experience. J Thorac Cardiovasc Surg 2000;120:99-107.

10. McCurry KR, Shearon TH, Edwards LB, et al. Lung transplantation in the United States, 1998-2007. Am J Transplant 2009; 9:942-958.

11. Thabut G, Christie JD, Ravaud P, et al. Survival after bilateral versus single lung transplantation for patients with chronic obstructive pulmonary disease: A retrospective analysis of registry data. Lancet 2008;371:744-751.

12. Nwakanma LU, Simpkins CE, Williams JA, et al. Impact of bilateral versus single lung transplantation on survival in recipients 60 years of age and older: Analysis of United Network for Organ Sharing database. J Thorac Cardiovasc Surg 2007;133:541-547.

13. Botha, P, Trivedi D, Searl CP, et al. Differential pulmonary vein gases predict primary graft dysfunction. Ann Thorac Surg 2006;82:1998-2002.

14. Norgaard MA, Olsen PS, Svendsen UG, Pettersson G. Revascularization of the bronchial arteries in lung transplantation: An overview. Ann Thorac Surg 1996;62:1215-1221.

15. FitzSullivan E, Gries CJ, Phelan P, et al. Reduction in airway complications after lung transplantation with novel anastomotic technique. Ann Thorac Surg 2010;92:309-315.

16. Aigner C, Jaksch P, Seebacher G, et al. Single running suture—the new standard technique for bronchial anastomoses in lung transplantation. Eur J Cardiothorac Surg 2003;23:488-493.

17. Schmidt F, McGiffin DC, Zorn G, et al. Management of congenital abnormalities of the donor lung. Ann Thorac Surg 2001;72:935-937.

18. Casula RP, Stoica SC, Wallwork J, Dunning J. Pulmonary vein augmentation for single lung transplantation. Ann Thorac Surg 2001;71:1373-1374.

19. Oto T, Rabinov M, Negri J, et al. Techniques of reconstruction for inadequate donor left atrial cuff in lung transplantation. Ann Thorac Surg 2006;81:1199-1204.

20. Sakamoto T, Yamashita C, Okada M. Efficacy of initial controlled perfusion pressure for ischemia-reperfusion injury in a 24-hour preserved lung. Ann Thorac Cardiovasc Surg 1999;5:21-26.

21. Barnard JB, Davies O, Curry P, et al. Size matching in lung transplantation: An evidence-based review. J Heart Lung Transplant 2013;32:849-860.

22. Yusen RD, Christie JD, Edwards LB, et al. The Registry of the International Society for Heart and Lung Transplantation: Thirtieth adult lung and heart-lung transplant report—2013; focus theme: Age. J Heart Lung Transplant 2013;32:965-978.

23. Taghavi S, Jayarajan SN, Komaroff E, et al. Single-lung transplantation can be performed with acceptable outcomes using selected donors with heavy smoking history. J Heart Lung Transplant 2013;32:1005-1012.

16

Bilateral sequential lung transplantation: Technical aspects

MARA B. ANTONOFF AND G. ALEXANDER PATTERSON

Although lung transplantation was first successfully applied as a strategy for end-stage lung disease in 1983, bilateral lung transplantation was not introduced until the late 1980s. Since then, the ideal operative approach has continued to evolve.[1-3] In this chapter the technical pearls of bilateral sequential lung transplantation are outlined, and additional details directed toward avoiding of pitfalls are provided along with lessons that we have learned over time.

PREPARATION AND CONSIDERATIONS

Choice of bilateral transplantation

Details regarding the choice of single-lung versus bilateral sequential lung transplantation are addressed elsewhere. In general, it is fairly well accepted that patients with septic lung disease, particularly cystic fibrosis and bronchiectasis, require bilateral lung transplants to remove the entire focus of sepsis and prevent soiling of the allograft lung.[3] However, patients with diseases such as emphysema tend to have favorable outcomes with either single-lung or bilateral lung transplants.[4,5] Considerations for single-lung as opposed to bilateral transplantation may be based on age,

size, and comorbid conditions, with bilateral lung transplantation emphasized for those who are younger, are more fit, and have greater stature. At our institution we have used bilateral sequential lung transplantation as our procedure of choice for most patients with end-stage lung disease.

Preoperative consideration of cardiopulmonary bypass

The decision whether to use cardiopulmonary bypass is based on data obtained from pulmonary artery catheterization, arterial blood gas analysis, and transesophageal echocardiography (TEE). The potential need for cardiopulmonary bypass should be considered in advance, with careful discussions involving the operating surgeons, anesthesia team, and perfusionist. In some cases, severe clinical findings may lead to a decision to use bypass early; regardless, the resources required for cardiopulmonary bypass must be on standby for every bilateral lung transplantation case. Hemodynamic instability, inability to adequately oxygenate or ventilate with one lung, dramatic increases in pulmonary arterial pressure with unilateral pulmonary artery clamping, and deterioration of right ventricular function are all potential reasons for cardiopulmonary bypass.[3] To minimize perioperative hemorrhage, every attempt should be made to complete as much of the dissection as possible and achieve optimal hemostasis on the chest wall before systemic heparinization and initiation of bypass.

Laterality sequence

The decision regarding which lung should be implanted first is based on the quantitative ventilation-perfusion scan (V/Q scan).[3] The lung with the lesser contribution to ventilation and perfusion should be removed first. This approach allows greater success with single-lung ventilation because the more functional native lung is relied on during transplantation of the more diseased lung and ventilation through the new donor lung during the dissection and implantation of the second lung. This strategy helps in avoiding cardiopulmonary bypass. Furthermore, if an event mandating abortion of the procedure were to occur before both lungs had been implanted, replacing the more diseased lung with a transplant first would be advantageous.

KEY STEPS

Anesthesia and operating room conduct

A cardiothoracic anesthesiologist with specific experience in lung isolation strategies, fiberoptic bronchoscopy, and use and interpretation of TEE images plays a critical role in the successful conduct of this procedure.[6] The use of epidural catheters for intraoperative and postoperative analgesia must be considered thoughtfully because of the need to always be prepared for the possibility of cardiopulmonary bypass and concomitant systemic heparinization.[6,7] We have found that if the latter are needed, our anesthesia pain service can place epidural catheters for analgesic optimization in the early postoperative period after stabilization of hemodynamics and bypass-related coagulopathy.

After induction of anesthesia the patient is intubated, with the type of tube depending on the need for preoperative bronchoscopy. For patients with cystic fibrosis, active pulmonary infection, or any other type of septic lung disease, a large single-lumen tube is placed initially to facilitate therapeutic bronchoscopy and thorough suctioning and clearance of secretions.[8] For patients with emphysema, restrictive disease, or pulmonary hypertension, this step is rarely required, and a standard left-sided double-lumen tube can be placed at initial intubation.

Central venous access is obtained when a pulmonary arterial catheter and both radial and femoral arterial lines are placed.[8,9] A TEE probe is used for an initial evaluation and left in place for ongoing assessment throughout the operative procedure.[10] In particular, attention should be directed toward determining the need for cardiopulmonary bypass on the basis of right ventricular function; it can be used to identify any intracardiac shunts, assess arterial and venous anastomoses, check for air, and assist with weaning from cardiopulmonary bypass.

Minimizing intravenous fluids can be helpful in reducing postoperative respiratory insufficiency; to this end, we administer vasopressors as needed to avoid excessive volume resuscitation while remaining cognizant of the need to maintain end-organ perfusion.[6] In addition to having a wide variety of vasoactive and inotropic medications, the anesthesia team should have access to nitric oxide and epoprostenol for management of pulmonary hypertension and refractory hypoxia[7] and should administer them carefully only after a thorough evaluation for any anastomotic or technical sources of such difficulties.

Patients are placed in a supine position with both arms tucked. A thermistor Foley catheter with temperature probe is placed to allow careful measurement of both urine output and bladder temperature. Forced-air heating blankets are used to maintain normothermia or, in cases involving cardiopulmonary bypass, to facilitate rewarming as appropriate.

Incision and initial dissection

For bilateral lung transplants, three basic options for incisions exist: bilateral anterolateral thoracotomy with or without sternal division and median sternotomy. Our preferred method of access for bilateral sequential lung transplantation is bilateral anterolateral thoracotomy without sternal division; we have found it to be a safe approach that facilitates adequate exposure without risk for the problems commonly observed with sternal healing.[11] Others have found that this approach minimizes operative trauma, improves postoperative functional recovery, and prevents potential spread of unilateral complications to the other pleural cavity.[12] For this technique, the skin incision follows the inframammary crease from the lateral edge of the sternum to the anterior axillary line. Because of the extent of the lateral aspect of these incisions, care should be taken during preparation and draping to ensure sterility and isolation from the tucked arm and bed linens. The breast tissue is elevated and may be tacked to the superior aspect of the operative field with a silk stitch to facilitate exposure. The pectoralis major muscle is divided, and the chest cavities are entered at the bilateral fourth intercostal spaces. Each of the internal mammary arteries are identified, ligated, and divided. It is possible to preserve the internal mammary arteries; however, doing so requires division of a short segment of the costal cartilage at the medial edge of the fourth rib so that the rib can be retracted upward without putting excessive tension on the internal mammary vascular bundle.[7] Before retractors are placed, the intercostal spaces are opened laterally and from within the pleural space to the edges of the paraspinal muscles.

A variation on this incision, known as the clamshell, includes a transverse sternotomy connecting the bilateral anterolateral thoracotomies. The addition of transverse sternotomy enhances exposure, which can be of great utility in providing access to cannulation sites for cardiopulmonary bypass. It also provides improved visualization of the hilum, which is an important asset in cases involving cardiomegaly or a particularly small thoracic cavity.[7] However, this approach mandates division of the internal mammary vasculature, requires sternal wiring during closure, and may result in greater postoperative sternal complications.[11]

Median sternotomy is a third approach to bilateral lung transplantation. This incision provides outstanding access to the intrapericardial structures. It can be useful with recipients who have large breasts, which can pose an additional challenge to exposure via anterolateral thoracotomy. In a retrospective review comparing median sternotomy with a clamshell incision for bilateral lung or heart-lung transplantation, patients undergoing sternotomy were found to have fewer wound complications.[13]

Back-table donor lung preparation

Donor procurement processes are outlined in Chapter 10. For the purposes of discussing the technical aspects of the bilateral lung transplantation, we will proceed under the premise that the organs will arrive at the operating room en bloc in accordance with well-accepted standardized approaches to thoracic organ procurement.[14-16] Separation of the two lungs on the back table is performed in an ice slush bath. The donor esophagus is removed, followed by the donor aorta. The posterior pericardium is sharply divided, and the left atrium is carefully split between the left and right pulmonary veins. The main pulmonary artery is divided at the bifurcation, after which the left bronchus is cut close to the carina by using a sharp No. 15 blade and leaving the carina with the right lung.

The donor bronchi are then further divided more distally while leaving just one ring proximal to the upper lobe orifice, and great care is taken to minimize proximal peribronchial dissection. We have found that decreasing the amount of potentially ischemic tissue implanted from the donor bronchus can reduce posttransplant airway complications and that shortening the donor bronchus to the level of the lobar carina decreases the tissue at risk for ischemia.[17] The right and left pulmonary arteries are also trimmed back to their first branches.

Cardiopulmonary bypass

Cardiopulmonary bypass is used selectively; the need for it is carefully evaluated before initiation of the operation, and a second assessment is performed before the recipient pneumonectomy. Cardiopulmonary bypass is specifically indicated for children in whom a double-lumen endotracheal tube cannot be placed, for concomitant cardiac procedures, and most patients with severe pulmonary hypertension.[6,7] If any of these situations exist, the procedure may be initiated after the dissection at the back table but before explantation of the native lung. Cardiopulmonary bypass is also indicated if hemodynamic instability or pulmonary hypertension,

hypoxemia, or hypercapnia refractory to initial interventions develops in the patient at any point during the operation.[3] Inadequate left hilar exposure has occasionally been cited as the sole indication for cardiopulmonary bypass; however, we have reported the use of a suction heart-positioning device to allow lifting of the heart to improve left hilar exposure. This technique makes it possible to continue the operation without bypass in cases with no additional indications for its use.[18]

Explantation

Before either of the recipient's lungs is removed, back-table preparation of the donor lungs should be completed. All adhesiolysis, hemostasis, and bilateral hilar dissections should also be performed in advance to allow expeditious removal of the second lung and minimize the time during which either lung is exposed to the entire cardiac output.[3,7] As discussed earlier, the lung with poorer function should be explanted first to optimize tolerance of single-lung ventilation.

In patients with small pleural spaces (e.g., pulmonary fibrosis), exposure can be improved by placing a traction suture through the fibrous portion of the diaphragm and bringing it out through a planned chest tube site.[7] The importance of meticulous hemostasis throughout adhesiolysis and dissection cannot be overemphasized inasmuch as mild bleeding becomes particularly problematic following systemic heparinization.[6] The inferior pulmonary ligament is divided. The hilar structures are dissected, with great care taken to protect the phrenic and vagus nerves. The pulmonary arteries and veins are dissected beyond their first bifurcations to ensure preservation of as much length as possible for subsequent anastomoses. In general, we favor vascular staple loads on the central side of the ligated vessels, with ties used peripherally. On the right side, the pulmonary artery transection should be approximately 1 cm beyond the truncus anterior branch, and on the left, it should be divided just beyond the second branch to the left upper lobe.[7] In addition to optimizing the length of pulmonary artery available for subsequent anastomosis, this strategy also downsizes the recipient pulmonary artery, which may provide a better donor-recipient size match.[6] Moreover, the first ligated branch of the recipient artery can serve as an anatomic landmark for orientation during the anastomosis.

Pulmonary veins are similarly divided at secondary branch points. Peribronchial dissection is carried out while taking great care to control bleeding from any bronchial arteries. The mainstem bronchus is divided sharply just proximally to the upper lobe takeoff.[6,19] After the specimen has been passed out of the field, the thoracic cavity is meticulously examined for adequacy of hemostasis.

The hilar structures are sequentially prepared for anastomosis to the donor lung. The native pulmonary artery stump is grasped with a Duval clamp, dissected centrally to improve length, and retracted medially. The native pulmonary veins are then grasped as well, and the pericardium around the veins is opened. A 0 silk retraction stitch is placed in the recipient bronchus to facilitate subsequent anastomosis.

Anastomoses and reperfusion

The order of anastomoses commences with the bronchus, followed by the pulmonary artery and then the pulmonary vein. The donor lung is placed over ice slush in the empty thoracic cavity, and it is covered with a cold lap pad.

Before the bronchial anastomosis is initiated, the anesthesiologist is asked to advance a small-caliber suction catheter into the ipsilateral recipient airway, which assists in keeping the field clean.[6] After a number of iterations and significant evolution, our current practice includes an end-to-end bronchial anastomosis created with two strands of 4-0 polydioxanone (PDS) suture in a running fashion.[3,20] The anastomosis is initiated on the membranous portion of the bronchus; it is subsequently run along the anterior cartilaginous portion of the airway by using a second suture to prevent a purse-string effect. In cases involving a significant size mismatch between the bronchi, the membranous portion is completed in a running fashion, whereas the cartilaginous part is approximated with simple interrupted 3-0 sutures.[6] The peribronchial tissues are then brought together with a running stitch to provide coverage to the anterior aspect of the anastomosis, where it will be in proximity to the pulmonary vascular anastomoses. Although we recommend inclusion of this step, others have described its omission with reasonable success.[6,19]

A vascular clamp is placed proximally on the recipient pulmonary artery. The staple line is resected, and the recipient and donor pulmonary arteries are trimmed to minimize distortion and kinking. A 5-0 polypropylene stitch is run in a continuous fashion to create an end-to-end arterial anastomosis.[3,6]

The venous anastomosis is initiated by opening the pericardium around the native pulmonary veins. A Satinsky clamp is placed centrally on the left atrium, the venous staple lines are cut off, and the bridge between the two pulmonary veins is slit open to create a single pulmonary venoatrial orifice.[3] A 4-0 polypropylene suture is used for a continuous running anastomosis, with the stitches placed via a mattress technique to optimize apposition of the intima from the donor to the recipient. This strategy facilitates exclusion of potentially thrombogenic atrial muscle from the anastomosis.[7]

De-airing is performed before the stitch used for the venous anastomosis is tied. A few breaths are given to the operative side, and the arterial clamp is transiently opened, after which the atrial clamp is released. Once the venous suture line has been tightened and the knot secured, all clamps are definitively removed.

All the aforementioned steps are repeated for the contralateral side after hemodynamic stability and adequacy of oxygenation and ventilation have been ensured.

Preparation for closure

Hemostasis is carefully confirmed. If cardiopulmonary bypass has been used, weaning and decannulation are performed according to standard technique. The patient is assessed for stability and appropriateness of chest closure.

Any concern for the development of primary graft dysfunction, as potentially demonstrated by marked hypoxia, pulmonary edema, elevated pulmonary artery pressure, or poor compliance, mandates immediate investigation for reversible causes.[19] Mechanical and anastomotic problems must be identified and corrected immediately, with particular attention directed toward ruling out technical issues with venous outflow. The anastomoses should be visually inspected for kinking, and TEE should be used specifically to examine pulmonary vein flow. Direct pressures across the anastomoses can also be measured.

Although we do not routinely perform quantitative perfusion scans in the postoperative setting, we have a low threshold for their selective use in evaluating for perfusion deficits. In fact, if significant concern exists, such scans can be performed in the operating room before transfer to the intensive care unit (ICU). Not all sources of graft dysfunction are easily correctable; for example, the dysfunction may be caused by humoral injury resulting from circulating anti-donor antibodies. If reversible causes cannot be found, treatment of primary graft dysfunction is largely supportive, with institution of venovenous extracorporeal membrane oxygenation (VV-ECMO) considered early if pulmonary edema is severe or O_2 need is excessive.[19] Temporary use of ECMO may permit resuscitation of the injured lung and help avoid injury secondary to barotrauma and high FIO_2.[19]

Closure

Once it has been determined that the patient is appropriately stable for chest closure, the diaphragmatic stay sutures are released. Two 24 to 28 French drains are placed on each side, with one tube placed apically and the other in a diaphragmatic location. The retraction stitches placed in the breasts are also released. If a transverse sternotomy was performed, two figure-of-eight wires are placed. Heavy monofilament absorbable sutures are inserted in a figure-of-eight fashion to reapproximate the ribs.[3,6] The muscle layers of the chest wall are closed with No. 1 absorbable braided suture followed by running stitches of 2-0 and 4-0 absorbable sutures for the dermis and subcuticular closure, respectively.

It should be noted that delayed chest closure following lung transplantation serves as a viable option and has been used with acceptable outcomes for reasons such as coagulopathy, hemodynamic instability, or oversized donor lung grafts.[21] We have selectively applied this strategy with plans for washout and closure over the ensuing 24 to 48 hours. Options for temporary closure include packing the chest as appropriate and whip-stitching the skin closed with nylon suture or applying a large adhesive dressing.

Bronchoscopy

After closure, the double-lumen endotracheal tube is exchanged for a single-lumen tube. Flexible fiberoptic bronchoscopy is performed by the operative team to clear the airway of blood and secretions, as well as to perform a preliminary evaluation of the anastomoses.[3,6]

TRANSITION TO POSTOPERATIVE CARE

The patient is subsequently transported to the ICU while still intubated. Care of the lung recipient in the immediate postoperative period focuses on ventilatory and hemodynamic support, with consideration of potential weaning if appropriate.[22] Details of early postoperative care and ICU management are outlined in Chapter 25.

POTENTIAL COMPLICATIONS AND PITFALLS

Native emphysematous disease

In patients with emphysema, it is important to avoid hyperinflation of the native lungs throughout the preparatory steps such as induction and line placement, as well as during dissection of the lung. If hypotension occurs before the chest is opened, positive pressure ventilation should be disconnected, thereby allowing intrathoracic pressure to return to normal.

Native septic disease

As already mentioned, with any patients whose indication for transplantation is septic lung disease, preoperative bronchoscopy performed by using an adult bronchoscope through a single-lumen tube is a critical step. Every attempt should be made to thoroughly clear the airways of purulent secretions, which helps reduce the need for cardiopulmonary bypass. Samples from both donor and recipient airways should be cultured to help direct postoperative antimicrobial therapy.

Damage or abnormalities in procured lungs

When both heart and lungs are being procured from the same donor for separate transplant recipients, efforts are made to equitably divide the left atrial cuff; in some circumstances, however, the donor lungs may arrive with an insufficient atrial cuff or injuries to the pulmonary vein orifices. In the case of a short cuff, our preference is to anastomose each individual recipient vein to the respective donor orifice and leaving the donor atrial cuff intact.[6] Alternatively, the superior and inferior veins in the recipient can be fashioned into a common orifice that can be anastomosed to the donor atrial cuff (Figure 16.1).[23] Another option that has been described for the left side involves performing the venous anastomosis to the left atrial appendage.[24] For extreme circumstances of left atrial cuff loss, reconstruction techniques involving the use of donor pericardium (Figure 16.2), superior vena cava, or pulmonary artery have been described.[25,26]

Of the pulmonary veins, the right inferior is the most frequently injured during procurement because of its proximity during division of the inferior vena cava and division of the left atrium.[14] For a lacerated pulmonary venous orifice we recommend repair, which should include identification and oversewing of small venous branches beyond the orifice.[6]

Less common are technically relevant injuries to the donor pulmonary arteries. The right pulmonary artery is more likely to be injured as a result of its course behind the superior vena cava and the aorta; however, it is significantly longer than the left pulmonary artery, and injuries at this point can usually just be trimmed away.[14] For lacerations to

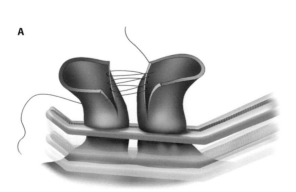

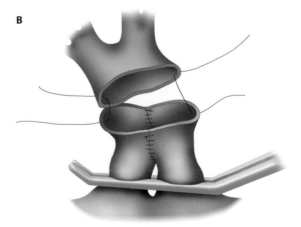

Figure 16.1 When the recipient atrial cuff is short, particularly on the left side, the two veins can be fashioned into one opening **(A)** for anastomosis to the donor atrial cuff **(B)**.

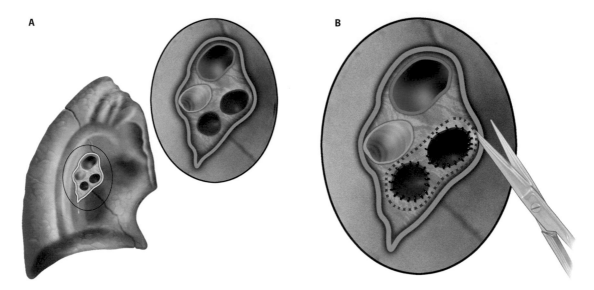

Figure 16.2 Creation of a new atrial cuff after suboptimal harvest. **(A)** The superior and inferior pulmonary veins are separated completely. **(B)** The intima of each vein is attached to the pericardium, after which the pericardium is incised to reconstruct an atrial cuff.

the distal right pulmonary artery or the truncus anterior or for the rare injury to the left pulmonary artery, holes can be repaired primarily with 5-0 suture or patched with donor cava, azygous vein, or extra segments of pulmonary artery.[6]

Congenital anomalies are also occasionally seen in the donor lungs, and the transplanting surgical team must be prepared to handle these anatomic variations. For donors with anomalous pulmonary venous drainage, techniques involving the use of autologous pericardium and donor iliac vein to reroute pulmonary venous return to the atrial cuff or recipient pulmonary vein have been described.[14,27] In the case of left-sided aberrant pulmonary veins, it may be possible to perform direct anastomosis to the left atrial appendage, with care taken to avoid injury to the circumflex artery during clamping of the appendage.[28]

Donor airway anomalies, including upper lobe segmental and lobar bronchi coming directly off the trachea, may also be seen. For segmental bronchi we have found that the bronchial orifice can be oversewn, after which standard implantation techniques can be used because of collateral airflow to the segment in question.[6] Reimplantation of anomalous segmental bronchi has been described, however.[27] In situations involving a complete lobar bronchus arising from the trachea, inclusion of the upper lobe in the implantation requires incorporation of the bronchus intermedius and upper lobe bronchus into a modified anastomosis with the recipient bronchus (Figure 16.3).[29]

Size-mismatched lungs

If lungs are oversized and this fact is recognized on the back table, lobectomy (discussed in detail in Chapter 18) can be performed. However, if the size mismatch is not realized until after implantation, appropriate wedge resections can be performed, with stapling devices used to target the lingula and right middle lobe. Such strategies have demonstrated efficacy in our experience, as well as in that of others.[30]

Perioperative hemorrhage

Excessive bleeding may be related to the large raw surface area created after explantation of septic lungs or lungs previously subjected to pleurodesis, and it can be severely exacerbated by the anticoagulation required for cardiopulmonary bypass. This potentially devastating problem can result in excessive transfusion needs, high-volume resuscitation, and exposure to large quantities of blood products, which have ongoing implications for hemodynamic stability and pulmonary function. However, such difficulties can typically be avoided with meticulous attention to stopping all surgically correctable bleeding—ideally, before initiation of cardiopulmonary bypass—and aggressive correction of coagulopathies. The chest wall and diaphragmatic surface

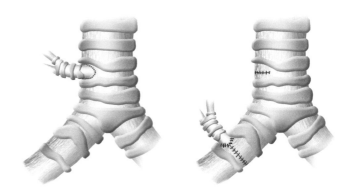

Figure 16.3 Incorporation of an anomalous segmental right upper lobe bronchus into the anastomosis.

should be carefully inspected when exposure is best for any sources of bleeding. In the setting of ongoing bleeding, delayed chest closure as described earlier can be used.

Pulmonary arterial or venous anastomotic problems

Issues with the vascular anastomoses may include persistent pulmonary hypertension, unexplained hypoxemia, pulmonary edema, or abnormal findings on intraoperative TEE. As already stated, nuclear perfusion scans can be performed immediately postoperatively in the ICU—or even in the operating room—to identify any issues related to flow to either lung. Gradients can be identified by comparing pressures on either side of the anastomosis intraoperatively or by contrast angiography postoperatively. Surgical correction must be performed if clinically relevant gradients exist.

Technically unsatisfactory bronchial anastomosis

Poor-quality bronchial anastomoses can be readily identified in the operating room during postimplantation bronchoscopy. In circumstances of inaccurate alignment or inadequate airway caliber, immediate revision should be performed. These problems will not improve with surveillance bronchoscopy and should be fixed before leaving the operating room.

Primary graft dysfunction

Indications of primary graft dysfunction may include a compromised Pao_2/Fio_2 ratio in the first 48 hours, accompanied by a finding of panlobar infiltrates on postoperative chest radiographs. In general, strategies for its management include aggressive cardiopulmonary support, use of positive end-expiratory pressure, diuresis, inhaled nitric oxide, aerosolized prostacyclin, and if the patient is unresponsive to treatment, ECMO and retransplantation. Although such management strategies are discussed in detail in Chapter 14, some key actions to avoid primary graft dysfunction should be mentioned here: ensure the absence of donor infection, aspiration, and contusion; pay careful attention to appropriate cold storage strategies; limit hyperinflation during and after procurement; implement optimal lung preservation strategies; and minimize ischemic times through detailed and accurate communication with the procurement team followed by expeditious operative conduct.

RESULTS

Significant progress in lung transplantation has been made in the last 25 years; 1-year patient and allograft survival rates are now comparable to the results seen with heart and liver transplants.[19] Our lung transplantation results at Washington University with the majority of our recipients undergoing bilateral lung transplantation have been

reported.[8,31] During the period from 1988 to 2012, 1251 transplants were performed in our institution (1216 primary transplants and 35 retransplants), with bilateral procedures accounting for 1038 (83.0%).[7] With experience, our outcomes have been optimized: the reported overall hospital mortality rate of 6.2% during our first 13 years decreased to only 3.9% during the period from 1995 to 2000.[7,31] Our functional outcomes have been excellent, with marked improvement in spirometry and 6-minute walk test results.[7]

Sequential bilateral lung transplantation is our procedure of choice for end-stage pulmonary disease. Over the years, adaptations and improvements in technique have optimized our approach to this procedure, and we have seen simultaneous advances in immunosuppression, organ preservation, and critical care.[6,32] The use of marginal and non–heart-beating donors and implementation of ex vivo lung perfusion have the potential to expand our donor pool, and research efforts continue to address the management of chronic rejection.[7,22,32-34] Although strategies for procurement and preservation, immunosuppression, and postoperative care will undoubtedly continue to evolve and improve outcomes, we cannot overemphasize the importance of meticulous attention to technical detail and application of experiential wisdom in the successful execution of this operation.

REFERENCES

1. Cooper JD. The evolution of techniques and indications for lung transplantation. Ann Surg 1990;212:249-255; discussion 255-256.
2. Cooper JD, Pearson FG, Patterson GA, et al. Technique of successful lung transplantation in humans. J Thorac Cardiovasc Surg 1987;93:173-181.
3. Meyers BF, Patterson GA. Bilateral lung transplantation. Oper Tech Thorac Cardiovasc Surg 1999;4:162-175.
4. Patterson GA, Maurer JR, Williams TJ, et al. Comparison of outcomes of double and single lung transplantation for obstructive lung disease. The Toronto Lung Transplant Group. J Thorac Cardiovasc Surg 1991;101:623-631; discussion 631-632.
5. Sundaresan RS, Shiraishi Y, Trulock EP, et al. Single or bilateral lung transplantation for emphysema? J Thorac Cardiovasc Surg 1996;112:1485-1494; discussion 1494-1495.
6. Puri V, Patterson GA. Adult lung transplantation: Technical considerations. Semin Thorac Cardiovasc Surg 2008;20:152-164.
7. Brown L, Puri V, Patterson GA. Lung Transplantation. In Sellke F, del Nido P, Swanson S, eds. Sabiston and Spencer Surgery of the Chest, 9th ed. St. Louis: Elsevier; 2015.
8. Meyers BF, Lynch J, Trulock EP, et al. Lung transplantation: A decade of experience. Ann Surg 1999;230:362-370; discussion 370-371.

9. Triantafillou A. Anesthetic considerations. In Patterson GA, ed. Lung transplantation: Current Topics in General Thoracic Surgery. Amsterdam: Elsevier Science;1995:171-190.

10. Serra E, Feltracco P, Barbieri S, et al. Transesophageal echocardiography during lung transplantation. Transplant Proc 2007;39:1981-1982.

11. Meyers BF, Sundaresan RS, Guthrie T, et al. Bilateral sequential lung transplantation without sternal division eliminates posttransplantation sternal complications. J Thorac Cardiovasc Surg 1999;117:358-364.

12. Taghavi S, Bîrsan T, Seitelberger R, et al. Initial experience with two sequential anterolateral thoracotomies for bilateral lung transplantation. Ann Thorac Surg 1999;67:1440-1443.

13. Macchiarini P, Ladurie FL, Cerrina J, et al. Clamshell or sternotomy for double lung or heart-lung transplantation? Eur J Cardiothorac Surg 1999;15:333-339.

14. Parekh K, Patterson GA. Technical considerations in adult lung transplantation. Semin Thorac Cardiovasc Surg 2004;16:322-332.

15. Pasque MK. Standardizing thoracic organ procurement for transplantation. J Thorac Cardiovasc Surg 2010;139:13-17.

16. de Perrot M, Keshavjee S. Lung preservation. Semin Thorac Cardiovasc Surg 2004;16:300-308.

17. van Berkel V, Guthrie TJ, Puri V, et al. Impact of anastomotic techniques on airway complications after lung transplant. Ann Thorac Surg 2011;92:316-320; discussion 320-311.

18. Lau CL, Hoganson DM, Meyers BF, et al. Use of an apical heart suction device for exposure in lung transplantation. Ann Thorac Surg 2006;81:1524-1525.

19. Davis RD. Bilateral sequential lung transplantation. Oper Tech Thorac Cardiovasc Surg 2007;12:57-72.

20. Aigner C, Jaksch P, Seebacher G, et al. Single running suture—the new standard technique for bronchial anastomoses in lung transplantation. Eur J Cardiothorac Surg 2003;23:488-493.

21. Shigemura N, Orhan Y, Bhama JK, et al. Delayed chest closure after lung transplantation: Techniques, outcomes, and strategies. J Heart Lung Transplant 2014;33:741-748.

22. Yeung JC, Keshavjee S. Overview of clinical lung transplantation. Cold Spring Harb Perspect Med 2014;4:a015628.

23. Robert JH, Murith N, de Perrot M, et al. Lung transplantation: How to perform the venous anastomosis when clamping is too distal. Ann Thorac Surg 2000;70:2164-2165.

24. Massad MG, Sirois C, Tripathy S, et al. Pulmonary venous drainage into the left atrial appendage facilitates transplantation of the left lung with difficult exposure. Ann Thorac Surg 2001;71:1046-1047.

25. Casula RP, Stoica SC, Wallwork J, Dunning J. Pulmonary vein augmentation for single lung transplantation. Ann Thorac Surg 2001;71:1373-1374.

26. Oto T, Rabinov M, Negri J, et al. Techniques of reconstruction for inadequate donor left atrial cuff in lung transplantation. Ann Thorac Surg 2006;81:1199-1204.

27. Schmidt F, McGiffin DC, Zorn G, et al. Management of congenital abnormalities of the donor lung. Ann Thorac Surg 2001;72:935-937.

28. Khasati NH, MacHaal A, Thekkudan J, et al. An aberrant donor pulmonary vein during lung transplant: A surgical challenge. Ann Thorac Surg 2005;79:330-331.

29. Sekine Y, Fischer S, de Perrot M, et al. Bilateral lung transplantation using a donor with a tracheal right upper lobe bronchus. Ann Thorac Surg 2002;73:308-310.

30. Noirclerc M, Shennib H, Giudicelli R, et al. Size matching in lung transplantation. J Heart Lung Transplant 1992;11:S203-S208.

31. Cassivi SD, Meyers BF, Battafarano RJ, et al. Thirteen-year experience in lung transplantation for emphysema. Ann Thorac Surg 2002;74:1663-1669; discussion 1669-1670.

32. Machuca TN, Cypel M, Keshavjee S. Advances in lung preservation. Surg Clin North Am 2013;93:1373-1394.

33. Steen S, Sjoberg T, Pierre L, et al. Transplantation of lungs from a non–heart-beating donor. Lancet 2001;357:825-829.

34. Venuta F, Diso D, Anile M, et al. Evolving techniques and perspectives in lung transplantation. Transplant Proc 2005;37:2682-2683.

17

Heart-lung transplantation: Technical aspects

MATTHIAS LOEBE, XIANG WEI, AND DEWEI REN

INTRODUCTION

Combined heart-lung transplantation was first applied clinically by Bruce Reitz and Norman Shumway at Stanford University on March 9, 1981.[1] The recipient was a 43-year-old woman with primary pulmonary hypertension. At the time, en bloc transplantation of a heart and lung was believed to be the only option to treat end-stage lung disease.[2] Attempts at transplanting isolated lungs had failed because of bronchial anastomotic problems.[3] In the following years a large number of patients around the world received combined heart-lung transplants for chronic obstructive pulmonary disease,[4] cystic fibrosis,[5] pulmonary fibrosis, or other end-stage lung disease. At one point, domino transplantation was suggested for patients who had normal cardiac function but needed lung replacement.[6] The heart was subsequently transplanted into a heart-only recipient.[4] In the 1990s this practice changed when single- and sequential double-lung transplantation proved to be a safe and valuable therapy.[3] Today, en bloc heart and lung transplantation is reserved for patients with severe heart disease and end-stage lung disease. This category of patients may include those in whom one disease (for example, sarcoidosis or pulmonary hypertension[7]) has destroyed both the heart and lung and those with end-stage heart disease (such as ischemic disease) together with end-stage lung disease (such as chronic obstructive pulmonary disease) of separate origin. Finally, Eisenmenger syndrome develops in a significant number of patients with congenital heart disease and may require a combined heart-lung transplant.[8] Combined heart-lung transplantation has also been suggested for Kartagener syndrome because of the complex anatomy. We and others have successfully used sequential double-lung transplantation in these cases.[9]

PREOPERATIVE EVALUATION

In our institution it has become practice for candidates to undergo evaluation by both the cardiology and pulmonology services and also be seen and evaluated by the transplant surgery service. Testing includes the usual heart transplant workup involving left and right heart catheters, echocardiography, a computed tomography (CT) scan of the chest, and so forth. Among other procedures, the lung transplantation workup includes a 6-minute walk test, lung function test, and perfusion-ventilation scintigraphy.

We would be very concerned about patients who have had multiple previous chest surgeries, such as shunts, ligation of ductus, or multiple valve replacements. The CT scan should be carefully studied for extracardiac malformations, abnormalities that would complicate the vascular anastomoses, or collaterals that would lead to extensive chest wall bleeding.

The function of the extrathoracic organs is reviewed, and a psychosocial evaluation is performed to ensure the long-term success of a transplant procedure.

DONOR MANAGEMENT

Donors for combined heart-lung transplantation are managed according to the protocols for thoracic organ retrieval. Fluid administration should be restricted to the minimum necessary. Cardiac function is assessed in the standard manner. Evaluation of the donor's lung function is based on oxygenation, chest radiography findings, and ventilator parameters, as with any lung donor. The heart-lung blocks should not be oversized for the recipient, whereas blocks from smaller donors are very acceptable in heart-lung transplantation.

Procurement includes bronchoscopy, as well as examination of radiographs and the results of the standard laboratory tests and separate analyses of blood gases from left and right pulmonary veins.[10]

SURGERY

Donor operation

The chest is opened through a midline incision and sternotomy. The pericardium is opened wide and the heart is inspected for contusion, calcification, or regional wall motion abnormalities. Both pleural cavities are opened completely, and the lungs are inspected carefully by lifting them from the chest cavity to see as much of the back of the lungs as possible.

The aorta, pulmonary artery, and superior vena cava are isolated. A heavy tie is placed around the superior vein. Purse-string sutures are placed on the aorta and the pulmonary artery. We use 4-0 polypropylene (Prolene) suture for this. After heparin has been given, the aorta and pulmonary artery are cannulated for perfusion solution. Prostaglandin solution is injected into the pulmonary artery. The superior vena cava is tied down, the inferior vena cava opened, the aorta cross-clamped, perfusion started, and the left atrial appendage opened wide. Ice is put on the heart and both pleural cavities are extensively irrigated with ice water. Ventilation is maintained with low tidal volumes. Care is taken to avoid overdistention of the left ventricle as a result of the infusion of large volumes of lung preservation solution. If heart perfusion is completed while the lung solution is still running, surface cooling for the heart is provided. We like to cut down on the pleura on both sides while the preservation solution is still running.

When the infusion has been completed, ventilation is stopped and the aortic arch is dissected free. The head vessels are transected and the trachea is visualized. The pericardium is cut along the base of the diaphragm; the pleura is separated from the descending aorta on the left and from the spine on the right. The endotracheal tube is then pulled back and the lung inflated to a mid-inspiratory level. The trachea is stapled with three staple lines, one cephalad and two toward the heart-lung block. The heart-lung block is then removed by transecting the residual tissue and brought to the back table.

On the back table a cannula is inserted into the pulmonary veins through the opened left atrial appendage; 1 to 2 L of lung preservation solution is administered retrograde. The opening in the pulmonary artery where the perfusion cannula was initially placed is opened with forceps to evacuate the clots being washed out by retrograde flushing. Next, the heart-lung block is put in a plastic bag filled with saline solution. Two more bags, each with cold saline solution, are used to package the donor organ.

Recipient operation

POSITIONING AND ANESTHESIA

The recipient is placed in a supine position with oral single-lumen intubation as for standard open heart surgery. The patient is prepared and draped as for heart transplantation.

The chest is opened through a midline sternotomy. The pericardium and both pleural cavities are opened. The lungs are inspected for adhesions, which are transected. The pulmonary artery is completely freed from the aorta. The pulmonary veins are identified at their exit through the pericardium, and the pericardium is carefully incised around them. Care is taken to not injure the phrenic nerve. When the anatomy is clearly visualized, heparin is given and the patient is placed on cardiopulmonary bypass with cannulation of the ascending aorta and separate cannulation of the superior and inferior venae cavae. Tape is placed around the superior and inferior venae cavae (Figure 17.1). We like to use CO_2 insufflation in the field to prevent air embolization.

EXCISION OF THE NATIVE HEART AND LUNGS

The aorta is cross-clamped and the heart is excised. The surgeon excises the lungs again while making sure that the nerves are not damaged. Placing an umbilical tape around the residual pericardium facilitates visualization. The pulmonary artery is removed in its entirety. Next, the

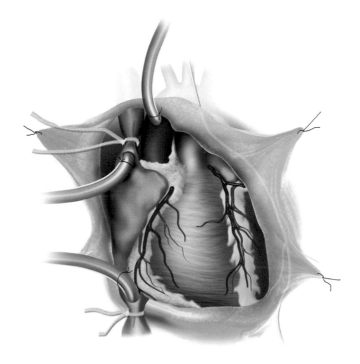

Figure 17.1 Exposure and cannulation for combined heart-lung transplantation. The ascending aorta is cannulated, as are the superior and inferior venae cavae; after extracorporeal circulation is initiated, the veins are occluded with umbilical tape.

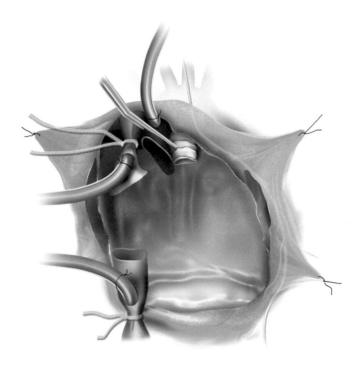

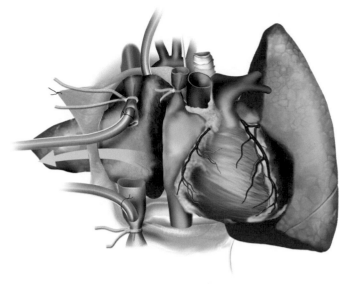

Figure 17.3 The right lung is slipped underneath the right atrium and through the pericardial window into the right pleural space.

Figure 17.2 After the heart and lungs have been excised, the nerves in the anterior and posterior mediastinum are preserved. A big window for placing the lungs into the pleural cavities is created on the left and right sides of the pericardium.

empty pericardium is examined. The right and left main bronchi are inspected to the carina. All sources of bleeding are addressed, and branches of the bronchial arteries are clipped. On the left side care is taken to not injure the descending aorta or its branches and the recurrent laryngeal nerve. The trachea is cut off right at the carina (Figure 17.2). Although total hemostasis in the posterior mediastinum is absolutely essential, we try to preserve as much surrounding tissue as possible to have good coverage of the tracheal anastomosis later. Care is also taken to preserve the vagus nerve (for this reason we do not put any ice inside the recipient's chest during the implantation procedure).[11]

IMPLANTATION

The donor heart-lung block is removed from the ice box and from the plastic bags. The implanting surgeon inspects the organs one more time. The left atrial appendage is closed with 4-0 Prolene suture. The trachea is shortened to approximately two to three rings above the carina, and the lungs are suctioned out. The heart-lung block is then moved into the operative field and placed in the chest. The pericardial bridge and the phrenic nerve are lifted, and the lungs are slipped through the gap into the left and right pleural cavities (Figure 17.3). Care is taken to not twist the lungs.

The trachea is anastomosed with 3-0 polydioxanone suture (PDS). The membranous part is connected with a running suture and the cartilaginous part with interrupted

sutures (Figure 17.4). Surrounding fat tissue may be fixed to the trachea with single stiches. Next, the right atrium is connected to the residual right recipient atrium by using 3-0 Prolene extra-long (Figure 17.5). Alternatively, a bicaval anastomosis can be created with 4-0 Prolene, which is our preferred approach today. Finally, the aorta is anastomosed with 4-0 Prolene running suture (Figure 17.6). The

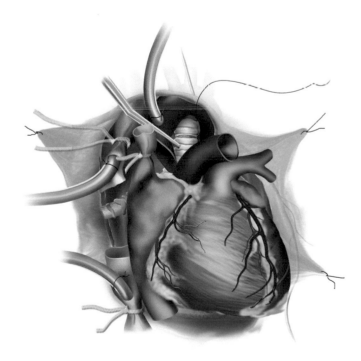

Figure 17.4 The trachea is anastomosed first with 3-0 polydioxanone suture (PDS). The back side (membranous part) of the trachea is sutured with running suture and the front (cartilaginous) part with interrupted suture.

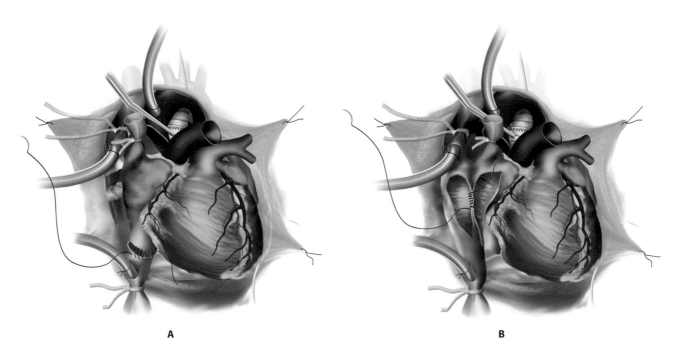

A   **B**

Figure 17.5 **(A)** The superior and inferior venae cavae are anastomosed with 4-0 polypropylene (Prolene) suture (a bicaval technique). **(B)** Alternatively, the right atrium is anastomosed to the recipient's atrium by using 3-0 Prolene running suture (a biatrial technique).

lung is suctioned out, steroids are administered, the tape is removed, and the heart is carefully drained of any residual air. The aortic cross-clamp is removed. At this point a vent drain can be inserted into the pulmonary artery at the cannulation site.

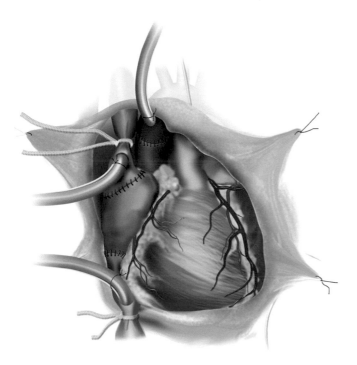

Figure 17.6 The aorta is anastomosed with a 4-0 running suture. Before this anastomosis is completed, the heart is extensively de-aired.

After reperfusion, the patient is weaned from cardiopulmonary bypass. Temporary pacing wires are placed on the atrium and ventricle. After protamine has been administered and hemostasis achieved, chest tubes are inserted: two tubes into each pleural cavity and one or two tubes into the mediastinum. Before the chest is closed in usual fashion, we like to inspect the posterior surface of the chest cavities for hemostasis one more time. Blood will collect deep inside the chest, and bleeding may be overlooked during standard inspection. Again, good hemostasis in the posterior mediastinum and on the chest walls is absolutely essential for success of the procedure. Achieving good hemostasis can be very challenging, especially in cases involving a redo or chronic inflammation. Extensive blood and volume replacement after combined heart-lung transplantation can lead to severe compromise of both heart and lung function and should therefore be minimized.

POSTOPERATIVE MANAGEMENT

Patients undergo postoperative management according to the guidelines for lung transplantation.[3,12,13] Bronchoscopy is performed at the end of surgery or on arrival in the intensive care unit. In some patients, right heart dysfunction may develop as a result of reperfusion of the lung and ischemia of the heart.[14] We are generous with the application of inhaled nitric oxide in heart-lung recipients. Fluid is restricted as in lung transplantation. Immunosuppression follows the protocol for lung transplantation.[13,14] Monitoring for rejection is based on the results of lung function tests and lung biopsy if needed.[15,16]

REFERENCES

1. Reitz BA, Wallwork JL, Hunt SA, et al. Heart-lung transplantation: Successful therapy for patients with pulmonary vascular disease. N Engl J Med 1982;306:557-564.

2. Reitz BA. The first successful combined heart-lung transplantation. J Thorac Cardiovasc Surg 2011;141:867-869.

3. Loebe M. Lung transplantation. Curr Opin Organ Transplant 2014;19:453-454.

4. Khaghani A, Banner N, Ozdogan E, et al. Medium-term results of combined heart and lung transplantation for emphysema. J Heart Lung Transplant 1991;10:15-21.

5. Madden BP, Hodson ME, Tsang V, et al. Intermediate-term results of heart-lung transplantation for cystic fibrosis. Lancet 1992;339:1583-1587.

6. Yacoub MH, Banner NR, Khaghani A, et al. Heart-lung transplantation for cystic fibrosis and subsequent domino heart transplantation. J Heart Transplant 1990;9:459-466.

7. O'Meara N, Clarke R, Gearty G, et al. Primary pulmonary hypertension: Treatment with heart-lung transplantation. Ir Med J 1987;80:174-175.

8. Yusen RD, Edwards LB, Kucheryavaya AY, et al. The registry of the International Society for Heart and Lung Transplantation: Thirty-first adult lung and heart-lung transplant report—2014; focus theme: Retransplantation. International Society for Heart and Lung Transplantation. J Heart Lung Transplant 2014;33:1009-1024.

9. Deuse T, Reitz BA. Heart-lung transplantation in situs inversus totalis. Ann Thorac Surg 2009;88:1002-1003.

10. Loebe M. Multiple-organ transplantation from a single donor. Tex Heart Inst J 2011;38:555-558.

11. Naik-Mathuria B, Jamous F, Noon GP, et al. Severe gastroparesis causing splenic rupture: A unique, early complication after heart-lung transplantation. Tex Heart Inst J 2006;33:508-511.

12. Deuse T, Sista R, Weill D, et al. Review of heart-lung transplantation at Stanford. Ann Thorac Surg 2010;90:329-337.

13. Bolman RM 3rd, Shumway SJ, Estrin JA, Hertz MI. Lung and heart-lung transplantation. Evolution and new applications. Ann Surg 1991;214:456-468.

14. Huddleston CB, Richey SR. Heart-lung transplantation. J Thorac Dis 2014;6:1150-1158.

15. McGregor CG, Baldwin JC, Jamieson SW, et al. Isolated pulmonary rejection after combined heart-lung transplantation. J Thorac Cardiovasc Surg 1985;90:623-626.

16. Wahlers T, Khaghani A, Martin M, et al. Frequency of acute heart and lung rejection after heart-lung transplantation. Transplant Proc 1987;19:3537-3538.

18

Lobar lung transplantation from living donors

HIROSHI DATE

INTRODUCTION

Living donor lobar lung transplantation (LDLLT) was introduced by Starnes and colleagues as an alternative form of treatment for patients who experience a decline in physical condition and have limited life expectancy. In the beginning a single donor was used, and successful living donor single-lobe transplantation was reported.[1] However, subsequent experience with single-lobe transplantation was not satisfactory. It is for this reason that Starnes' group developed bilateral LDLLT, in which two healthy donors donate their right or left lower lobes (Figure 18.1).[2,3] Because only two lobes are transplanted, LDLLT seems to be best suited for children and small adults, and in the group's experience it has been applied almost exclusively in patients with cystic fibrosis.[3] However, LDLLT is now well known to be applicable in cases of restrictive, obstructive, infectious, and hypertensive lung disease in both pediatric and adult patients when the size matching is acceptable.[4-6]

Although LDLLT began in the United States, its use there has decreased because of the recent change by the Organ Procurement and Transplantation Network in the urgency-benefit allocation system for cadaveric donor lungs. During the past several years, reports on LDLLT have come almost exclusively from Japan, where the average waiting time for a cadaveric lung is longer than 2 years.[7] In addition to the Japanese experience, small numbers of cases involving LDLLT have been reported from England,[8] Brazil,[9] and China.[10] The results of bilateral LDLLT have been as good as or better than those of conventional cadaveric lung transplantation (CLT).

RECIPIENT SELECTION

Candidates for LDLLT should be younger than 65 years and have progressive lung disease. All recipients should fulfill the criteria for conventional CLT. Because of the possible serious complications during donor lobectomy, LDLLT should be indicated only for critically ill patients who are unlikely to survive the long wait for cadaveric lungs. On the other hand, if the recipient were too sick, performing two lobectomies on two healthy donors would not be justified. In our experience with LDLLT, all patients were oxygen dependent, 59% were bedbound, and 11% were being supported by a ventilator at the time of transplantation. Whether LDLLT can be performed on patients already receiving ventilator support or requiring retransplantation is controversial. The St. Louis group reported that for retransplantation, LDLLT provided better survival than conventional CLT did.[11] The perioperative mortality rate after retransplantation was only 7.7% in patients who underwent LDLLT versus 42.3% in those who underwent CLT. Okayama,[12] Fukuoka,[13] and Kyoto[14,15] universities reported successful LDLLT for ventilator-dependent patients. We successfully performed LDLLT on nine patients who had been supported by a ventilator for as long as 7 months. The University of Southern California (USC) group reported that of the 123 patients on whom it performed LDLLT, those who required preoperative ventilator

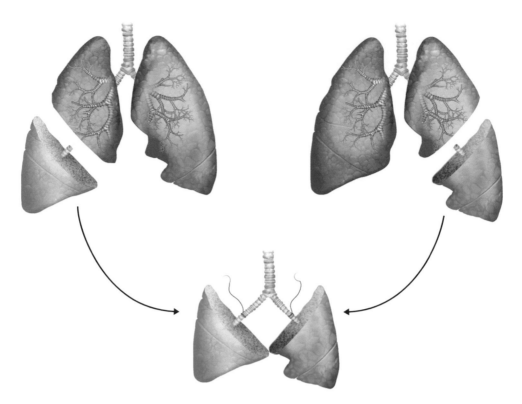

Figure 18.1 Bilateral living donor lobar lung transplantation. The right and left lower lobes from two healthy donors are implanted in a recipient in place of whole right and left lungs, respectively.

support had significantly worse outcomes and those undergoing retransplantation had an increased risk for death.[16] The Okayama group reported successful LDLLT in two patients who received extracorporeal membrane oxygenation (ECMO) support.[17] With both patients, ECMO was used as a bridge to LDLLT for 2 days, and both were successfully weaned from cardiopulmonary bypass (CPB) support in the operating room immediately after transplantation.

Cystic fibrosis represents the most common indication for LDLLT in the United States because only two lobes are transplanted during the procedure and patients with cystic fibrosis are usually small. The distribution of diagnoses considered indications for LDLLT in Japan is quite unique. Cystic fibrosis is a very rare disease here. We have accepted various lung disease, including hypertensive, restrictive, obstructive, and infectious lung disease, as indications for LDLLT. In our experience, interstitial pneumonia, bronchiolitis obliterans syndrome (BOS), and pulmonary hypertension are the three major indications. Most patients with interstitial pneumonia were receiving systemic corticosteroid therapy, most patients with BOS had previously undergone hematopoietic stem cell transplantation (HSCT) for various malignancies such as leukemia, and the patients with idiopathic pulmonary arterial hypertension were receiving high-dose epoprostenol.

DONOR SELECTION

The eligibility criteria for living lobar lung donation at Kyoto University are summarized in Table 18.1. Although

immediate family members (relatives within the third degree by consanguinity or a spouse) have been the only donors in our institution, non-Japanese institutions have accepted extended family members and unrelated individuals.[16] Extraction of more than one lobe from the donor should be prohibited.

Table 18.1 Eligibility criteria for living lung donation (Kyoto University)

Medical criteria
Age 20-60 years
ABO blood type compatible with the recipient's
Relatives within the third degree by consanguinity or a spouse
No significant past medical history
No recent viral infection
No significant abnormalities visible on echocardiography or electrocardiography
No significant ipsilateral pulmonary pathology on computed tomography
Arterial oxygen pressure ≥80 mm Hg (room air)
Forced vital capacity/forced expiratory volume in the first second of respiration ≥85% predicted
No previous ipsilateral thoracic surgery
No active tobacco smoking
Social and ethical criteria
No significant mental disorders proved by a psychiatrist
No ethical issues or concerns about donor motivation

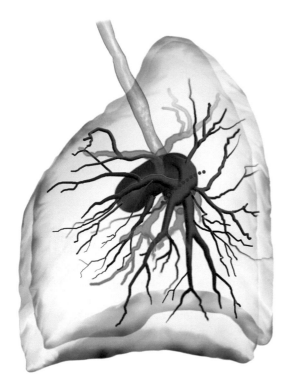

Figure 18.2 Three-dimensional computed tomography angiography in a left donor. The red dotted line shows the planned oblique line for cutting the pulmonary artery to preserve lingular branches.

Potential donors should be competent, willing to donate without coercion, medically and psychosocially suitable, fully informed of the risks and benefits of being a donor, and fully informed of the risks and benefits for and alternative treatment available to the recipient. In our institution, potential donors are interviewed at least three times to give them multiple opportunities to ask questions, reconsider donation, or withdraw as a donor.

The preoperative workup consists of posterior-anterior and left lateral chest radiography, high-resolution computed tomography (CT) of the chest (at maximal inspiration and expiration), formal pulmonary function tests and analysis of room-air blood gases, electrocardiography, and Doppler echocardiography. Three-dimensional multidetector CT angiography is used to confirm the pulmonary arterial and venous anatomy (Figure 18.2).[18] The completeness of pulmonary fissures is carefully evaluated by high-resolution CT. Although HLA matching is not required for donor selection, a prospective crossmatch is performed to rule out the presence of anti-HLA antibodies.

After a suitable donor pair has been found, the donor who is larger and has better vital capacity is selected for donation of the right lower lobe; the other is selected for removal of the left lower lobe.

SIZE MATCHING

Appropriate size matching between donor and recipient is important in LDLLT. It is often inevitable that small grafts are used during LDLLT involving implantation of only two lobes. Excessively small grafts may cause high pulmonary artery pressure, which results in lung edema.[19] A pleural space problem may increase the risk for empyema. Overexpansion of the donor lobes may contribute to obstructive physiology by early closure of small airways.[20] On the other hand, an adult lower lobe might be too big for small children. Using oversized grafts could cause high airway resistance, atelectasis, and hemodynamic instability by the time of chest closure.[21]

Functional size matching

For "functional size matching" we use forced vital capacity (FVC) of the graft.[22] We previously proposed a formula to estimate graft FVC on the basis of the donor's measured FVC and the number of pulmonary segments being implanted.[5] Given that the right lower lobe consists of 5 segments, the left lower lobe 4, and the whole lung 19, the total FVC of the two grafts is estimated by the following equation.

Total FVC of the two grafts = (Measured FVC of the right donor × 5/19) + (Measured FVC of the left donor × 4/19)

If the total FVC of the two grafts is more than 45% of the recipient's predicted FVC (calculated from a knowledge of height, age, and sex), we accept the size disparity regardless of the recipient's diagnosis.

Total FVC of the two grafts/Predicted FVC of the recipient > 0.45

The recipient's mean measured FVC at 6 months after LDLLT has been well correlated with the estimated graft FVC.[22] In contrast, we found no significant correlation between the recipient's predicted FVC and the recipient's measured FVC. These results indicate that the amount of lung tissue implanted, not recipient-related factors such as diagnosis, determines recipient FVC.

Anatomic size matching

For "anatomic size matching" three-dimensional CT (3D-CT) volumetry is performed for both the donor and recipient.[18,23] CT images are obtained by using a multidetector CT scanner during a single respiratory pause at the end of maximum inspiratory effort. The upper and lower thresholds of anatomic size matching have not yet been determined. We have accepted a wide range of volume ratios between the donor's lower lobe graft and the recipient's chest cavity. We found that when the ratio is within 40% to 160%, the recipient's ability to adapt to undersized or oversized grafts is remarkable.

SURGICAL TECHNIQUE

Three surgical teams and a back-table team are required to perform bilateral LDLLT. They communicate with each other closely to minimize graft ischemic time. The recipient and the right-side donor are brought to the operating room at the same time. The left-side donor is brought to the operating room 30 minutes later.

Donor lobectomy

The most common procedure involves a right lower lobectomy from a larger donor and a left lower lobectomy from a smaller donor. After induction of general anesthesia, donors are intubated with a left-sided double-lumen endotracheal tube. Fiberoptic bronchoscopy is performed to determine whether lower lobectomy is feasible. Adequate length for closure on the donor bronchus and for anastomosis in the recipient is left. The donors are placed in the lateral decubitus position and a posterolateral thoracotomy is performed though the fifth intercostal space. Fissures are developed by using linear stapling devices. The pericardium surrounding the inferior pulmonary vein is opened circumferentially. Dissection in the fissure is carried out to isolate the pulmonary artery to the lower lobe and define the anatomy of the pulmonary arteries to the middle lobe in the right-side donor and to the lingular segment in the left-side donor. If the branches of the middle lobe artery and lingular artery are small, they are ligated and divided. However, if these branches are large enough, arterioplasty with an autopericardial patch should be performed.[24]

Intravenous prostaglandin E_1 is administered to decrease the systolic blood pressure by 10 to 20 mm Hg, and 5000 units of heparin and 500 mg of methylprednisolone are administered intravenously. After vascular clamps have been placed in the appropriate positions, the pulmonary vein, pulmonary artery, and bronchus are divided in that order. The vascular stumps are closed with 5-0 polypropylene running suture. The bronchus is closed with 4-0 polypropylene interrupted suture. The bronchial stump is covered with pedicled pericardial fat tissue.

On the back table, the lobes are flushed both antegrade and retrograde with preservation solution from a bag positioned about 50 cm above the table. The lobes are gently ventilated with room air during the flush.

Recipient implantation

Recipients are anesthetized and intubated with a single-lumen endotracheal tube in children and left-sided double-lumen endotracheal tube in adults. A "clamshell" incision is used, and both chest cavities are entered through the fourth intercostal space. The sternum is notched at the level of transection by aiming the sternal saw at a 45-degree angle and cutting toward the midpoint to facilitate postoperative sternal adaptation.

To reduce blood loss, as many of the pleural and hilar dissections as possible are performed before heparinization. The ascending aorta and right atrium are cannulated after heparinization, and patients are placed on standard CPB. After the bilateral pneumonectomy, the hilum is prepared

to facilitate subsequent implantation. The chest is irrigated with warm saline solution containing antibiotics.

The right lower lobe is implanted first, followed by implantation of the left lower lobe. The bronchus, pulmonary vein, and pulmonary artery are anastomosed consecutively. The bronchial anastomosis is begun with running 4-0 polydioxanone suture for the membranous portion and completed with simple interrupted suture or a running suture for the cartilaginous portion. We use end-to-end anastomosis when the bronchi are the same size and a telescoping technique when a discrepancy in bronchial size is obvious. Bronchial wrapping is not used except in patients receiving high-dose steroid therapy. The venous anastomosis is performed between the donor inferior pulmonary vein and the recipient superior pulmonary vein; running 6-0 polypropylene suture is used. The pulmonary arterial anastomosis is completed in end-to-end fashion with running 6-0 polypropylene suture.

Just before the bilateral implantations are completed, 500 mg to 1 g of methylprednisolone is administered intravenously and nitric oxide inhalation is initiated at 20 ppm. After both lungs have been reperfused and ventilated, the patient is gradually weaned from CPB.

The alternative strategy for cardiopulmonary support during the recipient's portion of LDLLT is to provide ECMO via the femoral artery and vein. ECMO allows less heparin use, which seems to reduce perioperative bleeding.[25] This strategy is especially useful when extensive pleural adhesions are found. The activated clotting time is maintained at around 200 seconds. We have used ECMO instead of CPB in most LDLLT procedures since 2012.

STRATEGIES FOR DEALING WITH SIZE MISMATCH IN LDLLT

Oversized graft

For small children, an adult lower lobe might be too big. Use of oversized grafts could lead to the development of high airway resistance, atelectasis, and hemodynamic instability by the time of chest closure.[21] To overcome these problems we have developed several techniques, including performing single-lobe transplantation with or without contralateral pneumonectomy, delaying chest closure, and downsizing the graft.

Single LDLLT from a single living donor can be performed for selected small recipients. We retrospectively investigated 14 critically ill patients who had undergone single LDLLT at three lung transplant centers in Japan.[26] Their 3- and 5-year survival rates were 70% and 56%, respectively. The survival rate of these 14 patients was significantly worse than that of a group of 78 patients who underwent bilateral LDLLT during the same period. Single LDLLT provides acceptable results for sick patients who would soon die otherwise. However, bilateral LDLLT appears to be the better option if two living donors are found.

We reported successful right lower lobe transplantation and simultaneous left pneumonectomy in an 8-year-old girl who was being supported by a ventilator.[15] The graft, which was donated by her mother, was estimated to be 200% larger than the girl's right chest cavity.

It has been reported that delayed chest closure can be used safely after cadaveric bilateral lung transplantation. This technique can be applied to LDLLT.[27] The oversized graft volume is expected to decrease during the waiting period as a result of improvement in pulmonary edema, and the dimensions of the recipient's right heart are expected to decrease because of the reduction in afterload following LDLLT.

We reported another strategy for oversized grafts: downsizing the graft on the back table. A 15-year-old boy with BOS underwent successful bilateral LDLLT that involved resectioning of the superior segment of the oversized right lower lobe graft that had been obtained from his father.[18]

Undersized graft

When grafts are too small, the limited amount of vascular bed might cause high pulmonary artery pressure and thus lead to lung edema.[19] Intrathoracic dead space can remain and cause complications such as postoperative bleeding, persistent air leakage, and empyema. Moreover, hyperinflation of the grafted lungs may result in insufficient respiratory dynamics or hemodynamic collapse after LDLLT.[20]

We reported a successful LDLLT in which the problem of a very large size mismatch between donor lungs and recipient chest cavity was solved by sparing the bilateral native upper lobes.[28] The recipient, a 44-year-old man with BOS, was 17 cm taller than his donors, his sister and his wife. With regard to functional size matching, the estimated FVC of the graft was 45.7% of the recipient's predicted FVC. With respect to anatomic size matching, the volume ratio of the graft was only 22% in the right side and 36% in the left side. Sparing the native upper lobes provided a chest cavity adequate for small grafts. Candidates for this approach should have no infection in the spared lobes and minimum pleural adhesion with well-developed interlobar fissures. In view of these factors, a space-occupying noninfectious disease, such as BOS, would be an ideal indication for this procedure. Pulmonary fibrosis, pulmonary artery hypertension, emphysema, and lymphangioleiomyomatosis may also be possible indications.

POSTOPERATIVE MANAGEMENT

The patient is kept intubated for at least 3 days to maintain optimal expansion of the implanted lobes. We use pressure-limited ventilation and keep the maximal ventilation pressure lower than 25 cm H_2O. Fiberoptic bronchoscopy is performed every 12 hours during intubation to assess donor airway viability and suction any retained secretions. Bedside postoperative pulmonary rehabilitation is initiated as soon as possible.

Postoperative immunosuppression consists of triple-drug therapy with cyclosporine (CSA) or tacrolimus, mycophenolate mofetil (MMF), and corticosteroids. Induction cytolytic therapy is not used. The combination of CSA, MMF, and a steroid is chosen for patients with infectious lung disease, pediatric patients, and those receiving a steroid; the combination of tacrolimus, MMF, and a steroid is selected for other patients. Except for 125 mg of methylprednisolone administered during the first 3 days, all immunosuppressants are given via a nasal tube inserted to the proximal jejunum. With careful monitoring of daily serum creatinine, CSA and tacrolimus trough levels are often reduced to below the target range.

We judge acute rejection on the basis of radiographic and clinical findings without transbronchial lung biopsy because the risk for pneumothorax and bleeding after transbronchial lung biopsy may be higher after LDLLT. Because the two lobes are donated by different donors, acute rejection is usually seen unilaterally. Early acute rejection episodes are characterized by dyspnea, low-grade fever, leukocytosis, hypoxemia, and a diffuse interstitial infiltrate that is visible on chest radiographs and CT scans. A trial bolus dose of 500 mg methylprednisolone is administered, and various clinical signs are carefully observed. If acute rejection is indeed the problem, two additional daily bolus doses of methylprednisolone are given. If acute rejection is encountered more than three times, CSA is replaced by tacrolimus.

OUTCOME FOR LIVING DONORS

Successful LDLLT depends largely on good donor outcome. In our experience, all donors have returned to their previous lifestyles without any restrictions. However, long-term outcomes for live donors have not been well documented because they are generally monitored for only 1 year. More studies are needed to understand the long-term results of living lung donors.

Perioperative complications in living donors

Relatively high morbidity after lobectomy has been described in previous reports, but no perioperative mortality has been reported.[29,30] Morbidity rates have varied from 20% to 60%, depending on the definition of complications. Common complications are pleural effusion, bronchial stamp fistulas, hemorrhage, and arrhythmia. The Vancouver Forum Lung Group summarized the world experience of approximately 550 living lung donors in 2006.[31] Approximately 5% experienced complications requiring surgical or bronchoscopic intervention.

The relatively high morbidity after living donor lobectomy in comparison to that with standard lobectomy may be explained by three technical differences between the two surgical procedures. First, the circumferential incision into the pericardium surrounding the inferior pulmonary vein may increase the risk for arrhythmias and pericarditis. Second, the oblique transection of the right lower lobe bronchus may increase the risk for bronchial fistula and stenosis.

Third, administration of heparin may increase the risk for bleeding during the perioperative period.

Psychological outcome for living donors

Massachusetts General Hospital (MGH) reported that living lung donors enjoyed generally satisfactory physical and emotional health.[32] Donors reported positive feelings about donation; however, they wished for greater recognition and appreciation by the transplant team and the recipient. The Okayama group reported that the average quality of life of the living lung donors was better than that of the general population.[33] However, a fatal outcome for the recipient had a significant impact on the donor's mental health. Interestingly, a significant correlation of mental health scores between the paired donors existed. In a prospective study we reported that living donors' health-related quality of life and dyspnea worsened postoperatively.[34]

Pulmonary function of living donors

The MGH group reported that mean donor FVC decreased by 16% ± 3%.[32] The postdonation FVC value was higher than the preoperatively predicted value. We prospectively evaluated pulmonary function 3, 6, and 12 months after donor lobectomy.[35] During the first year after donor lobectomy, FVC and forced expiratory volume in the first second of respiration (FEV_1) values recovered steadily to about 90% of the preoperative values.

OUTCOME FOR THE LDLLT RECIPIENT

Only three groups have summarized recipient outcomes. In 2004 the USC group published its 10-year experience with 123 LDLLT recipients, including 39 children.[16] In the group's series, retransplantation and mechanical ventilation were identified as risk factors for mortality. The 1-, 3-, and 5-year survival rates were 70%, 54%, and 45%, respectively. The St. Louis group reported similar results for 38 pediatric LDLLT recipients.[36] We (the Okayama University Group) reported on 43 LDLLTs with a 5-year survival rate of 87.6% during a follow-up lasting between 1 and 98 months.[37]

As of August 2014, the author had accumulated experience with LDLLT in 96 patients (47 at Okayama University and 49 at Kyoto University). They included 64 females and 32 males ranging from 6 to 64 years of age (average age 33.3 years). Twenty-four were children and 72 were adults.

The LDLLT recipients' diagnoses before transplantation are listed in Table 18.2. We accepted various diseases, including restrictive, obstructive, vascular, and infectious lung diseases. Interstitial pneumonia, BOS, and pulmonary hypertension were the three major indications. All 96 patients were very sick and required oxygen inhalation therapy preoperatively. Fifty-seven (59%) were bedbound and 11 (11%) were being supported with a ventilator.

Bilateral LDLLT was performed on 82 patients, and single LDLLT was performed on 14 small patients. Six early deaths

Table 18.2 Diagnoses for living donor lobar lung transplantation

Diagnoses	Number
Interstitial pneumonia	36
Bronchiolitis obliterans syndrome	24
Pulmonary hypertension	21
Bronchiectasis	6
Lymphangioleiomyomatosis	4
Retransplantation	2
Cystic fibrosis	1
Emphysema	1
Eosinophilic granuloma	1
Total	96

occurred, thus resulting in a hospital mortality rate of 6.3%. The causes of early death were graft failure resulting from excessively small grafts in two cases, infection in two, acute rejection in one, and heart failure in one. Twelve late deaths occurred during a follow-up period of 1 to 190 months. The causes of late death were BOS in four cases, posttransplant lymphoproliferative disorder in three, cachexia in two, encephalitis in one, and unknown cause in two. The 5- and 10-year survival rates were 83.0% and 76.5%, respectively (Figure 18.3).

The question of whether two pulmonary lobes can provide sufficient long-term pulmonary function and clinical outcome for recipients has recently been answered. The USC group reported that in adult recipients surviving more than 3 months after transplantation, LDLLT provided intermediate- and long-term pulmonary function and exercise capacity comparable to that provided by bilateral CLT.[38] We have observed similar results in our LDLLT recipients. The measured recipient FVC ultimately reached 123% of the graft FVC estimated for two donor lobes (calculated on the basis of the donor FVC and number of segments implanted) at 36 months after LDLLT.[39]

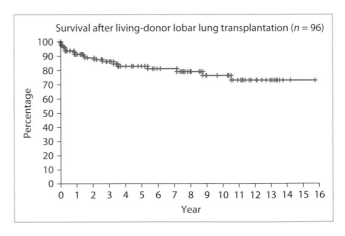

Figure 18.3 Survival after living donor lobar lung transplantation (N = 96). The 5- and 10-year survival rates were 83.0% and 76.5%, respectively.

Of the patients on the waiting list for a lung transplant, those with interstitial pneumonia have been shown to have the highest mortality rate while awaiting cadaveric donors. Patients with interstitial pneumonia have small chest cavities because of the nature of their restrictive lung disease, which we believe is rather beneficial for lobar implantation.[40] In two of these patients interstitial pneumonia was associated with dermatomyositis.[41] We have accepted patients who were receiving systemic corticosteroid therapy consisting of prednisone in doses as high as 50 mg/day. Excellent bronchial healing of all anastomoses was observed. Various factors, such as short donor bronchus, high blood flow in the small grafts implanted, and well-preserved lung parenchyma with short ischemic time, may contribute to the better oxygen supply to the donor bronchus, which in turn results in excellent bronchial healing after LDLLT. These data support the option of LDLLT in patients with advanced idiopathic interstitial pneumonia and interstitial pneumonia associated with collagen disease.

Of our 24 patients with BOS with or without pulmonary fibrosis, 21 underwent LDLLT after HSCT for hematopoietic diseases such as leukemia.[42] Despite medical advances in the field of HSCT, chronic, progressive, and irreversible pulmonary complications, such as BOS and pulmonary fibrosis, remain a significant and leading cause of death. Of note, one report described several patients who underwent LDLLT after HSCT involving the same living donor,[43] which gives the recipient advantages in terms of immunologic predominance. A Japanese group summarized its experience with 19 patients who had undergone LDLLT after HSCT.[44]

Of 21 patients with pulmonary hypertension, 15 had idiopathic pulmonary arterial hypertension (IPAH), 3 had pulmonary venoocclusive disease, 2 had Eisenmenger syndrome, and 1 had pulmonary capillary hemangiomatosis.

All the patients with IPAH except one were receiving high-dose intravenous epoprostenol with inotropic support. Most were in World Health Organization class IV and bedbound. Obvious concerns existed regarding whether pulmonary hypertension would develop because only two lobes were being implanted and they would be receiving the patient's entire cardiac output. We first reported successful LDLLT in an adult patient with IPAH.[45] Although a limited amount of lung tissue is implanted, pulmonary arterial pressure becomes nearly normal soon after LDLLT, thus validating the premise that two adult lobes have the functional capacity to handle the cardiac output of both adult and pediatric recipients with pulmonary hypertension (including IPAH), pulmonary venoocclusive disease, pulmonary capillary hemangiomatosis, and Eisenmenger syndrome.[46,47] Chest radiography shows dramatic improvement after LDLLT because of a reduction in right ventricular afterload (Figure 18.4).

COMPARISON WITH CADAVERIC LUNG TRANSPLANTATION

Table 18.3 compares the advantages and disadvantages of LDLLT with those of CLT. In general, the ischemic time for LDLLT is much shorter than that for CLT. In our experience the ischemic time for the right graft averages 151 ± 5 minutes as opposed to 121 ± 4 minutes for the left graft. Although only two lobes are transplanted, LDLLT seems to be associated with less frequent primary graft failure. We believe that use of a "small but perfect graft" gives LDLLT a big advantage.

Experienced centers have recently reported the incidence of bronchial complications in CLT to be about 5%. Contraindications to CLT include current high-dose

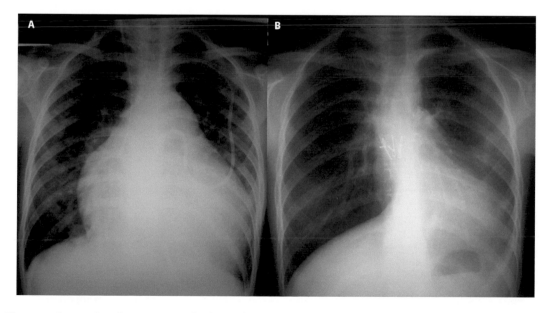

Figure 18.4 Chest radiographs of a patient with idiopathic pulmonary arterial hypertension. **(A)** Before transplantation marked cardiomegaly was present. **(B)** Two months after bilateral living donor lobar lung transplantation, a well-expanded lobe filled the chest cavities, thus leaving no detectable dead space and no cardiomegaly.

Table 18.3 Comparison between LDLLT and CLT

Indicator	LDLLT	CLT
Waiting time	Short	Long
Schedule	Controllable	Uncontrollable
Ischemic time	Short	Long
Graft size	Small	Full
Primary graft failure	Infrequent	10% to 20%
Infection transmitted from graft	Infrequent	Frequent
Number of teams	3	2
Rate of bronchial complications	Rare	5%
Chronic rejection	Often unilateral	Major cause of death

Note: CLT, cadaveric lung transplantation; LDLLT, living donor lobar lung transplantation.

systemic corticosteroid therapy because it may increase airway complications; however, low-dose corticosteroid therapy (prednisone in a dose of 20 mg/day or lower) before transplantation is acceptable. We have accepted patients receiving high-dose corticosteroid therapy (doses of prednisone as high as 50 mg/day) systemically as candidates for LDLLT. Of the 178 anastomoses performed, 171 (96%) demonstrated excellent bronchial healing.[48] Various factors, such as a short donor bronchus, high blood flow in the small grafts implanted, and well-preserved lung parenchyma with a short ischemic time, may contribute to better oxygen supply to the donor bronchus, thus resulting in excellent bronchial healing in LDLLT.

BOS has been the major obstacle after CLT. The USC group suggested that LDLLT was associated with a lower incidence of BOS, especially in pediatric patients. The group also indicated that the shorter ischemic time in LDLLT could explain the reduced incidence of BOS. BOS developed in 10 (25%) of our first 40 LDLLT recipients who survived longer than 6 months. Interestingly, unilateral BOS developed in 7 of the 10 recipients and the decline in their FEV_1 value stopped within 9 months. Transplanting two lobes obtained from two different donors appears to be beneficial in the long term because the unaffected contralateral lung may function as a reservoir in the event of development of unilateral BOS.[49]

REFERENCES

1. Starnes VA, Lewiston NJ, Luikart H, et al. Current trends in lung transplantation: Lobar transplantation and expanded use of single lungs. J Thorac Cardiovasc Surg 1992;104:1060-1068.
2. Starnes VA, Barr ML, Cohen RG. Lobar transplantation: Indications, technique, and outcome. J Thorac Cardiovasc Surg 1994;108:403-411.
3. Starnes VA, Barr ML, Cohen RG, et al. Living-donor lobar lung transplantation experience: Intermediate results. J Thorac Cardiovasc Surg 1996;112:1284-1291.
4. Starnes VA, Barr ML, Schenkel FA, et al. Experience with living-donor lobar lung transplantation for indications other than cystic fibrosis. J Thorac Cardiovasc Surg 1997;114:917-921.
5. Date H, Aoe M, Nagahiro I, et al. Living-donor lobar lung transplantation for various lung diseases. J Thorac Cardiovasc Surg 2003;126:476-481.
6. Date H, Aoe M, Sano Y, et al. Improved survival after living-donor lobar lung transplantation. J Thorac Cardiovasc Surg 2004;128,933-940.
7. Sato M, Okada Y, Oto T, et al. The Japanese Society of Lung and Heart-Lung Transplantation. Registry of the Japanese Society of Lung and Heart-Lung Transplantation: Official Japanese lung transplantation report, 2014. Gen Thorac Cardiovasc Surg 2014;62:594-601.
8. Camargo SM, Camargo Jde J, Schio SM, et al. Complications related to lobectomy in living lobar lung transplant donors. J Bras Pneumol 2008;34:256-263.
9. Chen QK, Jiang GN, Ding JA, et al. First successful bilateral living-donor lobar lung transplantation in China. Chin Med J (Engl) 2010;123:1477-1478.
10. Mohite PN, Popov AF, Yacoub MH, Simon AR. Live related donor lobar lung transplantation recipients surviving well over a decade: Still an option in times of advanced donor management. J Cardiothorac Surg 2013;8:37-41.
11. Kozower BD, Sweet SC, de la Morena M, et al. Living donor lobar grafts improve lung retransplantation survival. J Thorac Cardiovasc Surg 2006;131:1142-1147.
12. Toyooka S, Yamane M, Oto T, et al. Favorable outcomes after living-donor lobar lung transplantation in ventilator-dependent patients. Surg Today 2008;38:1078-1082.
13. Shiraishi T, Hiratsuka M, Munakata M, et al. Living-donor single-lobe lung transplantation for bronchiolitis obliterans in a 4-year-old boy. J Thorac Cardiovasc Surg 2007;134:1092-1093.
14. Shoji T, Bando T, Fujinaga T, Date H. Living-donor single-lobe lung transplant in a 6-year-old girl after 7-month mechanical ventilator support. J Thorac Cardiovasc Surg 2010;139:e112-e113.
15. Sonobe M, Bando T, Kusuki S, et al. Living-donor, single-lobe lung transplantation and simultaneous contralateral pneumonectomy in a child. J Heart Lung Transplant 2011;30:471-474.
16. Starnes VA, Bowdish ME, Woo MS, et al. A decade of living lobar lung transplantation. Recipient outcomes. J Thorac Cardiovasc Surg 2004;127:114-122.
17. Miyoshi K, Oto T, Okazaki M, Yamane M, et al. Extracorporeal membrane oxygenation bridging to living-donor lobar lung transplantation. Ann Thorac Surg 2009;88:e56-e57.
18. Chen F, Fujinaga T, Shoji T, et al. Perioperative assessment of oversized lobar graft downsizing in

living-donor lobar lung transplantation using three-dimensional computed tomographic volumetry. Transpl Int 2010;23:e41-e44.

19. Fujita T, Date H, Ueda K, et al. Experimental study on size matching in a canine living-donor lobar lung transplant model. J Thorac Cardiovasc Surg 2002;123:104-109.

20. Haddy SM, Bremner RM, Moore-Jefferies EW, et al. Hyperinflation resulting in hemodynamic collapse following living donor lobar transplantation. Anesthesiology 2002;97:1315-1317.

21. Oto T, Date H, Ueda K, et al. Experimental study of oversized grafts in a canine living-donor lobar lung transplantation model. J Heart Lung Transplant 2001;20:1325-1330.

22. Date H, Aoe M, Nagahiro I, et al. How to predict forced vital capacity after living-donor lobar-lung transplantation. J Heart Lung Transplant 2004;23:547-551.

23. Chen F, Kubo T, Shoji T, et al. Comparison of pulmonary function test and computed tomography volumetry in living lung donors. J Heart Lung Transplant 2011;30:572-575.

24. Chen F, Miwa S, Bando T, Date H. Pulmonary arterioplasty for the remaining arterial stump of the donor and the arterial cuff of the donor graft in living-donor lobar lung transplantation. Eur J Cardiovasc Surg 2012;42:e138-e139.

25. Ius F, Kuehn C, Tudorache I, et al. Lung transplantation on cardiopulmonary support: Venoarterial extracorporeal membrane oxygenation outperformed cardiopulmonary bypass. J Thorac Cardiovasc Surg 2012;144:1510-1516.

26. Date H, Shiraishi T, Sugimoto S, et al. Outcome of living-donor lobar lung transplantation using a single donor. J Thorac Cardiovasc Surg 2012;144:710-715.

27. Chen F, Matsukawa S, Ishii H, et al. Delayed chest closure assessed by transesophageal echocardiogram in single-lobe lung transplantation. Ann Thorac Surg 2011;92:2254-2257.

28. Fujinaga T, Bando T, Nakajima D, et al. Living-donor lobar lung transplantation with sparing of bilateral native upper lobes: A novel strategy. J Heart Lung Transplant 2011;30:351-353.

29. Bowdish ME, Barr ML, Schenkel FA, et al. A decade of living lobar lung transplantation. Perioperative complications after 253 donor lobectomies. Am J Transplant 2004;4:1283-1288.

30. Yusem RD, Hong BA, Messersmith EE, et al. Morbidity and mortality of live lung donation: Results from the RELIVE study. Am J Transplant 2014;14:1846-1852.

31. Barr ML, Belghiti J, Villamil FG, et al. A report of the Vancouver Forum on the care of the live organ donor. Lung, liver, pancreas, and intestine data and medical guidelines. Transplantation 2006;81:1373-1385.

32. Prager LM, Wain JC, Roberts DH, Ginns LC. Medical and psychologic outcome of living lobar lung transplant donors. J Heart Lung Transplant 2006;25:1206-1212.

33. Nishioka M, Yokoyama C, Iwasaki M, et al. Donor quality of life in living-donor lobar lung transplantation. J Heart Lung Transplant 2011;30:1348-1351.

34. Chen F, Oga T, Sakai H, et al. A prospective study analyzing one-year multidimensional outcomes in living lung transplant donors. Am J Transplant 2013;13:3003-3009.

35. Chen F, Fujinaga T, Shoji T, et al. Outcomes and pulmonary function in living lobar lung transplant donors. Transpl Int 2012;25:153-157.

36. Sweet SC. Pediatric living donor lobar lung transplantation. Pediatr Transplant 2006;10:861-868.

37. Date H, Yamane M, Toyooka S, et al. Current status and potential of living-donor lobar lung transplantation. Front Biosci 2008;13:1433-1439.

38. Bowdish ME, Pessotto R, Barbers RG, et al. Long-term pulmonary function after living-donor lobar lung transplantation in adults. Ann Thorac Surg 2005;79:418-425.

39. Yamane M, Date H, Okazaki M, et al. Long-term improvement in pulmonary function after living-donor lobar lung transplantation. J Heart Lung Transplant 2007;26;687-692.

40. Date H, Tanimoto Y, Yamadori I, et al. A new treatment strategy for advanced idiopathic interstitial pneumonia: Living-donor lobar lung transplantation. Chest 2005;128;1364-1370.

41. Shoji T, Bando T, Fujinaga T, et al. Living-donor lobar lung transplantation for interstitial pneumonia associated with dermatomyositis. Transpl Int 2010;23:e10-e11.

42. Yamane M, Sano Y, Toyooka S, et al. Living-donor lobar lung transplantation for pulmonary complications after hematopoietic stem cell transplantation. Transplantation 2008;86:1767-1770.

43. Oshima K, Kikuchi A, Mochizuki S, et al. Living-donor single lobe lung transplantation for bronchiolitis obliterans from mother to child following previous allogeneic hematopoietic stem cell transplantation from the same donor. Int J Hematol 2009;90:540-542.

44. Chen F, Yamane M, Inoue M, et al. Less maintenance immunosuppression in lung transplantation following hematopoietic stem cell transplantation from the same living donor. Am J Transplant 2011;11:1509-1516.

45. Date H, Nagahiro I, Aoe M, et al. Living-donor lobar lung transplantation for primary pulmonary hypertension in an adult. J Thorac Cardiovasc Surg 2001;122:817-818.

46. Date H, Kusano KF, Matsubara H, et al. Living-donor lobar lung transplantation for pulmonary arterial

hypertension after failure of epoprostenol therapy. J Am Coll Cardiol 2007;50;523-527.

47. Aokage K, Date H, Okazaki M, et al. Living-donor lobar lung transplantation and closure of atrial septal defect for adult Eisenmenger's syndrome. J Heart Lung Transplant 2009;28:1107-1109.

48. Toyooka S, Yamane M, Oto T, et al. Bronchial healing after living-donor lobar lung transplantation. Surg Today 2009;39:938-943.

49. Shinya T, Sato S, Kato K, et al. Assessment of mean transit time in the engrafted lung with ^{133}Xe lung ventilation scintigraphy improves diagnosis of bronchiolitis obliterans syndrome in living-donor lobar lung transplant recipients. Ann Nucl Med 2008;22:31-39.

19

Technical aspects of redo lung transplantation and lung transplantation after previous thoracotomy

SHELLY BANSAL AND JOHN A. ODELL

> The two biggest decisions in surgery are when not to operate and when to reoperate. Both these decisions are derived from long personal experience and the knowledge of those that have gone before.
>
> *John A. Odell*

INTRODUCTION

This chapter deals with the technical aspects of redo lung transplantation, as well as the technical aspects of lung transplantation after previous thoracic surgery. The number of cases requiring retransplantation is increasing, and many patients who are being considered for transplantation have had previous operations on the chest. This chapter does not debate the ethics or opposing views associated with the decision to retransplant: the utilitarian view that allocation of organs should be prioritized versus the egalitarian view that equal opportunity should be provided to those in need. Many of these views are tempered by the attitudes of the individual transplant unit. For example, many would take the view that patients who have already received a transplant have had their opportunity and it is now time to offer donor lungs to someone else. Others would argue that we cannot blame patients for failure of the transplanted organ and that the commitment to continue treatment must be honored even if doing so necessitates retransplantation.

The easier, less controversial part of this chapter deals with lung transplantation after previous chest surgery. The ethical debate is not as critical as the decision to retransplant; nevertheless, a cavalier or blasé attitude in the presence of a previous scar on the chest should not exist. The surgeon should carefully review the previous operative notes, evaluate the imaging results, and anticipate difficulties that may affect the operation.

RETRANSPLANTATION

The data

With the improvement in early morbidity after primary lung transplantation, long-term outcomes have improved; yet survival after a retransplant still does not match that after a primary transplant. Failure of the transplanted organ does occur and may necessitate retransplantation, with bronchiolitis obliterans syndrome (BOS) being the most common cause and other reasons for failure including primary graft dysfunction, airway complications, and technical issues.[1]

The International Society for Heart and Lung Transplantation reviewed the registry database for outcomes and questioned the appropriateness of retransplantation.[2] The reviewed data set included information on 47,647 lung transplant patients, 3.9% of whom received retransplants. Half of all patients undergoing retransplantation were less than 3 years from their initial operation and almost 25% had undergone retransplantation within 1 year. According to the review, outcomes for retransplantation are significantly worse than those for primary lung transplantation (1-year survival rates of 43% and 80%, respectively).

The registry confirmed that adults who underwent retransplantation continued to have lower rates of survival and higher rates of early mortality. The median survival time was 2.5 years, with a 1-year conditional survival time of 6.3 years. Era effect was noted in the cohort, with improved survival in the most recent era, which again reflects improved posttransplant care. Transplant-free interval continued to be a significant predictor of outcome; outcome after a transplant-free interval longer than 5 years was equivalent to that after a primary transplant. Risk factors for retransplantation included single-lung transplantation, performance of the procedure during the later transplant era, female sex, younger recipient age, older donor age, and greater recipient height.

Morbidity after retransplantation remains a concern in this cohort because of the long-term effects of immunosuppression. Primary transplants and retransplants were characterized by similar rates of rejection in the first year, and approximately 50% of recipients in both groups had BOS at 5 years. Retransplantation was associated with higher rates of hypertension and renal dysfunction than after primary transplantation; however, rates of diabetes and hyperlipidemia after both procedures were similar.

It is these sobering figures that create hesitancy to reoperate and fuel the fire of those advocating against retransplantation. Nevertheless, data suggesting acceptable long-term outcomes after retransplantation in specific patient populations do exist.

The Hannover Thoracic Transplant Program reviewed its experience with redo lung transplants and compared the results with those of primary lung transplants.[3] Of the 614 transplants performed, 54 were redo lung transplants, including 34 for chronic graft failure. Early and late survival rates in the BOS group were similar to those of patients who received primary transplants. More importantly, freedom from BOS was similar in patients who had received primary lung transplants and those who had received retransplants. A similar finding was noted by the Vienna group, which documented 30-day, 1-year, and 5-year survival rates similar to those reported by the Hannover group.[4] Their conclusion was that if no medical contraindication to lung transplantation exists, retransplantation can be offered to those with BOS with the expectation of acceptable long-term survival.

Patients with early need for retransplantation

Acute graft dysfunction after transplantation can be alarming; however, medical options, including extracorporeal support and mechanical ventilation, do exist, and retransplantation remains in the management algorithm. Aigner and colleagues reviewed their experience with redo transplantation for primary graft dysfunction. Time to transplantation averaged 26 ± 27 days.[4] The 30-day, 1-year, and 5-year survival rates in the group were dismal: 52.2%, 34.8%, and 29%, respectively. Interestingly, patients with primary graft dysfunction did not see a benefit from the era effect (transplants performed in the observation period before 2001 as compared with those performed after 2002), and outcomes remained poor.

Critically ill transplant patients

A 1996 review from the Pulmonary Retransplant Registry demonstrated patients' preoperative ambulatory status and center volume as predictors of survival.[5] A more recent review of 230 patients from the registry revealed that two factors, immobility (odds ratio = 1.93 [1.31 to 2.83]; $P < .001$) and preoperative mechanical ventilation (odds ratio = .53 [.37 to .74]; $P < .001$), were predictors of poor survival irrespective of center volume. In the recent review, two additional factors contributed to improved outcomes after retransplantation: transplant-free interval (>2 years) and era effect, which probably reflected improvements in posttransplant care after a primary transplant. The group confirmed what we suspected: critically ill patients who are undergoing reoperation, being supported by a ventilator, and immobile will do poorly.[6]

Our experience

Over the last 5 years we have performed 22 redo lung transplants at the Mayo Clinic. The median age at retransplantation was 59 years, and the median lung allocation score was 42. The most common indication for retransplantation in our cohort was BOS ($n = 15$), with secondary indications being primary graft dysfunction ($n = 3$) and other disease ($n = 4$). Of the 22 patients, 20 underwent redo double-lung transplantation. Finally, our findings were similar to those reported in the current literature, including a 3-year actuarial survival rate of 53%.

TECHNICAL ASPECTS OF REDO LUNG TRANSPLANTATION

The previous operative notes should be carefully reviewed for the surgical approach and any difficulties encountered. Posttransplantation course should also be reviewed; procedures performed to remove pleural fluid or complications that may have developed (e.g., stent placement in the bronchi) should be taken into account. The computed tomography scan and perfusion scan may indicate where potential difficulties may be encountered during reoperation.

Our own personal approach at retransplantation is to perform a standard posterolateral thoracotomy if possible rather than use an anterior approach because doing so allows better access to the hilar structures, where difficulties are anticipated. The more difficult side should be operated on first, thus allowing much of the dissection to be completed while the donor lungs are in transit and hence lessening the ischemic time for the second implanted lung. In similar fashion, if the patient has had a previous single-lung transplant and is to have a bilateral retransplant, the side requiring reoperation is worked on first. Most patients with BOS are able to tolerate single-lung ventilation. If perfusion to the lungs is similar, we tend to complete all procedures on the right lung first because doing so allows easy access for central cannulation for cardiopulmonary bypass. Another reason for operating on the right lung first is that the phrenic nerve on the right is more susceptible to damage because of its anatomic position, thus necessitating careful dissection in this area. When the left side is operated on, the femoral area is cleaned and draped in case peripheral cannulation becomes necessary. When the first transplant has been completed, the patient is turned to the opposite side and a similar posterolateral thoracotomy is performed. Should the patient need cardiopulmonary support, we would make a clamshell incision.

Because the allograft is usually adherent to the previous point of entry, excision of the rib or entry into a lower rib space may avoid adhesions; however, immunosuppressive therapy usually limits inflammatory changes at the pleural level. The costophrenic recess often contains adhesions that limit the size of the chest cavity and will need to be "freed." These adhesions do not attach to the lung and may be missed if not anticipated. Hilar dissection poses a larger challenge. Frequently, the pulmonary artery and bronchus are adherent to each other and previous use of hemostatic agents may have altered the anatomy in this area. Two techniques may be available. If any difficulties are encountered when encircling the hilar vessels, the surgeon should not hesitate to use an intrapericardial approach; on the right the pulmonary artery can be encircled between the superior vena cava and the ascending aorta. The second technique available is cardiopulmonary bypass, which may help decompress tense vessels and prevent the unmanageable bleeding that is possible during dissection.

The lung is excised after the donor lungs are in the operating room. Stents in the bronchi are easily removed once the bronchus is open. The bronchus is generally trimmed to healthy tissue, including removal of the previous suture line. The pulmonary artery is trimmed to the previous suture line (this thickened area seems stronger and tends to remain open, thereby making the anastomosis easier). Excess tissue is usually present at the pulmonary veins, and this area will need to be trimmed appropriately. Great care should be taken to achieve hemostasis before the anastomosis is started. This part of the procedure is critical because bleeding posterior to the hilum may be difficult to access after completion of the transplant. Once the anastomoses have been completed and the clamps removed, hemostasis should again be carefully obtained before the lung is inflated.

Retransplantation after single-lung transplantation

Another likely scenario is retransplantation after single-lung transplantation. Common causes of failure include overexpansion of the native lung, which then impinges on the donor lung, and chronic graft failure. Whether to replace both the native and donor lung, only the native lung, or only the donor lung is unclear. If failure was caused by infection, retransplantation of both lungs will probably be needed, in which case the perfusion scan and complexity of dissection will dictate which lung to remove first.

The reason that single-lung transplantation was initially performed should be reviewed. Was it because of previous thoracotomy, because of pleurodesis, or for some other reason? In the case of hyperexpansion of the native lung, it is the native lung that should be replaced with a transplant, and preparations for cardiopulmonary bypass are made in case oxygenation of the allograft is unsuccessful. A small review from Thailand included three single-lung retransplants. In their case of a patient with emphysema and native lung hyperexpansion, the authors chose to replace the native lung. In the other two cases they replaced the donor lung because of previous contralateral operations.[7]

Multiple strategies for retransplantation after a single-lung transplant exist. When a retransplant strategy is being chosen, two facts should be noted: first, the patients are older than at the time of the primary transplant and may now have additional comorbid conditions; second, a survival benefit exists for most patients who receive a double-lung transplant. A review of 390 cases of retransplantation included in the United Network for Organ Sharing (UNOS) data set (2005 to 2010) demonstrated variability in the surgical approach after a single-lung transplant.[8] In this series, 46 patients underwent ipsilateral retransplantation, 54 underwent contralateral retransplantation, and 70 underwent bilateral lung transplantation. Aigner's series of 46 patients exhibited a similar variety of retransplantation strategies. Both studies demonstrated the same inconsistency in retransplantation strategy (unlike the case in our own retransplantation experience), and neither looked at outcomes solely on the basis of approach. Our own personal approach is to replace both lungs with transplants if possible.

LUNG TRANSPLANTATION AFTER PREVIOUS THORACOTOMY

This report does not address patients who have undergone a lung biopsy. Because most of these procedures involve a video-assisted thoracoscopic (VATS) approach or a small open thoracotomy, the effect of lung biopsy during the operation is minimal.

Lung transplantation after lung volume reduction surgery

This situation occurs quite frequently. Lung volume reduction surgery (LVRS) for upper zone emphysema may be performed by using a median sternotomy, thoracotomy, or VATS approach. In an effort to reduce air leakage, which is the major complication associated with LVRS, virtually every center uses some form of buttressing. If the procedure is performed with a median sternotomy, the buttress strips tend to lie medially against the mediastinum; if it is performed through a VATS approach, the strips will lie against the chest wall. In some instances the surgeon will perform a pleurectomy, pleural tent, or pleurodesis in an effort to reduce air leakage.

Lung transplantation after LVRS is not considered difficult, but care should be taken during the dissection for two reasons. First, diathermy should be used with caution if high oxygen concentrations are involved because in patients with severe emphysema, freeing adhesions can lead to significant air leakage and risk of fire. Second, care should be taken during dissection in the areas of buttressing, especially close to the mediastinum, because it makes the phrenic nerve vulnerable to damage. Our approach in such situations is to leave the buttress behind. In general, the lungs are largely emphysematous and bleeding is not an issue; in fact, collapsing the lung makes the dissection easier.

The literature concerning risk is variable. According to a report from Pittsburgh, rates of postoperative bleeding requiring reexploration and renal dysfunction requiring dialysis were higher in patients with LVRS before lung transplantation. Five-year survival rates did not differ significantly (59.7% in patients with LVRS before lung transplantation versus 66.2% in patients with lung transplantation alone). In multivariate analysis, age older than 65 years, prolonged cardiopulmonary bypass time, and severe pulmonary hypertension were significant predictors of mortality ($P < .05$). The authors concluded that although LVRS remains a viable option as a bridge to lung transplantation in selected patients, unsuccessful LVRS before lung transplantation can impart substantial morbidity and compromised functional capacity after lung transplantation. LVRS should not be considered as a bridge to transplantation for all lung transplant candidates.[9]

In the largest series (from Seattle) comparing lung transplantation for chronic obstructive airway disease (COPD) after LVRS with lung transplantation alone, patients undergoing lung transplantation after LVRS had longer operative times (mean of 4.4 versus 5.6 hours; $P = .020$) and longer lengths of stay (mean of 17.6 versus 29.1 days; $P = .005$). Thirty-day mortality and major morbidity were similar. The posttransplant survival rate was reduced for transplantation after LVRS (median, 49 months; 95% confidence interval [CI], 16 to 85 months) compared with transplantation alone (median, 96 months; 95% CI, 82 to 106 months; $P = .008$). The composite benefit of the combined procedures, defined as a bridge from LVRS to transplantation of 55 months and posttransplantation survival of 49 months (total of 104 months), was comparable to that for patients who underwent either procedure alone.[10]

Lung transplantation after lobectomy

Lobectomy before lung transplantation is usually performed for inflammatory lung conditions such as cystic fibrosis or immobile cilia syndrome. Because of impaired pulmonary drainage, the lower lobes are the ones generally removed in these circumstances. The other common reason for lobectomy, namely, lung cancer, is a contraindication for transplantation. Usually, the lobectomy had been performed years beforehand because no one would consider such a resection with limited lung function. This latent period often results in a smaller chest cavity with crowded ribs and an elevated hemidiaphragm. The transplant plan typically calls for performing transplantation on the side with the lesser perfusion first, but after a lobectomy, the smaller chest cavity complicates the process. One issue is that the donor lungs need to be size-matched or downsized by wedge resection or lobectomy. Second, the issue of which side to operate on first needs to be decided. If the surgeon proceeds with transplantation on the lobectomy side, the allograft may be compressed and possibly atelectatic; if downsized, the allograft will need to cope with oxygenation while the contralateral lung is being transplanted. On the other hand, if the nonlobectomy side is chosen for transplantation first, will oxygenation of the residual lung be possible while the lung transplant is taking place? These decisions are often difficult and will be governed by specific circumstances.

The net result of the scenarios outlined is that cardiopulmonary bypass support is more likely. The easiest incision for placing a patient on cardiopulmonary bypass is the clamshell, and it is the recommended incision unless the surgeon is fairly confident that bypass will not be necessary.

The extent of adhesions resulting from the previous operation and the underlying infectious disease will vary. As part of accommodation to the previous lobectomy, the hemidiaphragm rises and the lateral aspects become adherent to the chest wall; the mediastinum shifts in a similar manner, and adhesions form between the pericardium and the anterior chest wall. Importantly, these accommodative adhesions must be freed to restore the chest cavity to a more normal larger size. Fortunately, these adhesions are easily freed by sweeping one's hands along the costophrenic recesses. The surgeon should be certain that hemostasis has been achieved before implantation of the lungs because evaluation for bleeding in the posterior aspects of a small chest cavity after the lungs have been implanted is very difficult.

Occasionally, we have not downsized lungs on the lobectomy side and have been surprised at how rapidly the chest cavity accommodates—the chest cavity enlarges and the

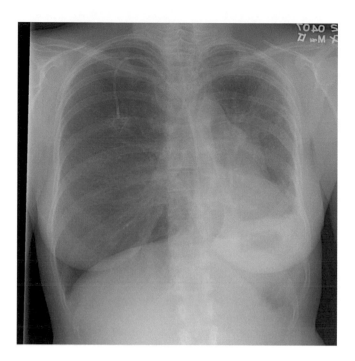

Figure 19.1 Pretransplantation chest radiograph of a patient with immobile ciliary syndrome and previous left lower lobectomy.

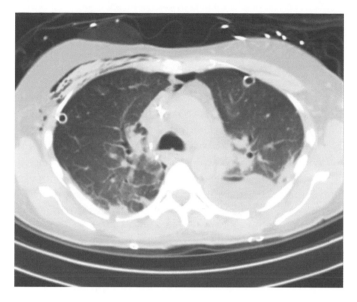

Figure 19.2 Patient with immobile ciliary syndrome and previous left lower lobectomy after bilateral double-lung transplantation. Note that the mediastinum has shifted to the center.

mediastinum shifts to a central position. The downside of this approach is that before accommodation occurs, atelectasis is more common and patients require ventilation longer, often with positive end-expiratory pressure (Figures 19.1, 19.2, and 19.3).

Lung transplantation after pneumonectomy

The reasons for previous pneumonectomy and subsequent lung transplantation are similar to those for previous lobectomy. Pneumonectomy usually follows an operation for inflammatory lung diseases. We have, however, performed the operation for adenocarcinoma in situ (that patient is still alive 10 years after a single-lung transplant). Others have reported similar experience with nine patients (two previous pneumonectomies).[11]

The main issue is obvious. Should a bilateral lung transplant or a single-lung transplant on the side remaining be performed? Both these situations have been reported previously[12-15]; however, only one bilateral lung transplantation after pneumonectomy has been reported to our knowledge.[15] The patient had a right upper lobectomy on the donor lung to cope with the smaller size of the right side of the chest.

With regard to a bilateral lung transplant after previous pneumonectomy, the operation is probably possible only after a right pneumonectomy because in the case of a left pneumonectomy, the bronchial stump will be short and difficult to access in the aortopulmonary window. One theoretical possibility for overcoming the problem of previous left pneumonectomy is a tracheal anastomosis. To our knowledge this scenario has not been reported.

The operation of single-lung transplantation after pneumonectomy is associated with significant risks. In 2009 Le Pimpec-Barthes reviewed a series of 14 cases collected from different centers in Europe.[14] The in-hospital mortality rate was 29% (4 of 14 patients) with 2 patients dying of perioperative difficulties secondary to mediastinal shift. Bronchiectasis not related to cystic fibrosis and pneumonectomy in childhood was associated with better results.[14] In this series all patients had severe mediastinal shift and two had postpneumonectomy empyema (one with a fistula), two were being supported by a ventilator, and

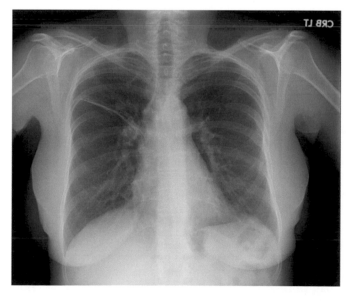

Figure 19.3 Patient with immobile ciliary syndrome and left lower lobectomy 6 years earlier after bilateral double-lung transplantation. Note that the mediastinum has shifted to the center.

postpneumonectomy syndrome was suspected in one of the latter two. All patients had pulmonary edema during the postoperative period. Sakiyalak and Vigneswaran reported a patient in whom postpneumonectomy syndrome developed after lung transplantation.[13]

On the basis of the aforementioned experience, severe mediastinal shift is a risk factor for intraoperative challenges and mortality. Cannulation for cardiopulmonary bypass is difficult and venous drainage from the femoral route is suboptimal. Postpneumonectomy syndrome caused by stretching of the anastomoses appears to be common. In our limited experience we had no complications or difficulties; however, in our patient the mediastinum was in a central position. Our recommendation for patients with severe mediastinal shift would be a clamshell incision and placement of tissue expanders within the pneumonectomy space to shift the mediastinum to a central position. This strategy will facilitate cannulation for cardiopulmonary bypass and probably reduce the incidence of postpneumonectomy syndrome.

Readers should be aware of two case reports in which a contralateral donor lung was transplanted into patients.[16,17] In one report the patient had previously undergone right pneumonectomy, and at the donor operation it was discovered that the intended single left lung could not be used.[16] The donor left lung was turned so that the posterior surface faced anteriorly. The bronchial anastomosis was made by suturing the membranous portion of the donor bronchus to the cartilaginous ring of the recipient. The pulmonary artery was mobilized so that its length made the anastomosis possible, and no problem with the venous anastomosis existed.

Lung transplantation after cardiac surgery

The issues associated with lung transplantation after cardiac surgery are related to difficulty with central cannulation for cardiopulmonary bypass, avoidance of damage to bypass grafts, and scarring around the right pulmonary veins if venting of the left ventricle or mitral valve procedures have been performed. None of these issues are insurmountable.

After previous coronary bypass grafting, a clamshell incision is not as great a concern as might be suspected. Initial limited dissection around the sternum is performed before division, and with care grafts are unlikely to be damaged. The computed tomographic coronary angiogram should be carefully perused to determine the position of bypass grafts. Care should be taken with grafts lying on the pulmonary veins.

With respect to the internal mammary artery grafts and adherence to the lungs, one approach chosen has been to staple the lung adherent to the graft and simply leave the small portion of lung adherent to the graft behind.[18] This approach lessens damage to the graft and to the phrenic nerve.

REFERENCES

1. Warnecke G, Haverich A. Lung re-transplantation: Review. Curr Opin Organ Transplant 2012;17:485-489.
2. Yusen RD, Edwards LB, Kucheryavaya AY, et al. The Registry of the International Society for Heart and Lung Transplantation: Thirty-first adult lung and heart-lung transplant report—2014; focus theme: Retransplantation. J Heart Lung Transplant 2014;33:1009-1024.
3. Strueber M, Fischer S, Gottlieb J, et al. Long-term outcome after pulmonary retransplantation. J Thorac Cardiovasc Surg 2006;132:407-412.
4. Aigner C, Jaksch P, Taghavi S, et al. Pulmonary retransplantation: Is it worth the effort? A long-term analysis of 46 cases. J Heart Lung Transplant 2008;27:60-65.
5. Novick RJ, Stitt LW, Al-Kattan K, et al. Pulmonary retransplantation: Predictors of graft function and survival in 230 patients. Pulmonary Retransplant Registry. Ann Thorac Surg 1998;65:227-234.
6. Kawut SM, Lederer DJ, Keshavjee S, et al. Outcomes after lung retransplantation in the modern era. Am J Respir Crit Care Med 2008;177:114-120.
7. Sakornpant P, Kasemsarn C, Yottasurodom C. Retransplantation after single lung transplantation. Transplant Proc 2008;40:2617-2619.
8. Kilic A, Beaty CA, Merlo CA, et al. Functional status is highly predictive of outcomes after redo lung transplantation: An analysis of 390 cases in the modern era. Ann Thorac Surg 2013;96:1804-1811; discussion 1811.
9. Shigemura N, Gilbert S, Bhama JK, et al. Lung transplantation after lung volume reduction surgery. Transplantation 2013;96:421-425.
10. Backhus L, Sargent J, Cheng A, et al. Outcomes in lung transplantation after previous lung volume reduction surgery in a contemporary cohort. J Thorac Cardiovasc Surg 2014;147:1678-1683.e1.
11. Samano MN, Waisberg DR, Villiger LE, et al. Bilateral lung transplantation in asymmetric thorax: Case reports. Transplant Proc 2008;40:872-874.
12. Zorn GL Jr, McGiffin DC, Young KR Jr, et al. Pulmonary transplantation for advanced bronchioloalveolar carcinoma. J Thorac Cardiovasc Surg 2003;125:45-48.
13. Sakiyalak P, Vigneswaran WT. Postpneumonectomy syndrome in single lung transplantation recipient following previous pneumonectomy. Ann Thorac Surg 2003;75:1023-1025.
14. Le Pimpec-Barthes F, Thomas PA, Bonnette P, et al. Single-lung transplantation in patients with previous contralateral pneumonectomy: Technical aspects and results. Eur J Cardiothorac Surg 2009;36:927-932.

15. Ris HB, Krueger T, Gonzalez M, et al. Successful bilateral lung transplantation after previous pneumonectomy. Ann Thorac Surg 2011;91:1302-1304.

16. Couetil JP, Argyriadis PG, Tolan MJ, et al. Contralateral lung transplantation: A left lung implanted in the right thorax. Ann Thorac Surg 2001;72:933-935.

17. Chen JY, Zheng MF, Jing ZH, et al. Case report: A left donor lung implanted in the recipient's right thorax for the therapy of pulmonary fibrosis. Transplant Proc 2006;38:1535-1537.

18. Halkos ME, Sherman AJ, Miller JI Jr. Preservation of the lima pedicle after cardiac surgery in left upper lobectomy. Ann Thorac Surg 2003;76:280-281.

20

Lung transplantation for idiopathic pulmonary fibrosis

JOSHUA C. GRIMM, LEANN L. SILHAN, AND ASHISH S. SHAH

INTRODUCTION

Idiopathic pulmonary fibrosis (IPF) is a diffuse parenchymal disease that results in oxygen dependence, severe disability, and ultimately death, with a median survival time of 3 to 5 years after diagnosis. Although several pharmacologic avenues are available to slow the progression of this aggressive disease, lung transplantation (LTx) remains the only option to improve survival and quality of life because failure in medical management is exceedingly common.[1] Preoperative optimization is paramount to maximize patient benefit following surgery and requires the concerted efforts of both medical and surgical staff. This chapter outlines the basic pathophysiology of IPF, the surgical considerations required when approaching this disease, and the expected short- and long-term outcomes following LTx.

NATURAL HISTORY AND DIAGNOSIS

IPF is the most common type of interstitial lung disease (ILD), with histology findings consistent with usual interstitial pneumonia (UIP). It results in chronic and progressive destruction of the lung parenchyma and, ultimately, in death from respiratory failure in nearly 40% of patients.[2,3] During the final stages of the disease process, pulmonary hypertension and concomitant right heart failure (cor pulmonale) result in hypoxemia refractory to oxygen therapy, which can complicate medical management aimed at aggressive diuresis because the dysfunctional right ventricle will become progressively preload dependent.

The incidence of IPF has been estimated at 7 to 16 per 100,000, and it increases with advancing age.[4,5] Its insidious onset can therefore be confused with an age-related decline in pulmonary function. Most cases are sporadic and manifested clinically as progressive exertional dyspnea and, often, a nonproductive cough. Other more subtle physical examination findings include fine bibasilar crackles and finger clubbing in approximately 50% of patients.[6] Because many other lung conditions share a similar symptom profile, accurate diagnosis is paramount in formulating a focused treatment strategy. IPF accounts for 20% to 50% of all interstitial lung disease (ILD).[6,7] Other types of ILD are treated differently and generally have a better prognosis, which makes establishing the correct diagnosis necessary for therapeutic and prognostic planning.

The procedure for evaluating presumed IPF was recently outlined in the American Thoracic Society's 2013 consensus statement, which redefined the findings on high-resolution computed tomography (CT) scan (UIP, possible UIP, and inconsistent with UIP) and lung biopsy (UIP, possible UIP, probable UIP, and not UIP) to reflect their association with a correct diagnosis.[2] First, other identifiable causes of lung disease, such as connective tissue disease or hypersensitivity pneumonitis, should be excluded because they can have a pattern consistent with UIP. In patients with radio-graphic findings typical of IPF (subpleural, basilar predominant reticulation, honeycombing, and bronchiectasis with an absence of features inconsistent with a UIP pattern), a definitive lung biopsy is unnecessary. This statement was substantiated by a study demonstrating that the ability of experts to confidently and accurately diagnose IPF from a combination of CT and clinical findings was approximately 80% (confirmed by subsequent parenchymal biopsy).[8]

However, in patients with atypical radiographic findings, surgical lung biopsy is an option to help make a definitive diagnosis, and it may be pursued in select cases. A mini-thoracotomy or a video-assisted approach is used to harvest biopsy samples from various segments of the affected lung. Bronchoscopy with transbronchial biopsy may be adequate for diagnosis of some forms of ILD such as hypersensitivity pneumonitis, sarcoidosis, or organizing pneumonia; however, it is almost always inadequate for the diagnosis of other types of ILD, including IPF or nonspecific interstitial pneumonia. Histologic examination of tissue from patients with IPF demonstrates patchy subpleural fibrosis with "honeycombing degeneration" adjacent to normal-appearing lung tissue.[9]

The typical physiologic changes associated with progression of IPF are reductions in compliance, diffusion capacity for carbon monoxide (D_{LCO}), forced vital capacity (FVC), and total lung capacity on pulmonary function testing. Because the disease is fibrotic, diminished compliance results in a relatively normal ratio of forced expiratory volume in the first second of respiration to FVC (FEV_1/FVC). This pattern holds true except in cases involving a concomitant obstructive process such as in combined pulmonary fibrosis and emphysema, in which case the ratio may be decreased in response to both a restrictive and obstructive pattern. Combined pulmonary fibrosis and emphysema may also lead to a deceptive preservation of vital capacity with a severe reduction in diffusion capacity. Response to therapy can be evaluated on the basis of serial measurements, and the decision to proceed to transplantation can be considered.[10]

INDICATIONS FOR TRANSPLANTATION AND BRIDGING STRATEGIES

Patients in whom IPF has been diagnosed have the highest relative waiting list mortality and, accordingly, should be promptly referred to a transplant center for evaluation, perhaps even before all available medical options have been exhausted.[11] As a result of implementation of the current lung allocation score (LAS) model, which assigns priority to patients with a greater degree of debility, the percentage of cases with IPF as the indication for LTx rose from 15% in 2000 to 37% in 2009 (Figure 20.1).

Indications for transplantation

Accordingly, patient selection is crucial to ensure acceptable outcomes. Current guidelines for LTx in patients with IPF

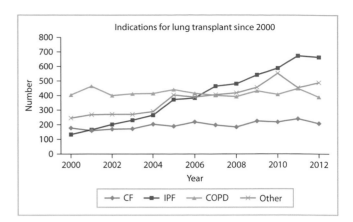

Figure 20.1 Indications for lung transplantation since 2000. Note the increase in lung transplantation for a diagnosis of IPF during the past decade. Based on the United Network for Organ Sharing Standard Transplant Analysis and Research Files through August 2013. CF, cystic fibrosis; COPD, chronic obstructive pulmonary disease; IPF, idiopathic pulmonary fibrosis.

include confirmation of the diagnosis and any of the following clinical findings:

- D_{LCO} less than 39% of the predicted value.
- A decrease in FVC greater than 10% over a 6-month period.
- A decrease in pulse oximetry below 88% during the 6-minute walk test.
- Findings of advanced disease (honeycombing) on high-resolution CT scan.[12,13]

Delaying referral for LTx until the aforementioned criteria have been satisfied has inherent disadvantages. Although earlier studies demonstrated worse outcomes in patients experiencing a decline in pulmonary function, more recent data have shown similarly poor outcomes in individuals with relatively normal function.[13] Therefore, predicting which patients will benefit most from LTx is complicated. Although LTx offers results superior to those of medical management alone, several strict contraindications to transplantation exist, including the following:

- Malignancy in the 2 preceding years (with the exception of some forms of cutaneous neoplasm).
- Active extrapulmonary infection, such as human immunodeficiency syndrome or untreated hepatitis C.
- Severe dysfunction of extrapulmonary organ systems (heart-lung transplantation should be considered in individuals with coronary disease not amenable to revascularization or intervention or in those with substantial left ventricular dysfunction).
- Chest deformity limiting surgical exposure.
- Untreatable psychiatric condition and lack of a reliable social network.
- Documented medical nonadherence.
- Active substance abuse within the preceding 6 months.

Mechanical ventilation and extracorporeal membrane oxygenation

Several important adjuncts must be considered before performing LTx in patients with a deteriorating clinical course. Most patients with end-stage IPF require home supplemental oxygen to maintain their baseline level of function. In cases of acute decompensation, more aggressive measures are often necessary. Several studies have examined the use of mechanical ventilation and rescue extracorporeal membrane oxygenation (ECMO) support in this setting.[14,15]

ECMO in the form of venoarterial or venovenous cannulation (depending on the presence of concomitant cardiac dysfunction or severe pulmonary hypertension) can be used to support potential LTx candidates until an appropriate donor is identified.[16,17] Small institutional studies have demonstrated inferior short-term survival in patients who are bridged to LTx with ECMO.[17] Bridged patients who survive for 1 year can experience acceptable long-term survival; therefore, patient selection is paramount to reduce perioperative mortality and ensure more favorable results.[16,18] Differentiating between fulminant respiratory failure and an acute but transient exacerbation may be important in understanding this phenomenon. Although the latter might respond favorably to a short period of ECMO as a means of regaining baseline function or while awaiting an organ, the former most likely constitutes a different clinical entity. That successful bridging strategies should incorporate intense physical rehabilitation while patients are receiving advanced mechanical support is becoming increasingly clear.[19]

Mechanical ventilation before LTx appears to confer a survival disadvantage in patients with end-stage IPF.[14] As when ECMO is used, determining the reason for ventilatory support is crucial because it might predict patients' probability of recovery before or following transplantation. In critically ill patients who have a high LAS and are already on the waiting list for an organ, however, mechanical ventilation should not necessarily preclude transplantation.

Bridging patients with IPF to LTx is a legitimate, albeit labor-intensive and high-risk strategy. Currently, ECMO-supported patients are given high priority for organs in the United States. Future studies will better clarify effective management during the bridging period, as well as the patient-specific factors associated with acceptable outcomes.

GRAFT CONSIDERATIONS

Single-lung versus bilateral lung transplantation

The decision to perform single LTx versus bilateral LTx in a patient with IPF remains controversial. An early longitudinal study with good long-term follow-up demonstrated no functional (as measured by the 6-minute walk distance or FEV$_1$) or survival advantage following double LTx.[20] In fact, a large review of the United Network for Organ Sharing (UNOS) database found that patients older than 60 years with a primary diagnosis of IPF should undergo single LTx. It was postulated that the higher perioperative mortality associated with bilateral LTx was related to technical complexity and prolonged graft ischemia.[21]

More recently, however, the trend has been toward bilateral LTx.[22] This practice has been supported by both single-institution and large database studies, which have identified single LTx as an independent predictor of mortality in patients with IPF.[23,24] Moreover, this benefit appears to be further amplified in critically ill patients with a higher mean LAS.[25] A single-institution experience suggested that rates of bronchiolitis obliterans syndrome (BOS) are lower in patients who undergo bilateral LTx.[26] Other data have demonstrated that if BOS does ultimately develop, its course is shorter and milder after double LTx than after single LTx.[27]

However, patients with IPF who are listed for bilateral LTx have longer wait times. Thus, some centers have actually favored single LTx to minimize death or disease progression while patients are on the waiting list.[28] Our current institutional practice has evolved to using single or double LTx as organs become available, even in the setting of pulmonary hypertension.

Size matching

Graft selection based on donor-to-recipient size matching is an important consideration in LTx.[29] Because patients with IPF have significantly reduced thoracic volume, finding appropriately sized donors can be challenging. Several methods for determining acceptable donor size exist.[30] Given the restraints of the thoracic cavity, optimal donor and recipient size matching is more relevant to bilateral LTx than to single LTx. The consequences of an oversized donor can be catastrophic. However, several surgical techniques, such as aggressive lung reduction and lobar transplantation, allow utilization of nearly all donor organs despite size mismatches. Using smaller donors may also create a long-term problem. Donor and recipient matches resulting in a higher predicted total lung capacity (pTLC) ratio (i.e., the donor's pTLC divided by the recipient's pTLC) appears to be associated with improved survival.[29] After stratification for single and bilateral LTx, it appears that the benefit is most notable in patients who have undergone bilateral LTx.[29]

INTRAOPERATIVE STRATEGIES

Bilateral sequential lung transplantation

After induction of anesthesia the patient is intubated with a double-lumen endotracheal tube when possible. Femoral and radial arterial lines are commonly used for monitoring blood pressure, as well as for providing access in case balloon pump placement or ECMO cannulation proves necessary. Access to the thoracic cavity is obtained via bilateral anterolateral thoracotomies through the fourth or

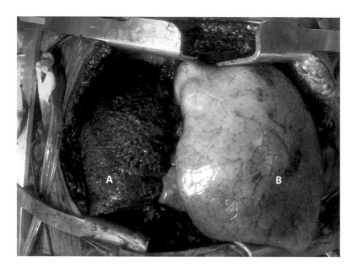

Figure 20.2 Double-lung transplantation. Photo demonstrates the native lung (**A**) and the first transplanted lung (**B**).

fifth intercostal space across the sternum. Alternatives to this "clamshell" approach are median sternotomy, bilateral posterolateral thoracotomy, and sternum-sparing bilateral anterolateral thoracotomy. After the retrosternal mediastinal adhesions have been cleared, the inferior and superior pulmonary veins and the pulmonary artery are isolated. Once the donor lungs have arrived in the operating room, the more poorly perfused lung (based on the preoperative ventilation-perfusion scan) is removed from the thoracic cavity.

The recipient's pulmonary vessels are dissected into the pericardium to simplify the anastomoses. First, the airway is sewn in continuous or interrupted fashion by using either a telescoping or end-to-end technique. The pulmonary artery is anastomosed first, followed by the pulmonary veins. The graft is then inflated with room air and allowed to reperfuse slowly over a period of 10 to 15 minutes (Figure 20.2). The other lung is then approached in an identical fashion. In patients with IPF, however, the left-sided dissection can be more challenging because of the orientation of the heart. To improve exposure and minimize cardiac instability, the pericardium can be fully incised to the right and the left ventricle medially displaced. Maintaining cardiovascular stability might necessitate proceeding with the left lung first or using central cardiopulmonary bypass (CPB) or ECMO. After both lungs have been reperfused and the patient has been stabilized, chest tubes are inserted and the incision is closed in layers. A final bronchoscopy can confirm the integrity of the anastomosis and identify any airway obstruction or lobar torsion, if present.

Cardiopulmonary bypass

Although CPB is not required during LTx, it may be essential in patients who experience hemodynamic instability or refractory hypoxemia following single-lung isolation. Pulmonary hypertension, which is common in patients

with IPF, is a major risk factor for CPB.[31] Some programs use CPB in all bilateral LTx procedures as standard practice. Occasionally, CPB or ECMO will be necessary for single LTx as well. The cannulation strategy should be determined before surgery. Our institutional practice is to use a blood prime and central cannulation with CPB. We also perform modified ultrafiltration after implantation. Although CPB has been associated with an increased risk for bleeding and primary graft dysfunction (PGD), our rates of the latter remain lower than 10%.

Concomitant procedures

Recent studies have demonstrated that patients requiring cardiac surgery at the time of LTx experience morbidity and mortality equivalent to that of patients not requiring cardiac surgery.[32] These concomitant procedures usually necessitate CPB, although off-pump coronary artery bypass grafting can easily be performed. If patients require extensive cardiac reconstruction, some consideration should be given to en bloc heart-lung transplantation.

POSTOPERATIVE CONSIDERATIONS

Perioperative management

Postoperative management of patients after LTx entails balancing allograft protection and global perfusion. Transplanted lungs are susceptible to early tissue edema and injury resulting in decreased compliance. Strategies to avoid progression of this process include maintenance of low central venous pressure and aggressive diuresis during the immediate perioperative period, with hemodynamic support provided by vasopressive agents. At our institution, mechanical ventilation is performed by using a pressure control mode with a positive end-expiratory pressure of 8 cm H_2O and target tidal volume of 8 mL/kg. These parameters may vary depending on the size of the donor and chest wall compliance. Additionally, the fraction of inspired oxygen (FIO_2) is minimized, and we use inhaled nitric oxide liberally. We routinely maintain patients on room air as tolerated and believe that it decreases the development of PGD.

Hemodynamic stability is maintained principally with epinephrine and judicious fluid administration. Once the patient is stable, an epidural catheter is inserted for pain control and the patient is weaned from the ventilator. With good allograft function most patients can be quickly switched to minimal settings (pressure support of 5 cm H_2O and positive end-expiratory pressure of 5 cm H_2O). Patients with IPF frequently have poor chest wall mechanics and may require an additional 24 to 48 hours to be successfully extubated. Toilet bronchoscopy is routinely performed before removal of the endotracheal tube. In patients who require prolonged ventilation, we perform early tracheostomy. Given the degree of pharyngeal dysfunction after LTx, all patients undergo a video fluoroscopic swallow study before the initiation of oral feeding.[33] Early mobilization, nutrition, and renal protection are critical in avoiding perioperative complications and death after transplantation.

Complications

Postoperative infection is the most common complication following LTx, and it is associated with significant morbidity and mortality.[34] Sepsis, which occurs in 15.2% of patients with IPF, accounts for 60% of the 6-month mortality.[35]

Acute rejection is another common complication; approximately 36% of all patients who undergo LTx have at least one episode within the first year after transplantation.[36] The vast majority of these cases have a cellular cause and require transbronchial biopsy for confirmation. Treatment for humoral rejection includes high-dose steroids, plasmapheresis, anti-CD20 antibody (rituximab), and intravenous immunoglobulin G. Repeated episodes of acute rejection have been demonstrated to possibly increase the risk for the development of BOS, which affects up to 74% of all patients within 10 years after LTx.[36]

Unfortunately, BOS is a major determinant of long-term outcomes, and patients with IPF seem to have a predisposition for its development. The reason for this relationship may be its association with PGD, which, occurs in 10% to 25% of all transplant recipients.[37-39]

Long-term outcomes

Patients undergoing LTx for IPF have worse survival than do patients with most other types of end-stage lung disease (Figure 20.3). The reason for this difference has not been fully elucidated; however, several aspects of the disease process appear to negatively influence postoperative mortality. Patients with IPF tend to be older and have a greater

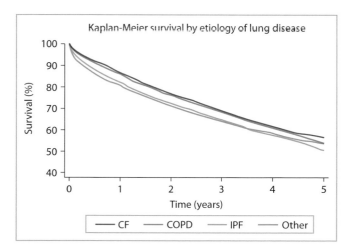

Figure 20.3 Kaplan-Meier 5-year survival by cause of lung disease. Note that IPF has the lowest survival when compared with the other indications for lung transplantation. Based on United Network for Organ Sharing Standard Transplant Analysis and Research Files through August 2013. CF, cystic fibrosis; COPD, chronic obstructive pulmonary disease; IPF, idiopathic pulmonary fibrosis.

incidence of several comorbid conditions such as obesity, hypertension, and hyperlipidemia. Permanent alterations in chest wall physiology result in deterioration of pulmonary mechanics, even after LTx. Furthermore, IPF represents a progressive process with an unremitting course. This process is evident following single LTx, after which the native lung suffers further pulmonary decline in the face of a contralateral transplant.[40,41] The native lung is also at increased risk for malignancy and infections.

CONCLUSION

LTx for IPF offers patients a viable option for better quality of life and survival than can be achieved by medical management alone. Patients with known IPF should be referred to a transplant center early in the disease process to optimize their medical condition and undergo an evaluation for LTx. Patients with IPF present unique and complex challenges in both the preoperative and postoperative settings. Fibrotic lung disease is an increasingly common indication for transplantation, and additional efforts to improve outcomes are needed.

REFERENCES

1. Elicker BM, Golden JA, Ordovas KG, et al. Progression of native lung fibrosis in lung transplant recipients with idiopathic pulmonary fibrosis. Respir Med 2010;104:426-433.
2. Raghu G, Collard HR, Egan JJ, et al. An official ATS/ERS/JRS/ALAT statement: Idiopathic pulmonary fibrosis: Evidence-based guidelines for diagnosis and management. Am J Respir Crit Care Med 2011;183:788-824.
3. Navaratnam V, Fleming KM, West J, et al. The rising incidence of idiopathic pulmonary fibrosis in the U.K. Thorax 2011;66:462-467.
4. Fernandez Perez ER, Daniels CE, Schroeder DR, et al. Incidence, prevalence, and clinical course of idiopathic pulmonary fibrosis: A population-based study. Chest 2010;137:129-137.
5. Raghu G, Weycker D, Edelsberg J, et al. Incidence and prevalence of idiopathic pulmonary fibrosis. Am J Respir Crit Care Med 2006;174:810-816.
6. Nalysnyk L, Cid-Ruzafa J, Rotella P, Esser D. Incidence and prevalence of idiopathic pulmonary fibrosis: Review of the literature. Eur Respir Rev 2012;21:355-361.
7. Coultas DB, Zumwalt RE, Black WC, Sobonya RE. The epidemiology of interstitial lung diseases. Am J Respir Crit Care Med 1994;150:967-972.
8. American Thoracic Society/European Respiratory Society International Multidisciplinary Consensus Classification of the Idiopathic Interstitial Pneumonias. This joint statement of the American Thoracic Society (ATS), and the European Respiratory Society (ERS) was adopted by the ATS

board of directors, June 2001, and by the ERS Executive Committee, June 2001. Am J Respir Crit Care Med 2002;65:277-304.

9. Cool CD, Groshong SD, Rai PR, et al. Fibroblast foci are not discrete sites of lung injury or repair: The fibroblast reticulum. Am J Respir Crit Care Med 2006;174:654-658.

10. Crystal RG, Fulmer JD, Roberts WC, et al. Idiopathic pulmonary fibrosis. Clinical, histologic, radiographic, physiologic, scintigraphic, cytologic, and biochemical aspects. Ann Intern Med 1976;85:769-788.

11. Steinman TI, Becker BN, Frost AE, et al. Guidelines for the referral and management of patients eligible for solid organ transplantation. Transplantation 2001;71:1189-1204.

12. Flaherty KR, Travis WD, Colby TV, et al. Histopathologic variability in usual and nonspecific interstitial pneumonias. Am J Respir Crit Care Med 2001;164:1722-1727.

13. Orens JB, Estenne M, Arcasoy S, et al. International guidelines for the selection of lung transplant candidates: 2006 update—a consensus report from the Pulmonary Scientific Council of the International Society for Heart and Lung Transplantation. J Heart Lung Transplant 2006;25:745-755.

14. Stern JB, Mal H, Groussard O, et al. Prognosis of patients with advanced idiopathic pulmonary fibrosis requiring mechanical ventilation for acute respiratory failure. Chest 2001;120:213-219.

15. Kim DS, Park JH, Park BK, et al. Acute exacerbation of idiopathic pulmonary fibrosis: Frequency and clinical features. Eur Respir J 2006;27:143-150.

16. Javidfar J, Brodie D, Iribarne A, et al. Extracorporeal membrane oxygenation as a bridge to lung transplantation and recovery. J Thorac Cardiovasc Surg 2012;144:716-721.

17. Bittner HB, Lehmann S, Rastan A, et al. Outcome of extracorporeal membrane oxygenation as a bridge to lung transplantation and graft recovery. Ann Thorac Surg 2012;94:942-949; author reply 949-950.

18. Camboni D, Philipp A, Lubnow M, et al. Support time–dependent outcome analysis for veno-venous extracorporeal membrane oxygenation. Eur J Cardiothorac Surg 2011;40:1341-1346; discussion 1346-1347.

19. Hoopes CW, Kukreja J, Golden J, et al. Extracorporeal membrane oxygenation as a bridge to pulmonary transplantation. J Thorac Cardiovasc Surg 2013;145:862-867; discussion 867-868.

20. Meyers BF, Lynch JP, Trulock EP, et al. Single versus bilateral lung transplantation for idiopathic pulmonary fibrosis: A ten-year institutional experience. J Thorac Cardiovasc Surg 2000;120:99-107.

21. Meyer DM, Edwards LB, Torres F, et al. Impact of recipient age and procedure type on survival after lung transplantation for pulmonary fibrosis. Ann Thorac Surg 2005;79:950-957; discussion 957-958.

22. Taylor DO, Edwards LB, Boucek MM, et al. Registry of the International Society for Heart and Lung Transplantation: Twenty-second official adult heart transplant report—2005. J Heart Lung Transplant 2005;24:945-955.

23. Weiss ES, Allen JG, Merlo CA, et al. Survival after single versus bilateral lung transplantation for high-risk patients with pulmonary fibrosis. Ann Thorac Surg 2009;88:1616-1625; discussion 1625-1626.

24. Mason DP, Brizzio ME, Alster JM, et al. Lung transplantation for idiopathic pulmonary fibrosis. Ann Thorac Surg 2007;84:1121-1128.

25. Russo MJ, Iribarne A, Hong KN, et al. High lung allocation score is associated with increased morbidity and mortality following transplantation. Chest 2010;137:651-657.

26. Neurohr C, Huppmann P, Thum D, et al. Potential functional and survival benefit of double over single lung transplantation for selected patients with idiopathic pulmonary fibrosis. Transpl Int 2010;23:887-896.

27. Lama VN, Murray S, Lonigro RJ, et al. Course of FEV(1) after onset of bronchiolitis obliterans syndrome in lung transplant recipients. Am J Respir Crit Care Med 2007;175:1192-1198.

28. Nathan SD, Shlobin OA, Ahmad S, et al. Comparison of wait times and mortality for idiopathic pulmonary fibrosis patients listed for single or bilateral lung transplantation. J Heart Lung Transplant 2010;29:1165-1171.

29. Eberlein M, Reed RM, Bolukbas S, et al. Lung size mismatch and survival after single and bilateral lung transplantation. Ann Thorac Surg 2013;96:457-463.

30. Mason DP, Batizy LH, Wu J, et al. Matching donor to recipient in lung transplantation: How much does size matter? J Thorac Cardiovasc Surg 2009;137:1234-1240.

31. Fang A, Studer S, Kawut SM, et al. Elevated pulmonary artery pressure is a risk factor for primary graft dysfunction following lung transplantation for idiopathic pulmonary fibrosis. Chest 2011;139:782-787.

32. Parekh K, Meyers BF, Patterson GA, et al. Outcome of lung transplantation for patients requiring concomitant cardiac surgery. J Thorac Cardiovasc Surg 2005;130:859-863.

33. Atkins BZ, Petersen RP, Daneshmand MA, et al. Impact of oropharyngeal dysphagia on long-term outcomes of lung transplantation. Ann Thorac Surg 2010;90:1622-1628.

34. Vicente R, Morales P, Ramos F, et al. Perioperative complications of lung transplantation in patients with emphysema and fibrosis: Experience from 1992-2002. Transplant Proc 2006;38:2560-2562.

35. de Perrot M, Chaparro C, McRae K, et al. Twenty-year experience of lung transplantation at a single center: Influence of recipient diagnosis on long-term survival. J Thorac Cardiovasc Surg 2004;127:1493-1501.

36. Christie JD, Edwards LB, Aurora P, et al. The Registry of the International Society for Heart and Lung Transplantation: Twenty-sixth official adult lung and heart-lung transplantation report—2009. J Heart Lung Transplant 2009;28:1031-1049.

37. Barr ML, Kawut SM, Whelan TP, et al. Report of the ISHLT Working Group on Primary Lung Graft Dysfunction part IV: Recipient-related risk factors and markers. J Heart Lung Transplant 2005;24:1468-1482.

38. Lee JC, Christie JD, Keshavjee S. Primary graft dysfunction: Definition, risk factors, short- and long-term outcomes. Semin Respir Crit Care Med 2010;31:161-171.

39. Diamond JM, Lee JC, Kawut SM, et al. Clinical risk factors for primary graft dysfunction after lung transplantation. Am J Respir Crit Care Med 2013;187:527-534.

40. Lok SS, Smith E, Doran HM, et al. Idiopathic pulmonary fibrosis and cyclosporine: A lesson from single-lung transplantation. Chest 1998;114:1478-1481.

41. Wahidi MM, Ravenel J, Palmer SM, McAdams HP. Progression of idiopathic pulmonary fibrosis in native lungs after single lung transplantation. Chest 2002;121:2072-2076.

Lung transplantation for emphysema and α_1-antitrypsin deficiency

WALTER WEDER AND ILHAN INCI

INTRODUCTION

Chronic obstructive pulmonary disease (COPD), including emphysema, is the most common indication for lung transplantation in adults.[1] Together, COPD and α_1-antitrypsin deficiency (α_1-ATD) account for 40% of all lung transplants performed worldwide.[1] Although more than 14,000 lung transplants were performed through June 2012, questions regarding the appropriate timing of the procedure in the natural progression of emphysema, the type of procedure that should be used, and the quality of life afterward still exist.[1,2]

HISTORICAL ASPECTS

The first lung transplant for emphysema was performed in 1972; it did not provide long-term survival.[3] The single-lung transplants that were performed thereafter were complicated by hyperinflation of the native lung, anastomotic problems, rejection, and infection.[3-5]

The introduction of cyclosporine as an effective immunosuppressive agent encouraged the transplantation community to perform transplants. In 1988, on the basis of their extensive research in the field of transplantation, Patterson and associates from Toronto General Hospital performed the first en bloc bilateral lung transplant in a patient with emphysema and α_1-ATD.[6] The group subsequently reported on its six successful transplantation cases.[7]

Single-lung transplantation (SLT), which was thought to create complications resulting from native lung hyperinflation, was also reported as being successful.[8,9] In 1990, Pasque and colleagues from Washington University in St. Louis reported the technical details of bilateral sequential lung transplantation, which supplanted the en bloc procedure.[10]

RECIPIENT SELECTION

The primary aim of lung transplantation is to provide a survival benefit and improved quality of life. Lung transplantation is indicated for patients who have end-stage lung disease and for whom maximal medical therapy is failing or no effective medical therapy exists.[11]

Two of the main challenges remaining in lung transplantation are recipient selection and timing of lung transplantation to ensure maximal benefit to the recipient, as well as appropriate allocation of scarce organs.[3] Although most centers apply the widely accepted guidelines reported by the International Society for Heart and Lung Transplantation (ISHLT), individual center differences do exist.[3,11,12]

Because long-term survival is possible for most patients with emphysema, deciding which patient should be listed for a lung transplant could be difficult.[3] Lung transplantation is a major surgery, and like other types of major surgery it is not free of complications or mortality. For this reason, choosing a recipient whose expected survival is at least comparable to that without surgery is extremely important.[3] In the recent ISHLT registry data, the conditional median survival time for patients surviving to 1 year was 6.9 years for patients with emphysema and 8.7 years for patients with α_1-ATD.[1] Studies from Vestbo and associates and Nishimura and colleagues have shown minimal decline in lung function for up to 5 years.[13,14]

Forced expiratory volume in the first second of respiration (FEV_1) has often been reported to be an established prognostic indicator for survival of patients with emphysema.[3] However, different 2-year survival rates, ranging from 44% to 90%, have been reported in patients with an FEV_1 less than 30% predicted.[3,15-18] In addition, for patients with α_1-ATD, Seersholm and colleagues reported a 2-year survival rate of 50% when FEV_1 is 15% predicted.[19] However, severity of airway obstruction is not the only factor that affects the natural progression of emphysema. The other factors are patient age, hypoxemia, hypercapnia, pulmonary hypertension, low body mass index (BMI), poor exercise capacity, magnitude of dyspnea, and severity of emphysema.[2,3,13,20,21]

Unfortunately, these factors have limited weight in defining a patient's prognosis. To overcome this limitation, Celli and colleagues assembled some of these factors into a multidimensional scoring system to predict survival in patients with emphysema.[22] They named it the BODE index, and they included the following four factors that might predict an increased risk for death in patients with emphysema: BMI (B), airflow obstruction measured by FEV_1 (O), dyspnea score (D), and exercise capacity measured by the 6-minute walk test (6MWT) (E).[22] BODE index scores range from 0 to 10, with a higher score indicating a higher risk for death.[2,22] As an example, patients with a BODE score between 7 and 10 (the highest quartile) had a risk for death of 50% at 3 years and 80% at 4 years.[22] Because the survival rate of patients in this quartile is lower than that after lung transplantation, patients in this subgroup should be considered for transplantation.[3] In patients in the less severe BODE quartiles, waiting might be more appropriate unless other mitigating factors not accounted for in the index (e.g., pulmonary hypertension) are present.[3] Martinez and coworkers found that an increase in BODE index greater than 1 point over a 6- to 24-month period was associated with a doubling of the risk for death.[23] The recent ISHLT guidelines (published in 2006) include the BODE score as a criterion when listing patients for transplantation because of emphysema.[11] Patients with a BODE score higher than 5 are recommended for referral.[11,22] ISHLT guidelines recommend listing patients with a BODE score of 7 to 10 or at least one of the following: (1) history of hospitalization for exacerbation associated with acute hypercapnia (Pco_2 >50 mm Hg), (2) pulmonary hypertension or cor pulmonale despite oxygen therapy, or (3) FEV_1 less than 20% and either a diffusing capacity for carbon monoxide (D_{LCO}) less than 20% or a homogeneous distribution of emphysema.[11]

Early referral for patients who do not meet the aforementioned criteria is also recommended because it might allow the transplant team to identify and address factors that could compromise the patients' future candidacy, such as ongoing smoking, extremes of weight, poor functional status, severe osteoporosis, excessive corticosteroid use, and coronary artery disease.[2]

Lung transplantation is a complex treatment option with a significant risk for perioperative morbidity and mortality. The ISHLT guidelines regarding absolute contraindications are as follows[11]: malignancy in the last 2 years, with the exception of cutaneous squamous and basal cell tumors; untreatable advanced dysfunction of another major organ (e.g., heart, liver, or kidney); incurable chronic extrapulmonary infection, including chronic active hepatitis B virus, hepatitis C virus, and human immunodeficiency virus; significant chest wall or spinal deformity; documented nonadherence to or inability to follow through with medical therapy, office follow-up, or both; untreatable psychiatric or psychological condition associated with an inability to cooperate or comply with medical therapy; absence of a consistent or reliable social support system; and substance (e.g., alcohol, tobacco, or narcotic) addiction that is either active or has occurred within the last 6 months.

The widely accepted relative contraindications reported by ISHLT are as follows[11]: age older than 65 years (older patients have less optimal survival[1] that is most likely associated with comorbid conditions; hence, recipient age should be a factor in candidate selection); critical or unstable clinical condition (e.g., shock, mechanical ventilation, or extracorporeal membrane oxygenation [ECMO]); severely limited functional status with poor rehabilitation potential; colonization with highly resistant or highly virulent bacteria, fungi, or mycobacteria; severe obesity defined as a BMI exceeding 30 kg/m^2; severe or symptomatic osteoporosis[24]; and mechanical ventilation. Transplantation may be successful in carefully selected candidates without other acute or chronic organ dysfunction who are being supported by mechanical ventilation and are able to actively participate in a meaningful rehabilitation program. Other medical conditions that have not resulted in end-stage organ damage, such as diabetes mellitus, systemic hypertension, peptic ulcer disease, or gastroesophageal reflux, should be optimally treated before transplantation. Patients with coronary artery disease may undergo percutaneous intervention before transplantation or coronary artery bypass grafting concurrent with the transplantation procedure.[25]

ECMO AND OTHER ARTIFICIAL LUNG DEVICES AS A BRIDGE TO LUNG TRANSPLANTATION

In many patients with end-stage lung disease, refractory hypercapnia or hypoxemia will develop despite maximal ventilatory support; therefore, extracorporeal life support is their only chance to survive until a compatible donor lung becomes available.[26] In the last decade, improvements in lung transplantation outcomes and patient selection, better understanding of ventilator-associated lung injury, and improvements in artificial lung device technologies have made it possible to bridge these sick patients to a successful lung transplant.[26,27] Despite limited experience, ECMO is no longer a contraindication to lung transplantation: the 1- and 2-year survival rates of patients who have been bridged to transplantation with ECMO are comparable to those of patients who underwent lung transplantation without pre-operative support.[27-29]

LUNG VOLUME REDUCTION SURGERY AS A BRIDGE TO LUNG TRANSPLANTATION

Lung volume reduction surgery (LVRS) is a successful pal-liative surgical therapy for carefully selected patients with advanced emphysema.[30] Although experience with LVRS has increased over the last few years, selection of patients for LVRS is still a matter of controversy when the distribution of emphysema is not heterogeneous, and selection processes differ widely between centers.[31-35] On the basis of early work from Brantigan[36] and a review by Cooper and colleagues,[37] the recommendation regarding LVRS is that it be performed as a nonanatomic resection of the most severely destroyed, functionless tissue to reduce lung volume by 20% to 30%. During the 1990s, this author and others began offering LVRS by video-assisted thoracoscopic surgery as a suitable procedure.

LVRS significantly improves lung function and quality of life, with the best results seen 3 to 6 months postopera-tively. The National Emphysema Treatment Trial (NETT) group found greater improvement in function in the cohort treated with LVRS than in the group that received medical therapy, especially when LVRS was performed in patients with predominantly upper lobe emphysema and a rela-tively good baseline exercise capacity versus in those with non–upper lobe emphysema and a low baseline exercise capacity.[38-40]

Our group has observed relevant symptomatic and func-tional improvements in both heterogeneous and homoge-neous emphysema. The maximal values were observed 3 to 6 months after the operation, with a subsequent decline toward preoperative levels in subsequent years.[41] FEV_1 increased from 27% to 45% predicted in the group with het-erogeneous emphysema and from 27% to 35% in the group with homogeneous emphysema and remained significantly improved for up to 3 years and 2 years, respectively. Total lung capacity (TLC) decreased from 7.77 ($\pm$1.5) L to 7.14 ($\pm$1.4) L and residual volume (RV) decreased from 5.31 ($\pm$1.3) L to 4.15 ($\pm$1.07) L at 3 months after LVRS ($P < .001$), thus resulting in a reduction in the RV/TLC ratio from 0.68 ($\pm$0.07) to 0.58 ($\pm$0.08) ($P < .001$) in the group with homo-geneous emphysema and from 0.67 ($\pm$0.09) to 0.52 ($\pm$0.11) ($P < .001$) in the group with heterogeneous emphysema.[42] A recent study from the authors' clinic demonstrated that in selected patients with end-stage emphysema who are poten-tial candidates for lung transplantation, LVRS could allevi-ate symptoms and improve lung function and quality of life to a degree allowing postponement of transplantation for up

to 4 to 5 years. Additionally, primary LVRS had no adverse impact on outcome after lung transplantation and did not influence patients' candidacy for transplantation.[43]

In patients with α_1-ATD, LVRS is less effective than in those involving smoking-related emphysema. On the basis of our own experience, we conclude that LVRS can be rec-ommended to selected symptomatic patients who have advanced emphysema associated with severe hyperinflation provided their FEV_1 and DLCO values are not less than 20% of the predicted values, their CT scans do not show vanish-ing lungs, and the resected lung volume is substantial.[41-43]

SURGICAL APPROACH

The surgical options for patients with emphysema are SLT, bilateral lung transplantation (BLT), and heart-lung trans-plantation (performed exceedingly rarely in cases involving significant cardiac pathology). Patients with secondary pul-monary hypertension can undergo BLT without any cardiac decompensation.[3,44-46] It has also been reported that patients with pulmonary hypertension can even undergo SLT with-out any increase in the rate of primary graft dysfunction (PGD) and with improved pulmonary hemodynamics in the early posttransplantation period.[45,46]

SLT can be performed via an anterolateral or posterolat-eral thoracotomy incision. BLT was initially performed via a clamshell incision (bilateral transsternal thoracotomy).[3] At many centers the clamshell incision has been replaced by bilateral anterolateral thoracotomy without transverse sternotomy.[47-49]

CHOICE OF PROCEDURE

According to the latest ISHLT registry report, bilateral lung transplant recipients have a median survival time of 6.9 years, whereas single-lung transplant recipients have a median survival time of 4.6 years.[1] These survival times increase to 9.6 years in bilateral lung transplant recipients and to 6.5 years in single-lung transplant recipients who survive the first year following their transplant.[1]

Also according to the recent ISHLT registry report, 14,784 lung transplants were performed for emphysema (n = 12,602) and α_1-ATD (n = 2182) from January 1995 to June 2012.[1] SLT was performed in 49.8% and BLT in 33%. Between 1997 and 2001 only approximately 28% of the transplants performed for emphysema were bilateral. Beginning in 2013, the percentage of bilateral lung transplants increased steadily and reached 72% in 2011.[1]

After a publication by Stevens and colleagues that pre-sented a semiquantitative analysis of ventilation and perfu-sion distribution in two single-lung transplant recipients with native lung emphysema, many centers became con-cerned that SLT for emphysema would result in severe ventilation-perfusion mismatching and failure of the allograft.[50] In their paper perfusion was directed preferen-tially to the allograft whereas the highly compliant emphyse-matous lung received the preponderance of ventilation, thus leading to progressive hyperinflation of the native lung and significant abnormalities in gas exchange.[50] However, these cases involved allograft injury, which might have resulted in the reported abnormalities.[50] Despite this report, in the early 1990s surgeons started performing SLT with good results.[51,52] If graft function is adequate, both ventilation and perfusion are preferentially directed to the allograft.[2]

BLT is preferred by most centers because native lung hyperinflation might be responsible for the poorer results with SLT.[52,53] However, SLT is characterized by shorter total ischemia and operation times, thus leading to its lower perioperative morbidity and mortality rates.[54] Supporters of SLT also emphasize that it reduces the donor organ shortage and decreases waiting list morbidity and mortality.[54]

In a retrospective study Sundaresan and colleagues reported the outcomes of their patients with emphysema who underwent lung transplantation.[55] Recipients who underwent BLT and those who underwent SLT had comparable morbidity and mortality rates. In this series the overall hospital mortality rate was 6.2%.[55] The researchers did not find any difference between the recipients of single versus bilateral lung transplants in terms of hospital stay, intensive care unit stay, or duration of mechanical ventilation. However, the 5-year survival rate with BLT was 53% as compared to 41% with SLT.[55] In another study, Cassivi and coworkers reported 5-year survival rates of 66.7% with BLT and 44.9% with SLT.[56] Delgado and associates from Spain demonstrated a similar cumulative 5-year survival rate: excluding preoperative mortality, survival rates were 54% overall, 59% for SLT, and 56% for BLT. The frequency of bronchiolitis obliterans syndrome (BOS) was 34% after SLT and 42% after BLT. Acute rejection episodes and perioperative complication rates were also comparable between the SLT and BLT groups.[57]

Thabut and colleagues aimed to compare survival after SLT and BLT in patients with emphysema by analyzing data from the ISHLT registry.[58] They analyzed data for 9883 patients with emphysema, 3525 (35.7%) of whom underwent BLT and 6358 (64.3%) SLT between 1987 and 2006. The median survival after either type of lung transplantation for patients with emphysema was 5.0 years (95% confidence interval [CI] = 4.8 to 5.2 years). The proportion of patients who underwent BLT increased from 101 of 467 (21.6%) in 1993 to 345 of 614 (56.2%) in 2006. Median survival time after BLT was longer than after SLT: 6.4 years (6.02 to 6.88 years) versus 4.6 years ($P < .0001$). The pretransplantation characteristics of the patients who underwent SLT and BLT differed, but regardless of the method used to adjust for baseline differences, BLT was associated with longer survival than was SLT: the hazard ratio (HR) ranged from 0.83 (0.78 to 0.92) with analysis of covariance to 0.89 (0.80 to 0.97) with propensity-based matching. However, when compared with SLT, BLT provided little additional benefit for patients 60 years and older (HR = 0.95; CI = 0.81 to 1.13). These authors concluded that BLT leads to longer survival than SLT does in patients with emphysema, especially in those who are younger than 60 years.[58]

Meyer and colleagues analyzed 2260 lung transplant recipients (1835 single-lung transplants and 425 bilateral lung transplants) with emphysema who were included in the ISHLT/United Network for Organ Sharing thoracic registry between January 1991 and December 1997.[59] For patients younger than 50 years, the 30-day, 1-year, and 5-year survival rates after SLT were 93.6%, 80.2%, and 43.6%, respectively, as opposed to 94.9%, 84.7%, and 68.2%, respectively, after BLT. For patients aged 50 to 60 years, the respective survival rates were 93.5%, 79.4%, and 39.8% after SLT versus 93.0%, 79.7%, and 60.5% after BLT. For those older than 60 years, the SLT survival rates were 93.0%, 72.9%, and 36.4% compared with 77.8% and 66.0% for the BLT group. The multivariate model showed a higher risk ratio for mortality in patients aged 40 to 57 years who received SLT versus BLT. The authors concluded that SLT might offer acceptable early survival for patients with end-stage respiratory failure. However, long-term survival data favor BLT in recipients until approximately age 60. The authors' data suggest that the BLT approach offers a significant survival advantage to recipients younger than 60 years.[59] The superiority of BLT over SLT has also been shown in a multicenter study.[60] From these studies it can be concluded that BLT provides short-term results similar to those of SLT but superior intermediate- and long-term results.[61]

In addition to the survival advantage shown in previous studies, other facts support performing BLT in patients with emphysema.[61] Hyperinflation of the native lung was reported to occur in 5% to 15% of patients and often required independent lung ventilation or LVRS.[62-65] Pneumonia in the native lung occurred in 10% to 20% of patients, with the mortality rate in those with this complication reaching 20%.[66,67] Development of lung cancer in the native lung was reported in approximately 2% to 3% of patients.[68,69]

On the other hand, Hadjiliadis and Angel reported that SLT might be beneficial for patients with emphysema if severe PGD develops.[61] These patients might still have a functioning emphysematous lung that could potentially sustain them while their PGD resolves.[61]

FUNCTIONAL OUTCOMES

Lung transplantation dramatically improves most physiologic parameters of patients with emphysema.[70] FEV_1 and forced vital capacity improve, whereas TLC and RV tend to normalize; in addition, the need for oxygen disappears and the carbon dioxide level normalizes.[70] Distance during the 6MWT also improves dramatically.[51,55,56,71,72] Lung function improves dramatically in patients with COPD following both SLT and BLT; as expected, patients who undergo BLT experience greater improvement. Following SLT, FEV_1 typically increases to 40% to 60% predicted, whereas following BLT, it typically exceeds 80% predicted.[55,72,73]

Despite the differences in 6MWT distance, studies have not demonstrated a significant difference in measures of daily physical activity after SLT as opposed to after BLT.[74,75] In addition, exercise performance as assessed by the age-adjusted parameter of maximum oxygen consumption was also comparable between SLT and BLT.[76,77]

The effect of type of procedure on the development of BOS attracted the attention of several investigators; these studies failed to detect a difference in the incidence of BOS between recipients of single- versus bilateral lung transplants.[51,55,72] However in one study, Hadjiliadis and associates demonstrated increased freedom from BOS after BLT at both 3 and 5 years.[78] They also reported increased survival after a diagnosis of BOS in the BLT group. This difference was attributed to the increased pulmonary reserve conferred by BLT.[78]

QUALITY OF LIFE

Following lung transplantation, quality of life improves significantly in recipients with emphysema. Although no prospective trial has assessed the same group of patients before and after transplantation in longitudinal fashion,[70] the changes that have been reported in cross-sectional studies are highly significant.[75,79] In another study, a survival analysis showed that although patients with emphysema may have had a worse lung transplantation survival rate, their quality-of-life–adjusted years were better after lung transplantation.[80]

COMPLICATIONS

Complications following lung transplantation can occur immediately after surgery or days or weeks later. Clinical suspicion and close follow-up of these patients are the strategies to reduce morbidity and mortality in those who survive the procedure.[81] The main complications following lung transplantation can be divided into three major groups that are also valid for emphysema recipients: (1) surgical complications, (2) immunologic complications, and (3) side effects of immunosuppressive drugs. In this chapter, we focus on the surgical complications and their management following lung transplant surgery. Vascular complications following lung transplantation occur as a result of inadequate anastomotic technique. Anastomotic leaks are usually corrected during the operation. Pulmonary venous complications usually develop in the early postoperative period in the form of unilateral pulmonary edema and respiratory failure. They may result from anastomotic stenosis or thrombosis. External compression of the anastomosis by a clot, pericardial fat, or an omental flap used for coverage of the bronchial anastomosis can also impair venous outflow.[81] Persistent pulmonary hypertension and unexplained hypoxemia can occur as a result of stenosis at the pulmonary artery anastomosis. This problem may be detected by a nuclear perfusion scan, which will demonstrate the unsatisfactory flow to a single-lung graft or unequal distribution of flow in a bilateral lung transplant recipient.[81] Transesophageal echocardiography is also valuable in detecting stenosis, especially on the right side. Pulmonary angiography can be used as a confirmatory test and also helps show the anatomic details.

Treatment options include noninvasive approaches such as balloon dilatation, stent implantation, and open surgical revision.[82,83]

Airway complications

Pulmonary transplantation is unique among all solid-organ transplants in that the systemic arterial blood supply is generally not restored during engraftment. For this reason, anastomotic complications have been attributed primarily to ischemia of the donor bronchus.[84] Rejection,[85] intense immunosuppressive therapy,[86] invasive infections,[87] and inadequate organ preservation[84] are additional factors that have been identified as being associated with compromised airway healing. The rate of anastomotic problems following lung transplantation has dropped from 80% before 1983[88] to 2.6%.[89,90] Bronchial ischemia is reported to be a significant risk factor for the development of airway complications.[91] The viability of the donor bronchus is initially dependent on retrograde low-pressure collaterals derived from the pulmonary artery because the bronchial arterial circulation is lost during harvest of the donor lungs.[85] Several techniques have been proposed to protect the bronchial anastomosis: keeping the donor bronchus as short as possible and wrapping the anastomosis with vascularized pedicles,[84] direct revascularization of donor bronchial arteries,[92] and double antegrade and retrograde flush perfusion of the donor lungs at the time of harvest.[93] During acute rejection episodes, microcirculation may be significantly impaired because of an increase in pulmonary vascular resistance and decrease in pulmonary collateral blood supply.[94]

We firmly believe that surgical technique is paramount for subsequent successful healing of the bronchial anastomosis.[95,96] The surgical approach for performing the anastomosis may vary among transplant centers. Telescoping, end-to-end anastomosis with a running suture for the membranous part and interrupted sutures for the cartilaginous part, and end-to-end anastomosis with a single running suture are used most often.[97-99] Some centers have reported changing their anastomotic technique from telescoping to end-to-end single suture because of a high airway complication rate.[100,101] Others have used telescoping or a modified telescoping technique from the beginning of their program with a low complication rate.[91,100] In fact, in most studies telescoping has been demonstrated to be an independent risk factor for airway complications.[90,97,100] We have not modified our technique since our program was established in 1992. Furthermore, we think that resection of the donor bronchus down to the lobar carina in an oblique plane while keeping the peribronchial tissue intact is a critical step in performing the bronchial anastomosis.[95,96]

Pleural space complications are common in the early postoperative period after lung transplantation. In the early experience of some centers, the rate of postoperative hemorrhage requiring reoperation after heart-lung and en bloc double-lung transplants was about 25%. The underlying pulmonary disease usually leads to dense pleural adhesions, which can cause hemorrhage during recipient pneumonectomy. The use of cardiopulmonary bypass (CPB) in some transplant cases can also increase bleeding resulting from anticoagulation.

Primary graft dysfunction

PGD is a form of acute lung injury that follows the sequence of events inherent in the lung transplantation process, including brain death of the donor, pulmonary ischemia, preservation of donor tissue, transplantation, and reperfusion of donor tissue in the recipient.[101] PGD typically occurs within 72 hours after lung transplantation and is characterized by poor oxygenation, low pulmonary compliance, interstitial or alveolar edema, increased pulmonary vascular resistance, pulmonary infiltrates visible on a chest radiograph, and acute alveolar injury as revealed by diffuse alveolar damage on pathologic analysis.[102] PGD affects about 10% to 25% of lung transplant recipients and is the leading cause of early posttransplantation morbidity and mortality.[102-108] Thirty-day mortality rates are up to eightfold higher in patients with severe PGD than in those without PGD.

The pathogenesis of PGD is complex. Generation of reactive oxygen species during the ischemia-reperfusion process plays an important role in the development of PGD.[101] In addition to the direct injury from reactive oxygen species on the pulmonary endothelium and epithelium, inflammatory cascades are initiated, adhesion molecules are upregulated, and procoagulant factors that contribute to lung injury are increased.[109-111] Donor-acquired risk factors,[112] such as prolonged mechanical ventilation, aspiration pneumonitis or pneumonia, trauma, and hemodynamic instability after brain death, have not been shown to contribute to the development of PGD, although theoretical bases for an association between such risk factors and PGD do exist. Recipient factors such as age, sex, race, body weight, underlying hepatic or renal impairment, left-sided heart disease, diabetes, and medication (steroids, inotropes) use before surgery are not directly associated with an increased risk for PGD.[113]

In addition, a history of previous thoracic surgery or pretransplantation mechanical ventilation has not been shown to be directly associated with PGD. The association between PGD and CPB is also controversial: in a study of lung transplant recipients without a diagnosis of pulmonary arterial hypertension, the need for CPB was predictive of worse early outcomes and early death[114]; however, others have shown that the use of CPB was not an independent risk factor for PGD and that patients had similar early outcomes when CPB was not dictated by pulmonary hypertension or other factors.[103,115] Treatment of PGD is mainly supportive. Treatment strategies are low-stretch ventilation for the prevention of barotrauma and avoidance of excessive fluid administration (negative fluid balance), pulmonary vasodilatation (prostaglandin, inhaled nitric oxide),[116-121] ECMO,[122,123] surfactant replacement,[124,125] and urgent retransplantation. Other experimental therapeutic strategies such as administration of N-acetylcysteine and p38 and c-jun kinase inhibitors are promising.[126-128]

THE ZURICH EXPERIENCE

From November 1992 to August 2013, 108 consecutive lung transplants for emphysema (77 for COPD and 31 for α_1-ATD) were performed at Zurich University Hospital. The median recipient age was 56.6 years (range = 31 to 68). The 30-day mortality rate was 3.7%. The 1- and 5-year survival rates of recipients with COPD and those with α_1-ATD were comparable (91% and 70% versus 84% and 72%, respectively; $P = .87$, log-rank test).

The 1- and 5-year survival rates for recipients younger than 60 years were significantly better than those for recipients 60 years and older (91% and 79% versus 84% and 54%; $P = .05$, log-rank test). Since 2007, 1- and 5-year survival rates for these two age groups were 96% and 92% versus 86% and 44%, respectively ($P = .04$, log-rank test). Use of ECMO or CPB during transplantation, waiting list time, sex, size reduction, BMI, and diagnosis of COPD or α_1-ATD had no significant influence on survival rates in univariate analysis. Age at transplantation (≥ 60) was a risk factor in univariate analysis (HR = 2.1, 95% CI = 1.09 to 4.09, $P = .02$). In multivariate analysis (Cox regression, backward stepwise) unilateral lung transplantation was an independent risk factor for mortality (HR = 0.04, 95% CI = 0.01 to 0.2).

REFERENCES

1. Yusen RD, Christie JD, Edwards LB, et al. International Society for Heart and Lung Transplantation. The Registry of the International Society for Heart and Lung Transplantation: Thirtieth adult lung and heart-lung transplant report—2013; focus theme: Age. J Heart Lung Transplant 2013;32:965-978.
2. Shah RJ, Kotloff RM. Lung transplantation for obstructive lung diseases. Semin Respir Crit Care Med 2013;34:288-296.
3. Patel N, Criner GJ. Transplantation in chronic obstructive pulmonary disease. COPD 2006;3:149-162.
4. Veith FJ, Koerner SK, Attai LA, et al. Single-lung transplantation in emphysema. Lancet 1972;1:1138-1139.
5. Veith FJ, Koerner SK, Siegelman SS, et al. Single lung transplantation in experimental and human emphysema. Ann Surg 1973;178:463-476.
6. Patterson GA, Cooper JD, Goldman B, et al. Technique of successful clinical double-lung transplantation. Ann Thorac Surg 1988;45:626-633.
7. Cooper JD, Patterson GA, Grossman R, Maurer J. Double-lung transplant for advanced chronic obstructive lung disease. Am Rev Respir Dis 1989;139:303-307.
8. Mal H, Andreassian B, Pamela F, et al. Unilateral lung transplantation in end-stage pulmonary emphysema. Am Rev Respir Dis 1989;140:797-802.

9. Trulock EP, Egan TM, Kouchoukos NT, et al. Single lung transplantation for severe chronic obstructive pulmonary disease. Washington University Lung Transplant Group. Chest 1989;96:738-742.

10. Pasque MK, Cooper JD, Kaiser LR, et al. Improved technique for bilateral lung transplantation: Rationale and initial clinical experience. Ann Thorac Surg 1990;49:785-791.

11. Orens JB, Estenne M, Arcasoy S, et al. International guidelines for the selection of lung transplant candidates: 2006 update—a consensus report from the Pulmonary Scientific Council of the International Society for Heart and Lung Transplantation. J Heart Lung Transplant 2006;25:745-755.

12. American Thoracic Society. International guidelines for the selection of lung transplant candidates. Am J Respir Crit Care Med 1998;158:335-339.

13. Vestbo J, Edwards LD, Scanlon PD, et al. Changes in forced expiratory volume in 1 second over time in COPD. N Engl J Med 2011;365:1184-1192.

14. Nishimura M, Makita H, Nagai K, et al. Annual change in pulmonary function and clinical phenotype in chronic obstructive pulmonary disease. Am J Respir Crit Care Med 2012;185:44-52.

15. Anthonisen NR. Prognosis in chronic obstructive pulmonary disease: Results from multicenter clinical trials. Am Rev Respir Dis 1989;140:S95-S99.

16. Renzetti AD Jr, McClement JH, Litt BD. The Veterans Administration cooperative study of pulmonary function. 3. Mortality in relation to respiratory function in chronic obstructive pulmonary disease. Am J Med 1966;41:115-129.

17. Boushy SF, Thompson HK Jr, North LB, et al. Prognosis in chronic obstructive pulmonary disease. Am Rev Respir Dis 1973;108:1373-1383.

18. Hodgkin JE. Prognosis in chronic obstructive pulmonary disease. Clin Chest Med 1990;11:555-569.

19. Seersholm N, Kok-Jensen A, Dirksen A. Survival of patients with severe alpha 1-antitrypsin deficiency with special reference to non-index cases. Thorax 1994;49:695-698.

20. Martinez FJ, Kotloff R. Prognostication in chronic obstructive pulmonary disease: Implications for lung transplantation. Semin Respir Crit Care Med 2001;22:489-498.

21. Traver GA, Cline MG, Burrows B. Predictors of mortality in chronic obstructive pulmonary disease: A 15-year follow-up study. Am Rev Respir Dis 1979;119:895-902.

22. Celli BR, Cote CG, Marin JM, et al. The body-mass index, airflow obstruction, dyspnea, and exercise capacity index in chronic obstructive pulmonary disease. N Engl J Med 2004;350:1005-1012.

23. Martinez FJ, Han MK, Andrei AC, et al. National Emphysema Treatment Trial Research Group. Longitudinal change in the BODE index predicts mortality in severe emphysema. Am J Respir Crit Care Med 2008;178:491-499.

24. Kanasky WF Jr, Anton SD, Rodrigue JR, et al. Impact of body weight on long-term survival after lung transplantation. Chest 2002;121:401-406.

25. Parekh K, Meyers BF, Patterson GA, et al. Outcome of lung transplantation for patients requiring concomitant cardiac surgery. J Thorac Cardiovasc Surg 2005;130:859-863.

26. Marcello C, Keshavjee S. Extracorporeal life support as a bridge to lung transplantation. Clin Chest Med 2011;32:245-251.

27. Toyoda Y, Bhama JK, Shigemura N, et al. Efficacy of extracorporeal membrane oxygenation as a bridge to lung transplantation. J Thorac Cardiovasc Surg 2013;145:1065-1970; discussion 1070-1071.

28. Lafarge M, Mordant P, Thabut G, et al. Experience of extracorporeal membrane oxygenation as a bridge to lung transplantation in France. J Heart Lung Transplant 2013;32:905-913.

29. Fuehner T, Kuehn C, Hadem J, et al. Extracorporeal membrane oxygenation in awake patients as bridge to lung transplantation. Am J Respir Crit Care Med 2012;185:763-768.

30. Weder W, Thurnheer R, Stammberger U, et al. Radiologic emphysema morphology is associated with outcome after surgical lung volume reduction. Ann Thorac Surg 1997;64:313-319; discussion 319-320.

31. Criner GJ, Cordova FC, Furukawa F, et al. Prospective randomized trial comparing bilateral lung volume reduction surgery to pulmonary rehabilitation in severe chronic obstructive pulmonary disease. Am J Respir Crit Care Med 1999;160:2018-2027.

32. Fujimoto T, Teschler H., Hillejan L, et al. Long-term results of lung volume reduction surgery. Eur J Cardiothorac Surg 2002;21:483-488.

33. Ciccone AM, Meyers BF, Guthrie TJ, et al. Long-term outcome of bilateral lung volume reduction in 250 consecutive patients with emphysema. J Thorac Cardiovasc Surg 2003;125:513-525.

34. Pompeo E, Marino M, Nofroni I, et al. Reduction pneumoplasty versus respiratory rehabilitation in severe emphysema: A randomized study. Pulmonary Emphysema Research Group. Ann Thorac Surg 2000;70:948-953.

35. Weder W, Tutic M, Bloch KE, Lung volume reduction surgery in nonheterogeneous emphysema. Thorac Surg Clin 2009;19:193-199.

36. Brantigan OC, Kress MB, Mueller EA, The surgical approach to pulmonary emphysema. 1961. Chest 2009;136(Suppl 5):e30.

37. Cooper JD, Patterson GA, Sundaresen RS, et al. Results of 150 consecutive bilateral lung volume reduction procedures in patients with severe emphysema. J Thorac Cardiovasc Surg 1996;112:1319-1330.

38. National Emphysema Treatment Trial Research Group. Patients at high risk of death after lung-volume-reduction surgery. N Engl J Med 2001;345):1075-1083.

39. National Emphysema Treatment Trial Research Group. A randomized trial comparing lung-volume-reduction surgery with medical therapy for severe emphysema. N Engl J Med 2003;348:2059-2073.

40. Naunheim KS, Wood DE, Mohsenifar Z, et al. Long-term follow-up of patients receiving lung-volume-reduction surgery versus medical therapy for severe emphysema by the National Emphysema Treatment Trial Research Group. Ann Thorac Surg 2006;82:431-443.

41. Bloch KE, Georgescu CL, Russi EW, Weder W. Gain and subsequent loss of lung function after lung volume reduction surgery in cases of severe emphysema with different morphologic patterns. J Thorac Cardiovasc Surg 2002;23:845-854.

42. Weder W, Tutic M, Lardinois D, et al. Persistent benefit from lung volume reduction surgery in patients with homogeneous emphysema. Ann Thorac Surg 2009;87:229-236; discussion 236-237.

43. Tutic M, Lardinois D, Imfeld S, et al. Lung-volume reduction surgery as an alternative or bridging procedure to lung transplantation. Ann Thorac Surg 2006;82:208-213.

44. Marinelli WA, Hertz MI, Shumway SJ, et al. Single lung transplantation for severe emphysema. J Heart Lung Transpl 1992;11:577-582; discussion 582-583.

45. Bjortuft O, Simonsen S, Geiran OR, et al. Pulmonary haemodynamics after single-lung transplantation for end-stage pulmonary parenchymal disease. Eur Respir J 1996;9:2007-2011.

46. Boujoukos AJ, Martich GD, Vega JD, et al. Reperfusion injury in single-lung transplant recipients with pulmonary hypertension and emphysema. J Heart Lung Transplant 1997;16:439-448.

47. Kaiser LR, Pasque MK, Trulock EP, et al. Bilateral sequential lung transplantation: The procedure of choice for double-lung replacement. Ann Thorac Surg 1991;52:438-445; discussion 445-446.

48. Taghavi S, Bîrsan T, Seitelberger R, et al. Initial experience with two sequential anterolateral thoracotomies for bilateral lung transplantation. Ann Thorac Surg 1999;67:1440-1443.

49. Meyers BF, Sundaresan RS, Guthrie T, et al. Bilateral sequential lung transplantation without sternal division eliminates posttransplantation sternal complications. J Thorac Cardiovasc Surg 1999;117:358-364.

50. Stevens PM, Johnson PC, Bell RL, et al. Regional ventilation and perfusion after lung transplantation in patients with emphysema. N Engl J Med 1970;282:245-249.

51. Levine SM, Anzueto A, Peters JI, et al. Medium term functional results of single-lung transplantation for end stage obstructive lung disease. Am J Respir Crit Care Med 1994;150:398-402.

52. Mal H, Brugière O, Sleiman C, et al. Morbidity and mortality related to the native lung in single lung transplantation for emphysema. J Heart Lung Transplant 2000;19:220-223.

53. Venuta F, Boehler A, Rendina EA, et al. Complications in the native lung after single lung transplantation. Eur J Cardiothorac Surg 1999;16:54-58.

54. Aziz F, Penupolu S, Xu X, He J. Lung transplant in end-staged chronic obstructive pulmonary disease (COPD) patients: A concise review. J Thorac Dis 2010;2:111-116.

55. Sundaresan RS, Shiraishi Y, Trulock EP, et al. Single or bilateral lung transplantation for emphysema? J Thorac Cardiovasc Surg 1996;112:1485-1494.

56. Cassivi SD, Meyers BF, Battafarano RJ, et al. Thirteen-year experience in lung transplantation for emphysema. Ann Thorac Surg 2002;74:1663-1639.

57. Delgado M, Borro JM, De La Torre MM, et al. Lung transplantation as the first choice in emphysema. Transplant Proc 2009;41:2207-2209.

58. Thabut G, Christie JD, Ravaud P, et al. Survival after bilateral versus single lung transplantation for patients with chronic obstructive pulmonary disease: A retrospective analysis of registry data. Lancet 2008;371:744-751.

59. Meyer DM, Bennett LE, Novick RJ, Hosenpud JD. Single vs bilateral, sequential lung transplantation for end-stage emphysema: Influence of recipient age on survival and secondary end-points. J Heart Lung Transplant 2001;20:935-941.

60. Hadjiliadis D, Chaparro C, Gutierrez C, et al. Impact of lung transplant operation on bronchiolitis obliterans syndrome in patients with chronic obstructive pulmonary disease. Am J Transplant 2006;6:183-189.

61. Hadjiliadis D, Angel LF. Controversies in lung transplantation: Are two lungs better than one? Semin Respir Crit Care Med 2006;27:561-566.

62. Weill D, Torres F, Hodges TN, et al. Acute native lung hyperinflation is not associated with poor outcomes after single lung transplant for emphysema. J Heart Lung Transplant 1999;18:1080-1087

63. Malchow SC, McAdams HP, Palmer SM, et al. Does hyperexpansion of the native lung adversely affect outcome after single lung transplantation for emphysema? Preliminary findings. Acad Radiol 1998;5:688-693

64. Moy ML, Loring SH, Ingenito EP, et al. Causes of allograft dysfunction after single lung transplantation for emphysema: Extrinsic restriction versus intrinsic obstruction. Brigham and Women's Hospital Lung Transplantation Group. J Heart Lung Transplant 1999;18:986-993.

65. Mal H, Brugiere O, Sleiman C, et al. Morbidity and mortality related to the native lung in single lung transplantation for emphysema. J Heart Lung Transplant 2000;19:220-223.

66. Hadjiliadis D, Ahya VN, Christie JD, et al. Early results of lung transplantation after implementation of the new lung allocation score. J Heart Lung Transplant 2006;25:1167-1170.

67. McAdams HP, Erasmus JJ, Palmer SM. Complications (excluding hyperinflation) involving the native lung after single-lung transplantation: Incidence, radiologic features, and clinical importance. Radiology 2001;218:233-241.

68. Collins J, Kazerooni EA, Lacomis J, et al. Bronchogenic carcinoma after lung transplantation: Frequency, clinical characteristics, and imaging findings. Radiology 2002;224:131-138.

69. von Boehmer L, Draenert A, Jungraithmayr W, et al. Immunosuppression and lung cancer of donor origin after bilateral lung transplantation. Lung Cancer 2012;76:118-122.

70. Mora JI, Hadjiliadis D. Lung volume reduction surgery and lung transplantation in chronic obstructive pulmonary disease. Int J Chron Obstruct Pulmon Dis 2008;3:629-635.

71. Bavaria JE, Kotloff R, Palevsky H, et al. Bilateral vs single lung transplantation for chronic obstructive pulmonary disease. J Thorac Cardiovasc Surg 1997;113:520-522.

72. Pochettino A, Kotloff RM, Rosengard BR, et al. Bilateral versus single lung transplantation for chronic obstructive pulmonary disease: Intermediate-term results. Ann Thorac Surg 2000;70:1813-1818.

73. Gaissert HA, Trulock EP, Cooper JD, et al. Comparison of early functional results after volume reduction or lung transplantation for chronic obstructive pulmonary disease. J Thorac Cardiovasc Surg 1996;111:296-306.

74. Bossenbroek L, ten Hacken NH, van der Bij W, et al. Cross-sectional assessment of daily physical activity in chronic obstructive pulmonary disease lung transplant patients. J Heart Lung Transplant 2009;28:149-155.

75. Gerbase MW, Spiliopoulos A, Rochat T, et al. Health-related quality of life following single or bilateral lung transplantation: A 7-year comparison to functional outcome. Chest 2005;128:1371-378.

76. Levy RD, Ernst P, Levine SM, et al. Exercise performance after lung transplantation. J Heart Lung Transplant 1993;12:27-33.

77. Williams TJ, Patterson GA, McClean PA, et al. Maximal exercise testing in single and double lung transplant recipients. Am Rev Respir Dis 1992;145:101-105.

78. Hadjiliadis D, Davis RD, Palmer SM. Is transplant operation important in determining posttransplant risk of bronchiolitis obliterans syndrome in lung transplant recipients? Chest 2002;122:1168-1175.

79. Anyanwu AC, McGuire A, Rogers CA, et al. Assessment of quality of life in lung transplantation using a simple generic tool. Thorax 2001;56:218-222.

80. Singer LG, Gould MK, Glidden DV, et al. Effect of lung transplantation on quality-adjusted survival in emphysema. J Heart Lung Transplant 2002;21:154S.

81. Inci I, Weder W. Managing surgical complications. In Vignesvaran WT, Garrity ER Jr, eds. Lung Transplantation. London: Informa Healthcare; 2010:249-265.

82. Clark SC, Levine AJ, Hasan A, et al. Vascular complications of lung transplantation. Ann Thorac Surg 1996;61:1079-1082.

83. Fadel BM, Abdulbaki K, Nambiar V, et al. Dual thrombosis of the pulmonary arterial and venous anastomotic sites after single lung transplantation: Role of transesophageal echocardiography in diagnosis and management. J Am Soc Echocardiogr 2007;20:438.e9-e12.

84. Shennib H, Massard G. Airway complications in lung transplantation. Ann Thorac Surg 1994;57:506-511.

85. Takao M, Katayama Y, Onoda K, et al. Significance of bronchial mucosal blood flow for the monitoring of acute rejection in lung transplantation. J Heart Lung Transplant 1991;10:956-967.

86. Lima O, Cooper JD, Peters WJ, et al. Effects of methylprednisolone and azathioprine on bronchial healing following lung autotransplantation. J Thorac Cardiovasc Surg 1981;82:211-215.

87. Kshettry VR, Kroshus TJ, Hertz MI, et al. Early and late complications after lung transplantation: Incidence and management. Ann Thorac Surg 1997;63:1576-1583.

88. Wildevuur CRH, Benfield JR. A review of 23 human lung transplants by 20 surgeons. Ann Thorac Surg 1970;9:489-515.

89. Ruttmann E, Ulmer H, Marchese M, et al. Evaluation of factors damaging the bronchial wall in lung transplantation. J Heart Lung Transplant 2005;24:275-281.

90. Van De Wauwer C, Van Raemdonck D, Verleden GM, et al. Risk factors for airway complications within the first year after lung transplantation. Eur J Cardiothorac Surg 2007;31:703-701.

91. Alvarez A, Algar J, Santos F, et al. Airway complications after lung transplantation: A review of 151 anastomoses. Eur J Cardiothorac Surg 2001;19:381-387.

92. Baudet EM, Dromer C, Dubrez J, et al. Intermediate-term results after en bloc double-lung transplantation with bronchial arterial revascularization. J Thorac Cardiovasc Surg 1996;112:1292-1300.

93. Alvarez A, Salvatierra A, Lama R, et al. Preservation with a retrograde second flushing of Eurocollins in clinical lung transplantation. Transplant Proc 1999;31:1088-1090.

94. Calhoon JH, Grover FL, Gibbons WJ, et al. Single lung transplantation. Alternative indications and technique. J Thorac Cardiovasc Surg 1991;101:816.

95. Weder W, Inci I, Korom S, et al. Airway complications after lung transplantation: Risk factors, prevention and outcome. Eur J Cardiothorac Surg 2009;35:293-298.

96. Inci I, Weder W. Airway complications after lung transplantation can be avoided without bronchial artery revascularization. Curr Opin Organ Transplant 2010;15:578-681.

97. Date H, Trulock EP, Arcidi JM, et al. Improved airway healing after lung transplantation. An analysis of 348 bronchial anastomoses. J Thorac Cardiovasc Surg 1995;110:1424-1432.

98. Schmid RA, Boehler A, Speich R, et al. Bronchial anastomotic complications following lung transplantation: Still a major cause of morbidity? Eur Respir J 1997;10:2872-2875.

99. Herrera JM, McNeil KD, Higgins RS, et al. Airway complications after lung transplantation: Treatment and long-term outcome. Ann Thorac Surg 2001;71:989-999.

100. Murthy SC, Blackstone EH, Gildea TR, et al. Impact of anastomotic airway complications after lung transplantation. Ann Thorac Surg 2007;84:401-409.

101. Lee JC, Christie JD. Primary graft dysfunction. Proc Am Thorac Soc 2009;6:39-46.

102. Christie JD, Carby M, Bag R, et al. Report of the ISHLT working group on primary lung graft dysfunction: Part II. Definition. J Heart Lung Transplant 2005;24:1454-1459.

103. Christie JD, Bavaria JE, Palevsky HI, et al. Primary graft failure following lung transplantation. Chest 1998;114:51-60.

104. King RC, Binns OA, Rodriguez F, et al. Reperfusion injury significantly impacts clinical outcome after pulmonary transplantation. Ann Thorac Surg 2000;69:1681-1685.

105. Christie JD, Kotloff RM, Pochettino A, et al. Clinical risk factors for primary graft failure following lung transplantation. Chest 2003;124:1232-1241.

106. Arcasoy SM, Kotloff RM. Lung transplantation. N Engl J Med 1999;340:1081-1091.

107. Christie JD, Sager JS, Kimmel SE, et al. Impact of primary graft failure on outcomes following lung transplantation. Chest 2005;127:161-165.

108. Arcasoy SM, Fisher A, Hachem RR, et al. Report of the ISHLT working group on primary lung graft dysfunction: Part V. Predictors and outcomes. J Heart Lung Transplant 2005;24:1483-1488.

109. Christie JD, Kotloff RM, Ahya VN, et al. The effect of primary graft dysfunction on survival after lung transplantation. Am J Respir Crit Care Med 2005;171:1312-1316.

110. Christie JD, Van Raemdonck D, de Perrot M, et al. Report of the ISHLT working group on primary lung graft dysfunction: Part I. Introduction and methods. J Heart Lung Transplant 2005;24:1451-1453.

111. Miotla JM, Jeffery PK, Hellewell PG. Platelet-activating factor plays a pivotal role in the induction of experimental lung injury. Am J Respir Cell Mol Biol 1998;18:197-204.

112. Serrick C, Adoumie R, Giaid A, Shennib H. The early release of interleukin-2, tumor necrosis factor-alpha and interferon-gamma after ischemia reperfusion injury in the lung allograft. Transplantation 1994;58:1158-1162.

113. Moreno I, Vicente R, Ramos F, et al. Determination of interleukin-6 in lung transplantation: Association with primary graft dysfunction. Transplant Proc 2007;39:2425-2426.

114. de Perrot M, Bonser RS, Dark J, et al. Report of the ISHLT working group on primary lung graft dysfunction: Part III. Donor-related risk factors and markers. J Heart Lung Transplant 2005;24:1460-1467.

115. Barr ML, Kawut SM, Whelan TP, et al. Report of the ISHLT working group on primary lung graft dysfunction: Part IV. Recipient-related risk factors and markers. J Heart Lung Transplant 2005;24:1468-1482.

116. Szeto WY, Kreisel D, Karakousis GC, et al. Cardiopulmonary bypass for bilateral sequential lung transplantation in patients with chronic obstructive pulmonary disease without adverse effect on lung function or clinical outcome. J Thorac Cardiovasc Surg 2002;124:241-249.

117. Shargall Y, Guenther G, Ahya VN, et al. Report of the ISHLT working group on primary lung graft dysfunction: Part VI. Treatment. J Heart Lung Transplant 2005;24:1489-1500.

118. Adatia I, Lillehei C, Arnold JH, et al. Inhaled nitric oxide in the treatment of postoperative graft dysfunction after lung transplantation. Ann Thorac Surg 1994;57:1311-1318.

119. Date H, Triantafillou AN, Trulock EP, et al. Inhaled nitric oxide reduces human lung allograft dysfunction. J Thorac Cardiovasc Surg 1996;111:913-919.

120. Macdonald P, Mundy J, Rogers P, et al. Successful treatment of life-threatening acute reperfusion injury after lung transplantation with inhaled nitric oxide. J Thorac Cardiovasc Surg 1995;110:861-863.

121. Fiser SM, Kron IL, McLendon Long S, et al. Early intervention after severe oxygenation index elevation improves survival following lung transplantation. J Heart Lung Transplant 2001;20:631-636.

122. Meyers BF, Sundt TM III, Henry S,. Selective use of extracorporeal membrane oxygenation is warranted after lung transplantation. J Thorac Cardiovasc Surg 2000;120:20-26.

123. Smedira NG, Moazami N, Golding CM, et al. Clinical experience with 202 adults receiving extracorporeal membrane oxygenation for cardiac failure: Survival at five years. J Thorac Cardiovasc Surg 2001;122:92-102.

124. Kermeen FD, McNeil KD, Fraser JF, et al. Resolution of severe ischemia-reperfusion injury post–lung

transplantation after administration of endobronchial surfactant. J Heart Lung Transplant
2007;26:850-856.

125. Amital A, Shitrit D, Raviv Y, et al. The use of surfactant in lung transplantation. Transplantation
2008;86:1554-1559.

126. Inci I, Zhai W, Arni S, et al. N-Acetylcysteine attenuates lung ischemia-reperfusion injury after lung
transplantation. Ann Thorac Surg 2007;84:240-246.

127. Chamogeorgakis TP, Kostopanagiotou GG, Kalimeris
CA, et al. Effect of N-acetyl-L-cysteine on lung isch-
aemia reperfusion injury in a porcine experimental
model. ANZ J Surg 2008;78:72-77.

128. Wolf PS, Merry HE, Farivar AS, et al. Stress-activated
protein kinase inhibition to ameliorate lung ischemia reperfusion injury. J Thorac Cardiovasc Surg
2008;135:656-665.

22

Lung transplantation for cystic fibrosis and bronchiectasis

JOHN H. DARK

INTRODUCTION

The diagnoses of cystic fibrosis (CF) and bronchiectasis in lung recipients represent a challenge to transplantation. Both conditions involve a huge bacterial load in the lungs, often with resistant organisms and persistence of infection in the upper airways. Previous surgery, be it pleurodesis or lobectomy, may add to the postinflammatory pleural adhesions. Finally, nonpulmonary comorbid conditions—diabetes, malabsorption, and liver dysfunction in patients with CF and background immunodeficiency in patients with bronchiectasis—may dominate the posttransplant phase. Such patients are some of the most challenging but most rewarding to treat with lung transplantation.

Cystic fibrosis

CF is the most common lethal disease in the white population. It affects approximately 1 in 3000 births in northern and western Europe, and the incidence in white Americans is similar. The highest incidence occurs in the Republic of Ireland, where it affects 1 in 1400 births. By contrast, the incidence is 1 in 4000 to 10,000 in Latin Americans and 1 in 15,000 to 20,000 in African-Americans, and it falls to 1 in 350,000 in Japan.[1]

The lung is involved in a cycle of infection and destruction that progresses to bronchiectasis and chronic lung damage. As many as 98% of children show either culture or serologic evidence of *Pseudomonas aeruginosa* infection by the age of 3 years. At least 80% of deaths in patients with CF are the result of respiratory failure.

On the other hand, the outlook for patients has been improving markedly over recent decades. In the United States, life expectancy improved from 31 to 37 years during the first decade of this century. It has been suggested that a child born in the United Kingdom with CF now has a life expectancy of at least 50 years.[2] One result of these changes is that whereas many candidates in the early days of lung transplantation were children or teenagers, we are presently performing transplants on mature adults, even into their 40s and 50s. One can now imagine a day when patients with CF may be "too old" for transplantation!

Furthermore, the scene may change dramatically in the future. As rapid and easy prenatal diagnosis becomes available, modification of the cellular pathways may become possible. Even though direct gene insertion has been a huge disappointment, the example of a drug such as ivacaftor, which is very effective in a small subset of patients with a specific and rare mutation, opens the prospect of effective reversal of the cellular problem in the not too distant future.[3]

CF is a heterogeneous disease that is caused partly by different mutations in the gene that encodes the CF transmembrane conductance regulator (CFTR) protein. But even with the same mutation, which is termed F508del and occurs in two thirds of Europeans, the disease's severity varies to a large extent. Some of this variation is due to quality of care; however, interactions with other gene polymorphisms also exist.

203

As might be expected with a fatal respiratory disease affecting young adults, CF has been prominent among pretransplantation diagnoses for many years. In the most recent report of the Registry of the International Society for Heart and Lung Transplantation (ISHLT), which contains information on almost 50,000 transplants in the years 1995 to 2013, CF accounted for 16% of all transplants and 24% of bilateral lung transplants.[4] Fourteen percent of all heart lung-transplants were for CF, but whereas heart-lung transplants accounted for up to 20% of transplants performed on patients in the mid-1990s, only a handful are being performed today.

The situation is different in pediatrics, where 70% of lung transplants in the 11- to 17- year-old group were for CF. The preponderance of lung transplants performed for CF occur in Europe, where approximately 75% of all lung transplants in those younger than 18 years are performed for the disease.[5]

This transatlantic difference is seen in adults too (and it might be expected, given the different population distributions). In the latest Organ Procurement and Transplantation Network/Scientific Registry of Transplant Recipients (OPTN/SRTR) report, CF is grouped with "immunodeficiency disorders," which accounted for only 14% of the almost 2000 lung transplants performed in the United States in 2013.[6]

Bronchiectasis

Despite its heterogeneity, CF constitutes a single diagnosis. In contrast, the label *bronchiectasis*, or more correctly albeit laboriously *non-CF bronchiectasis*, encompasses a range of septic lung conditions. The label is applied to those with dilated airways visible by high-resolution computed tomography, recurrent infections, and sputum production, and it is much more common in the elderly. In up to half of all patients, bronchiectasis develops following a destructive infection such as pneumonia, measles, tuberculosis, or allergic bronchopulmonary aspergillosis, but in such cases the problem tends to be self-limited and rarely requires transplantation. Some candidates will have bronchiectasis linked to other lung pathology such as emphysema, which determines the severity of illness. Most patients with this diagnosis who reach transplantation have immunodeficiency or one of the congenital disorders grouped as primary ciliary dyskinesia.[7]

The numbers of such cases are much smaller than those involving lung transplantation in a patient with CF. Thus, in the ISHLT registry report bronchiectasis that was not CF accounted for just 2.7% of all lung transplants and 4% of bilateral lung transplants.[4] The numbers of lung transplantation cases involving immunodeficiency or ciliary dyskinesia are not recorded separately.

In practice, many of the technical or surgical problems in patients with bronchiectasis who reach transplantation are the same as in those with CF: inflammatory adhesions and spillage of purulent secretions. The conditions linked with ciliary dysfunction, such as Kartagener syndrome, bring their own specific, but easily solved, problems.

Disease progression is not as consistent as with CF, and prognostic markers cannot automatically be applied. However, the most important difference occurs in cases involving a nonrespiratory disease in the background. Thus, immunodeficiency severe enough to cause end-stage lung failure brings with it a range of other posttransplant problems.

PATIENT SELECTION

The ISHLT has very recently updated the consensus document on selection of lung transplant candidates (the previous document dates from 2006).[8] The document deals with general considerations in determining acceptability, as well as the specifics of both referral and listing. It is fully up to date, benefits from expertise from around the world, and covers the field of selection very well. The acceptability of candidates in general and those with CF in particular is discussed.

In addition to the indications for lung transplantation, the evidence regarding a number of relative contraindications is widely discussed. Some of these—colonization with pan-resistant or highly resistant organisms and previous surgery—are particularly relevant to CF and are discussed at length later.

Detailed criteria for referral to a transplant center are provided in Box 22.1. After assessment, a very clear set of criteria are used for timing listing; they are presented in Box 22.2.

BOX 22.1: Timing of referrals

- An FEV_1 value that has fallen to 30% predicted or a patient who has advanced disease and a rapidly falling FEV_1 value despite optimal therapy (particularly a female patient), or is infected with nontuberculous mycobacterial disease or *Burkholderia cepacia* complex with or without diabetes
- 6-minute walk distance <400 m
- Development of pulmonary hypertension in the absence of a hypoxic exacerbation (as defined by systolic PAP >35 mm Hg measured by echocardiography or mean PAP >25 mm Hg measured by right-heart catheterization)
- Clinical decline characterized by increasing frequency of exacerbations associated with any of the following:
  - An episode of acute respiratory failure requiring noninvasive ventilation
  - Increasing antibiotic resistance and poor clinical recovery from exacerbations
  - Worsening nutritional status despite supplementation
  - Pneumothorax
- Life-threatening hemoptysis despite bronchial embolization

Note: FEV_1, forced expiratory volume in the first second of respiration; PAP, pulmonary arterial pressure.

SPECIAL CONSIDERATIONS DURING SELECTION

Pretransplant colonization

ASPERGILLUS

One area of considerable concern is colonization of potential recipients by pan-resistant or multiresistant organisms. Two concerns exist: spillage into the pleural space at the time of transplantation or into the newly implanted lung. The latter may occur at the time of transplantation in the absence of rigorous separation of the two airways or later, perhaps from the trachea or nasal sinuses.

Many potentially serious infections can be avoided or their effects minimized by carefully planned prophylactic treatment. For instance, pretransplantation *Aspergillus* colonization is very common, but invasive aspergillosis is rare. *Aspergillus* cultured from the airway at the time of surgery is a risk factor for invasive aspergillosis, particularly at the site of the bronchial anastomosis. Identifying such patients before transplantation is worthwhile because it allows focused administration of antifungal prophylaxis. Although it does not eliminate the problem, such a policy largely prevents death or serious airway problems.[9]

An additional problem in recipients with positive *aspergillus* cultures is the finding of a cavity containing an aspergilloma (Figure 22.1). Great care must be taken when removing such lungs to avoid spillage and the possibility of fungal empyema in the posttransplantation phase.

BURKHOLDERIA CEPACIA

One of the most debated areas is carriage of *B. complex* (BCC). The organism is associated with faster decline in patients with CF, as a result of which it is present in a disproportionately high percentage of potential transplant recipients. The strain *Burkholderia cenocepacia*, which was previously called genomovar III, is now well established as being the real problem. In a series from Duke,[10] the 1-year survival rate for recipients with non–*B. cenocepacia* BCC was the same as that for patients with no BCC detected, but the rate for patients with *B. cenocepacia* was down to 29%.

Our group encountered the same outcomes. Of 216 patients, 22 were infected with BCC before transplantation, including 12 with *B. cenocepacia* infection. Patients with non–*B. cenocepacia* BCC had the same survival rate as did recipients without BCC. However, the group with *B. cenocepacia* had a mortality rate at 1 year of 75%, with eight of nine patients dying of sepsis and BCC bacteremia.[11]

As a result, we no longer accept *B. cenocepacia*–colonized patients, and this is the case with many but not all centers. A laudable suggestion is that teams accepting such patients do so within the framework of an active research program examining novel approaches.[8]

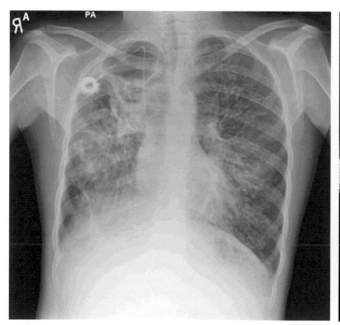
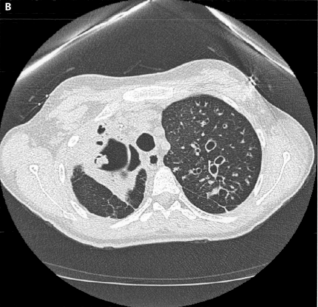

Figure 22.1 (A) Plain chest radiograph of the apical cavity in a patient with cystic fibrosis. (B) Computed tomography scan of the same patient showing an aspergilloma within the cavity.

MYCOBACTERIUM ABSCESSUS

Mycobacterium abscessus is another organism associated with more rapid disease progression; hence, it is being seen in increasing numbers of patients. No consensus regarding the acceptability of such candidates exists, but numerous anecdotal descriptions of multiple postoperative recurrences, typically in the form of chest wall masses and unremitting wound destruction, do exist. Only one series has been reported; consequently, little evidence on which to base advice is available. It is suggested that treatment be well established before transplantation. Eradication is possible but may take as long as 2 years. Disease that continues to progress before transplantation despite treatment should be regarded as a contraindication, and patients who are not tolerant of treatment similarly should not be accepted.[8] The whole field of nontuberculous mycobacteria in patients with CF has recently been reviewed.[13]

PREVIOUS SURGERY AND THE ASYMMETRIC CHEST

Pneumothorax is a specific problem that occurs in up to 20% of patients with CF. It is a marker of poor prognosis and can precipitate respiratory failure. At the other end of the spectrum, lung resection is now relatively uncommon in patients with CF; its impact on the disease is small, and better ways of controlling massive hemoptysis are available. Such patients are still encountered, although their resection was usually performed many years in the past. Lung resection procedures may be more common in patients with non-CF bronchiectasis and were perhaps performed before the disease's generalized nature was recognized.

Early reports[14] suggested no increased risk associated with previous surgery, but publication bias undoubtedly existed. We examined the specific issue of pleurodesis for pneumothorax in patients with CF and found more bleeding and longer operations but no impact on survival.[15] Although pleural thickening can be identified on a radiograph or computed tomography scan, we found radiologic appearance to be a poor predictor of surgical difficulty. Another specific report on recipients with CF came to the same conclusion.[16]

A much larger recent report identified older patients and long bypass as risk factors for death.[17] Our conclusion was that the pneumothorax should be treated in its own right, by the most effective method, and regardless of future lung transplantation–related considerations. We advise avoiding pleurectomy if at all possible.

If a resection has been performed or long-standing lobar collapse is present, the hemithoraces may be of very different sizes. During short-term loss of volume the mediastinum will centralize, so standard lung-sizing approaches can be taken. However, if a major size difference exists, the donor lung is best reduced via an anatomic approach: a lobectomy may be required to fit the donor lung in the "small" side without having too small a lung on the other (Figure 22.2).

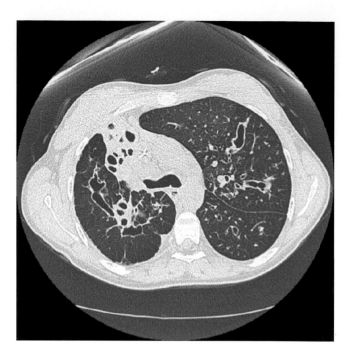

Figure 22.2 Moderate chest asymmetry, which is a situation best dealt with by a donor lobectomy on the right and oversized single lung on the left.

In cases involving extreme size differences, fitting any sort of lung into the space may be difficult and possibly compounded by hilar rotation (Figure 22.3). Faced with this problem, we have on a few occasions performed a pneumonectomy followed immediately by a single-lung transplant on the other side.[18] A principal requirement is that function on the small side be so limited that the patient will remain stable throughout the initial pneumonectomy.

At the far end of the spectrum are patients with a long-ago pneumonectomy. Anecdotes and one series exist.[19] The group of 14 patients studied in the series was assembled from a number of centers over an 18-year period; the best outcomes occurred in those with non-CF bronchiectasis and a pneumonectomy during childhood. Particular attention must be paid to the bypass cannulation strategy and siting of incisions.

SURGICAL EVOLUTION

From the beginning, it was acknowledged that patients with CF and bronchiectasis would require removal of both lungs and would be challenging candidates. The first successful lung transplants were the single-lung transplants reported by the Toronto group in 1985; they were performed for fibrotic disease with no infection. In that era, only combined heart-lung transplants provided removal of both lungs, and patients with CF were represented in early series on both sides of the Atlantic.[20,21] The experience with use of this procedure for a patient with bronchiectasis in Toronto prompted evolution of en bloc double-lung transplants.

The double-lung transplant proved to be an evolutionary dead end, but it did establish the principle that removal of

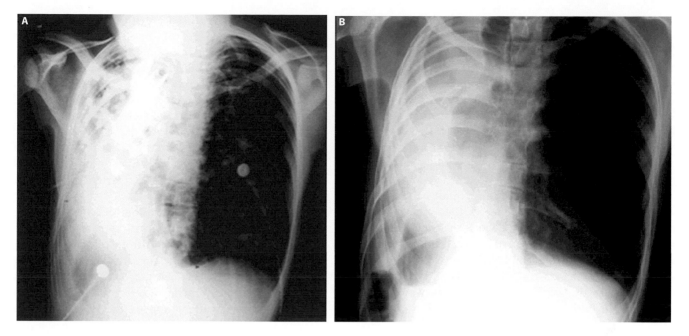

Figure 22.3 (**A**) Plain chest radiograph of a grossly shrunken right hemithorax and severe mediastinal shift. The patient underwent synchronous right pneumonectomy and left single-lung transplant. (**B**) A late postoperative chest radiograph of the same patient with further mediastinal shift and obliteration of the right pleural space.

the heart (as in heart-lung transplantation) was not essential, and even a disadvantage. This method was tempered by the "domino" procedure, in which the healthy heart of a recipient with CF was transplanted into a cardiac recipient and the patient with CF received a heart-lung transplant.[21] Although economy of donor organs was achieved, surgical and logistic difficulties were encountered, and of course the CF patient received a denervated allograft heart. The heart-lung transplant did at least almost guarantee airway healing. Nonetheless, after the setbacks of en bloc double-lung transplantation, surgical techniques evolved from the bibronchial approach described by the French to the now-accepted bilateral or single-sequential lung transplantation technique that was first described by Kaiser, Pasque, and others from St. Louis.[22]

CURRENT SURGERY

The standard approach now is to perform a bilateral or single sequential lung transplant via a "clamshell" incision. This incision gives wonderful access to the whole of the pleural space, as can be seen in Figure 22.4. The adjective *sequential* in the name of the procedure refers to removal of one lung, followed by implantation, then removal of the other lung, and implantation of the second lung as the final stage.

A left-sided double-lumen endotracheal tube is used in all recipients except small teenagers and children. Standard monitoring is used together with transesophageal echocardiography. The latter technique allows monitoring of the right ventricle during one-lung anesthesia, can give warning of potential air embolism after reperfusion of the lung,

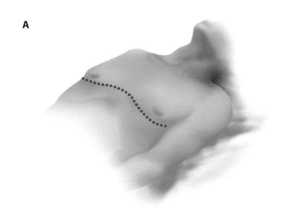

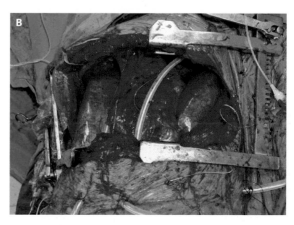

Figure 22.4 A clamshell incision gives superb access to the entirety of both pleural spaces.

and confirms unobstructed flow from the pulmonary veins at the completion of the transplant.

The incision should be made through the fifth intercostal space, thereby providing direct access to the hilum of the lung. If cardiopulmonary bypass is not being used, some prefer to keep the pleura of the side not being operated on intact. An unintended parenchymal air leak from the second lung can be a major problem.

As first described, the procedure was performed without cardiopulmonary bypass. However, a heart-lung machine is essential in some circumstances (e.g., during a lobar transplant); it can provide some advantage in all patients, and it has been the approach of choice in the author's center since 1991.[23] The approach developed at the center includes removal of both lungs, exclusion of the trachea, and simultaneous reperfusion. The first implanted lung is kept cool, but not reperfused, in the chest while the second lung is being implanted. The advantages of cardiopulmonary bypass are summarized in Table 22.1.

The procedure's disadvantages are of course the potentially greater bleeding, the need for clotting products, and (as shown in a recent major paper) a significantly increased risk for primary graft dysfunction.[24] Placement of an epidural catheter is often delayed for 24 hours while clotting abnormalities are reversed.

An alternative to a full conventional cardiopulmonary bypass in patients who require intraoperative support is to use a closed extracorporeal membrane oxygenation–type circuit, which entails lower doses of heparin, much less blood trauma, and less activation of inflammatory cytokines. Although rigorous comparison is lacking, there would appear to be less bleeding, less lung injury, and a shorter stay in the intensive therapy unit.[25]

The fundamental steps of the transplantation procedure are the same regardless of whether cardiopulmonary bypass is used. Pleural adhesions are freed and the vascular structures ligated and divided. In cases involving septic lung disease, our custom has been to staple the bronchus before removing the lung. Great care must be taken to avoid spillage of secretions during the explantation; the old lung must be completely removed from the operative field as soon as possible.

Table 22.1 Advantages of cardiopulmonary bypass

- Use of a single-lumen endotracheal tube, which results in much easier clearance of viscid secretions, especially in smaller patients
- Complete isolation of the airway, thereby allowing tracheal lavage with antiseptics
- Avoidance of any risk of cross-contamination from the old lung to the new lung
- Simultaneous pressure-controlled reperfusion of both lungs without the dependent lung taking all the pulmonary blood flow

Irrigation of the pleural space with a powerful antiseptic, both after lung removal and at completion of the procedure, may reduce the risk for infection of the pleural space and empyema. We have found the antiseptic Taurolin to be particularly effective in this setting.[26]

Great care must be taken to avoid vagal injury. We divide the bronchus relatively distally and dissect the vagus nerve off the posterior wall while avoiding electrocautery in its vicinity and keeping the nerve well clear of subsequent suture lines. The hilum is often a mass of inflamed lymph nodes and large feeding bronchial arteries. Meticulous attention to hemostasis is vital.

The bronchus is usually anastomosed first, with care taken to keep the donor bronchus as short as possible: because it depends on collaterals from within the lung for blood supply, it should be as close to the parenchyma as possible. We use monofilament nonabsorbable suture, but others use braided absorbable material; the choice of suture probably does not matter provided that the principles of preservation of the surrounding tissues and use of a short donor airway are adhered to.[27]

End-to-end anastomoses of the pulmonary artery and donor and recipient left atria are followed by de-airing of the graft, which is usually performed via an antegrade approach through the still-open venous anastomosis. Effort should be made to achieve intima-to-intima apposition at the atrial junction by using an inverting suture technique. Reperfusion pressure should be modest, and evidence suggests that initial ventilation with room air is an advantage.[24]

Closure is achieved by wiring the sternal edges together, after which numerous pericostal stitches approximate the ribs. Pain control can be a particular problem with this very extensive incision, and use of either an epidural catheter or bilateral paravertebral cannulas for continuous delivery of local anesthetic solutions is almost mandatory.

LOBAR TRANSPLANTS

Many patients with CF and bronchiectasis are smaller than average, and small size is a risk factor for death on the waiting list in many registries.[6] An alternative is to transplant a smaller lung. Reduction may be performed nonanatomically, but the best results appear to be provided by anatomic lobectomies in the donor lung. A number of well-described series are available, and in the hands of experienced groups, outcomes are the same as with full-size lungs.[28] We have found that a donor with *double* the predicted total lung capacity of the recipient is required for successful bilateral lobar transplants.

In some parts of the world, again to deal with the issue of smaller recipients' poor access to donor lungs, living donor lung transplants have been performed. Such transplants are associated with significant ethical issues[29] but represent an interesting surgical challenge. A group in Los Angeles has accumulated the largest experience with living donor transplants in all age groups.[30] Although donor morbidity was generally minimal, the 1-year survival rate was not as good as that of similar patients undergoing conventional cadaveric transplants. A large experience with children in the United States was described by Sweet in 2006,[31] but since the introduction of the lung allocation score in the United States in 2005, such activity has largely ceased. It continues in Japan, with very good results indeed,[32] but is not really relevant to CF.

LUNG-LIVER TRANSPLANTATION

CF-related liver disease is the third most common cause of death in the population of patients with CF, and it is frequently found in candidates seeking lung transplantation. With the current selection criteria, including the need for good synthetic function despite abnormal liver function test results, outcomes are identical to those for the general population of patients with CF. The presence of portal hypertension, even with known varices, is not a contraindication in our hands provided that synthetic function is maintained.

Nonetheless, despite not having reached the liver transplantation stage, a percentage of candidates have such poor function that they are unlikely to survive lung transplantation without hepatic decompensation. In this setting, satisfactory outcomes are achieved by performing a liver transplant from the same donor immediately after completion of the lung transplant.[33] Such transplants are not as good as standard transplants (although the numbers are small), and the rationale for combined procedures has been questioned.[34]

We have performed such operations only on otherwise relatively low-risk recipients and have obtained gratifying results. Having the liver accompany the lung has not been seen to protect against acute rejection.

ISSUES SPECIFIC TO BRONCHIECTASIS

Only one major center has reported a specific series involving non-CF bronchiectasis.[35] In many patients with this condition, the diagnosis was either idiopathic or related to a childhood infection. The transplant considerations were therefore similar to those with CF.

A small group of patients had a background of hypogammaglobulinemia. Because this disorder is controlled by regular immunoglobulin supplements, such patients make entirely acceptable candidates for a transplant. In our limited experience, the postoperative infections have been no different from those affecting other lung transplant patients.

Finally, most series include a handful of patients with ciliary dyskinesia (immotile cilia syndrome). The largest experience, though still anecdotal, involves Kartagener syndrome, which includes situs inversus, as well as possible cardiac defects.[36] The initial reports described heart-lung transplantation,[37] which may still be required in the event of significant intracardiac defects that are not amenable to easy repair. However, a bilateral lung transplant involving insertion of the lungs into the appropriate hemithorax and anatomic "correction" at the hilum is perfectly possible.[38]

A set of very rare primarily airway problems, such as Williams-Campbell[39] and Mounier-Kuhn[40] syndromes, which involve a cartilage defect causing airway collapse and recurrent infection, have been successfully treated with lung transplantation, but the decision making must be individualized. In particular, persistent tracheal collapse is a contraindication because lung transplantation will not fix the issue.

RESULTS

Recipients who receive a lung transplant for CF have some of the best long-term survival prospects despite their many surgical and infectious disease–related problems. They have the best 5- and 10-year outcomes of all recipients in the ISHLT registry regardless of the specific diagnosis prompting transplantation.[4] Recipients with CF are relatively young and accustomed to taking numerous medications. Any poor compliance has already been identified.

Our own series was published in 2008[41]; our 176 patients at that time (we now have more than 250) had a median survival time in excess of 10 years (Figure 22.5), and currently, survival time is greater than 11 years.

Despite past doubts about the overall benefit of lung transplantation in children with CF,[42] series from specific centers with extensive experience have demonstrated excellent outcomes. The group in Vienna reported a 5-year survival rate of 70% in the recent era.[43]

CONCLUSION

Patients with CF and non-CF bronchiectasis are among the most challenging but also the most satisfying to treat. They bring selection problems and technical difficulties but have the best long-term outcomes. In the future we will see an older population as general care improves, and some cohorts will perhaps never reach transplantation. For the moment, however, they remain central to the science and art of lung transplantation.

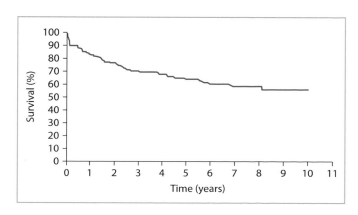

Figure 22.5 Late survival after lung transplantation for cystic fibrosis.

REFERENCES

1. O'Sullivan BP, Freedman SD. Cystic fibrosis. Lancet 2009;373:1891-1904.
2. Dodge JA, Lewis PA, Stanton M, Wilsher J. Cystic fibrosis mortality and survival in the UK: 1947-2003. Eur Respir J 2007;29:522-526.
3. Massie J, Castellani C, Grody WW. Carrier screening for cystic fibrosis in the new era of medications that restore CFTR function. Lancet 2014;383:923-925.
4. Yusen RD, Edwards LB, Kucheryavaya AY, et al. The Registry of the International Society for Heart and Lung Transplantation: Thirty-first adult lung and heart-lung transplant report—2014; focus theme: Retransplantation. J Heart Lung Transplant 2014;33:1009-1024.
5. Benden C, Goldfarb SB, Edwards LB, et al. The Registry of the International Society for Heart and Lung Transplantation: Seventeenth official pediatric lung and heart-lung transplantation report—2014; focus theme: Retransplantation. J Heart Lung Transplant 2014;33:1025-1033.
6. Valapour M, Skeans MA, Heubner BM, et al. OPTN/SRTR 2012 annual data report: Lung. Am J Transplant 2014;14(Suppl 1):139-165.
7. McDonnell MJ, Ward C, Lordan JL, Rutherford RM. Non–cystic fibrosis bronchiectasis. QJM 2013;106:709-715.
8. Weill D, Benden C, Corris PA, et al. A consensus document for the selection of lung transplant candidates: 2014—an update from the Pulmonary Transplantation Council of the International Society for Heart and Lung Transplantation. J Heart Lung Transplant 2015;34:1-15.
9. Luong ML, Chaparro C, Stephenson A, et al. Pretransplant *Aspergillus* colonization of cystic fibrosis patients and the incidence of post–lung transplant invasive aspergillosis. Transplantation 2014;97:351-357.
10. Alexander BD Petzold EW, Reller LB et al. Survival after lung transplantation of cystic fibrosis patients infected with *Burkholderia cepacia* complex. Am J Transplant 2008;8:1025-1030.
11. De Soyza A, Meachery G, Hester KL et al. Lung transplantation for patients with cystic fibrosis and *Burkholderia cepacia* complex infection: A single-center experience. J Heart Lung Transplant 2010;29:1395-1404.
12. Lobo LJ Chang LC, Esther CR Jr. Lung transplant outcomes in cystic fibrosis patients with pre-operative *Mycobacterium abscessus* respiratory infections. Clin Transplant 25:1447-1455.
13. Qvist T, Pressler T, Hoiby N, Katzenstein TL. Shifting paradigms of nontuberculous mycobacteria in cystic fibrosis. Respir Res 2014;15:41.
14. Dusmet M, Winton TL, Kesten S, Maurer J. Previous intrapleural procedures do not adversely affect lung transplantation. J Heart Lung Transplant 1996;15:249-254.
15. Curtis HJ, Bourke SJ, Dark JH, Corris PA. Lung transplantation outcome in cystic fibrosis patients with previous pneumothorax. J Heart Lung Transplant 2005;24:865-869.
16. Rolla M, Anile M, Venuta F, et al. Lung transplantation for cystic fibrosis after thoracic surgical procedures. Transplant Proc 2011;43:1162-1163.
17. Shiegmura N, Bhama J, Gries CJ, et al. Lung transplantation in patients wih prior cardiothoracic surgical procedures. Am J Transplant 2012;12:1249-1255.
18. Forty J, Hasan A, Gould FK, et a;. Single lung transplantation with simultaneous contralateral pneumonectomy for cystic fibrosis. J Heart Lung Transplant 1994;13:727-730.
19. Le Pimpec-Barthes F, Thomas PA, Bonnette P, et al. Single-lung transplantation in patients with previous contralateral pneumonectomy: Technical aspects and results. Eur J Cardiothorac Surg 2009;36:927-932.
20. Frist WH, Fox MD, Campbell PW, et al. Cystic fibrosis treated with heart-lung transplantation: North American results. Transplant Proc 1991;23:1205-1206.
21. Yacoub MH BN, Khaghani A et al. Heart lung transplantation for cystic fibrosis and subsequent domino heart transplantation. J Heart Transplant 1990;9:459-467.
22. Kaiser LR, Pasque MK, Trulock EP, et al. Bilateral sequential lung transplantation: The procedure of choice for double-lung replacement. Ann Thorac Surg 1991;52:438-445; discussion 445-446.
23. Hasan A, Corris PA, Healy M, et al. Bilateral sequential lung transplantation for end stage septic lung disease. Thorax 1995;50:565-566.
24. Diamond JM, Lee JC, Kawut SM, et al. Clinical risk factors for primary graft dysfunction after lung transplantation. Am J Respir Crit Care Med 2013;187:527-534.
25. Machuca TN, Collaud S, Mercier O, et al. Outcomes of intraoperative ECMO versus cardiopulmonary bypass for lung transplantation. J Thorac Cardiovasc Surg 2015;149:1152-1157.
26. Perry JD, Riley G, Johnston S, et al. Activity of disinfectants against gram-negative bacilli isolated from patients undergoing lung transplantation for cystic fibrosis. J Heart Lung Transplant 2002;21:1230-1231.
27. Colquhoun IW, Gascoigne AD, Au J, et al. Airway complications after pulmonary transplantation. Ann Thorac Surg 1994;57:141-145.
28. Mitilian D, Sage E, Puyo P, et al. Techniques and results of lobar lung transplantations. Eur J Cardiothorac Surg 2014;45:365-369; discussion 369-370.

29. Wells WJ, Barr ML. The ethics of living donor lung transplantation. Thorac Surg Clin 2005;15:519-525.

30. Barr ML, Schenkel FA, Bowdish ME, Starnes VA. Living donor lobar lung transplantation: Current status and future directions. Transplant Proc 2005;37:3983-3986.

31. Sweet S. Paediatric living donor lobar lung transplantation. Pediatr Transplant 2006;10:861-868.

32. Date H, Sato M, Aoyama A, et al. Living-donor lobar lung transplantation provides similar survival to cadaveric lung transplantation even for very ill patients. Eur J Cardiothorac Surg 2014;47:967-973.

33. Barshes NR, DiBardino DJ, McKenzie ED, et al. Combined lung and liver transplantation: The United States experience. Transplantation 2005;80:1161-1167.

34. Wolf JH, Sulewski ME, Cassuto JR, et al. Simultaneous thoracic and abdominal transplantation: Can we justify two organs for one recipient? Am J Transplant 2013;13:1806-1816.

35. Beirne PA, Banner NR, Khaghani A, et al. Lung transplantation for non–cystic fibrosis bronchiectasis: A 13 year experience. J Heart Lung Transplant 2005;24:1530-1535.

36. Tkebuchava T, Niederhauser U, Weder W, et al. Kartagener's syndrome: Clinical presentation and cardiosurgical aspects. Ann Thorac Surg 1996;62:1474-1479.

37. Rabago G, Copeland JG 3rd, Rosapepe F, et al. Heart-lung transplantation in situs inversus. Ann Thorac Surg. 1996;62:296-298.

38. Sidney Filho LA, Machuca TN, Camargo Jde J, et al. Lung transplantation without the use of cardiopulmonary bypass in a patient with Kartagener syndrome. J Bras Pneumol 2012;38: 806-809.

39. Burguete SR, Levine SM, Restrepo MI, et al. Lung transplantation for Williams-Campbell syndrome with a probable familial association. Respir Care 2012;57:1505-1508.

40. Eberlein M, Geist LJ, Mullan BF, et al. Long-term success after bilateral lung transplantation for Mounier-Kuhn syndrome: A physiological description. Ann Am Thorac Soc 2013;10:534-537.

41. Meachery G, De Soyza A, Nicholson A. Outcomes of lung transplantation for cystic fibrosis in a large UK cohort. Thorax 2008;63:725-731.

42. Liou TG, Cahill BC. Pediatric lung transplantation for cystic fibrosis. Transplantation 2008;86:636-637.

43. Gruber S, Eiwegger T, Nachbaur E, et al. Lung transplantation in children and young adults: A 20-year single-center experience. Eur Respir J 2012;40:462-469.

23

Lung transplantation for pulmonary hypertension

STÉPHANE COLLAUD AND MARC DE PERROT

INTRODUCTION

Pulmonary hypertension (PH) is not a disease per se but a medical condition that develops as an adaptive response to increased resistance of downstream blood flow. It is defined as a mean pulmonary arterial pressure (PAP) of 25 mm Hg or higher at rest, as assessed by right-heart catheterization.[1] If uncontrolled, PH is a life-threatening condition with a poor prognosis related to secondary right ventricular failure.

Diagnosis of PH is often delayed because its early symptoms, including fatigue or dyspnea on exertion, are nonspecific. As the disease evolves, symptoms and clinical signs of right ventricular failure, such as angina or syncope on exertion or ascites and peripheral edema, appear.

The World Health Organization (WHO) classification of PH into five groups is based on similarities in pathophysiologic mechanisms, clinical findings, and therapeutic approach. It was last updated in 2013 (Table 23.1).[2,3] The previous classification of PH as primary (without an identified

cause) or secondary (with an identified cause) should no longer be used.

When PH is suspected, investigation should be aimed at confirming the diagnosis and clarifying its cause. Figure 23.1 depicts the algorithm for diagnosis and treatment of PH that has been suggested by the European Society of Cardiology and the European Respiratory Society in their recent guidelines.[1]

TREATMENT OF PATIENTS WITH PULMONARY HYPERTENSION

Baseline assessment

Assessment of disease severity, in terms of both exercise capacity and hemodynamics, is of paramount importance because it will serve as a baseline for evaluating response to treatment throughout the disease's progression. Stratification of impairment in exercise capacity is best performed by using the WHO functional classification

Table 23.1 Updated World Health Organization classification of pulmonary hypertension

1. PAH
    1.1. Idiopathic PAH
    1.2. Heritable PAH
        1.2.1. BMPR2
        1.2.2. ALK1, ENG, SMAD9, CAV1, KCNK3
        1.2.3. Unknown
    1.3. Drug and toxin induced
    1.4. Associated with
        1.4.1. Connective tissue disease
        1.4.2. HIV infection
        1.4.3. Portal hypertension
        1.4.4. Congenital heart disease
        1.4.5. Schistosomiasis
1'. Pulmonary venoocclusive disease, pulmonary capillary hemangiomatosis, or both
1". Persistent pulmonary hypertension of the newborn
2. Pulmonary hypertension resulting from left-heart disease
    2.1. Left ventricular systolic dysfunction
    2.2. Left ventricular diastolic dysfunction
    2.3. Valvular disease
    2.4. Congenital or acquired left-heart inflow/outflow tract obstruction and congenital cardiomyopathies
3. Pulmonary hypertension resulting from lung disease, hypoxia, or both
    3.1. Chronic obstructive pulmonary disease
    3.2. Interstitial lung disease
    3.3. Other pulmonary diseases with mixed restrictive and obstructive pattern
    3.4. Sleep-disordered breathing
    3.5. Alveolar hypoventilation disorders
    3.6. Chronic exposure to high altitude
    3.7. Developmental lung diseases
4. Chronic thromboembolic pulmonary hypertension
5. Pulmonary hypertension with unclear multifactorial mechanisms
    5.1. Hematologic disorders: chronic hemolytic anemia, myeloproliferative disorders, splenectomy
    5.2. Systemic disorders: sarcoidosis, pulmonary histiocytosis, lymphangioleiomyomatosis
    5.3. Metabolic disorders: glycogen storage disease, Gaucher disease, thyroid disorders
    5.4. Others: tumoral obstruction, fibrosing mediastinitis, chronic renal failure, segmental pulmonary hypertension

Source: Adapted from Simonneau G, Gatzoulis MA, Adatia I, et al. Updated clinical classification of pulmonary hypertension. J Am Coll Cardiol 2013;62(Suppl 25):D34-D41.

Note: ALK-1, activin receptor–like kinase; BMPR2, bone morphogenic protein receptor type II; CAV1, caveolin-1; ENG, endoglin; HIV, human immunodeficiency virus; KCNK3, potassium channel subfamily K member 3; PAH, pulmonary arterial hypertension; SMAD9, mothers against decapentaplegic homolog 9.

(Table 23.2), as well as the 6-minute walk test. Hemodynamic parameters relevant to pulmonary circulation are estimated initially by echocardiography and subsequently confirmed by right-heart catheterization.

Medical therapy

Initial medical treatment of PH is known as primary therapy, and in patients whose PH meets the criteria of WHO classification groups 2 through 5, it targets the underlying cause. In the case of persistent PH or in symptomatic patients with group 1 PH, specific treatment of PAH is considered. Treatment for PAH aims at treating the actual PH. Drugs available include prostanoids (e.g., epoprostenol, treprostinil, and iloprost), endothelin receptor antagonists (e.g., bosentan, ambrisentan, and macitentan), phosphodiesterase-5 inhibitors (e.g., sildenafil and tadalafil), soluble guanylate cyclase stimulants (e.g., riociguat), and rarely, calcium channel blockers (e.g., nifedipine and diltiazem). Combination therapy with two agents having different mechanisms of action is generally used in cases in which single-drug therapy has failed.

Creation of a right-to-left shunt

Atrial septostomy and Potts shunt are part of the armamentarium for palliative treatment of patients with PH. Atrial septostomy consists of creating a right-to-left shunt, which

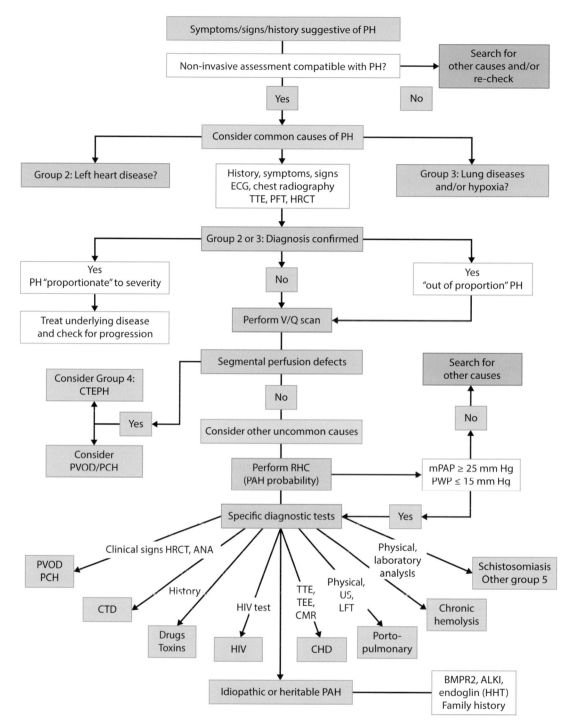

Figure 23.1 Diagnostic algorithm. ALK1, activin receptor–like kinase 1; ANA, antinuclear antibodies; BMPR2, bone morphogenetic protein receptor 2; CHD, congenital heart disease; CMR, cardiac magnetic resonance; CTD, connective tissue disease; CTEPH, chronic thromboembolic pulmonary hypertension; ECG, electrocardiography; Group, clinical group (see Table 23.4); HHT, hereditary hemorrhagic telangiectasia; HIV, human immunodeficiency virus; HRCT, high-resolution computed tomography; LFT, liver function tests; mPAP, mean pulmonary arterial pressure; PAH, pulmonary arterial hypertension; PCH, pulmonary capillary hemangiomatosis; PFT, pulmonary function test; PH, pulmonary hypertension; PVOD, pulmonary veno-occlusive disease; PWP, pulmonary wedge pressure; RHC, right-heart catheterization; TEE, transesophageal echocardiography; TTE, transthoracic echocardiography; US, ultrasonography; V/Q scan, ventilation-perfusion lung scan.

allows increased systemic cardiac output and therefore end-organ oxygen delivery, albeit while sacrificing the absolute value of peripheral oxygen saturation. In contrast to atrial septostomy, which connects the right and left atria, a Potts shunt connects the left pulmonary artery to the descending aorta, thereby limiting the hypoxemia to the lower part of the body.[4,5] The Potts shunt has been particularly successful in palliating pediatric patients with suprasystemic PH.

Table 23.2 World Health Organization functional classification of pulmonary hypertension

Class	Description
I	Patients with asymptomatic PH
II	Patients with PH and symptoms during ordinary physical activity
III	Patients with PH and symptoms during less than ordinary physical activity
IV	Patients with PH resulting in an inability to carry out any physical activity without symptoms. Symptoms may be present at rest. Presence of sign of right-sided heart failure

Source: Adapted from Rich S. Primary pulmonary hypertension: Executive summary. Evian, France: World Health Organization; 1998.

Note: PH, pulmonary hypertension; Symptoms include fatigue, dyspnea, chest pain, syncope.

Transplantation

Transplantation improves both the survival and quality of life of patients with end-stage lung disease. Transplantation for PH is considered when patients with PH in WHO classification groups 1, 3, 4, and 5 are unresponsive to medical therapy.[2] This chapter focuses mainly on the surgical treatment of patients with group 1 PH because their surgical management is the most challenging.

Patients with group 1 PH who have pulmonary venoocclusive disease and pulmonary capillary hemangiomatosis should be referred for transplantation assessment as soon as the diagnosis is established because no other viable medical therapy is available.[1] Patients with group 3 PH (PH resulting from lung disease, hypoxia, or both) or group 5 PH (PH with unclear multifactorial mechanisms) are discussed elsewhere in this book. Timing for referral and indications for transplantation follow the criteria for the primary underlying disease. In principle, patients with group 4 PH (chronic thromboembolic PH) can also be candidates for transplantation; however, thanks to the current success of pulmonary endarterectomy, transplantation is now indicated for very few such patients.[6] Hence, all patients with a new diagnosis of PH should have a ventilation-perfusion scan performed and in the presence of mismatched perfusion defects be seen by an experienced surgical center to determine the feasibility of pulmonary endarterectomy.

PULMONARY ARTERIAL HYPERTENSION

WHO classification group 1 defines patients with pulmonary arterial hypertension (PAH). PAH is idiopathic, heritable, and induced by drugs or toxins or associated with connective tissue disease, human immunodeficiency virus (HIV), portal hypertension, congenital heart disease, or schistosomiasis. The surgically relevant entities in group 1 are reviewed later. Patients with PAH related to HIV or schistosomiasis are not currently candidates for transplantation.

Medical therapy for patients with most types of PAH consists of advanced therapy targeting the actual PH. Tremendous recent progress in advanced medical therapy has led to a decrease in patient referrals to transplant centers.[6] However, because PAH will typically progress despite therapy, lung or combined heart-lung transplantation remains the therapy of choice for patients who are unresponsive to medical treatment. In a study from the Toronto Lung Transplant Program, 11% of nearly 3000 referred patients had PAH.[7] The most common indications for transplantation were idiopathic pulmonary arterial hypertension, followed by PAH associated with connective tissue disease and PAH associated with congenital heart disease.

Biology, pathology, and physiology of pulmonary arterial hypertension

PAH probably develops because of a combination of environmental factors and genetic predisposition to pulmonary vascular disease. Environmental factors may include additional acquired genetic mutation, viral infection (including HIV), a chronic inflammatory condition (connective tissue disease), drugs (appetite suppressants), and variations in the hemodynamics of the pulmonary circulation (congenital systemic-to-pulmonary shunts). Mutations with a role in PAH have been found in genes encoding for bone morphogenetic protein receptor type II (BMPR2), activin receptor–like kinase 1 (ALK1), 5-hydroxytryptamine transporter (5HTT), endoglin (ENG), mothers against decapentaplegic homolog 9 (SMAD9), caveolin-1 (CAV1), and potassium channel subfamily K member 3 (KCNK3).[8-14] Genetic predisposition and exposure to environmental factors probably lead to dysregulation of the microenvironment of the lung, which in turn results in an imbalance between agents with promitotic or vasoconstrictive (endothelin) and antimitotic or vasodilatative (nitric oxide, prostacyclin) effects.[15] Indeed, an increase in the production of endothelin, as well as a lack of nitric oxide and prostacyclin production, has been suggested in different studies.[16-21] Consequently, vasoconstriction and vascular remodeling occur, which in turn leads to increased pulmonary vascular resistance (PVR) and PH.

The association between increased PVR and PH is well described by the following adaptation of the modern form of Ohm's law to hemodynamics:

$$Pressure\ variations = Flow \times Resistance$$

Therefore, an increase in pulmonary resistance results in PH in patients with idiopathic and heritable PAH, PAH related to connective tissue disease, HIV infection, or Eisenmenger syndrome. An increase in pulmonary flow (at least initially) results in PH in patients with PAH associated with portal hypertension or congenital heart defects. Indeed, the increase in pulmonary flow is due to portal-to-systemic and systemic-to-pulmonary shunts for PAH, which are related to portal hypertension and congenital heart defects, respectively.

Idiopathic and heritable pulmonary arterial hypertension

Idiopathic PAH accounts for 39% of all PAH and is therefore the most common type.[22] Idiopathic PAH is diagnosed in the absence of evidence of a risk factor or a family history of PAH; therefore, diagnosis of idiopathic PAH is a diagnosis of exclusion.[1] Patients of both sexes and all ages can be affected, but women in their 30s to 60s are at higher risk.[22] In the results of an analysis of data in a national registry, no features differentiating patients with idiopathic PAH from those with hereditary PAH were found except for the fact that despite their similar hemodynamic impairments, those with hereditary PAH had better exercise tolerance.[23]

Germline mutation in BMPR2, which is a member of the transforming growth factor β (TGF-β) signaling pathway, is detected in up to 80% of patients with heritable PAH.[23] Gene transmission is autosomal dominant with incomplete penetrance.[8] Other forms of heritable PAH lack BMPR2 mutations. In patients with PAH related to hereditary hemorrhagic telangiectasia or Osler-Weber-Rendu syndrome, mutations of the *ALK1* (a type I receptor of the TGF-β superfamily) and *ENG* genes were found.[24]

Drug- and toxin-induced pulmonary arterial hypertension

Many drugs are thought to play a role in the development of PAH. In their recent guidelines for the diagnosis and treatment of PH, the European Society of Cardiology and the European Respiratory Society have stratified the risk posed by different drugs and toxins for the development of PAH (Table 23.3).[1] Notably, despite the fact that reversibility of PAH after withdrawal of appetite suppressants is uncommon, treatment of such patients by transplantation is the exception.

Pulmonary arterial hypertension associated with congenital heart disease

The most common congenital heart defects are congenital systemic-to-pulmonary shunts (or left-to-right shunts). They include atrial septal defects, ventricular septal defects, atrioventricular septal defects, and patent ductus arteriosus. In cases of delayed or no repair, a left-to-right shunt creates chronic volume (and pressure) overload into the pulmonary circulation. It induces shear stress that disrupts the vascular endothelium. Endothelial dysfunction results in the activation of vascular remodeling, which in turn leads to increasing PVR and progression of PH. When PVR reaches systemic vascular resistance, inversion of the shunt occurs and it becomes a pulmonary-to-systemic (or right-to-left) shunt. The symptoms and clinical signs associated with this shunt inversion define Eisenmenger syndrome.

Table 23.3 Updated level of risk posed by drugs and toxins known to induce pulmonary arterial hypertension

Definite
- Aminorex
- Fenfluramine
- Dexfenfluramine
- Toxic rapeseed oil
- Benfluorex

Possible
- Cocaine
- Phenylpropanolamine
- St. John's wort
- Chemotherapeutic agents
- Selective serotonin reuptake inhibitors
- Pergolide

Likely
- Amphetamines
- L-Tryptophan
- Methamphetamines

Unlikely
- Oral contraceptives
- Estrogen
- Cigarette smoking

Source: From Galie N, Hoeper MM, Humbert M, et al. Guidelines for the diagnosis and treatment of pulmonary hypertension: The Task Force for the Diagnosis and Treatment of Pulmonary Hypertension of the European Society of Cardiology (ESC) and the European Respiratory Society (ERS), endorsed by the International Society of Heart and Lung Transplantation (ISHLT). Eur Heart J 2009;30:2493-2537.

Pulmonary arterial hypertension associated with portal hypertension

PAH associated with portal hypertension defines portopulmonary hypertension (POPAH). POPAH is most commonly associated with liver cirrhosis, but other cause of portal hypertension are described. It is a rare condition that is found in up to 6% of patients with portal hypertension.[25]

Although the mortality associated with liver transplantation is related to the severity of PAP, liver transplantation does not usually reverse POPAH.[26,27] Therefore, a combined lung-liver transplantation is to be considered if PAP does not respond to targeted medical therapy.

Pulmonary arterial hypertension associated with connective tissue disease

Scleroderma (or systemic sclerosis) is the connective tissue disease most frequently associated with PAH. PAH has been found in 7% to 12% of a population with scleroderma.[28,29] Systemic lupus erythematosus, mixed connective tissue disease, rheumatoid arthritis, primary Sjögren syndrome, and dermatomyositis may all be associated with PAH.

Patients with connective tissue disease (especially scleroderma) may be offered lung transplantation for end-stage lung disease. However, patient selection plays an important role because of the potential multiorgan involvement in the disease, which would preclude candidacy for transplantation.

TIMING OF REFERRAL AND LISTING FOR LUNG TRANSPLANTATION

The timing of listing of patients with PAH for lung transplantation remains particularly challenging because of the difficulty of predicting the resilience of the right ventricle and the wait time until surgery. In general, patients who remain in functional class III or IV despite having received maximal medical therapy should be listed for transplantation. Patients with refractory right ventricular failure despite initiation of intravenous prostacyclin therapy and patients with pulmonary venoocclusive disease or pulmonary capillary hemangiomatosis should also be listed for transplantation.

The timing of referral for pretransplantation evaluation varies by transplant center. However, proceeding with earlier rather than later referral is recommended because predicting patients' clinical course in response to medical therapy can be difficult. Early referral will give patients and the transplant center time to review the assessment process and detect potential problems. In our own practice in Toronto, we have recommended that the lung transplantation referral be performed when patients are being considered for intravenous prostacyclin therapy. Patients who respond to intravenous therapy adequately will not be listed. However, this early referral allows us to proceed to listing rapidly if the response to intravenous therapy is not as good as expected. In addition, early referral allows us to consider extracorporeal life support (ECLS) even on an urgent basis because the patient will already be familiar with the option of transplantation.

BRIDGE TO LUNG TRANSPLANTATION

Because of the difficulty of determining the optimal timing for listing of patients with PAH, the mortality rate of patients with PAH while on the waiting list has been high (approximately 20%). Since implementation of the lung allocation score in the United States in 2005, the rate of mortality while on the waiting list has remained high for patients with idiopathic PAH because of the lack of specific markers for determining the severity of right ventricular failure during calculation of the lung allocation score.[30] Hence, options to bridge patients with PAH to lung transplantation have been particularly important. ECLS in particular has been able to dramatically reduce the waiting list mortality of patients with PAH over the past few years.

Balloon atrial septostomy

Balloon atrial septostomy entails creating an interatrial right-to-left shunt, thereby allowing decompression of the right heart and increasing left ventricular preload and

cardiac output.[31] This option can be particularly dangerous in patients with decompensated right-sided heart failure and has been largely abandoned in our institution since the 2006 implementation of ECLS as a bridge to transplantation for patients with PAH and severe ventricular failure refractory to inotropic support.[32]

Extracorporeal life support

ECLS for patients with PH should aim to support cardiac function without compromising oxygenation. Hence, the venoarterial extracorporeal membrane oxygenation (VA ECMO) and the pulmonary artery–left atrium (PA-LA) Novalung (Heilbronn, Germany) have been used successfully.[33] In general, once ECLS has been established, patients can be weaned off inotropic support, specific PH therapy drugs, or both. The required anticoagulation is provided with heparin and a target activated clotting time between 160 and 200 seconds until transplantation.

VA ECMO is used as a parallel circuit to the heart and lungs and leads to improvement in patients' hemodynamics and gas exchange. The cannulas are usually inserted under local anesthesia, with femoral access favored. Rarely, the internal jugular vein and axillary artery are used. Inflow and outflow cannulas are connected to a heparin-coated circuit driven by a centrifugal pump.

When connected between the pulmonary artery and left atrium, the Novalung device functions as a pumpless parallel circuit to the lungs only. It unloads the right ventricle, allows blood oxygenation as well as carbon dioxide removal, and increases cardiac output by increasing left ventricular filling. Insertion of femorofemoral VA-ECMO support under local anesthesia precedes the general anesthesia and sternotomy for PA-LA Novalung insertion. The outflow cannula is inserted into the main pulmonary arterial trunk and the inflow cannula into the left atrium through the right superior pulmonary vein. No pump is required because right ventricular contractions drive blood flow into the circuit.

The choice between the two ECLS modes varies according to centers' expertise. Table 23.4 provides the advantages and disadvantages of both the VA ECMO and PA-LA Novalung.[33] Use of ECLS has profoundly changed the fate of patients with PH who were bridged to transplantation. In our experience, the rate of mortality while on the waiting list for patients with idiopathic PAH decreased from 22% in the pre-ECLS era (1998 to 2005) to 0% with the routine use of ECLS (2006 to 2010), whereas posttransplantation survival remained similar.[32]

TRANSPLANTATION

Single-lung transplantation (SLT), bilateral lung transplantation (BLT), and heart-lung transplantation (HLT) have been described for the treatment of end-stage PH. SLT for PH has been largely abandoned because of the adverse early and late outcomes when compared with those of BLT or HLT, and BLT has become the procedure most commonly

Table 23.4 Characteristics of two extracorporeal life support modes used in patients with arterial hypertension as a bridge to transplantation

Characteristics	VA ECMO	PA-LA ECMO
Advantages	Local anesthesia	Pumpless
	Safe and fast	Long-term bridge
	Can be maintained after transplantation	Allows mobilization
Disadvantages	Arterial complications	General anesthesia
	No mobilization (except for right internal jugular vein and axillary artery cannulation)	Sternotomy required
		Normal left ventricular function required
Indications	Adult recipients	Pediatric or small recipients
	Predicted short waiting time	Predicted long waiting time
	Emergency cases	

Source: Modified from Granton J, Mercier O, De Perrot M. et al, Management of severe pulmonary arterial hypertension. Semin Respir Crit Care Med 2013;34:700-713.

Note: VA ECMO, venoarterial extracorporeal membrane oxygenation; PA-LA, pulmonary artery–left atrium extracorporeal membrane oxygenation.

performed for this indication. In the latest report of the International Society for Heart and Lung Transplantation registry, 87 single-lung transplants, 1073 bilateral lung transplants, and 890 heart-lung transplants were performed for idiopathic PAH between January 1995 and June 2012, thus representing 0.6% of all adult single-lung transplants, 4.6% of all adult bilateral lung transplants, and 27.5% of all adult heart-lung transplants, respectively.[34]

Indications for BLT or HLT vary among centers and depend on organ availability and clinical experience. In our center, HLT is considered for patients with evidence of severe left ventricular dysfunction (left ventricular ejection fraction less than 40%) on the echocardiogram, the presence of technical limitations to performance of BLT (such as complex uncorrectable cardiac defects), or both.[7] BLT is performed in all other patients, even if severe right ventricular failure is present. Indeed, BLT will generally lead to sustained recovery of right ventricular function. However, the choice between BLT and HLT is not always straightforward because the left ventricular function of patients with severe right ventricular failure may have been overestimated during evaluation of their echocardiograms in connection with low cardiac output.

The techniques of transplantation are largely described elsewhere.[35,36] Here, we will note that lung transplantation for PH is routinely performed while patients are on cardiopulmonary bypass or, more recently, while they are being supported with VA-ECMO. HLT is performed through clamshell or sternotomy incisions. In our experience, a clamshell incision is selected for use with patients in whom pleural adhesions, bleeding from large bronchial vessels in the posterior mediastinum, or both is anticipated.

POSTOPERATIVE MANAGEMENT

In addition to addressing patients' underlying disease, early care after transplantation focuses on cardiopulmonary management, immunosuppression to prevent rejection, and prophylaxis and treatment of infection. Postoperative management of patients with PH necessitates consideration of some important potential pathophysiologic complications, including right ventricular hypertrophy with a risk for outflow tract obstruction if patients are kept too dry (suicidal right ventricle), fluid overload resulting from severe preoperative right ventricular failure, and left ventricular dysfunction because of a sudden increase in cardiac output through the pulmonary vasculature. All three of these potential complications increase the risk for severe primary graft dysfunction (PGD), which has traditionally been a major problem after BLT for PAH. However, increasing knowledge and understanding of the pathophysiology of patients with PAH have resulted in substantial improvement in their care after transplantation.[7] A recent report from the Toronto Lung Transplant Program compared two different eras and found that the 30-day mortality rate for recipients with PAH decreased from 24% in 1997 to 2004 to 6% in 2005 to 2010.

After transplantation for a condition other than PH, patients can occasionally be extubated in the operating room or within the first few hours after surgery. For patients with PH, sedation and ventilatory support are generally maintained for at least 48 to 72 hours. This process is meant to stabilize hemodynamics and improve gas exchange while the systemic inflammatory response to surgery and cardiopulmonary bypass resolves. At this time, judicious fluid management is essential. Whereas fluid overload carries an increased risk for lung edema, fluid depletion leads to collapse of the hypertrophied right ventricular outflow tract. Careful intraoperative hemostasis is mandatory for easier postoperative fluid management, which is particularly important in patients with previous surgery (e.g., in those with congenital heart disease). From 48 to 72 hours after transplantation, when the systemic inflammatory response has resolved and capillary leak has decreased, interstitial fluid is redistributed into the vascular compartment, which could potentially lead to lung edema. Consequently, achieving a high negative fluid balance of up to 3 to 5 L in 24 hours is essential at this point. Patients with PAH and severe right ventricular failure will typically have a fluid overload of

10 to 15 L, which will be mobilized within 2 to 3 days after unloading of the right ventricle after the lung transplant. Therefore, using diuretics or ultrafiltration to maintain a targeted negative fluid balance of up to 10 to 15 L (depending on kidney function) for 3 to 4 days is recommended.

Right-heart function

The postoperative course after transplantation for PH is often determined by the function of the right heart. Lung transplantation leads to an immediate reduction in PAP and unloading of the right ventricle and allows increased cardiac output. In a prospective study evaluating patients in the operating room before and after transplantation, mean PAP decreased significantly from 76 ± 14 to 31 ± 11 mm Hg and the cardiac index increased from 2.1 ± 1.4 to 2.6 ± 0.6 L/min/m^2 in the group of patients with a pretransplantation systolic PAP of 75 mm Hg or higher.[37]

Despite the immediate decrease in right ventricular afterload after lung transplantation, various factors altering right ventricular output may trigger right ventricular failure and death. These factors include but are not limited to fluid overload resulting from an increase in right ventricular preload and PGD, pulmonary edema, antibody-mediated rejection (AMR), and atelectasis in response to an increase in right ventricular afterload. In addition, pneumonia and sepsis, as well as arrhythmia (especially atrial arrhythmia), may also decrease right ventricular function and precipitate its failure. Therefore, early detection and treatment of complications, as well as monitoring of right ventricular function, are crucial to minimizing postoperative morbidity and mortality after transplantation for PH.

Primary graft dysfunction

PGD is an injury to the lung that occurs within 72 hours after transplantation. It is characterized by severe hypoxemia and radiographic evidence of lung edema. Its pathophysiology is not understood completely; however, multiple factors from the donor and from the process of retrieval, preservation, and transplantation have been described as potentially affecting the occurrence of PGD.

PH was described as a risk factor for the development of PGD in several studies.[38-41] In another study supporting these results, a progressive increase in risk for PGD with increases in systolic PAP above 60 mm Hg was shown.[42] PGD is a diagnosis of exclusion, and the differential diagnosis includes lung edema resulting from other causes, pneumonia, and atelectasis.

Lung edema from causes other than primary graft dysfunction

ATRIAL CUFF STENOSIS

Rarely, pulmonary edema is the result of a technical problem such as stenosis of the atrial cuff. This complication appears at the time of reperfusion, when the pulmonary arterial clamp is removed. The diagnosis is suspected when lung edema is unilateral, and it can be confirmed by transesophageal echocardiography or intraoperative measurement of pressure in the pulmonary veins and left atrium. Early recognition of the pathology followed by takedown of the anastomosis and a repeat anastomosis is the only viable treatment.

LEFT VENTRICULAR FAILURE

Pulmonary edema secondary to left ventricular dysfunction may develop In patients with chronic PH. Left ventricular dysfunction can be caused by a transient reduction in left ventricular filling resulting from leftward displacement of the intraventricular septum by an enlarged and pressurized right ventricle.[33,43] On a more chronic basis, reduction of left ventricular filling causes left ventricular atrophy. At the time of transplantation, when the cardiac index increases in response to the drop in PVR, the atrophied left ventricle may be overwhelmed and fail, thus leading to pulmonary edema. Treatment is supportive and includes adequate management of fluid, administration of inotropes, and mechanical ventilation. Transesophageal echocardiography provides good evaluation of both volume status and heart function.

ANTIBODY-MEDIATED REJECTION

Massive lung edema after reperfusion associated with allograft dysfunction and the presence of donor-specific antibodies should evoke a diagnosis of AMR. It is considered hyperacute (within 24 hours) or acute (beyond 24 hours) AMR depending on the timing of lung edema after allograft reperfusion. In our center, routine preoperative screening for donor-specific antibodies followed by intraoperative plasmapheresis in cases of a positive virtual cross-match has led to a decreased incidence of AMR.

OUTCOME AFTER TRANSPLANTATION

Transplantation offers improvement in quality of life and survival for patients with end-stage lung disease.

Lung transplantation

Survival benefit varies by indication for lung transplantation. According to the most recent data from the International Society for Heart and Lung Transplantation registry, recipients in whom idiopathic PAH is diagnosed will have a lower 3-month survival rate (78%) than do patients with cystic fibrosis (90%), chronic obstructive pulmonary disease (90%), and interstitial lung disease (85%).[34] However, long-term survival of patients with idiopathic PAH is better than that of patients with most of the other underlying diseases. The 10-year survival rate of patients with idiopathic PAH was 36%; in contrast, those with cystic fibrosis, chronic obstructive pulmonary disease, and interstitial lung disease had 10-year survival rates of 44%, 25%, and 23%, respectively.[34] The early mortality has been linked to the specific characteristics of patients with idiopathic PAH, including preoperative right ventricular dysfunction, routine intraoperative use of cardiopulmonary bypass, and increased risk for PGD.[30]

Heart-lung transplantation

Early mortality after HLT is higher than for BLT but with a similar long-term benefit. In a large study that looked at 219 patients with PH between 1986 and 2008, the in-hospital mortality rates after HLT and BLT were 21.7% and 14.9%, respectively ($P = .24$).[43] This trend of increased mortality with HLT may be explained by the technical difficulty of the procedure. Indeed, in a comparative analysis of the major causes of death within the first 30 days after transplantation, a "technical" cause of death was identified in 21.9% of cases involving HLT as compared with only 11% involving BLT.[34] Long-term survival rates were good: 1-, 5-, 10-, and 15-year survival rates of 70%, 50%, 39%, and 26% for HLT versus 79%, 52%, 43%, and 30% for BLT.[43]

CONCLUSION

With its impact on the right ventricle, PH represents a unique entity in transplantation that requires special consideration. Adequate timing of referral of patients for transplantation assessment and use of ECLS will help decrease patient mortality while on the waiting list. Transplantation and immediate postoperative care for patients with PH should be provided in specialized centers to reduce postoperative morbidity and mortality.

REFERENCES

1. Galie N, Hoeper MM, Humbert M, et al. Guidelines for the diagnosis and treatment of pulmonary hypertension: The Task Force for the Diagnosis and Treatment of Pulmonary Hypertension of the European Society of Cardiology (ESC) and the European Respiratory Society (ERS), endorsed by the International Society of Heart and Lung Transplantation (ISHLT). Eur Heart J 2009;30:2493-2537.
2. Simonneau G, Robbins IM, Beghetti M, et al. Updated clinical classification of pulmonary hypertension. J Am Coll Cardiol 2009;54(Suppl 1):S43-S54.
3. Simonneau G, Gatzoulis MA, Adatia I, et al. Updated clinical classification of pulmonary hypertension. J Am Coll Cardiol 2013;62(Suppl 25):D34-D41.
4. Esch JJ, Shah PB, Cockrill BA, et al. Transcatheter Potts shunt creation in patients with severe pulmonary arterial hypertension: Initial clinical experience. J Heart Lung Transplant 2013;32:381-387.
5. Bhamra-Ariza P, Keogh AM, Muller DW. Percutaneous interventional therapies for the treatment of patients with severe pulmonary hypertension. J Am Coll Cardiol 2014;63:611-618.
6. Keogh AM, Mayer E, Benza RL, et al. Interventional and surgical modalities of treatment in pulmonary hypertension. J Am Coll Cardiol 2009;54(Suppl 1):S67-S77.
7. de Perrot M, Granton JT, McRae K, et al. Outcome of patients with pulmonary arterial hypertension referred for lung transplantation: A 14-year single-center experience. J Thorac Cardiovasc Surg 2012;143:910-918.
8. International PPH Consortium, Lane KB, Machado RD, et al. Heterozygous germline mutations in BMPR2, encoding a TGF-beta receptor, cause familial primary pulmonary hypertension. Nat Genet 2000;26:81-84.
9. Harrison RE, Flanagan JA, Sankelo M, et al. Molecular and functional analysis identifies ALK-1 as the predominant cause of pulmonary hypertension related to hereditary haemorrhagic telangiectasia. J Med Genet 2003;40:865-871.
10. Marcos E, Fadel E, Sanchez O, et al. Serotonin-induced smooth muscle hyperplasia in various forms of human pulmonary hypertension. Circ Res 2004;94:1263-1270.
11. McAllister KA, Grogg KM, Johnson DW, et al. Endoglin, a TGF-beta binding protein of endothelial cells, is the gene for hereditary haemorrhagic telangiectasia type 1. Nat Genet 1994;8:345-351.
12. Austin ED, Ma L, LeDuc C, et al. Whole exome sequencing to identify a novel gene (caveolin-1) associated with human pulmonary arterial hypertension. Circ Cardiovasc Genet 2012;5:336-343.
13. Nasim MT, Ogo T, Ahmed M, et al. Molecular genetic characterization of SMAD signaling molecules in pulmonary arterial hypertension. Hum Mutat 2011;32:1385-1389.
14. Ma L, Roman-Campos D, Austin ED, et al. A novel channelopathy in pulmonary arterial hypertension. N Engl J Med 2013;369:351-361.
15. Humbert M, Morrell NW, Archer SL, et al. Cellular and molecular pathobiology of pulmonary arterial hypertension. J Am Coll Cardiol 2004;43(Suppl 12):13S-24S.
16. Christman BW, McPherson CD, Newman JH, et al. An imbalance between the excretion of thromboxane and prostacyclin metabolites in pulmonary hypertension. N Engl J Med 1992;327:70-75.
17. Giaid A, Saleh D. Reduced expression of endothelial nitric oxide synthase in the lungs of patients with pulmonary hypertension. N Engl J Med 1995;333:214-221.
18. Giaid A, Yanagisawa M, Langleben D, et al. Expression of endothelin-1 in the lungs of patients with pulmonary hypertension. N Engl J Med 1993;328:1732-1739.
19. Archer SL, Djaballah K, Humbert M, et al. Nitric oxide deficiency in fenfluramine- and dexfenfluramine-induced pulmonary hypertension. Am J Respir Crit Care Med 1998;158:1061-1067.

20. Tuder RM, Cool CD, Geraci MW, et al. Prostacyclin synthase expression is decreased in lungs from patients with severe pulmonary hypertension. Am J Respir Crit Care Med 1999;159:1925-1932.

21. Bauer M, Wilkens H, Langer F, et al. Selective upregulation of endothelin B receptor gene expression in severe pulmonary hypertension. Circulation 2002;105:1034-1036.

22. Humbert M, Sitbon O, Chaouat A, et al. Pulmonary arterial hypertension in France: Results from a national registry. Am J Respir Crit Care Med 2006;173:1023-1030.

23. Fessel JP, Loyd JE, Austin ED. The genetics of pulmonary arterial hypertension in the post-BMPR2 era. Pulm Circ 2011;1:305-319.

24. Faughnan ME, Granton JT, Young LH. The pulmonary vascular complications of hereditary haemorrhagic telangiectasia. Eur Respir J 2009;33:1186-1194.

25. Krowka MJ, Swanson KL, Frantz RP, et al. Portopulmonary hypertension: Results from a 10-year screening algorithm. Hepatology 2006;44:1502-1510.

26. Le Pavec J, Souza R, Herve P, et al. Portopulmonary hypertension: Survival and prognostic factors. Am J Respir Crit Care Med 2008;178:637-643.

27. Krowka MJ, Plevak DJ, Findlay JY, et al. Pulmonary hemodynamics and perioperative cardiopulmonary-related mortality in patients with portopulmonary hypertension undergoing liver transplantation. Liver Transpl 2000;6:443-450.

28. Hachulla E, Gressin V, Guillevin L, et al. Early detection of pulmonary arterial hypertension in systemic sclerosis: A French nationwide prospective multi-center study. Arthritis Rheum 2005;52:3792-3800.

29. Mukerjee D, St George D, Coleiro B, et al. Prevalence and outcome in systemic sclerosis associated pulmonary arterial hypertension: Application of a registry approach. Ann Rheum Dis 2003;62:1088-1093.

30. Lordan JL, Corris PA. Pulmonary arterial hypertension and lung transplantation. Expert Rev Respir Med 2011;5:441-454.

31. Galie N, Corris PA, Frost A, et al. Updated treatment algorithm of pulmonary arterial hypertension. J Am Coll Cardiol 2013;62(Suppl 25):D60-D72.

32. de Perrot M, Granton JT, McRae K, et al. Impact of extracorporeal life support on outcome in patients with idiopathic pulmonary arterial hypertension awaiting lung transplantation. J Heart Lung Transplant 2011;30:997-1002.

33. Granton J, Mercier O, De Perrot M. Management of severe pulmonary arterial hypertension. Semin Respir Crit Care Med 2013;34:700-713.

34. Yusen RD, Christie JD, Edwards LB, et al. The Registry of the International Society for Heart and Lung Transplantation: Thirtieth adult lung and heart-lung transplant report—2013; focus theme: Age. J Heart Lung Transplant 2013;32:965-978.

35. Boasquevisque CH, Yildirim E, Waddel TK, Keshavjee S. Surgical techniques: Lung transplant and lung volume reduction. Proc Am Thorac Soc 2009;6:66-78.

36. Vouhe PR, Dartevelle PG. Heart-lung transplantation. Technical modifications that may improve the early outcome. J Thorac Cardiovasc Surg 1989;97:906-910.

37. Katz WE, Gasior TA, Quinlan JJ, et al. Immediate effects of lung transplantation on right ventricular morphology and function in patients with variable degrees of pulmonary hypertension. J Am Coll Cardiol 1996;27:384-391.

38. Whitson BA, Nath DS, Johnson AC, et al. Risk factors for primary graft dysfunction after lung transplantation. J Thorac Cardiovasc Surg 2006;131:73-80.

39. Boujoukos AJ, Martich GD, Vega JD, et al. Reperfusion injury in single-lung transplant recipients with pulmonary hypertension and emphysema. J Heart Lung Transplant 1997;16:439-448.

40. King RC, Binns OA, Rodriguez F, et al. Reperfusion injury significantly impacts clinical outcome after pulmonary transplantation. Ann Thorac Surg 2000;69:1681-1685.

41. Christie JD, Kotloff RM, Pochettino A, et al. Clinical risk factors for primary graft failure following lung transplantation. Chest 2003;124:1232-1241.

42. Kuntz CL, Hadjiliadis D, Ahya VN, et al. Risk factors for early primary graft dysfunction after lung transplantation: A registry study. Clin Tansplant 2009;23:819-830.

43. Fadel E, Mercier O, Mussot S, et al. Long-term outcome of double-lung and heart-lung transplantation for pulmonary hypertension: A comparative retrospective study of 219 patients. Eur J Cardiothorac Surg 2010;38:277-284.

24

Lung transplantation for connective tissue disorders

ABBAS ARDEHALI

Connective tissue disorders (CTDs), which are also referred to as collagen vascular diseases, comprise a heterogeneous group of systemic autoimmune disorders characterized by immune-mediated end-organ dysfunction. CTDs include systemic sclerosis (scleroderma), rheumatoid arthritis, systemic lupus erythematosus, primary Sjögren syndrome, polymyositis and dermatomyositis, mixed CTDs, and undifferentiated CTDs. Consensus statements on the criteria for diagnosis of each of the aforementioned disorders now exist.[1,2] A common feature uniting this heterogeneous group is autoimmune-mediated organ damage, with the lungs being a frequent target.[3] Lung involvement may include the parenchyma, pleura, airways, or vasculature and combinations thereof. All patients with CTDs are at risk for the development of interstitial lung disease (ILD); however, ILD is more likely to occur in patients with systemic sclerosis and rheumatoid arthritis than in those with other CTDs.[4] Many patients have a subclinical form of ILD that although evident on a high-resolution computed tomography (HRCT) scan, may remain asymptomatic for decades. The ILD associated with CTDs generally has a better prognosis than does idiopathic interstitial pneumonia of equivalent severity.[5] Which patients with CTD-associated lung diseases should receive therapy is unknown. No data to support initiation of any type of immunosuppressive therapies in patients with CTD and asymptomatic or mild ILD exist. In cases involving more severe forms of ILD or symptomatic patients, the following factors are usually considered when starting immunosuppressive therapies: severity of lung disease, rate of progression, underlying CTDs and extrapulmonary disease activity, patients' age and comorbid conditions, and likelihood of a response (assessed on the basis of radiographic patterns). Although these factors may reflect expert opinion and guidelines, little or no robust evidence-based data on when and how to treat patients with CTD and advanced or symptomatic ILD are available.[6] An exception is the body of data on patients with systemic sclerosis, who constitute a population that is discussed further in the following section. Patients with CTD refractory end-stage ILD are considered for lung transplantation. Historically, such patients were considered poor candidates for lung transplantation because of the systemic nature of their disease and the advanced stages of presentation (characterized by debilitation and overt immunosuppression). With the improved outcomes in lung transplantation and some success in the management of extrapulmonary diseases, lung transplantation is increasingly being considered for selected patients with CTDs who otherwise meet the criteria for lung transplantation. Most of the data on lung transplantation in cases involving CTDs concern patients with systemic sclerosis. Consequently, this chapter focuses on lung transplantation in patients with systemic sclerosis.

SYSTEMIC SCLEROSIS AND LUNG TRANSPLANTATION

Scleroderma is a Greek word meaning "hard skin." Scleroderma, or systemic sclerosis, is a systemic autoimmune disorder characterized by endothelial and fibroblast dysfunction that leads to excess collagen deposition and tissue fibrosis. This condition is classified into two classes on the basis of the extent of skin involvement: (1) diffuse cutaneous sclerosis and (2) limited cutaneous sclerosis. Systemic sclerosis, as the name implies, may involve any organ including the lung, the gastrointestinal tract, the kidneys, the heart, and of course the skin. Lung involvement in systemic sclerosis may be due to direct fibrotic involvement, which in turn leads to ILD with or without pulmonary hypertension. In addition, systemic sclerosis can also affect the pulmonary system indirectly by creating a predisposition to gastroesophageal reflux and aspiration, infections, chest wall involvement, or possibly cardiac involvement. Although more than 90% of patients with systemic sclerosis have interstitial parenchymal disease that would be evident by HRCT,[7] only one fourth of patients with systemic sclerosis will manifest clinically significant parenchymal lung disease within 3 years of diagnosis. As expected, these patients demonstrate a reduction in forced vital capacity and diffusing capacity of the lung for carbon monoxide on pulmonary function tests.

In addition to parenchymal lung involvement, pulmonary hypertension is also likely to develop in patients with systemic sclerosis. The incidence of pulmonary hypertension ranges from 13% to 35%.[8,9] Different classes of pulmonary vasodilator agents have been studied in patients with systemic sclerosis and pulmonary hypertension as part of larger studies. Although none of these studies have demonstrated a survival benefit, many have shown an improvement in patients' exercise tolerance.

TREATMENT OPTIONS

The treatments for patients with systemic sclerosis who have clinically significant ILD are limited. Although used historically, steroids have never been proved efficacious in cases of systemic sclerosis. In fact, data suggest that higher doses may be associated with scleroderma renal crisis.[10,11] Mycophenolate mofetil is being used for the treatment of patients with ILD with increasing frequency but without robust evidence.[12] A study of scleroderma lung disease has shown that in patients with acute symptomatic lung disease, 1 year of oral cyclophosphamide may improve symptoms and reduce skin thickness.[13] In general, patients with systemic sclerosis who have progressive or symptomatic ILD are usually treated with mycophenolate mofetil, cyclophosphamide, or both, depending on their tolerance profile and response. Associated pulmonary hypertension may be managed with the addition of a pulmonary vasodilator for symptomatic improvement. A progressive decline in pulmonary function test results or worsening of symptoms despite optimal medical therapy may lead to patients being considered for lung transplantation.

Like those with other CTDs, patients with systemic sclerosis have been considered poor candidates for lung transplantation because of the systemic nature of their disease (e.g., renal crisis) and concern regarding gastroesophageal reflux disease and risk for aspiration. In fact, many lung transplant centers have excluded patients with systemic sclerosis and significant gastroesophageal reflux, esophageal aperistalsis, or both. However, several reports in the past decade have shown that selected patients with systemic

sclerosis can undergo lung transplantation with acceptable outcomes.

GASTROINTESTINAL DISORDERS

Gastroesophageal motility disorders are present in nearly all patients with systemic sclerosis.[6] The subgroup of patients with ILD has a higher incidence of esophageal motility disorder, lower esophageal sphincter tone, and a higher frequency of reflux episodes. Furthermore, a correlation exists between the degree of gastroesophageal reflux episodes and progression of ILD (decline in the diffusing capacity of the lung for carbon monoxide).[14]

Awareness of the association between gastroesophageal reflux and chronic lung allograft dysfunction after lung transplantation is also increasing. Although controversial, some reports have shown a decreased incidence of chronic lung allograft dysfunction in patients (not those with systemic sclerosis) with gastroesophageal reflux disease who undergo lung transplantation and antireflux procedures.[15] Antireflux procedures are not well studied in patients with systemic sclerosis because the intrinsic esophageal dysmotility in this patient population can be adversely affected by the procedure.[16] Several case reports have described incomplete reflux procedures, such as partial Nissen fundoplication or a variant of Collis gastroplasty, in patients with systemic sclerosis to decrease the risk for aspiration, but with a high incidence of consequent dysphagia.[17-20] The role of antireflux procedures in patients with symptomatic gastroesophageal reflux diseases associated with systemic sclerosis has not been well defined.

Given the nearly universal presence of gastroesophageal reflux disease in patients with systemic sclerosis, many transplant centers have excluded this patient population from lung transplantation. In the few past decades, several reports have shown that selected patients with systemic sclerosis and gastroesophageal motility disorders can undergo lung transplantation with satisfactory outcomes.[21,22] The extent of gastroesophageal involvement that may be an exclusionary criterion is not explicitly described in these reports. However, with accumulating data indicating that gastroesophageal diseases in this patient population do not necessarily lead to shorter survival after lung transplantation, the general consensus is that lung transplantation can be safely offered to selected patients with systemic sclerosis. Each center may need to develop its own criteria (if any) for excluding patients with systemic sclerosis from candidacy for lung transplantation on the basis of the severity of their associated gastroesophageal disease. At UCLA, all potential candidates undergo dual-probe pH monitoring, esophageal manometry, esophagography or endoscopy, and gastric emptying studies. Patients with symptomatic gastroesophageal reflux diseases (i.e., documented aspiration) despite optimal medical therapy (high-dose H_2 receptor antagonist therapy) and lifestyle modifications are considered poor candidates for lung transplantation. Esophageal strictures, esophageal atonia or achalasia, and abnormal gastric emptying (less than 25% clearance at 90 minutes) are other contraindications to lung transplantation.

SELECTION CRITERIA FOR LUNG TRANSPLANTATION

Lung transplantation is a viable option for selected patients with systemic sclerosis–associated ILD at experienced centers (Table 24.1). Potential candidates must meet each center's general criteria for lung transplantation, such as age, other organ function, and psychosocial support. In addition, because systemic sclerosis is a systemic disease, ensuring the absence of any other active end-organ involvement (i.e., no active digital ischemia, creatinine clearance greater than 50 mL/min, and no renal crisis in the past 5 years) is imperative. An exception to this statement is the extent of gastrointestinal involvement, which is present in nearly every patient with systemic sclerosis. The extent of gastroesophageal motility disorder and reflux disease as criteria for exclusion from lung transplantation is a subject of controversy and varies depending on the transplant center (see earlier).

TIMING FOR LISTING

No clear guidelines on the timing of lung transplantation in patients with systemic sclerosis, ILD, or pulmonary hypertension exist. As for patients with other medical conditions, lung transplantation remains the last option and is offered only after all other therapies have been exhausted. Lung transplantation is offered to patients with systemic sclerosis who have extensive lung disease (HRCT evidence of involvement of more than 20% of the lung), demonstrate a marked decline in their pulmonary function test results, have failed medical treatment, remain symptomatic and oxygen dependent, and have a life expectancy of less than 2 years. Lung transplant candidates with systemic sclerosis and secondary pulmonary hypertension have usually been treated with optimal vasodilator therapies but remain symptomatic.

SURGICAL CONSIDERATIONS

Patients with systemic sclerosis can undergo single- or double-lung transplantation depending on recipient factors such as their age at initial evaluation and associated

Table 24.1 Lung transplantation criteria for patients with systemic sclerosis at UCLA

- Meets general criteria for lung transplantation at UCLA
- No active digital ischemia
- Creatinine clearance > 50 mL/min
- No history of renal crisis in past 5 years
- No evidence of ongoing aspiration

Note: UCLA, University of California at Los Angeles.

pulmonary hypertension. In a retrospective review, the 21 patients with systemic sclerosis who underwent single-lung transplantation had a 1-year survival rate of 61.9%, whereas the 16 patients who underwent double-lung transplantation had a 1-year survival rate of 75%.[23] In another report, 15 patients who underwent double-lung transplantation had a 1-year survival rate of 93%.[22] According to the currently available data, both single- and double-lung transplantation are reasonable strategies depending on recipient factors and institutional preferences. At UCLA, we favor double-lung transplantation in most patients with systemic sclerosis.

The perioperative care of lung transplant candidates with systemic sclerosis has several unique aspects. Although many of these aspects may reflect institutional biases, they may provide some guidelines for any center performing lung transplantation in this patient population. Because of the Raynaud phenomenon, we do not place radial arterial lines; instead, we favor a femoral arterial line for monitoring. Inserting a transesophageal probe may be problematic because of a small oral opening and possible esophageal strictures. We frequently use pediatric probes for intraoperative monitoring. Moreover, to ensure the absence of esophageal stricture, all lung transplant candidates undergo esophageal contrast imaging, endoscopy, or both before they are listed for a transplant. Obtaining a reliable oxygen saturation measurement in this patient population is usually challenging because of their thick digital skin. We must invariably place several monitors on the skin, face, and ear lobes to obtain a reliable measurement of oxygen saturation throughout the procedure. The lung transplantation procedure is performed in a manner similar to that with any other lung transplant patient, with special attention directed to dissection of the inferior pulmonary ligaments. Many patients with systemic sclerosis have a patulous esophagus, which can be inadvertently injured during this part of the procedure. Patients with systemic sclerosis have small and rigid thoracic cavities, thus making the lung transplantation procedure technically more challenging. Because of their "rubbery" skin, immunosuppressed lung transplant recipients with systemic sclerosis are at higher risk for wound complications. Aspiration precautions to minimize the risk for aspiration pneumonia, such as elevation of the head of the bed, remain an important part of the perioperative care of such patients.

After transplantation, all patients are cared for by a multidisciplinary team consisting of pulmonologists, rheumatologists, and other consultants as needed. We routinely administer angiotensin-converting enzyme inhibitors or angiotensin receptor blockers to decrease the incidence of possible "scleroderma renal crises."

OUTCOMES

Several reports in the past 2 decades have examined the short- and long-term clinical outcomes of lung transplantation in patients with systemic sclerosis. In 2000, Rosas and associates compared the short-term outcomes of nine patients with systemic sclerosis and those of a cohort of patients with other diagnoses who also underwent lung transplantation. The two cohorts' 4-year survival rates and rates of acute rejection and infection were similar.[23] A two-center collective experience found that the survival rate of highly selected patients with systemic sclerosis is similar to that of patients with idiopathic pulmonary fibrosis or pulmonary hypertension who undergo lung transplantation.[24] A UCLA report compared the outcomes of 14 patients with systemic sclerosis and those of 38 matched patients with idiopathic pulmonary fibrosis who had undergone lung transplantation.[22] Their 1-year mortality rates were 6.6% and 13.0%, respectively (P = .62). Rates of acute cellular rejection episodes were significantly higher in the group of recipients with systemic sclerosis; however, the other end points of bronchiolitis obliterans syndrome (BOS) and infections after 1 year of follow-up were similar in the two groups.

Sottile and colleagues reported on 23 patients with systemic sclerosis who had undergone lung transplantation; they compared this cohort with a matched group.[21] The 1- and 5-year survival rates of the two groups were similar, as was the incidence of BOS. The incidence of acute cellular rejection was lower in the group of patients with systemic sclerosis. Interestingly, esophageal dysfunction (defined as a DeMeester score higher than 14 or more than mild esophageal dysmotility) was not associated with worse outcomes.

In a recent analysis of the United Network for Organ Sharing (UNOS) registry, Depasquale and colleagues compared the largest cohort of patients with systemic sclerosis who had undergone lung transplantation with other lung transplant recipients.[25] Table 24.2 shows the characteristics and risk factors of patients with systemic sclerosis (n = 149) and without systemic sclerosis (n = 20,128) who had undergone lung transplantation. The patients with systemic sclerosis had a higher mean pulmonary arterial pressure, were more likely to be sensitized, had higher lung allocation scores, and were more likely to have undergone double-lung transplantation. Interestingly, the percentage of patients with systemic sclerosis who underwent lung transplantation increased markedly over time. The 1-month, 1-year, and 5-year post–lung transplantation survival rates of the patients with and without systemic sclerosis were similar (Figure 24.1). When the patients with systemic sclerosis were compared with patients with other diagnoses, the 5-year survival rates were again similar (Figure 24.2).

The leading cause of death after lung transplantation in patients with systemic sclerosis was infection (26%). Table 24.3 shows the causes of death in lung transplant recipients with or without systemic sclerosis. This report, along with other published studies, demonstrates that the outcomes of lung transplantation in selected patients with systemic sclerosis remain similar to those of other lung transplant recipients for up to 5 years.

FUTURE DIRECTIONS

Pulmonary involvement remains a leading cause of mortality in patients with CTDs and, more specifically, in patients with systemic sclerosis. Lung transplantation is a viable option for selected patients who meet the general criteria for lung transplantation and have inactive extrapulmonary disease. Patients with aspiration episodes despite optimal medical therapy and lifestyle modifications may be poor

Table 24.2 Lung transplant recipient demographics and characteristics: Comparison of recipients with or without the diagnoses of scleroderma

Recipient characteristics	Scleroderma (n = 149)	Nonscleroderma (n = 20,128)
Age, mean ± SD, yr	51 ± 10	52 ± 13
Sex, No. males (%)	67 (45%)	10,881 (54%)
Diabetes mellitus	5 (3%)	2334 (13%)
Serum creatinine, mean ± SD, mg/dL	0.9 ± 0.3	0.9 ± 0.9
Pulmonary arterial pressure, mean ± SD, mm Hg	33 ± 12	27 ± 12
Panel reactive antibodies ≥ 20%	149 (100%)	11,582 (58%)
No. listed by era		
1990–1994	0 (0%)	2805 (14%)
1995–1999	0 (0%)	4251 (21%)
2000–2004	12 (8%)	4450 (22%)
2005–2010	135 (91%)	8622 (43%)
Life support at transplant	24 (16.1%)	1210 (6.0%)
Lung allocation score, mean ± SD	47 ± 12	45 ± 16
Double-lung transplant, No. (%)	111 (74.5%)	10,687 (53%)

Source: From DePasquale EC, Ross D, Ardehali A. Lung Transplantation in Scleroderma? Abstract presented at the 34th Annual Meeting of the International Society for Heart and Lung Transplantation, April 11, 2014, San Diego, California.
Note: SD, standard deviation.

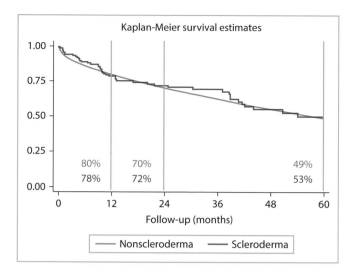

Figure 24.1 Kaplan-Meier survival curves for patients with or without scleroderma who have undergone lung transplantation. (From DePasquale EC, Ross D, Ardehali A. Lung Transplantation in Scleroderma. Abstract presented at the 34th Annual Meeting of the International Society for Heart and Lung Transplantation, April 11, 2014, San Diego, California.)

candidates for lung transplantation. Recent reports have demonstrated that selected patients with systemic sclerosis can undergo lung transplantation with satisfactory 1- and 5-year survival rates, thus further justifying continuing to offer this lifesaving treatment to such patients. Additional refinement of the selection criteria and optimal management of posttransplant gastrointestinal complications may further improve the outcome of lung transplantation in patients with systemic sclerosis.

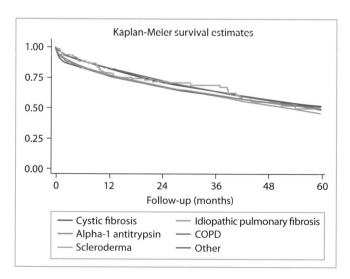

Figure 24.2 Kaplan-Meier survival curves for patients with different diagnoses who have undergone lung transplantation. (From DePasquale EC, Ross D, Ardehali A. Lung Transplantation in Scleroderma. Abstract presented at the 34th Annual Meeting of the International Society for Heart and Lung Transplantation, April 11, 2014, San Diego, California.)

Table 24.3 Causes of death in lung transplant recipients with or without the diagnoses of scleroderma, up to 5 years after transplantation

| | Death—overall (P = .453) | |
| | Scleroderma (n = 49) | Nonscleroderma (n = 11,340) |
Cause of death	no. (%)	no. (%)
Graft failure	2 (4%)	652 (6%)
Rejection	2 (4%)	1544 (14%)
Infection	13 (27%)	2609 (23%)
Cardiovascular	5 (10%)	642 (6%)
Malignancy	4 (8%)	853 (8%)
Multiorgan failure	2 (4%)	576 (5%)
Bronchiolitis obliterans syndrome	0 (0%)	348 (3%)
Respiratory failure	6 (12%)	1273 (11%)
Other	15 (31%)	2843 (25%)

Source: From DePasquale EC, Ross D, Ardehali A. Lung Transplantation in Scleroderma. Abstract presented at the 34th Annual Meeting of the International Society for Heart and Lung Transplantation, April 11, 2014, San Diego, California.

REFERENCES

1. Masi AT. Subcommittee for Scleroderma Criteria of the American Rheumatism Association Diagnostic and Therapeutic Criteria Committee. Preliminary criteria for the classification of systemic sclerosis (scleroderma). Arthritis Rheum 1980;23:581-590.
2. Aletaha D, Neogi T, Silman AJ, et al. Rheumatoid arthritis classification criteria: An American College of Rheumatology/European League Against Rheumatism collaborative initiative. Arthritis Rheum 2010;62:2569-2581.
3. Vij R, Strek ME. Diagnosis and treatment of connective tissue disease–associated interstitial lung disease. Chest 2013;143:814-824.
4. Fischer A, du Bois R. Interstitial lung disease in connective tissue disorders. Lancet 2012;380:689-698.
5. Park JH, Kim DS, Park IN, et al. Prognosis of fibrotic interstitial pneumonia: Idiopathic versus collagen vascular disease-related subtypes. Am J Respir Crit Care Med 2007;175:705-711.
6. Solomon JJ, Olson AL, Fischer A, et al. Scleroderma lung disease. Eur Respir Rev 2013;22:6-19.
7. Schurawitzki H, Stiglbauer R, Graninger W, et al. Interstitial lung disease in progressive systemic sclerosis: High-resolution CT versus radiography. Radiology 1990;176:755-759.
8. Battle RW, Davitt MA, Cooper SM, et al. Prevalence of pulmonary hypertension in limited and diffuse scleroderma. Chest 1996;110:1515-1519.
9. MacGregor AJ, Canavan R, Knight C, et al. Pulmonary hypertension in systemic sclerosis:

Risk factors for progression and consequences for survival. Rheumatology (Oxford) 2001;40:453-459.

10. Steen VD, Medsger TA Jr. Case-control study of corticosteroids and other drugs that either precipitate or protect from the development of scleroderma renal crisis. Arthritis Rheum 1998;41:1613-1619.

11. Teixeira L, Mouthon L, Mahr A, et al. Mortality and risk factors of scleroderma renal crisis; a French retrospective study of 50 patients. Ann Rheum Dis 2008;67:110-116.

12. Tzouvelekis A, Galanopoulos N, Bouros E, et al. Effect and safety of mycophenolate mofetil or sodium in systemic sclerosis-associated interstitial lung disease: A meta-analysis. Pulm Med 2012;2012:143637. doi: 10.1155/2012/146637.

13. Tashkin DP, Elashoff R, Clements PJ, et al. Cyclophosphamide versus placebo in scleroderma lung disease. N Engl J Med 2006;354:2655-2666.

14. Marie I, Dominique S, Levesque H, et al. Esophageal involvement and pulmonary manifestations in systemic sclerosis. Arthritis Rheum 2001;45:346-354.

15. Cantu E 3rd, Appel JZ 3rd, Hartwig MG. J. Maxwell Chamberlain Memorial Paper. Early fundoplication prevents chronic allograft dysfunction in patients with gastroesophageal reflux disease. Ann Thorac Surg 2004;78:1142-1151.

16. Gasper WJ, Sweet MP, Golden JA, et al. Lung transplantation in patients with connective tissue disorders and esophageal dysmotility. Dis Esophagus 2008;21:2150-655.

17. Henderson RD, Pearson FG. Surgical management of esophageal scleroderma. J Thorac Cardiovasc Surg 1973;66:686-692.

18. Orringer MB, Orringer JS, Dabich L, Zarafonetis CJ. Combined Collis gastroplasty: Fundoplication operations for scleroderma reflux esophagitis. Surgery 1981;90:624-630.

19. Poirier NC, Taillefar R, Topart P, Doranceau A. Antireflux operations in patients with scleroderma. Ann Thorac Surg 1994;58:66-72.

20. Mansour KA, Malone CE. Surgery for scleroderma of the esophagus: A 12-year experience. Ann Thorac Surg 1988;46:513-514.

21. Sottile PD, Iturbe D, Katsumoto TR, et al. Outcomes in systemic sclerosis–related lung disease after lung transplantation. Transplantation 2013;95:975-980.

22. Saggar R, Khanna D, Furst DE, et al. Systemic sclerosis and bilateral lung transplantation: A single centre experience. Eur Respir J 2010;36:893-900.

23. Rosas V, Conte JV, Yang SC, et al. Lung transplantation and systemic sclerosis. Ann Transplant 2000;5:38-43.

24. Schachna L, Medsger TA Jr, Dauber JH, et al. Lung transplantation in scleroderma compared with idiopathic pulmonary fibrosis and idiopathic pulmonary arterial hypertension. Arthritis Rheum 2006;54:3954-3961.

25. DePasquale EC, Ross D, Ardehali A. Lung Transplantation in Scleroderma. Abstract presented at the 34th Annual Meeting of the International Society for Heart and Lung Transplantation, April 11, 2014, San Diego, CA.

25

Posttransplantation critical care management

CESAR A. KELLER AND JOSÉ L. DÍAZ-GÓMEZ

INTRODUCTION

Lung transplantation is the best care alternative for providing a survival benefit and improved quality of life for qualified patients with end-stage lung and pulmonary vascular diseases that are refractory to standard medical and surgical therapies.

The 30th official report from the Registry of the International Society for Heart and Lung Transplantation stated that 3640 adult lung transplant procedures were performed in 2011 by 132 participating transplant centers.[1] Survival rates from 1988 to 1995 were 81% at 3 months and 70% at 1 year as compared with 90% and 81% for the period from 2004 to 2011. These improved survival rates are largely attributable to better recognition and management of complications during the immediate postoperative period and to improvements in organ preservation, surgical techniques, management of immunosuppression, prophylaxis, and treatment of infectious complications.[2]

Several issues contribute to the increased complexity of caring for lung transplant recipients in the intensive care unit (ICU), including a critical shortage of lung donors. Ideal donors are young (<55 years) with adequate oxygenation (Pao_2/Fio_2 >300), a minimal smoking history (<20 pack-years), and no sign of infiltrates on their chest radiographs. Less than 20% of multiorgan donors meet these

criteria. The increased demand for lung transplantation has resulted in the use of "extended criteria" donors who may be older, have a significant smoking history, or have some degree of atelectasis or infiltration on their chest radiographs. Although some studies have reported similar outcomes when marginal or extended donors are used,[3,4] others have described more complex and prolonged stays in the ICU, longer hospital stays, decreased lung function,[5] and increased early mortality.[6]

Current strategies to increase the donor pool may affect care required in the ICU. Such strategies include the use of donors after cardiac death[7,8] and ex vivo lung perfusion techniques, the reported survival outcomes of which are similar to those when brain-dead donors are used.[9] As experience in lung transplantation has increased, the tendency has been to accept marginal candidates for lung transplantation, such as older candidates or those with comorbid conditions.[10] Previously, mechanical ventilation was considered a contraindication to transplantation, but for patients with end-stage lung disease who are progressing to respiratory failure and require mechanical ventilation, lung transplantation constitutes the best chance for survival. Lung transplantation candidates who require mechanical ventilation receive the highest lung allocation scores and have the greatest probability of undergoing transplantation; their reported 1- and 2-year survival rates are 62% and 57%, respectively.[7] Today, increasing numbers of patients are undergoing transplantation while receiving support from a mechanical ventilator. In addition, increasing numbers of patients with progressive respiratory failure will reach surgery while being supported with venovenous (VV) or venoarterial (VA) extracorporeal membrane oxygenation (ECMO).[11] The main aim of this review is to address the practical aspects of managing lung transplant recipients in the ICU with consideration for their underlying diagnoses and also treating the multiple life-threatening complications that may arise during the immediate posttransplantation period.

ARRIVAL IN THE INTENSIVE CARE UNIT FROM THE OPERATING ROOM

Communication between cardiothoracic surgeons, anesthesiologists, critical care physicians, and physicians specializing in pulmonary transplantation is crucial to ensuring optimal care in the ICU. Critical and pertinent information needs to be made clearly available. Table 25.1 summarizes the relevant information on donors, recipients, and intraoperative events that will largely influence the postoperative outcome of transplant recipients. Primary graft dysfunction (PGD) following lung transplantation has been associated with multiple clinical factors. Donor-related risk factors include, but are not limited to, age (>45 years), race (Afro-American), sex (female), smoking history (>20 pack-years), prolonged mechanical ventilation, pneumonia, aspiration, multiple blood transfusions, head trauma, and hemodynamic instability. Recipient-related factors include obesity, idiopathic pulmonary hypertension, secondary pulmonary hypertension, idiopathic pulmonary fibrosis, and sarcoidosis. Intraoperative risks include single-lung transplantation, prolonged ischemia time, use of cardiopulmonary bypass, and blood transfusions.[12] Ischemia times greater than 330 minutes have been associated with increased mortality.[13] Reports from surgeons regarding pleural adhesions, difficulties during explantation of the native lungs, technical difficulties during the performance of bronchial or vascular anastomosis, the need to downsize donor lungs, challenges in maintaining hemodynamic stability in the operating

Table 25.1 Arrival in the ICU from the operating room: Relevant information pertinent to management in the ICU

Donor Information: Age, sex, cause of death, race
Standard donor: Age <55 years, ABO compatible, clear radiograph, PaO_2/FiO_2 >300 on PEEP of 5 cm H_2O, smoking history <20 pack-years, no chest trauma, no aspiration, clear sputum, negative bronchoscopy
Extended donor (by which criteria?): Age, long smoking history, presence of contusion, atelectasis, infiltrates, history of lung disease (asthma), prolonged mechanical ventilation, purulent secretions or infection
Type of donor: Donor after cardiac death or donor after ex vivo lung perfusion
Recipient information:
Clinical diagnosis: Indication for transplantation
Characteristics: Age, sex, race, functional status before transplantation, pulmonary artery pressure before transplantation, body mass index, mechanical ventilation before transplantation, ECMO before transplantation
Intraoperative information:
Type of procedure: Single-lung or double-lung or heart-lung transplant
Surgical approach: Sternotomy, posterior thoracotomy, clamshell incision, chest closure
Cardiopulmonary bypass: Pump time
Ischemia time: <330 minutes or >330 minutes
Intraoperative immunosuppression:
Induction therapy administered in the OR and timing: Steroids, calcineurin agents, purine antagonists, others
Prophylactic antibiotics given in the OR and timing
Administration of blood products and intravenous fluids and management of coagulopathy: Crystalloids, colloids, red packed cells, fresh frozen plasma, platelets, cryoprecipitates, intake-output balance
Use of vasodilator therapy for pulmonary hypertension: Prostacyclin, inhaled nitric oxide, nitroglycerin, others
Use of vasopressor therapy: Epinephrine, norepinephrine, phenylephrine (Neo-Synephrine), vasopressin, others
Use of inotropic therapy: Dopamine, dobutamine, milrinone, others
Pain control and sedation on arrival in ICU: Propofol, midazolam, fentanyl, hydromorphone, morphine
Technical Issues: Explantation of native lung or lungs, implantation of transplant lung or lungs, difficulties with bronchial or vascular anastomosis, reperfusion issues, ventilation and oxygenation following reperfusion, injury to the phrenic nerves, allograft size matching, donor lung downsizing, chest closure versus open chest after transplantation
OR postoperative information:
Airway control (single- or double-lumen tube)
Chest tube drainage (chest tube output, air leak)
Issues during transport to the OR to ICU

Note: ECMO, extracorporeal membrane oxygenation; ICU, intensive care unit; OR, operating room; PEEP, positive end-expiratory pressure.

room, the status of drainage tubes, whether closure of the chest cavity following organ implantation was possible, and patients' stability during transport are all pieces of information that are necessary to provide the best postoperative care in ICU.

INITIAL MANAGEMENT

Transplant recipients arrive at the ICU while they are still under the effects of sedation and analgesia, intubated, and receiving mechanical ventilation (usually in the pressure control mode or low–volume control mode with low positive end-expiratory pressure [PEEP] and a high FIO_2 setting) to be weaned as tolerated. Patients typically arrive with a pulmonary artery catheter and arterial line in place; chest tubes to drain pleural spaces; and an indwelling bladder catheter in place to fully monitor gas exchange, hemodynamics, output of pleural drainage, and urinary output. On arrival, patients undergo a full physical examination, evaluation of their hemodynamic parameters, and assessment of their peripheral circulation and perfusion. Evaluation of the position of their endotracheal tube, placement of their central and arterial lines and chest tube, and drainage and urinary output is essential. Patients are commonly hypothermic and require support from forced-air warming devices. Arterial and venous blood samples are obtained to monitor arterial blood gases, complete blood count, coagulation profile, renal profile, hepatic profile, and lactate levels.

Because of the administration of large doses of corticosteroids, postoperative hyperglycemia is common; patients are given an intravenous (IV) insulin drip to normalize their glycemic levels. Patients are placed with their head elevated at a 30-degree angle, protocols to avoid central line sepsis and ventilator-associated pneumonia are followed, and IV proton pump inhibitors are administered to minimize acid reflux.

In our program, bedside electrocardiography and portable chest radiography are performed along with ultrasound evaluation of the lungs (see the section on ultrasound).

Initial immunosuppression

Immunosuppressive management is initiated preoperatively and intraoperatively. Most protocols include the intraoperative use of methylprednisolone boluses of 10 mg/kg with or without preoperative or intraoperative administration of calcineurin inhibitors (tacrolimus or cyclosporine) and purine and pyrimidine synthesis inhibitors (mycophenolate or azathioprine). Depending on the individual center's protocols, patients may receive induction therapy to reduce the T cells' initial immune response to the transplanted organ. Lymphocyte depletion can be achieved by using polyclonal antibodies such as antithymocyte globulin (Thymoglobulin) or humanized monoclonal antibodies against interleukin-2 (IL-2) receptors, which inhibit IL-2–mediated proliferation and differentiation of T cells (basiliximab or daclizumab).

Other agents include humanized monoclonal complement-fixing anti-CD52 antibodies, which are present in virtually all lymphocytes. One such agent is alemtuzumab, which induces long-lasting lymphopenia (T and B cell). Induction therapy is controversial because of the long-term risks, such as opportunistic infections and posttransplantation lymphoproliferative disease.[14] A selective approach to administering induction therapy to patients at high risk for rejection, such as sensitized patients with preformed panel-reactive antibodies, Afro-American recipients, and others, while avoiding induction therapy for patients at high risk for infection and debilitated elderly subjects, is favored by our group.

Triple immunosuppressive therapy, including glucocorticoids combined with a calcineurin-inhibiting agent and purine and pyrimidine synthesis inhibitors, is continued in the ICU.[15] Methylprednisolone is given intravenously at an initial dose of 2 mg/kg every 12 hours for 48 hours, to be reduced by 0.5 mg/kg every 12 hours with progressive tapering. In addition, patients receive tacrolimus initially at 0.05 to 0.1 mg/kg/day via IV infusion. Alternatively, 1 to 2 mg can be administered sublingually every 12 hours until an oral route can be established. Doses are adjusted to reach serum trough levels of 8 to15 ng/mL. If used, cyclosporine is administered at an initial dose of 2 to 3 mg/kg/day by IV infusion, which is switched to 3 to 5 mg/kg every 12 hours orally to reach trough levels of between 250 and 350 ng/mL and obtain levels between 900 and 1200 ng/mL 2 hours following administration (C2 levels). Most commonly, the third immunosuppressive agent is mycophenolate mofetil (500 to 1000 mg given intravenously twice per day and switched to the oral route when possible). Alternatively, azathioprine (1 to 2 mg/kg intravenously or orally) is administered daily. Newer immunosuppressants such as sirolimus should be avoided in the early phase after lung transplantation because their capacity to inhibit fibroblast proliferation results in poor wound healing and can predispose patients to early anastomotic dehiscence with fatal consequences.[16] Patients will need to be monitored and managed for the multiple adverse effects associated with immunosuppression therapy that may follow induction therapy (for example, cytokine release syndrome and pulmonary edema after induction therapy, which can mimic PGD with noncardiogenic pulmonary edema, alveolar infiltrates, and hypoxemia). Other adverse events include leukopenia, thrombocytopenia, and increased susceptibility to opportunistic infections. Tacrolimus or cyclosporine may produce neurotoxicity (focal neurologic deficit, confusion, tremor, and posterior reversible encephalopathy syndrome), renal dysfunction, and nephrotoxicity. Mycophenolate and azathioprine may induce significant myelosuppression, gastrointestinal abnormalities, or hepatotoxicity.

Initial infection prophylaxis

The lung remains the most common site for initial infections. Predisposing factors include continuous exposure to the environment, impairment of mucus clearance mechanisms by airway ischemia and denervation impeding normal ciliary motion, cough reflexes impaired because of postoperative pain and sedation, and immune status weakened by immunosuppression. Preventive antimicrobial strategies reduce the consequences of acute infection. Antibacterial prophylaxis is initiated with a wide-spectrum protocol for the first 72 hours. In our center, the initial protocol includes cefepime, metronidazole, and vancomycin. Subsequent antimicrobial therapy is guided by results of the initial cultures. Patients with chronic infections (bronchiectasis, cystic fibrosis) receive prophylaxis based on the results of sputum cultures obtained before transplantation. Antifungal prophylaxis most commonly includes inhaled amphotericin with or without Iitraconazole. Most recently, protocols that include voriconazole to minimize the risk for invasive aspergillosis have been described.[17] Cytomegalovirus (CMV) is one of the main pathogens associated with lung transplantation in seropositive donors or recipients. Antiviral prophylaxis significantly reduces CMV disease and CMV infection. Prophylaxis includes IV ganciclovir followed by oral valganciclovir.[18] CMV-seronegative donors and recipients receive prophylaxis with acyclovir. *Pneumocystis jirovecii* prophylaxis is initiated when patients can tolerate oral medication with sulfamethoxazole and trimethoprim, which add protection against other infections such as *Listeria* species, *Toxoplasma gondii*, and *Nocardia*.

Imaging studies

Portable chest radiographs are reviewed for placement of an endotracheal tube, central lines, drainage tube, and a nasogastric tube. Images of the lungs are examined to ascertain the presence or absence of alveolar infiltrates and evidence of barotrauma (pneumothorax, pneumomediastinum, or subcutaneous emphysema), lung contusion, atelectasis, or consolidation. Images of the pleural spaces are studied for intrathoracic bleeding and pleural effusions, and images of the diaphragm are inspected for an abnormal position suggestive of diaphragmatic paralysis. In the case of patients who have received single-lung transplants, particularly those with chronic obstructive pulmonary disease (COPD), special attention is directed to assessing hyperinflation of the native lung after displacement of mediastinal structures toward the transplanted side. In special circumstances, non–contrast-enhanced chest computed tomography (CT) is performed to further define the pleural or mediastinal structures and look for the presence of hemothorax, postoperative bleeding, or possible anastomotic dehiscence. Contrast-enhanced CT is useful when conditions such as postoperative pulmonary emboli, stenotic pulmonary arterial anastomosis, or obstruction of the pulmonary veins are suspected. Bedside perfusion lung scans are used to define any regional perfusion defects that may occur with pulmonary arterial stenosis, which may indicate the need for additional complementary studies such as pulmonary angiography.

Bronchoscopy

Bronchoscopy is performed early to inspect the native airways and assess injury to the bronchial mucosae from the previous double-lumen intubation in the operating room. Anastomotic structures are inspected to assess integrity and patency and rule out dehiscence. The distal airways are inspected, bronchoalveolar lavage is performed to obtain fluid for culturing, and pulmonary toilet is performed to aspirate blood clots and secretions to avoid postoperative atelectasis.

ASSESSMENT AND MANAGEMENT OF HEMODYNAMICS AND GAS EXCHANGE

Management of lung transplant recipients in the ICU depends largely on their hemodynamic and gas exchange profile. Figure 25.1 shows a systematic approach for assessment and management of lung transplant recipients following monitoring of mixed venous saturation (Svo_2) as a physiologic marker of tissue hypoperfusion and hypoxemia.[19]

A declining Svo_2 in lung transplant recipients should prompt an immediate search for and correction of all the possible physiologic abnormalities causing tissue hypoperfusion and hypoxemia. The two main physiologic causes of declining Svo_2 in critically ill patients are factors inducing increased oxygen consumption (Vo_2) and factors resulting in decreased oxygen delivery (O_2D) to tissues.

Increased oxygen consumption

Posttransplant factors that commonly cause increased Vo_2 in lung transplant recipients include fever, agitation and pain, and increased work of breathing.

FEVER

Fever after a transplant is common and should trigger a search for the causal agent, including obtaining pertinent cultures and reviewing all possible clinical causes. Fever will be treated symptomatically with IV or enteral acetaminophen or by using forced-air cooling devices in addition to treating the specific cause of fever.

AGITATION AND PAIN

Initially, patients require infusion regimens with short-acting sedative agents (propofol and midazolam), from which they are to be weaned as their respiratory status improves. Pain control is essential because patients must be weaned from mechanical ventilation, be able to clear secretions by coughing and breathing deeply, and be able to tolerate early mobilization. The protocols include the use of opioids (fentanyl or hydromorphone via IV infusion) or a patient-controlled analgesia infusion pump. Epidural analgesia with infusion of local anesthetic (bupivicaine) alone or in combination with a narcotic facilitates weaning from mechanical ventilation while avoiding the adverse effects of systemic narcotics.[20] Other therapies include lidocaine patches

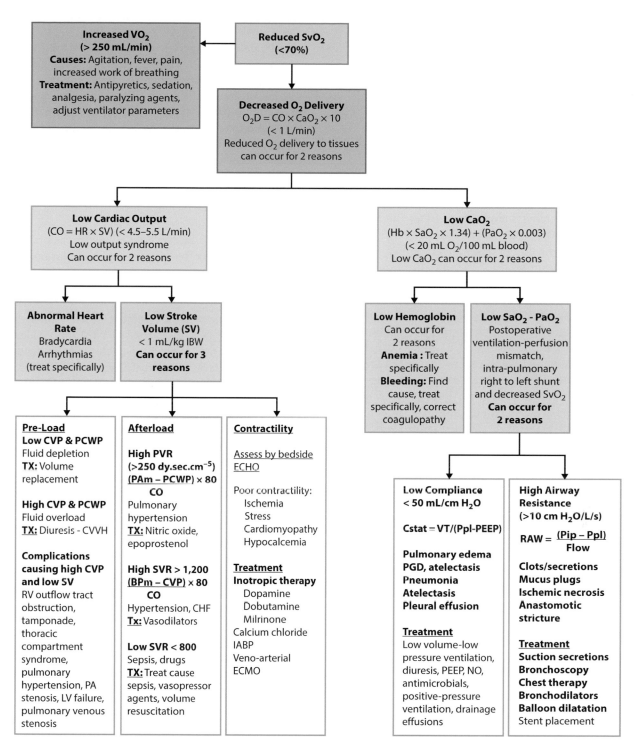

Figure 25.1 Hemodynamic monitoring after lung transplantation. BPm, beats per minute; CHF, congestive heart failure; CO, cardiac output; Cstat, static compliance; CVP, central venous pressure; CVVH, continuous veno-venous hemofiltration; HR, heart rate; ECHO, echocardiography; ECMO, extracorporeal membrane oxygenation; Hb, hemoglobin; IABP, intra-aortic balloon pump; IBW, ideal body weight; LV, left ventricular; NO, nitrous oxide; PAm, mean pulmonary arterial pressure; PA, pulmonary artery; PCWP, pulmonary capillary wedge pressure; PEEP, positive end-expiratory pressure; PGD, preimplantation genetic diagnosis; Pip, peak inspiratory pressure; Ppl, plateau pressure; PVR, pulmonary vascular resistance; RAW, resistance, airway; RV, right ventricular; SV, stroke volume; SVR, systemic vascular resistance; VT, ventricular tachycardia.

above and below the incision lines and IV acetaminophen. Nonsteroidal anti-inflammatory agents and cyclooxygenase-2 inhibitors are avoided because of the potential for renal dysfunction.

WORK OF BREATHING (MECHANICAL VENTILATION)

Patients will be ventilated with pressure control and pressure support modes to minimize barotrauma, with the aim being to maintain low pressure (a plateau airway pressure [Ppl] <35 mm Hg) and low tidal volume (VT) (6 to 8 mL/kg) with the lowest PEEP and FIO$_2$ settings possible to maintain SaO$_2$ higher than 90% and PaO$_2$ higher than 60 mm Hg. Most patients in whom PGD or other postoperative complications do not develop can be weaned from mechanical ventilation within 72 hours after transplantation; they can be transitioned from full ventilator support to pressure- or volume-synchronized intermittent mandatory pressure support ventilation, then to continuous positive airway pressure plus pressure support ventilation, and eventually to extubation. Noninvasive ventilation may be a useful supportive maneuver to reduce the work of breathing in patients with ICU myopathy, weak respiratory muscles, or dysfunctional diaphragms. Patients who do not tolerate early extubation or require reintubation as a result of hypercapnic or hypoxic respiratory failure will benefit from an early bedside percutaneous tracheostomy. Single-lung transplant recipients with COPD may require specific ventilator support to minimize hyperinflation of the native lung by using low respiratory rates and adjusted inspiratory-to-expiratory time ratios of 1:4 or longer, thereby allowing prolonged expiratory time. Monitoring of auto-PEEP helps avoid hyperinflation and thoracic tamponade. Prevention of postoperative atelectasis includes aggressive chest therapy, use of incentive spirometry, and removal of thick secretions and necrotic debris by bronchoscopy as needed.

Decreased oxygen delivery to tissues

O$_2$D to tissues depends on how much blood flows to tissues every minute (cardiac output [CO]) and how much oxygen is contained in the blood (arterial oxygen content [CaO$_2$]), which is calculated as O$_2$D = CO × CaO$_2$ × 10. Under resting conditions, the cardiopulmonary system delivers approximately 1 L of O$_2$ to tissues per minute. Decreased O$_2$D can occur for two reasons: decreased or inappropriate CO or CaO$_2$. CO is calculated as CO = heart rate × stroke volume (SV) (normal range, 4 to 6 L/min), and CaO$_2$ = (hemoglobin level × SaO$_2$/100 × 1.34) + (PaO$_2$ × 0.0031) (normal range = 18 to 20 mL O$_2$/100 mL blood).

DECREASED CARDIAC OUTPUT AND MANAGEMENT OF CARDIAC COMPLICATIONS

CO inadequate for the given physiologic demands can occur for two reasons: abnormal heart rate or inadequate SV.

Heart rate

Heart rate abnormalities are common in lung transplant recipients. Atrial arrhythmias, including atrial flutter, atrial fibrillation, and other organized types of atrial tachycardia, occur frequently after transplantation. Anastomosis of the donor left atrial tissue cuffs surrounding the pulmonary veins to the posterior wall of the recipient's left atrium electrically isolates the donor pulmonary veins; however, residual recipient pulmonary vein tissue may persist as part of the left atrial anastomosis, which in turn may result in an electroanatomic substrate for reentry.[21] Management of atrial arrhythmias includes direct current cardioversion in hemodynamically compromised patients, use of antiarrhythmic agents (β-blockers or amiodarone), or rate control strategies involving the use of atrioventricular node–blocking agents.

Stroke volume

SV is the volume of blood ejected from the ventricular cavity during every beat. A decreased SV (<1 mL/kg ideal body weight) may result from inadequate preload, inadequate afterload, or decreased contractility.

Preload

Preload is represented by the passive ventricular wall tension at the end of diastole. Contributing factors include compliance of the ventricles and pericardium, myocardial wall thickness, and an end-diastolic volume producing an end-diastolic filling pressure that is clinically measured as central venous pressure (CVP) on the right heart and pulmonary capillary wedge pressure (PCWP) on the left heart. Patients with low SV, CVP, and PCWP are commonly intravascularly volume-depleted, thus requiring volume resuscitation with crystalloids, colloids, or blood products as clinically indicated. Evidence of persistent volume depletion should trigger a search for intrathoracic bleeding. Posttransplant patients benefit from avoiding fluid overload because the lungs easily become edematous as a result of an inflammatory state that favors noncardiogenic pulmonary edema. Fluid overload commonly results in elevated PCWP and CVP. Such patients will benefit from diuresis (furosemide, bumetanide, acetazolamide, and other diuretics). Management of lung transplant recipients should include carefully seeking a negative fluid balance to minimize pulmonary edema while maintaining a cardiac output adequate to provide normal SvO$_2$. Renal failure secondary to volume depletion, hypoperfusion, and the use of calcineurin inhibitor agents and other nephrotoxic drugs may develop in such patients. Their management includes achieving optimal volume status and, when necessary, transient continuous VV hemofiltration and dialysis while their renal function recovers. Decisions about volume replacement, diuresis, or both should not be made solely on the basis of CVP or PCWP measurements because clinical conditions other than intravascular volume may change end-diastolic pressure. Clinical assessment, review of chest radiographs, and bedside echocardiography further complement hemodynamic parameters, thus allowing the best decisions about volume management.

Posttransplant complications other than volume overload characterized by elevated CVP and low SV include right ventricular outflow tract obstruction, thoracic or cardiac tamponade, thoracic compartment syndrome, pulmonary hypertension, stenosis of the pulmonary artery anastomosis, pulmonary embolism, left ventricular failure, and stenosis or thrombosis of the pulmonary veins.

Right Ventricular Outflow Tract Obstruction. This condition occurs in transplant recipients with previous right ventricular hypertrophy secondary to long-standing primary or secondary pulmonary hypertension; it develops following the sudden normalization of pulmonary vascular resistance (PVR) and postoperative reduction of end-diastolic right ventricular volume. Right ventricular outflow tract obstruction in lung transplant recipients occurs in the setting of a hypertrophied right ventricle; it is associated with reduced preload and the use of inotropic therapy. When this condition is suspected, bedside echocardiography is performed to look for end-systolic obliteration of the right ventricular outflow tract. Sequential measurements of CVP, systolic right ventricular pressure, and systolic pulmonary arterial pressure (PAP) are obtained and followed by a "pullback" of the pulmonary arterial catheter from the pulmonary artery into the right ventricle. A systolic gradient from the right ventricle to the pulmonary artery greater than 25 mm Hg, which is associated with hemodynamic instability, tachycardia, and hypotension, confirms the diagnosis. When this complication is present, fluid replacement is required; in such cases, we have successfully used volume replacement via the distal port of the pulmonary arterial catheter to preload the left ventricle distal to the obstruction. β-Blockers may help slow the heart rate to allow adequate diastolic filling. Inotropic agents should be avoided because they worsen this condition.[22]

Thoracic or Cardiac Tamponade. Causes of this condition include progressively edematous lungs, oversized lungs, intrathoracic or mediastinal bleeding compressing the right or left ventricle chest wall, tissue edema, increased PEEP or auto-PEEP, and elevated intrathoracic pressure resulting in diastolic collapse of the right, left, or both ventricles. Tamponade can also be associated with other posttransplant complications such as tension pneumopericardium and large pleural effusions.[23,24] Hemodynamic monitoring and bedside echocardiography show elevation of central pressure, equalization of central diastolic pressure (CVP, pulmonary artery diastolic pressure, and PCWP), systemic hypotension, tachycardia, and the presence of pulsus paradoxus, which is manifested as more than a 10–mm Hg decrease in systolic pressure during inspiration. A bedside echocardiogram may show diastolic collapse of the right atrium, right ventricle, or both with or without collapse of the left chambers and with or without pericardial effusion. Clinical recognition of this syndrome should be followed by immediate intervention, which may include drainage of

pericardial or pleural effusions or immediate opening of the chest cavity, surgical downsizing of the lungs, and aggressive treatment of fluid overload and edema. ECMO support may be required in refractory cases.[25]

Thoracic Compartment Syndrome. This condition, which occurs more commonly in patients requiring prolonged surgical intervention, is frequently complicated by coagulopathy and the requirement for a large infusion of blood products, which results in decreased lung compliance secondary to edema, oversized lungs, intrathoracic bleeding, or a combination thereof and raises mediastinal pressure, thereby leading to cardiac compression and hemodynamic collapse. It will be clinically recognized by high ventilator airway pressure, hypotension, poor tissue perfusion, progressive acidosis, and hypoxemia. This syndrome may occur immediately after chest closure or several hours later. Recognition of thoracic compression syndrome should be followed by surgical intervention to open the thoracic cavity and by delayed chest closure (Figure 25.2).

Pulmonary Hypertension. Elevated central pressure, persistent pulmonary hypertension (mean PAP >25 mm Hg) with normal PCWP, and a transpulmonary gradient (mean PAP - PCWP) higher than 15 mm Hg will frequently be present after transplantation as a result of intraoperative complications, the adverse effects of cardiopulmonary bypass, persistent posttransplant hypoxemia, acidosis, or a combination of PGD on the transplant side and persistent elevation of PVR from the native lung disease in single-lung transplant recipients. The preferred initial treatment includes inhaled vasodilator therapy with either inhaled nitric oxide (iNO) or inhaled prostacyclin.[26]

Stenosis of the Pulmonary Artery Anastomosis. The symptoms with stenosis of the pulmonary artery anastomosis will be similar to those with persistent pulmonary hypertension after transplantation. Clues suggesting this diagnosis include a history of intraoperative challenges during performance of the anastomosis, a history of size mismatch between a smaller donor and a larger recipient, a poor response to inhaled vasodilator therapy, and the finding of a significant gradient from proximal to distal PAP with a pulmonary arterial catheter. The diagnosis is established by stenotic pulmonary arteries visible on the CT angiography associated with low or absent regional perfusion on lung perfusion scans. The clinical symptoms of these patients can be dramatic and include early signs of right ventricular failure. Management includes pulmonary angiography with documentation of increased gradients (higher than 15 to 20 mm Hg) and deployment of a vascular stent. Surgical repair is seldom required; the incidence of serious anastomotic complications in lung transplant recipients is rare (<2% of cases).[27]

Pulmonary Embolism. Acute pulmonary embolism can occur in lung transplant recipients during the early postoperative period and cause systemic hypotension, pulmonary hypertension, right ventricular dysfunction, and elevated CVP in association with acute deterioration in gas exchange. In the absence of other acute complications that could

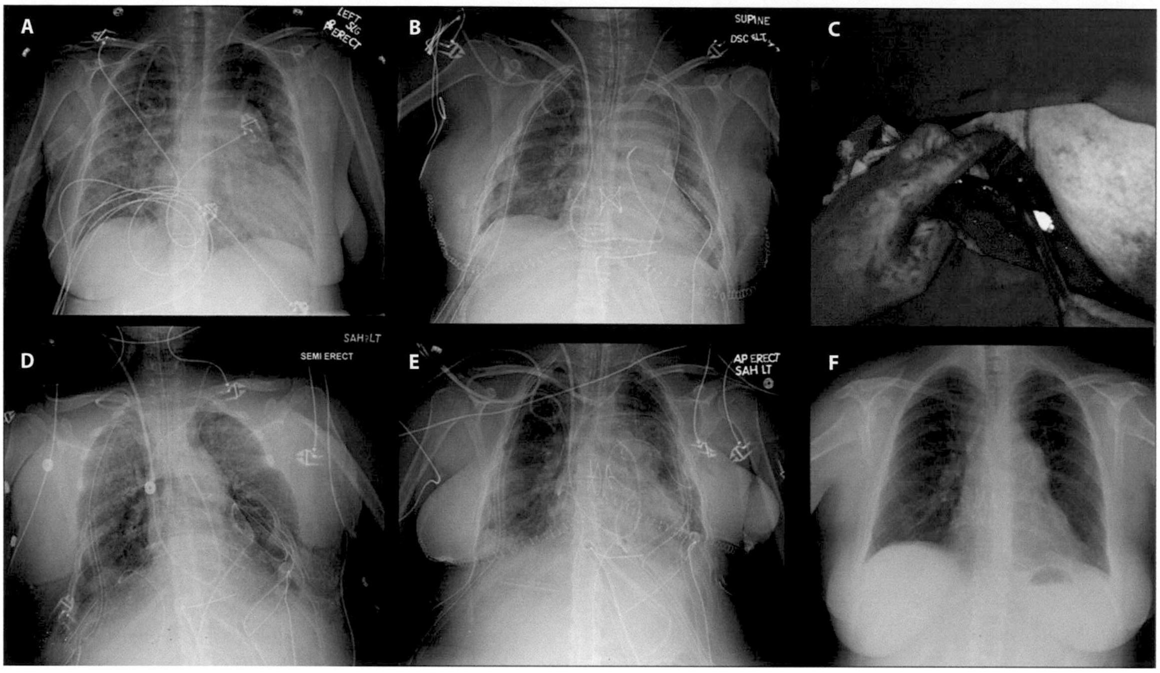

Figure 25.2 Thoracic compartment syndrome. **(A)** A 32-year-old woman with a history of idiopathic pulmonary arterial hypertension and anti-PR3 antibodies had severe pulmonary hypertension (mean pulmonary arterial pressure, 68 mm Hg) and hypoxemia (blood gas analysis results: pH = 7.14, $Paco_2$ = 48 to 64 mm Hg, Oxy-Max 15 LXO_2). The patient was given inhaled nitric oxide and was already being treated with bosentan, tadalafil, and intravenous treprostrinil before being listed for a double-lung transplant. **(B)** The patient arrived in the intensive care unit (ICU) after a double-lung transplant with cardiopulmonary bypass support after having received a large infusion of blood products in the operating room (OR). The patient was hemodynamically unstable with a systolic blood pressure of 75 mm Hg despite volume resuscitation and inotropic agents. Her chest radiograph showed postoperative changes and a wide upper mediastinum (arterial blood gas analysis results: pH = 7.14, $Paco_2$ = 46 to 64 mm Hg, Fio_2 = 1.0, and positive end-expiratory pressure (PEEP) = 10 cm H_2O with pressure control ventilation). The patient worsened suddenly (Pvo_2 = 19 mm Hg; Svo_2 = 36%; Sao_2 = 77%; and declining lung volume). A bedside echocardiogram showed an enlarged right ventricle with decreased function. A diagnosis of thoracic compartment syndrome was made. **(C)** The patient's clamshell incision was reopened in the ICU, and her chest was opened. An immediate improvement in her hemodynamics was noted: her Sao_2 increased to 100% and Svo_2 increased to 45%. The patient was stabilized and eventually returned to the OR, where large amounts of clot were removed from both hemithoraces. Sources of bleeding were found in multiple areas but mainly in the left hilar area. The bleeding was contained and the patient was left with her chest open, covered with sterile dressings, and returned to the ICU. **(D)** The radiograph shows postoperative changes and the image shows the open chest. The mediastinal structures appear normal and lungs are expanded. **(E)** Seventy-two hours later, the patient returned to the OR to have her clamshell incision closed with no hemodynamic or respiratory impairment. The patient required a tracheostomy and prolonged ventilatory support. She was discharged from the hospital 30 days after the transplant. **(F)** Radiograph of the patient 1-year after double-lung transplantation.

explain these findings, the index of clinical suspicion for pulmonary embolism should be high and prompt studies such as echocardiography to rule out intracardiac thrombosis, Doppler ultrasound of the upper and lower extremities, and CT angiography. Sources of thrombotic emboli include deep vein thrombosis of the upper and lower extremities (particularly in critically ill recipients supported by mechanical ventilation before transplantation), intracardiac clots in patients with arrhythmias, a stenotic pulmonary artery anastomosis, or unexpected emboli from the donor lungs.[28] Management can be challenging because full anticoagulation or thrombolytic therapy may be contraindicated in the early posttransplantation period, thus making open surgical embolectomy while the patient is undergoing cardiopulmonary bypass a viable therapeutic alternative.[29]

Left Ventricular Failure. Left ventricular failure after transplantation is rare because recipients are screened before transplantation to rule out significant left ventricular dysfunction. Transient left ventricular dysfunction (stress cardiomyopathy) can occur following hypoxemia, tachyarrhythmia, or multiorgan failure. Treatment will be directed mainly toward managing the primary cause of dysfunction.

Thrombosis or Stenosis of the Pulmonary Veins. This rare but acute, dramatic, and often fatal complication develops immediately after transplantation and is associated with persistent and dense pulmonary edema in the lung and a stenotic pulmonary vein anastomosis. Hemodynamic symptoms will include elevated PCWP (although left atrial pressure will be decreased and the echocardiogram will show a hyperdynamic volume-depleted left ventricle), elevated PAPl and CVP along with decreased SV, and severe arterial and mixed venous hypoxemia. Systemic hypotension and metabolic acidosis will be present. The diagnosis will be confirmed by transesophageal echocardiography and CT angiography. Aggressive supportive management and exploratory thoracic surgery that includes repair of a stenotic anastomosis or acute redo transplantation may be lifesaving (Figure 25.3).[30]

Afterload

Afterload is represented by the myocardial wall tension occurring at initial systolic ejection. The main factor related to myocardial wall tension during systolic ejection will be the PVR for the right heart and systemic vascular resistance (SVR) for the left heart. PVR is calculated as PVR = 80 × (mean PAP - PCWP)/CO (normal value, <250 dynes/sec/cm⁵). SVR = 80 × (mean blood pressure - CVP)/CO (normal range = 800 to 1200 dynes/sec/cm⁵). Posttransplant patients with abnormal SV secondary to pulmonary hypertension and increased PVR will benefit from vasodilator therapies such as inhaled nitric oxide, systemic pulmonary vasodilators (epoprostenol or treprostinil), phosphodiesterase inhibitors (sildenafil), or combinations thereof. Patients with an abnormal SV response and increased SVR will benefit from systemic vasodilator therapy (hydralazine, nitroprusside, calcium channel blocker, and others). Patients

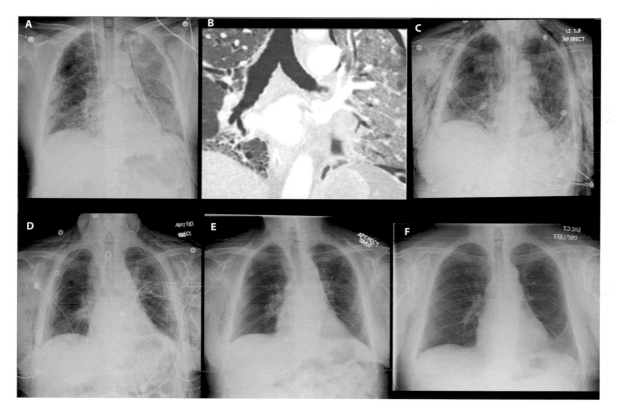

Figure 25.3 Stenosis of the pulmonary vein anastomosis. **(A)** A chest radiograph of a 58-year-old man shows interstitial changes in his native left lung that are consistent with idiopathic pulmonary fibrosis and a transplanted left single lung with pulmonary edema. The patient was clinically unstable with moderate pulmonary hypertension and an elevated pulmonary capillary wedge pressure (18 to 20 mm Hg). He had abundant and persistent pulmonary edema aspirated from his left lung. His arterial blood gas results were as follows: pH = 7.28 and Paco₂ = 37 to 74 mm Hg with mechanical ventilator support (a positive end-expiratory pressure [PEEP] setting of 12 cm H₂O and Fio₂ setting of 1.0). The recipient had small pulmonary veins, and the surgeon reported performing the pulmonary anastomosis by opening the pulmonary veins separately and suturing the two to provide a wider opening, after which the donor pulmonary vein was anastomosed to both veins. **(B)** A CT angiogram shows a tight focal stricture at the site of anastomosis of the transplanted left lung's superior and inferior pulmonary veins to the surgically created common pulmonary venous trunk on the left of the recipient heart. Additional postsurgical changes in the mediastinum, including a small pneumomediastinum and large left pneumothorax, are evident. Dense consolidation is diffusely present in the transplanted left lung. Transesophageal echocardiography also showed changes consistent with a stenotic pulmonary venous anastomosis. The patient was provided with ventilator support and inhaled nitric oxide and listed for a redo double-lung transplant. **(C)** A radiograph shows the patient with a tracheostomy in place after the development of bilateral pneumothoraces and extensive subcutaneous emphysema as a result of mechanical ventilator support with high PEEP. The patient remained hypoxic with a Pao₂/Fio₂ ratio lower than 100. **(D)** Twenty-three days after the initial left single-lung transplant, the patient received an uncomplicated double-lung transplant. **(E)** Chest radiograph taken 7 days after the double-lung transplant and removal of the tracheostomy. The patient was discharged from the hospital 7 days after the redo double-lung transplant and 30 days after the initial left single-lung transplant. **(F)** A chest radiograph shows the patient 1 year after the transplant.

with declining SV and decreased systemic pressure with decreased SVR should be evaluated for precipitant factors such as sepsis or adverse drug effects and treated accordingly. While the cause of reduced vascular resistance is being managed, patients will benefit from vasopressor agents such as norepinephrine, epinephrine, phenylephrine, vasopressin, or dopamine.

Contractility

The ability of the myocardium to contract depends on adequate blood and oxygen supply to the muscle. Many clinical circumstances alter contractility after transplantation, including metabolic or respiratory acidosis, hypoxemia, hypotension, and electrolytic imbalances such as hypocalcemia. When SV is abnormal, thus causing a decline in Svo_2, and poor contractility is suspected, a bedside echocardiogram complements the hemodynamic profile and helps establish an accurate diagnosis. If reduced contractility is diagnosed, inotropic agents (dobutamine, dopamine, milrinone) are administered to optimize CO while correcting the primary event resulting in myocardial dysfunction. Inotropic agents will be most effective if all electrolytic imbalances, volume depletion, and metabolic acidosis have been corrected. Patients refractory to medical therapy could require transient intra-aortic balloon pump support or VA ECMO support.

DECREASED ARTERIAL OXYGEN CONTENT

Decreased Cao_2 (18 to 20 mL O_2/100 mL or less) will contribute to decreased oxygenation of peripheral tissues and a consequent decline in Svo2. Decreased Cao_2 occurs for two reasons: reduced hemoglobin or reduced Sao_2.

Low hemoglobin

Low hemoglobin is related to two factors.

Anemia

Lung transplant recipients may have anemia because they were debilitated before transplantation. The cause of posttransplantation anemia must be identified and treated specifically.

Postoperative bleeding

Postoperative bleeding is a common complication. Hourly monitoring of vital signs, clinical evaluation, bedside radiography, serial hemoglobin testing, and analysis of hematocrit and coagulation profiles are part of the postoperative monitoring. Patients with persistent active bleeding (250 mL/hr) via chest tubes may need exploratory thoracotomy to remove clots and contain active sources of postoperative bleeding. Lack of bloody drainage via chest tubes should not dissuade the ICU physician from considering active bleeding as a cause of decompensation because tubes can become obstructed or may not be located in a position that allows effective drainage. Patients with active bleeding will have clinical and hemodynamic signs of hypovolemia with low CVP, pulmonary artery wedge pressure, and declining Svo_2;

they will have hypotension and changes in pulse pressure consistent with loss of volume, as well as declining Svo_2 resulting from low SV (decreased preload) and decreased Cao_2. Bedside radiographs and, when indicated, CT of the chest will show progressively larger pleural densities consistent with accumulation of blood and clots. Such patients will need aggressive correction of postoperative coagulopathy by the administration of blood products as indicated (transfusion of fresh frozen plasma, platelets, cryoprecipitate, and other products). While coagulopathy is being corrected (or afterward), thoracic exploration must be performed to evacuate accumulated blood and clots, identify sources of bleeding, contain areas of active bleeding, and replace chest tube drains.

Hematologic Complications. Patients requiring large infusions of packed red blood cells require frequent monitoring of the prothrombin time, partial thromboplastin time, fibrinogen, and platelets. Transfusion of fresh frozen plasma, cryoprecipitate, and platelets should be administered as indicated to prevent transfusion-induced coagulopathy. A large infusion of packed red blood cells may cause metabolic alkalosis and hypocalcemia secondary to citrate toxicity induced by the citrate present in stored blood products. Monitoring of ionized calcium and IV administration of calcium chloride will prevent or manage complications from hypocalcemia, such as myocardial dysfunction and hypotension. Administration of blood products can cause pulmonary edema resulting from volume overload or may induce transfusion-related acute lung injury secondary to leukocyte sequestration and priming in the lung microvasculature and subsequent activation of these leukocytes by preformed antileukocyte antibodies contained in the transfused product. Such complications will produce a new acute lung injury pattern with noncardiogenic pulmonary edema following the infusion of blood products, thus requiring further ventilatory support.[31]

Low Sao_2 and Pao_2 and pulmonary complications

After hypoxemia attributable to an intracardiac right-to-left shunt via a patent foramen ovale has been ruled out, a systematic review of postoperative hypoxemia, which can be caused by either ventilation-perfusion mismatch or an intrapulmonary right-to-left shunt resulting in low Svo_2, should be performed to explore two possible physiologic causes of hypoxic respiratory failure: decreased static lung compliance and increased airway resistance.

Decreased static lung compliance

Compliance of the respiratory system as a whole is conventionally measured by dividing the V_T by the difference between the Ppl measured at the airway opening during an occlusion at the end of inspiration and PEEP (V_T /[Ppl - PEEP]). Total PEEP should be used in patients with auto-PEEP. Decreased compliance (<50 mL/cm H_2O) will be present in cases involving abnormalities occurring at the level of the lung parenchyma and alveolar spaces, including in the setting of clinical conditions such as volume overload, cardiogenic or noncardiogenic pulmonary edema, interstitial pneumonitis, and all clinical conditions resulting in postoperative atelectasis or consolidation.

Pulmonary complications producing decreased compliance include the following: PGD; pneumonia; pulmonary edema; atelectasis, which may be secondary to extrinsic compression of lung tissue resulting from pleural complications; dysfunctional diaphragms; and other postoperative complications.

PGD is a severe type of acute ischemia-reperfusion injury that occurs within 72 hours of lung transplantation and results in noncardiogenic pulmonary edema similar to that with adult respiratory distress syndrome; it is characterized by the presence of diffuse alveolar infiltrates on chest radiographs and refractory hypoxemia that is best identified by Pao_2/Fio_2 ratios lower than 200 in cases of severe (grade 3) PGD. The diagnosis is established if no other causes of dysfunction, such as cardiogenic pulmonary edema, pneumonia, acute rejection, or pulmonary venous outflow obstruction, are present. When the results of histologic examination are available, diffuse alveolar damage will be present at the histologic level.[32,33] Severe PGD is associated with increased morbidity, mortality, and a higher probability of the development of bronchiolitis obliterans syndrome. Treatment is largely supportive and similar to that provided for acute respiratory distress syndrome (ARDS); it includes protective low-volume (6 mL/kg ideal body weight) and low-pressure ventilator support for prevention of barotrauma, use of PEEP for alveolar recruitment, avoidance of fluid overload and diuresis in the setting of alveolar-capillary leak, use of iNO, and endobronchial administration of exogenous surfactant via bronchoscopy. Refractory cases will benefit from ECMO.[32]

Pneumonia is diagnosed on the basis of the presence of areas of consolidation on chest radiographs, fever, leukocytosis, and purulent secretions associated with positive cultures in samples obtained by bronchoalveolar lavage. Management includes supportive measures, mechanical ventilation, and specific antimicrobial therapy guided by culture data.

Pulmonary edema is caused not only by PGD but also by volume overload, left-heart failure, or pulmonary venous anastomosis. As discussed elsewhere, management will be specific for each condition.

Atelectasis is the loss of lung volume resulting from the collapse of lung tissue. Lung tissue may collapse postoperatively as a result of poor inspiratory and cough efforts, which are limited because of postoperative pain, thereby resulting in bronchial obstruction in the form of mucus plugs or clots. Lung transplant recipients have impaired mucociliary clearance and thick secretions secondary to ischemic necrosis of the anastomosis and distal airways. Treatment includes adequate pain control, chest therapy, suctioning, and therapeutic bronchoscopy. Atelectasis may occur as a result of surfactant dysfunction, which increases surface tension and thereby induces alveolar collapse.

Endobronchial instillation of exogenous surfactant may help improve postoperative atelectasis. Compressive atelectasis may occur secondary to other problems such as pleural complications or diaphragmatic dysfunction.

Pleural complications resulting in compressive atelectasis include persistent pleural effusions, hemothorax, pneumothorax, and chylothorax. Thoracostomy chest tube drains are left in place until the transplanted lungs show full reexpansion and pleural drainage is less than 100 mL/day. Bleeding in the pleural cavity occurs more frequently as a result of traumatic lesions to the pleura during surgery and more commonly in patients requiring cardiopulmonary bypass. Those with large accumulations of blood in the pleural cavity require surgical exploration to remove blood from the pleural space, correct the cause of bleeding, and allow lung reexpansion.

Chylothorax is a rare complication that causes an accumulation of lymphatic fluid (chyle) in the pleural space; it is diagnosed by the milky appearance of fluid, high levels of triglycerides (>110 mg/dL), and the presence of chylomicrons. Chylothorax results from surgical disruption of the thoracic duct or its tributaries and leakage into the pleural space. Chylothorax is more likely to develop in patients who have received transplants for lymphangioleiomyomatosis because of leakage of chyle from dilated or torn mediastinal lymphatic vessels or from transdiaphragmatic flow of chylous ascites. High-output chylothorax is a challenge in the setting of added immune suppression, electrolytic imbalance, and malnutrition. Management includes prolonged drainage, IV hyperalimentation, an IV infusion of octreotide, thoracic duct ligation, and pleuroperitoneal or pleurovenous shunts.[34,35]

Other complications resulting in atelectasis include diaphragmatic dysfunction or paralysis, which occurs in 15% to 30% of lung transplant recipients as a result of mechanical trauma, stretch injury, or hypothermic injury to the phrenic nerves. It is more common in recipients with previous thoracic surgery or complex mediastinal pathology. Patients have elevated diaphragms on chest radiographs with abdominothoracic respiratory dissociation during spontaneous breathing, and they cannot be successfully weaned from positive pressure ventilation, as a result of which percutaneous tracheostomy placement and prolonged ventilator support are required. Unilateral diaphragmatic paralysis can be managed by surgical plication of the diaphragm. In some cases the dysfunctional diaphragm will recover function with time, as well as with physical and respiratory therapy.[36] Another cause of compressive atelectasis of the transplanted lung is hyperinflation of the native lung in single-lung transplant recipients with COPD. If supporting such patients with mechanical ventilation does not provide sufficient expiratory flow, progressive hyperinflation occurs and results in mediastinal shift and extrinsic compression of the graft. Management includes double-lumen intubation to provide independent lung ventilation, with the ventilator settings for the native lung selected to provide a prolonged expiratory time, minimal PEEP, and low V_T while the transplant side is managed with high PEEP and protective ventilation. Double-lumen intubation makes clearance of secretions difficult. In our program, cases refractory to independent lung ventilation have been managed with lung volume reduction surgery on the native lung to facilitate expansion of the transplanted lung.

Increased airway resistance and airway complications

Airway resistance is calculated as the difference between peak inspiratory pressure (PIP) minus Ppl during an occlusion at the end of inspiration divided by the airflow: airway resistance = (PIP - Ppl)/flow (normal range, 10 cm $H_2O/L/$ sec or less). Patients with increased airway resistance (>10 cm $H_2O/L/$sec) should be evaluated for endotracheal tube obstruction or tracheostomy, increased secretions, mucus plugging, anastomotic stenosis, or clot formation in the distal airways. Airway complications occurring after transplantation include ischemic necrosis, airway dehiscence, and bronchial stenosis.[37]

Ischemic Necrosis. During harvesting of the donor lung, the bronchial arterial circulation is lost and not reestablished. Microrevascularization will occur in the weeks following transplantation. During that period, low-pressure retrograde blood flow from poorly oxygenated pulmonary arterial circulation collaterals sustains the viability of the bronchial structures. Factors such as hypotension, low CO, hypoxemia, and others enhance ischemic necrosis and results in thick necrotic debris that requires extensive suctioning and débridement with therapeutic bronchoscopy until the ischemic necrosis is removed.

Airway Dehiscence. Some degree of ischemic necrosis develops in all transplant recipients. Some cases will progress to partial or, rarely, complete dehiscence. Patients with dehiscence exhibit dyspnea, failure to wean from mechanical ventilation, pneumothorax, pneumomediastinum, and subcutaneous emphysema. A CT scan will show bronchial wall defects and extraluminal air around the anastomotic area. A small dehiscence (<4 mm in diameter) is managed conservatively with antibiotics and temporary placement of uncovered self-expanding metal stents, which may promote the growth of granulation tissue and in turn help heal the dehiscence. Larger defects require open surgical repair in which muscle or pericardium is used to wrap the defect. In selected cases, retransplantation may be required.

Bronchial Stenosis. Stenotic lesions occur following ischemic necrosis, healing of dehiscence, or early bronchial infections. Stenotic lesions may be at the level of the bronchial anastomosis or in distal bronchial structures. Bronchial stenosis is a common complication of lung transplantation but is rarely present early after transplantation. It can range from mild, asymptomatic lesions to nearly complete occlusion of the airways with severe functional impairment. When present, it will be managed initially with balloon bronchoplasty, which allows airways to be dilated from 6 to as much as 15 mm in diameter. Lesions refractory to balloon dilatation can be managed with various

modalities of care such as cryotherapy, brachytherapy, argon plasma coagulation, or laser therapy in preparation for the deployment of temporary removable silicone stents or self-expanding uncovered metallic stents, which are typically left in place.

OTHER COMPLICATIONS FOLLOWING LUNG TRANSPLANTATION

Neurologic complications

In general, metabolic encephalopathy, posterior reversible encephalopathy syndrome (PRES), drug reaction involving eosinophilia and systemic symptoms, nosocomial bacterial infection, calcineurin inhibitor toxicity, perioperative stroke, and anoxic encephalopathy are the most relevant neurologic complications during the first month after lung transplantation.

The Mayo Clinic Lung Transplant Registry (1998 to 2008) has provided the largest retrospective study to date demonstrating an association between post–lung transplantation neurologic complications and a higher risk for death (hazard ratio = 7.2, 95% confidence interval = 3.5 to 14.6, P <.001). The neurologic complications are described as severe in 31% of cases. Encephalopathy, stroke, and seizures are the main causes of neurologic deficit in the early postoperative period. Perioperative anoxic or hypoxic encephalopathy, sepsis, metabolic encephalopathy, and medications (specifically cyclosporine and tacrolimus) are common. In this cohort, only older age and bilateral lung transplants have been identified as risk factors.[38] On rare occasion, air embolism has been found to be the cause of perioperative stroke after lung transplantation.[39] Sirolimus has also been implicated as a medication that can cause encephalopathy.

Post–lung transplantation patients characterized by an acute confusional state, focal neurologic deficit, or decreased level of consciousness require evaluation by a neurocritical care specialist or neurologist. A careful chart review is followed by an examination of the patient that emphasizes focal signs; brain CT and preferably magnetic resonance imaging with gadolinium contrast help in better characterizing the cause of perioperative encephalopathy. Furthermore, PRES is a condition related to cyclosporine or tacrolimus toxicity; it is characterized by areas of hyperintensity on T2-weighted and fluid-attenuated inversion recovery images of the subcortical white matter of the posterior temporal, parietal, and occipital lobes. Such areas represent vasogenic edema and clinical symptoms, including confusion, hypertension, seizures, and headache. Recognition of PRES is crucial to patient outcome and it is often reversible, but it can be associated with stroke and seizures. In cases of cyclosporine- or tacrolimus-related PRES, sirolimus and mycophenolate are valid alternatives.[40,41]

Early hyperammonemia and associated coma are well-described, potentially fatal complications after lung transplantation. Typically, hyperammonemia is characterized by encephalopathy, psychomotor agitation, seizures, or coma. The pathophysiology remains elusive. Treatment is supportive, and a high caloric intake is recommended. Discontinuation of exogenous nitrogen, increased caloric intake to suppress catabolism, alternative waste nitrogen agents (such as sodium benzoate or phenyl acetate), and hemodialysis to remove brain ammonia and glutamine are considered reasonable interventions in patients with secondary hyperammonemic coma. Aggressive management is pivotal to improving clinical outcomes because of the apparent existence of a point of irreversibility, after which efforts to decrease ammonia levels are ineffective.

Gastrointestinal complications

Gastrointestinal complications are the second most common cause of an emergency condition following lung transplantation. They can be associated with substantial morbidity and mortality, with reported rates ranging from 3.2% to 43% and 0% to 26%, respectively.[42-45] Furthermore, Lahon and colleagues reported a 7.4% incidence and 19% rate of direct mortality resulting from these early severe digestive complications after lung transplantation without cardiopulmonary bypass. The main risk factors were older age and bilateral lung transplantation.

These complications in the early postoperative phase can be tentatively classified as surgical and nonsurgical. Among the nonsurgical complications, gastroparesis, gastroesophageal reflux, dysphagia, ileus, mild gastrointestinal bleeding, and pancreatitis are commonly described. Pancreatitis may be relatively common after lung transplantation with cardiopulmonary bypass. However, most of these episodes are asymptomatic or subclinical and show an increase in the serum lipase level, amylase level, or both.

The main implications of ileus after lung transplantation are directly related to the decision to perform tracheal extubation, provide airway protection, and administer oral immunosuppressive medications. This complication is multifactorial, and its treatment remains supportive.[46,47] First, epidural analgesia is a valuable alternative to IV opioid analgesia once the coagulopathy has subsided. Second, repletion of hypomagnesemia and hypokalemia facilitates intestinal motility. Third, avoidance of medications that cause ileus, such as calcium channel blockers, is recommended. Fourth, laxatives are needed to allow daily stools, especially for distal obstruction syndrome in patients with cystic fibrosis once mechanical obstruction has been ruled out by contrast-enhanced CT of the abdomen. Finally, enterotomy and fecal disimpaction are possible interventions when the aforementioned measures have been unsuccessful.

The coexistence of gastrointestinal reflux disease increases the risk for both aspiration and subsequent bronchiolitis obliterans and rejection.[48] Utilization of duodenal or jejunal enteral nutrition and avoidance of gastric tubes are overemphasized.[49] Prokinetics and proton pump inhibitors are another measure to prevent reflux. In selective cases, surgical intervention to control reflux has been proposed.[50,51]

Assessment of swallowing function after tracheal extubation is a common practice to prevent aspiration and can improve the survival of lung transplant patients.[52]

Surgical gastrointestinal complications are less common (occurring in up to 17% of cases) but portend higher mortality if emergency intervention is required. Such complications include colon or diverticula perforation and appendicitis, which can be masked by immunosuppression and postoperative analgesia with opioids. One of the first reports of colonic perforation during corticosteroid therapy showed a mortality rate of 70%.[53] Thus, the index of suspicion should be high any time that a patient has a septic condition with nonspecific findings on the abdominal examination. Toxic megacolon is another *Clostridium difficile*–related complication necessitating exploratory laparotomy.[54]

ULTRASONOGRAPHIC ASSESSMENT OF PATIENTS FOLLOWING LUNG TRANSPLANTATION

In the postrecovery period, ultrasonography provides noninvasive, rapid, and accurate diagnostic information. Focused transthoracic echocardiography is better suited for the dynamic nature of the critically ill patients in the ICU than is formal echocardiography performed by cardiology services.[55] We have found the combined application of both focused echocardiography and lung ultrasonography to be very useful in the initial assessment of lung transplant patients with symptoms of shock, acute respiratory failure, or both.

Focused echocardiography following lung transplantation

Two point-of-care echocardiography protocols are commonly used with the critically ill patients (Figure 25.4A).[56]

The FEEL (focused echocardiographic evaluation in life support) examination. Echocardiography may distinguish "true" pulseless electrical activity (PEA) from pseudo-PEA. In pseudo-PEA, a coordinated cardiac contraction is found despite a PEA rhythm. Furthermore, identification and appropriate management of the following four treatable causes of cardiac arrest may be lifesaving in the perioperative period: (1) cardiac tamponade, (2) hypovolemia, (3) pulmonary embolism, and (4) severe left or right ventricular dysfunction (Figure 25.4B).[57-59]

The FATE (focused assessment with transthoracic echocardiography) examination. Focused transthoracic echocardiography is a form of qualitative point-of-care ultrasonography; it is noninvasive and performed at the bedside (Table 25.2). At a minimum, FATE includes qualitative assessment of left and right ventricular function, intravascular volume, and pleural effusion or hemothorax (Figure 25.4B). It supplements critical care evaluation in the perioperative setting. However, focused echocardiography does not replace a comprehensive echocardiogram performed by a cardiology specialist whenever quantitative analysis is needed. The main goal of the FATE examination

A

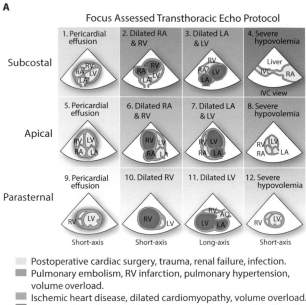

Focus Assessed Transthoracic Echo Protocol

Postoperative cardiac surgery, trauma, renal failure, infection.
Pulmonary embolism, RV infarction, pulmonary hypertension, volume overload.
Ischemic heart disease, dilated cardiomyopathy, volume overload.
Intravascular volume depletion, hemorrhage, aggressive diuresis, diarrhea.

B

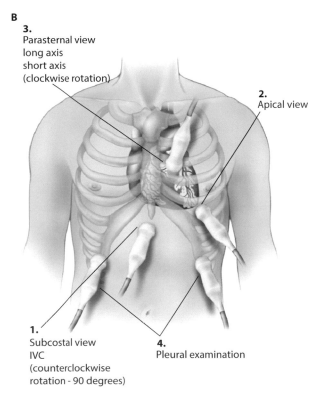

Figure 25.4 **(A)** The FATE (focused transthoracic echocardiography) protocol. **(B)** Echocardiography views: (1) subcostal view; (2) apical view; (3) parasternal view; and (4) pleural examination. (By permission of the Mayo Foundation for Medical Education and Research. All rights reserved.)

is to better characterize the state of shock or hypotension and pleural pathology (Figure 25.4B):

- Hypovolemia (inferior vena cava [IVC] diameter and distensibility index [see later]).

- Myocardial dysfunction (qualitative evaluation of the right ventricle and left ventricle).
- Pericardial effusion or tamponade.
- Pulmonary embolism (changes in acute right ventricular dysfunction).
- Pleural effusion (or hemothorax) and pneumothorax.[60]

The appropriate procedure for performing FATE includes acquisition of images, recognition of normal anatomy of the heart, fundamental knowledge of the more important pathologic conditions, and application of the findings to the clinical context. In emergency conditions, the first view obtained is the subcostal view (Figure 25.4A). For this view, the patient is placed in the supine position. In contrast, the left lateral position is advantageous for the study of parasternal and apical views.

Assessment of Volume Status. This form of assessment is used to visualize the IVC and measure the distensibility index (of patients receiving mechanical ventilatory support) by proceeding with a counterclockwise rotation from "3 o'clock to 12 o'clock" (90 degrees) from the initial subcostal view.

Distensibility index

$$= \frac{IVC_{max} \text{ (end inspiration)} - IVC_{min} \text{ (end exhalation)}}{IVC_{min} \text{ (end exhalation)}}$$
$$\times 100 \text{ (percentage)}$$

A distensibility index greater than 18% predicts fluid responsiveness with a positive predictive value of 93% and a negative predictive value of 92%. Patients should be well sedated or even paralyzed, receiving a V_T of 8 to 10 mL/kg, and maintaining a sinus rhythm. A false-negative result is defined as a V_T less than 8 mL/kg. If the patient has active breathing while receiving mechanical ventilatory support, a passive leg-raising test is advised.[61,62]

Finally, for patients who do not have an optimal subcostal view for visualization of the IVC, use of the maximal velocity (Vpeak) variation with respiration in the left ventricular outflow tract and pulsed wave Doppler is a very valuable technique for mechanically ventilated patients. A $V\Delta peak$ variation of greater than 12% predicts fluid responsiveness with a sensitivity of 100% and specificity of 89%.[63,64]

$$V\Delta peak = 100 \times \frac{(Vpeak_{max} - Vpeak_{min})}{(Vpeak_{max} - Vpeak_{min})/2}$$

Lung ultrasonography following lung transplantation

Lung ultrasound has very high yield in the immediate management of potential life-threatening conditions (severe pulmonary edema, large hemothorax, pneumothorax, and lung collapse) and a very high impact on clinical decision making after lung transplantation (Figure 25.5A and B).[65,66] We present these perioperative applications.

Table 25.2 Technique for the focused assessed transthoracic echocardiography (FATE) protocol

View	Transducer location	Approximate probe orientation marker	Depth	Helpful tips
Subcostal	2–3 cm below the xyphoid process or right upper quadrant if chest tubes are in place	3 o'clock	15–25 cm	Hold the transducer from the top angled between 10 and 40 degrees with the patient in a supine position
Subcostal inferior vena cava	From the previous view rotate the transducer 90 degrees counterclockwise	12 o'clock	16–24 cm	Keep the right atrium–IVC junction on the screen. Make sure that the merger of the IVC into right atrium is visible
Apical	Find the point of maximal impulse if feasible. Otherwise from the anterior axillar line to the nipple	3 o'clock	14–18 cm	Use gentle pressure to ensure good contact with the rib
Parasternal long-axis	3rd or 4th intercostal space	11 o'clock	12–20 cm (up to 24 if pleural or pericardial effusion present)	Ideally, use the left lateral decubitus position
Parasternal short-axis	Rotate 90 degrees clockwise from the parasternal long-axis view, so approximately 2 o'clock	2 o'clock	12–16 cm	With "rocking" movement of the probe: Aortic valve level: Hold the transducer facing slightly upward toward the patient's right shoulder Mitral valve level: Hold the transducer perpendicular to the chest wall Papillary muscle level: Hold the transducer facing slightly downward toward the patient's left flank

Note: IVC, inferior vena cava.

STEP 1: TECHNIQUE AND IDENTIFICATION OF NORMAL AND ABNORMAL SIGNS AND PATTERNS ON LUNG ULTRASONOGRAPHY WITH THE LINEAR PROBE

Assessment of patients with clinical symptoms indicative of pneumothorax and lung collapse

The first step of the examination (examination of lung/pleural sliding) should be performed with a higher-frequency linear probe (7.5 to 12 MHz). This linear transducer allows higher ultrasound resolution for structures that are closer to the probe (pleura). For this reason, one of the most relevant applications of focused lung ultrasonography is for the evaluation of patients in whom pneumothorax is suspected.

Technique

As described previously, the anterior chest wall can be divided into four quadrants when the patient is in a supine position (Figure 25.5B and Table 25.3).[67,68a]

Lung sliding

A sliding movement between the visceral and parietal pleura is described as the "lung sliding sign." This sign is useful to exclude pneumothorax. However, its absence does not confirm pneumothorax because other conditions, such as adhesions resulting from previous thoracic surgeries or severe ARDS, may make it more difficult to see normal "lung sliding" (Figure 25.5A).[68] Representation of this normal "lung sliding" in M-mode complements the sonographic evaluation. The resultant complex image, which includes the static thoracic wall, the dynamic pleural movement, and the lung parenchyma, provides a granular pattern that has been called the "seashore sign" because of its similarity to the appearance of beach sand. The absence of lung sliding on M-mode has been termed a "bar code sign." Its appearance differs from that of the normal "seashore sign" (Figures 25.5C and E).[69]

Lung point

The lung point is a useful sign for the diagnosis of partial pneumothorax. Furthermore, it indicates the point of

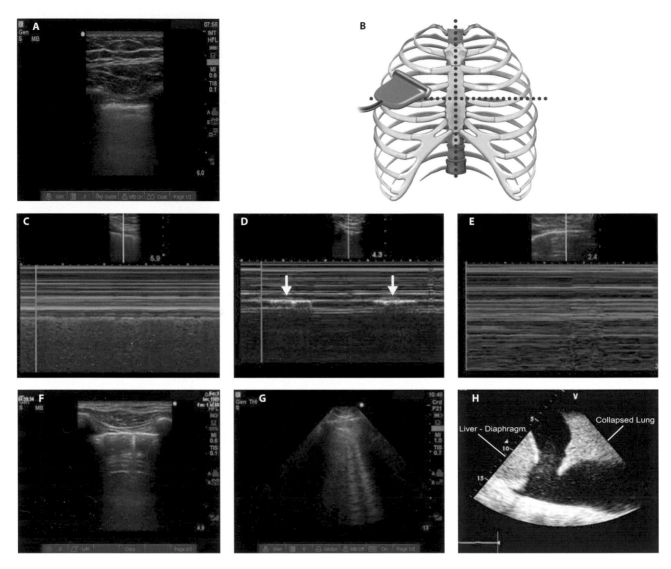

Figure 25.5 Lung ultrasound findings in the perioperative period. **(A)** Normal lung and pleural sliding visualized with a linear probe. The maximal depth is 6 cm. **(B)** Probe manipulation in four chest wall quadrants. The ultrasound examination should include each quadrant. **(C)** Normal lung and pleural sliding visualized by using a linear probe and M-mode. **(D)** M-mode representation of the lung point and partial pneumothorax (mix of a granular-normal pattern with arrows and horizontal-pneumothorax patterns). **(E)** Bar code sign and pneumothorax. **(F)** Representation of normal A-lines with a phased-array transducer; the lines have a horizontal orientation. **(G)** Representation of abnormal B-lines with a phased-array transducer; these lines have a vertical orientation. **(H)** Ultrasound appearance of a large right pleural effusion. The liver, diaphragm, and collapsed lung are labeled.

transition between normal sliding and absence of sliding. Use of M-mode (time-motion mode) can facilitate its recognition. This sign is considered very specific (98% to 100%) for pneumothorax. However, the examination of all quadrants must be extended to the lateral regions of the chest wall to rule out pneumothorax.

Lung pulse

The lung pulse is a useful sign for the diagnosis of lung collapse. Complete atelectasis facilitates interaction of the ultrasound beam with the beats of the heart at the pleural line on M-mode. The appearance of cardiac pulsation at the pleural line on M-mode and absence of lung sliding in

real-time two-dimensional ultrasonography characterizes the lung pulse sign (Figure 25.5D).[70]

STEP 2: TECHNIQUE AND IDENTIFICATION OF NORMAL AND ABNORMAL SIGNS AND PATTERNS IN FOCUSED LUNG ULTRASONOGRAPHY WITH THE PHASED-ARRAY PROBE

Clinical significance of A-lines

The second step in the examination (examination of the lung parenchyma) should be performed with the phased-array probe (2.5 to 4 MHz). Under normal conditions, the A-lines constitute the basic artifact of normal lungs. They are depicted as horizontal artifacts parallel to the pleural

Table 25.3 Technique of perioperative lung ultrasonography

Probe	Transducer location	Approximate probe orientation marker	Depth	Helpful tips and diagnostic implications
Linear probe	Any of the four anterior quadrants of the anterior chest wall Ensure good contact with two ribs (a rib shadow on each side of the screen monitor, called the *bat sign*, is visible)	12 o'clock	6 cm	Hold the transducer from the side (as a pen) at a 90-degree angle (perpendicular) to the anterior chest wall with the patient in a supine or semirecumbent position Diagnosis: • Pneumothorax • Lung collapse • Pleural effusion—pleurocentesis guidance
Phased-array probe	Any of the four anterior quadrants of the anterior chest wall Ensure good contact with two ribs (rib shadow on each side of the screen monitor, called the *bat sign*, is still visible but will be less noticeable)	12 o'clock	12–14 cm	Hold the transducer from the side (as a pen) at a 90-degree angle (perpendicular) to the anterior chest wall with the patient in a supine position. Diagnosis: • Alveolar interstitial pulmonary syndrome • Pleural effusion—passive atelectasis

In any case of an unclear image:
• Rule out the presence of subcutaneous emphysema or overlying obstruction (dressings, electrocardiography pads, etc.)
• Verify use of the correct probe, reposition the patient, use more gel

line and can be multiples of the distance between the skin and pleural line (Figure 25.5F). It is important to acknowledge that A-lines can be present in cases of pneumothorax when the sliding sign is absent.

Clinical significance of B-lines and alveolar interstitial syndrome

One of the most useful applications of lung ultrasonography is for the early detection of acute interstitial pulmonary edema. Furthermore, other causes of alveolar interstitial syndrome are ARDS, pneumonia, and chronic interstitial lung disease. Thus, serial application is helpful in determining changes in patients with previous findings associated with their underlying pathologic condition.[71,72] The ultrasound representation of this syndrome is the appearance of B-lines or "lung comets" (Figure 25.5G).[73,74] These lines represent diffuse involvement of the lung interstitium, as well as the alveolar air spaces, and thickening of interlobular septa. Alveolar interstitial syndrome is defined by a hyperechogenic, wedge-based signal that fans out from the lung-wall interface and is separated by a distance greater than 7 mm at the subpleural level. At least three lung comets between two ribs on one longitudinal scan must be identified (Figure 25.5G). It is important to mention that B-lines can be normally present in the dependent regions of the thorax (below the anterior axillary and below the fifth intercostal space).

The "gold standard" for diagnosing interstitial syndrome is CT of the chest, and its high level of comparability with lung ultrasound has been demonstrated (sensitivity = 87% to 97%, specificity = 87% to 96%).[75,76]

Ultrasound assessment of patients with signs of pleural effusions

Reliable recognition of pleural effusions is feasible with the use of a phased-array probe, which provides penetration and image depth adequate to assess the liver or spleen (left side), diaphragm, and lung bases. Usually, minimal fluid (which is evident as a "hypoechoic" image) is present between the base of the lung and the diaphragm (Figure 25.5H).[77,78] However, when the accumulation of fluid is more significant, the hypoechoic imaging is more evident and the collapsed lower lobe lung takes on the appearance of a hyperechoic structure (Figure 25.5H). Passive (compression) atelectasis can be noticed as a consequence of a large pleural effusion.

The nature and quantification of pleural effusion can be accurately assessed with lung ultrasonography. In fact, evidence indicates that ultrasonography provides higher sensitivity and specificity in this respect than chest radiography does.

The amount of pleural effusion can be estimated with a formula proposed by Balik:

$$V \text{ (mL)} = 20 \times Sep \text{ (mm)}$$

where V is the volume of pleural effusion and Sep is the distance between the two pleural layers.

To obtain better superficial resolution and assistance with needle manipulation in the chest wall, pleurocentesis should be guided by ultrasound with a linear probe.[77,78]

Limitations

First, subcutaneous emphysema prevents the ultrasound beam from reaching deeper structures (the pleura). Second, obese patients can be difficult to evaluate. Third, previous chest operations impede the assessment.

In summary, the evolving role of lung ultrasonography in perioperative patients improves the diagnosis of diseases of the lung and pleura. The ubiquitous availability and point-of-care use of ultrasound devices in the perioperative setting should encourage intensivists to acquire the skills and knowledge needed for lung ultrasound to provide better patient care.

EXTRACORPOREAL MEMBRANE SUPPORT FOLLOWING LUNG TRANSPLANTATION

PGD affects more than 30% of all lung transplant patients, and its severe symptoms, including refractory hypoxemia, are the main indication for ECMO following lung transplantation. In fact, ECMO is considered a reasonable and potentially lifesaving treatment option for patients with PGD who are not responding to conventional supportive therapy. Perhaps the most favorable clinical setting is an isolated occurrence of PGD and absence of infection or major comorbidity. The current incidence of ECMO support after lung transplantation in the study by Bermudez and colleagues was 7.6% during the first weeks after lung transplantation.[79]

Despite all the aforementioned supportive aspects of ECMO, uniform criteria for initiating it after lung transplantation do not exist. It is commonly used in the presence of a PIP of 35 cm H_2O and F_{IO_2} greater than 0.6, as well as in any case involving severe pulmonary edema.[80] Some publications encourage early use of ECMO support for PGD and consider it a bridge to recovery from PGD following lung transplantation; further investigations are needed to allow its better application in lung transplantation during the perioperative period, as well as to determine

its cost-effectiveness.[81] Late institution of ECMO (> 24 to 36 hours after lung transplantation) for PGD portend worse outcomes with higher mortality (even approaching 100%), particularly if ECMO is not initiated until 7 days after transplantation. Therefore, ECMO support should not be viewed as a "salvage" strategy, it should be implemented early (within 24 hours) to produce better outcomes.

Recent investigations demonstrate improved outcomes in patients with PGD who receive ECMO support, with 30-day and 1-year survival rates of 82% and 64%, respectively.[80]

ECMO is also useful as a bridge to retransplantation, which may actually be the only indication for prolonging ECMO support beyond 4 to 7 days because most of the patients who continue with this modality in the long term will not survive.[82] The average durations of ECMO among survivors in two different investigations were 2.8 and 5.0 days.[83] Moreover, some authors consider ECMO a futile therapy if it is extended more than 14 days in the clinical setting of PGD after lung transplantation.[79] Another proposed application of ECMO is for prophylaxis at the beginning of transplantation in patients at higher risk for PGD, such as those with an "oxygenation index" greater than 30 (oxygenation index = mean airway pressure × Pao_2/F_{IO_2}).[82] In a recent publication, Diamond and colleagues identified risk factors for grade 3 PGD. This risk factor profile can be helpful in improving preparedness for severe PGD.[84] VV ECMO is the preferred modality for PGD following lung transplantation. When compared with VA ECMO, VV ECMO has two major disadvantages: compromised coronary oxygenation and right ventricular overloading.[85] Furthermore, if the patient is concurrently in a state of shock, VA support can provide higher O_2D (Table 25.4).[86]

Generally, whenever concerns exist regarding full anticoagulation and hemorrhagic or neurologic complications associated with VA ECMO, VV ECMO appears to be the more attractive modality. However, when severe ventricular dysfunction or refractory shock occurs, VA ECMO provides better hemodynamic stability than does VV ECMO. Bermudez and colleagues described some potential disadvantages associated with VA ECMO, including limitation of bronchial arterial blood flow and increased hypoxic

Table 25.4 Physiologic differences between VV and VA ECMO support

Factor	VV ECMO	VA ECMO
O_2 delivery	Acceptable Pao_2	Excellent Pao_2
Pao_2 range	45-80 mm Hg	80-150 mm Hg
Blood flow	Pulsatile	Narrow pulse pressure
Pulmonary blood flow	Unaffected	Decreased
Coronary blood flow	Unaffected	Decreased
Limitation to oxygenation	Recirculation	Recovery of cardiac ejection
Cardiac effect	Mild improvement	Decreases preload, increases afterload
Mixed venous oxygen saturation	Is high by definition	Can decrease (<70%) in the case of recovering native heart function

Note: VA ECMO, venoarterial extracorporeal membrane oxygenation; VV ECMO, venovenous extracorporeal membrane oxygenation.

pulmonary vasoconstriction.[79] A clinical comparison of the VV and VA approaches is presented in Table 25.4.

Single cannulation for VV ECMO has a potentially promising role in patients who need more prolonged support as a bridge to transplantation.[87] Reasonable levels of mechanical ventilator support during VV ECMO, including lung-protective and rest levels of mechanical ventilator support, are a PiP of 20 to 25 cm H_2O, PEEP of 10 cm H_2O, and F_{IO_2} less than 0.30. Data on other ventilator modalities during ECMO are lacking.[80]

The most common complications during ECMO therapy in the early phase (48 to 72 hours) after lung transplantation are coagulopathy and bleeding. A multiple organ system failure remains the main cause of death.[80,85]

The University of Pittsburgh group has published its 15-year experience with ECMO support for early PGD; it reported 1- and 5-year survival rates of 40% and 25%, respectively, for the entire cohort. However, patients who survived PGD while receiving ECMO support had survival rates similar to those of patients who did not receive such support (1- and 5-year survival rates of 53.8% and 46.2%, respectively).[79]

REFERENCES

1. Yusen RD, Christie JD, Edwards LB, et al. The Registry of the International Society for Heart and Lung Transplantation: Thirtieth adult lung and heart-lung transplant report—2013; focus theme: Age. J Heart Lung Transplant 2013;32:965-978.
2. Lee JC, Diamond JM, Christie JD. Critical care management of the lung transplant recipient. Curr Respir Care Rep 2012;1:168-176.
3. Sundaresan S, Semenkovich J, Ochoa L, et al. Successful outcome of lung transplantation is not compromised by the use of marginal donor lungs. J Thorac Cardiovasc Surg 1995;109:1075-1079, discussion 1079-1080.
4. Bhorade SM, Vigneswaran W, McCabe MA, Garrity ER. Liberalization of donor criteria may expand the donor pool without adverse consequence in lung transplantation. J Heart Lung Transplant 2000;19:1199-1204.
5. Kawut SM, Reyentovich A, Wilt JS, et al. Outcomes of extended donor lung recipients after lung transplantation. Transplantation 2005;79:310-316.
6. Pierre AF, Sekine Y, Hutcheon MA, et al. Marginal donor lungs: A reassessment. J Thorac Cardiovasc Surg 2002;123:421-427; discussion, 427-428.
7. Mason DP, Thuita L, Alster JM, et al. Should lung transplantation be performed using donation after cardiac death? The United States experience. J Thorac Cardiovasc Surg 2008;136:1061-1066.
8. De Oliveira NC, Osaki S, Maloney JD, et al. Lung transplantation with donation after cardiac death donors: Long-term follow-up in a single center. J Thorac Cardiovasc Surg 2010;139:1306-1315.
9. Cypel M, Yeung JC, Machuca T, et al. Experience with the first 50 ex vivo lung perfusions in clinical transplantation. J Thorac Cardiovasc Surg 2012;144:1200-1206.
10. Pierre AF, Keshavjee S. Lung transplantation: Donor and recipient critical care aspects. Curr Opin Crit Care 2005;11:339-344.
11. Hammainen P, Schersten H, Lemstrom K, et al. Usefulness of extracorporeal membrane oxygenation as a bridge to lung transplantation: A descriptive study. J Heart Lung Transplant 2011;30:103-107.
12. Suzuki Y, Cantu E, Christie JD. Primary graft dysfunction. Semin Respir Crit Care Med 2013;34:305-319.
13. Thabut G, Mal H, Cerrina J, et al. Graft ischemic time and outcome of lung transplantation: A multicenter analysis. Am J Respir Crit Care Med 2005;171:786-791.
14. Hachem RR, Edwards LB, Yusen RD, et al. The impact of induction on survival after lung transplantation: An analysis of the International Society for Heart and Lung Transplantation Registry. Clin Transplant 2008;22:603-608.
15. Bhorade SM, Stern E. Immunosuppression for lung transplantation. Proc Am Thorac Soc 2009;6:47-53.
16. King-Biggs MB, Dunitz JM, Park SJ, et al. Airway anastomotic dehiscence associated with use of sirolimus immediately after lung transplantation. Transplantation 2003;75:1437-1443.
17. Husain S, Paterson DL, Studer S, et al. Voriconazole prophylaxis in lung transplant recipients. Am J Transplant 2006;6:3008-3016.
18. Zamora MR, Nicolls MR, Hodges TN, et al. Following universal prophylaxis with intravenous ganciclovir and cytomegalovirus immune globulin, valganciclovir is safe and effective for prevention of CMV infection following lung transplantation. Am J Transplant 2004;4:1635-1642.
19. Antonelli M, Levy M, Andrews PJ, et al. Hemodynamic monitoring in shock and implications for management. International Consensus Conference, Paris, France, 27-28 April 2006. Intensive Care Med 2007;33:575-590.
20. Rosenberg AL, Rao M, Benedict PE. Anesthetic implications for lung transplantation. Anesthesiol Clin North Am 2004;22:767-788.
21. See VY, Roberts-Thomson KC, Stevenson WG, et al. Atrial arrhythmias after lung transplantation: Epidemiology, mechanisms at electrophysiology study, and outcomes. Circ Arrhythm Electrophysiol 2009;2:504-510.
22. Denault AY, Chaput M, Couture P, et al. Dynamic right ventricular outflow tract obstruction in cardiac surgery. J Thorac Cardiovasc Surg 2006;132:43-49.
23. Lasocki S, Castier Y, Geffroy A, et al. Early cardiac tamponade due to tension pneumopericardium after bilateral lung transplantation. J Heart Lung Transplant 2007;26:1069-1071.

24. Kaplan LM, Epstein SK, Schwartz SL, et al. Clinical, echocardiographic, and hemodynamic evidence of cardiac tamponade caused by large pleural effusions. Am J Respir Crit Care Med 1995;151:904-908.

25. Denault A, Ferraro P, Couture P, et al. Transesophageal echocardiography monitoring in the intensive care department: The management of hemodynamic instability secondary to thoracic tamponade after single lung transplantation. J Am Soc Echocardiogr 2003;16:688-692.

26. Khan TA, Schnickel G, Ross D, et al. A prospective, randomized, crossover pilot study of inhaled nitric oxide versus inhaled prostacyclin in heart transplant and lung transplant recipients. J Thorac Cardiovasc Surg 2009;138:1417-1424.

27. Clark SC, Levine AJ, Hasan A, et al. Vascular complications of lung transplantation. Ann Thorac Surg 1996;61:1079-1082.

28. Oto T, Rabinov M, Griffiths AP, et al. Unexpected donor pulmonary embolism affects early outcomes after lung transplantation: A major mechanism of primary graft failure? J Thorac Cardiovasc Surg 2005;130:1446.

29. Yalamanchili K, Fleisher AG, Lehrman SG, et al. Open pulmonary embolectomy for treatment of major pulmonary embolism. Ann Thorac Surg 2004;77:819-823; discussion 823.

30. Schulman LL, Anandarangam T, Leibowitz DW, et al. Four-year prospective study of pulmonary venous thrombosis after lung transplantation. J Am Soc Echocardiogr 2001;14:806-812.

31. Bux J, Sachs UJ. The pathogenesis of transfusion-related acute lung injury (TRALI). Br J Haematol 2007;136:788-799.

32. Christie JD, Sager JS, Kimmel SE, et al. Impact of primary graft failure on outcomes following lung transplantation. Chest 2005;127:161-165.

33. Lee JC, Christie JD, Keshavjee S. Primary graft dysfunction: Definition, risk factors, short- and long-term outcomes. Semin Respir Crit Care Med 2010;31:161-171.

34. Ferrer J, Roldan J, Roman A, et al. Acute and chronic pleural complications in lung transplantation. J Heart Lung Transplant 2003;22:1217-1225.

35. Fremont RD, Milstone AP, Light RW, Ninan M. Chylothoraces after lung transplantation for lymphangioleiomyomatosis: Review of the literature and utilization of a pleurovenous shunt. J Heart Lung Transplant 2007;26:953-955.

36. Mogayzel PJ Jr, Colombani PM, Crawford TO, Yang SC. Bilateral diaphragm paralysis following lung transplantation and cardiac surgery in a 17-year-old. J Heart Lung Transplant 2002;21:710-712.

37. Santacruz JF, Mehta AC. Airway complications and management after lung transplantation: Ischemia, dehiscence, and stenosis. Proc Am Thorac Soc 2009;6:79-93.

38. Mateen FJ, Dierkhising RA, Rabinstein AA, et al. Neurological complications following adult lung transplantation. Am J Transplant 2010;10:908-914.

39. Erasmus DB, Alvarez F, Keller CA. Fatal arterial gas embolism in an adult 1 year after bilateral sequential lung transplantation. J Heart Lung Transplant 2008;27:692-694.

40. Pruitt AA, Graus F, Rosenfeld MR. Neurological complications of solid organ transplantation. Neurohospitalist 2013;3:152-166.

41. Sharma P, Eesa M, Scott JN. Toxic and acquired metabolic encephalopathies: MRI appearance. AJR Am J Roentgenol 2009;193:879-886.

42. Lahon B, Mordant P, Thabut G, et al. Early severe digestive complications after lung transplantation. Eur J Cardiothorac Surg 2011;40:1419-1424.

43. Goldberg HJ, Hertz MI, Ricciardi R, et al. Colon and rectal complications after heart and lung transplantation. J Am Coll Surg 2006;202:55-61.

44. Fuehner T, Welte T, Simon A, Gottlieb J. [Complications after lung transplantation. Part 1: Intensive medical and pneumologic complications.] Dtsch Med Wochenschr 2008;133:782-786.

45. Gautam A. Gastrointestinal complications following transplantation. Surg Clin North Am 2006;86:1195-1206, vii.

46. Vather R, O'Grady G, Bissett IP, Dinning PG. Postoperative ileus: Mechanisms and future directions for research. Clin Exp Pharmacol Physiol 2014;41:358-370.

47. Vather R, Trivedi S, Bissett I. Defining postoperative ileus: Results of a systematic review and global survey. J Gastrointest Surg 2013;17:962-972.

48. Leal S, Sacanell J, Riera J, et al. Early postoperative management of lung transplantation. Minerva Anestesiol 2014;80:1234-1245.

49. Kaltenbach T, Crockett S, Gerson LB. Are lifestyle measures effective in patients with gastroesophageal reflux disease? An evidence-based approach. Arch Intern Med 2006;166:965-971.

50. Castor JM, Wood RK, Muir AJ, et al. Gastroesophageal reflux and altered motility in lung transplant rejection. Neurogastroenterol Motil 2010;22:841-850.

51. Robertson AG, Ward C, Pearson JP, et al. Lung transplantation, gastroesophageal reflux, and fundoplication. Ann Thorac Surg 2010;89:653-660.

52. Atkins BZ, Petersen RP, Daneshmand MA, et al. Impact of oropharyngeal dysphagia on long-term outcomes of lung transplantation. Ann Thorac Surg 2010;90:1622-1628.

53. Miller CB, Malaisrie SC, Patel J, et al. Intraabdominal complications after lung transplantation. J Am Coll Surg 2006;203:653-660.

54. Paul S, Escareno CE, Clancy K, et al. Gastrointestinal complications after lung transplantation. J Heart Lung Transplant 2009;28:475-479.

55. Faris JG, Veltman MG, Royse C. Focused transthoracic echocardiography in the perioperative period. Anaesth Intensive Care 2011;39:306-307; author reply 307-308.

56. Breitkreutz R, Walcher F, Seeger FH. Focused echocardiographic evaluation in resuscitation management: Concept of an advanced life support-conformed algorithm. Crit Care Med 2007;35(Suppl 5):S150-S161.

57. Breitkreutz R, Price S, Steiger HV, et al. Focused echocardiographic evaluation in life support and peri-resuscitation of emergency patients: A prospective trial. Resuscitation 2010;81:1527-1533.

58. Prosen G, Krizmaric M, Zavrsnik J, Grmec S. Impact of modified treatment in echocardiographically confirmed pseudo-pulseless electrical activity in out-of-hospital cardiac arrest patients with constant end-tidal carbon dioxide pressure during compression pauses. J Int Med Res 2010;38:1458-1467.

59. Grmec S, Prosen G. Continuous capnography and focused echocardiographic evaluation during resuscitation—additional criteria for cessation of treatment out-of-hospital-cardiac arrest. Resuscitation 2010;81:1731; author reply 1732.

60. Saito Y, Donohue A, Attai S, et al. The syndrome of cardiac tamponade with "small" pericardial effusion. Echocardiography 2008;25:321-327.

61. Barbier C, Loubieres Y, Schmit C, et al. Respiratory changes in inferior vena cava diameter are helpful in predicting fluid responsiveness in ventilated septic patients. Intensive Care Med 2004;30:1740-1746.

62. Preau S, Saulnier F, Dewavrin F, et al. Passive leg raising is predictive of fluid responsiveness in spontaneously breathing patients with severe sepsis or acute pancreatitis. Crit Care Med 2010;38:819-825.

63. Lamia B, Ochagavia A, Monnet X, et al. Echocardiographic prediction of volume responsiveness in critically ill patients with spontaneously breathing activity. Intensive Care Med 2007;33:1125-1132.

64. Teboul JL, Monnet X. Prediction of volume responsiveness in critically ill patients with spontaneous breathing activity. Curr Opin Crit Care 2008;14:334-339.

65. Stefanidis K, Dimopoulos S, Nanas S. Basic principles and current applications of lung ultrasonography in the intensive care unit. Respirology 2011;16:249-256.

66. Xirouchaki N, Kondili E, Prinianakis G, et al. Impact of lung ultrasound on clinical decision making in critically ill patients. Intensive Care Med 2014;40:57-65.

67. Uchiyama H, Soejima Y, Taketomi A, et al. Successful adult-to-adult living donor liver transplantation in a patient with moderate to severe portopulmonary hypertension. Liver Transpl 2006;12:481-484.

68. Ueda K, Ahmed W, Ross AF. Intraoperative pneumothorax identified with transthoracic ultrasound. Anesthesiology 2011;115:653-655.

68a. Lichtenstein DA, Mezière GA, Lagoueyte JF, Biderman P, et al. A-lines and B-lines: Lung ultrasound as a bedside tool for predicting pulmonary artery occlusion pressure in the critically ill. Chest 2009;136(4):1014-1020. doi: 10.1378/chest.09-0001.

69. Lichtenstein DA, Menu Y. A bedside ultrasound sign ruling out pneumothorax in the critically ill. Lung sliding. Chest 1995;108:1345-1348.

70. Lichtenstein DA, Lascols N, Prin S, Meziere G. The "lung pulse": An early ultrasound sign of complete atelectasis. Intensive Care Med 2003;29:2187-2192.

71. Volpicelli G, Mussa A, Garofalo G, et al. Bedside lung ultrasound in the assessment of alveolar-interstitial syndrome. Am J Emerg Med 2006;24:689-696.

72. Copetti R, Soldati G, Copetti P. Chest sonography: A useful tool to differentiate acute cardiogenic pulmonary edema from acute respiratory distress syndrome. Cardiovasc Ultrasound 2008;6:16.

73. Picano E, Frassi F, Agricola E, et al. Ultrasound lung comets: A clinically useful sign of extravascular lung water. J Am Soc Echocardiogr 2006;19:356-363.

74. Agricola E, Bove T, Oppizzi M, et al. "Ultrasound comet-tail images": A marker of pulmonary edema: A comparative study with wedge pressure and extravascular lung water. Chest 2005;127:1690-1695.

75. Xirouchaki N, Magkanas E, Vaporidi K, et al. Lung ultrasound in critically ill patients: Comparison with bedside chest radiography. Intensive Care Med 2011;37:1488-1493.

76. Peris A, Tutino L, Zagli G, et al. The use of point-of-care bedside lung ultrasound significantly reduces the number of radiographs and computed tomography scans in critically ill patients. Anesth Analg 2010;111:687-692.

77. Balik M, Plasil P, Waldauf P, et al. Ultrasound estimation of volume of pleural fluid in mechanically ventilated patients. Intensive Care Med 2006;32:318-321.

78. Havelock T, Teoh R, Laws D, Gleeson F. Pleural procedures and thoracic ultrasound: British Thoracic Society Pleural Disease Guideline 2010. Thorax 2010;65(Suppl 2):ii61-ii76.

79. Bermudez CA, Adusumilli PS, McCurry KR, et al. Extracorporeal membrane oxygenation for primary graft dysfunction after lung transplantation: Long-term survival. Ann Thorac Surg 2009;87:854-860.

80. Hartwig MG, Walczak R, Lin SS, Davis RD. Improved survival but marginal allograft function in patients treated with extracorporeal membrane oxygenation after lung transplantation. Ann Thorac Surg 2012;93:366-371.

81. Wigfield CH, Lindsey JD, Steffens TG, et al. Early institution of extracorporeal membrane oxygenation for primary graft dysfunction after lung transplantation improves outcome. J Heart Lung Transplant 2007;26:331-338.

82. Shargall Y, Guenther G, Ahya VN, et al. Report of the ISHLT Working Group on Primary Lung Graft Dysfunction part VI: Treatment. J Heart Lung Transplant 2005;24:1489-1500.

83. Dahlberg PS, Prekker ME, Herrington CS, et al. Medium-term results of extracorporeal membrane oxygenation for severe acute lung injury after lung transplantation. J Heart Lung Transplant 2004;23:979-984.

84. Diamond JM, Lee JC, Kawut SM, et al. Clinical risk factors for primary graft dysfunction after lung transplantation. Am J Respir Crit Care Med 2013;187:527-534.

85. Heard ML, Davis J, Fontenberry JD. Principles and practice of venovenous and venoarterial extracorporeal membrane oxygenation. In Short BL, Williams L, eds. ECMO Specialist Training Manual, 3rd ed. Ann Arbor, MI: ELSO; 2010:59-75.

86. Sidebotham D, McGeorge A, McGuinness S, et al. Extracorporeal membrane oxygenation for treating severe cardiac and respiratory disease in adults: Part 1—overview of extracorporeal membrane oxygenation. J Cardiothorac Vasc Anesth 2009;23:886-892.

87. Bermudez CA, Rocha RV, Sappington PL, et al. Initial experience with single cannulation for venovenous extracorporeal oxygenation in adults. Ann Thorac Surg 2010;90:991-995.

26

Primary graft dysfunction

CATHERINE BORDERS,* JOHN ELLIS,* EDWARD M. CANTU III,† AND JASON D. CHRISTIE†

INTRODUCTION

Primary graft dysfunction (PGD) is a common complication with varying levels of severity that occurs within the first 72 hours following lung transplantation. PGD afflicts between 10% and 30% of lung transplant recipients, and those with grade 3 PGD have a high attributable mortality at 30 days, 90 days, and 1 year following lung transplantation.[1-10] In addition, PGD is associated with worse short- and long-term physical functioning and an increased risk for chronic lung allograft dysfunction. PGD is characterized clinically by impaired oxygenation, pulmonary edema, and radiographic evidence of diffuse pulmonary infiltrates in the absence of other identifiable causes. This review provides an update on current risk factors for PGD and summarizes studies focusing on the epidemiology, physiopathology, and molecular and genetic factors affecting PGD.

DEFINITION AND CLINICAL FEATURES

PGD is a multifactorial injury to the grafted lung and the leading cause of early posttransplantation respiratory failure, morbidity, and mortality.[4,5] PGD is manifested as a spectrum of injury ranging from mild to severe and is characterized by impaired oxygenation, decreased lung compliance, and diffuse radiographic pulmonary parenchymal opacities without any other verifiable cause.[1,3,9-15] PGD shares these clinical and pathologic features with other forms of acute respiratory

distress syndrome (ARDS).[2] Additional clinical manifestations of PGD may include intrapulmonary shunting and elevated pulmonary vascular resistance.[13]

PGD has previously been known as early graft dysfunction, primary graft failure, posttransplant ARDS, ischemia-reperfusion injury, reimplantation response and edema, reperfusion edema, and noncardiogenic pulmonary edema.[13,16] In the past, this lack of a standardized taxonomy led to inconsistencies in clinical and research efforts.[17,18] Therefore, in 2005 the International Society for Heart and Lung Transplantation (ISHLT) formulated a standardized classification and grading scheme for PGD that parallels those for ARDS. The ISHLT definition of PGD is based on the ratio of the arterial oxygen partial pressure to the inspired oxygen concentration (Pao_2/Fio_2 ratio) and the presence of radiographic infiltrates that are consistent with pulmonary edema assessed at several time points up to 72 hours after transplantation (Table 26.1).[13] Studies conducted after 2005 that have examined clinical outcomes and biomarkers of PGD severity have demonstrated the validity of the ISHLT's 2005 definition of PGD.[19,20] The definition has been used in studies of risk factors and therapies; however, in an effort to improve the 2005 ISHLT PGD definition and enhance its utility, several changes have been proposed (Table 26.2).[13,21-26]

The current definition of PGD is operational in that it gives consideration to the symptoms of PGD but not its heterogeneity.[13] A recent study of 1255 lung transplant recipients indicated the possible existence of distinct phenotypes of injury resolution in subjects with grade 3 PGD[27]—phenotypes that have been associated with different risk for death and frequency of known risk factors for PGD.[27] Therefore,

---

* These authors contributed equally to this work.

† These senior authors contributed equally to this work.

Table 26.1 ISHLT classification of primary graft dysfunction

Grade at T_0, T_{24}, T_{48}, T_{72}[a]	Infiltrates on chest radiographs consistent with pulmonary edema[b]	PaO_2/FIO_2[c]	Specific exceptions
0: no PGD	–	Any	
1: mild PGD	+	>300	Supported with a nasal cannula or $FIO_2 < .3$
2: moderate PGD	+	200–300	
3: severe PGD	+	<200	Any patients receiving ECMO or NO with $FIO_{22} > .5$ MV

Exclusion criteria: cardiogenic pulmonary edema, pneumonia and aspiration, hyperacute rejection, and pulmonary venous anastomotic obstruction

Source: Adapted from Christie JD, Carby M, Bag R, et al. Report of the ISHLT Working Group on Primary Lung Graft Dysfunction part II: Definition. A consensus statement of the International Society for Heart and Lung Transplantation. J Heart Lung Transplant 2005;24:1454-1459.

Note: ECMO, extracorporeal membrane oxygenation support; FIO_2, fraction of inspired oxygen; ICU, intensive care unit; ISHLT, International Society of Heart Lung Transplantation; MV, mechanical ventilator; NO, nitric oxide; PaO_2, partial arterial oxygen pressure (mm Hg); PGD, primary graft dysfunction.

[a] Time points for assessment: T_0 (0 to 6 hours of reperfusion or on arrival to the ICU), T_{24}, T_{48}, and T_{72}.

[b] Patients are not classified as having PGD without radiographic lung infiltrates.

[c] Blood gas measurement is ideally taken when patients are on MV (FIO_2, 1.0, positive end-expiratory pressure, 5 cm H_2O).

Table 26.2 Limitations and proposed refinements of the 2005 ISHLT primary graft dysfunction taxonomy

Issues	ISHLT PGD guidelines	Suggested revisions
Definition of time points	T_0, T_{24}, T_{48}, T_{72}	Add T_6 and T_{12} Early trends in P/F ratio can be added (% change in P/F from T_0 to T_{12})
Multiple blood gas analysis results available	Use worst P/F ratio	Use P/F ratio closest to the time point
Arterial line removed, no P/F ratio available	No suggestion	No suggestion
Type of transplant	Apply identically	Designate SLT and BLT separately
Unilateral infiltrates in BLT	No suggestion	Consider infiltrates present only if bilateral
Extubated patients	$FIO_2 \geq .3$: No suggestion $FIO_2 < .3$ (or supported by nasal cannula): Grade as 0 or 1 on basis of CXR	All extubated patients with CPAP included (grade 0 or 1 on basis of CXR)
Mode of ventilation and ventilator settings	Ideally, base P/F measurement on $FIO_2 = 1.0$ and PEEP = 5 cm H_2O	Mode and conditions of ventilation appended
Exclusion pathology can be missed clinically	No suggestion	No suggestion
Exclusion pathology can exist at the same time	No suggestion	No suggestion
Interobserver reliability of CXR reading	No suggestion	Inconsistency may be improved by training sessions
Changes in cardiac output	No suggestion	No suggestion

Source: Adapted from references 13, 21-26.

Note: BLT, bilateral lung transplantation; CPAP, continuous positive airway pressure support or other noninvasive mechanical ventilator support; CXR, chest radiograph; ISHLT, International Society of Heart Lung Transplantation; P/F ratio, ratio of PaO_2 (arterial oxygen tension, mm Hg)/FIO_2 (fraction of inspired oxygen); PEEP, positive end-expiratory pressure; PGD primary graft dysfunction; SLT, single-lung transplantation.

further refinement of the 2005 PGD definition and phenotyping within the syndrome may lead to improved risk stratification of lung transplant candidates, development of therapeutic interventions to combat PGD, and better understanding of the mechanisms underlying PGD.

CLINICAL RISK FACTORS

Many studies examining the clinical risk factors for PGD have been limited by small sample size, single-center design, and varied PGD phenotype. Although larger multicenter studies have been reported, they are limited by differences in the treatment and clinical management of both donors and recipients.[10,17,18,28] Despite these limitations, several clinical risk factors for the development of PGD have been consistently reported and can be classified as donor, recipient, and operative risk factors; they are summarized in Table 26.3.[1,5,10,17,18,28,29]

Donor risk factors

Donor-related risk factors include inherent and acquired variables. Inherent donor-related risk factors that have been associated with PGD include older age, female sex, Afro-American race, and smoking history.[1,5,17,28,29] Additionally, a study by Oto and colleagues suggested that recipients who

receive lungs from donors with evidence of pulmonary embolism may be at increased risk for the development of PGD after transplantation.[30] Acquired donor risk factors include primary and secondary injuries associated with their cause of death. Risk factors that have been identified as contributing to the development of PGD include those acquired before brain death (e.g., trauma) or in the hours thereafter (e.g., prolonged mechanical ventilation, aspiration, and hemodynamic instability).[1,5,17,28,29] Although these acquired conditions may be unmodifiable by the time that the lung donor is offered, some acquire donor-related risk factors may be mitigated through better matching strategies to identify compatible donor-recipient pairs. Additionally, ex vivo lung perfusion (EVLP) is a novel technology that has shown great promise as a means for better assessing and reconditioning donor lungs and possibly repairing some of the lung damage caused by donor-related risk factors (see Chapter 12).

In particular, the use of lungs from donors with a history of smoking has remained a major concern and controversy in the media.[31] A multi-institutional study of 1255 recipients found that smoking history is the major donor-related factor linked to the development of severe PGD, with an absolute increase in risk of 5%.[28] This figure is consistent with the findings of elevated mortality associated with donations from smokers in the United Kingdom.[32,33] However, a recent review of 232 lung transplants performed at a single

Table 26.3 Clinical risk factors for primary graft dysfunction

Category	Risk factor for PGD
Donor-inherent variables	Age >45 yr
	Age <21 yr
	Afro-American race
	Female sex
	History of smoking >20 p-yr or >10 p-yr, **any** current
Donor-acquired variables	Prolonged mechanical ventilation
	Aspiration
	Head trauma
	Hemodynamic instability after brain death
Recipient variables	**Body mass index >25 (obesity)**
	Female sex
	Diagnosis of idiopathic pulmonary hypertension
	Diagnosis of secondary pulmonary hypertension
	Diagnosis of idiopathic pulmonary fibrosis
	Diagnosis of sarcoidosis
	Elevated pulmonary arterial pressure at time of surgery
Operative variables	**Single-lung transplantation**
	Prolonged ischemic time
	Use of cardiopulmonary bypass
	Blood product transfusion >1 L
	High $F_{IO_2} \geq 0.4$ at reperfusion
	Use of intracellular (hyperkalemic)-type preservation solution (Euro-Collins)

Source: Adapted from references 1, 5, 17, 18, 28, 29. Boldface indicates PGD risk factors identified in Lung Transplant Outcomes Group multicenter study.

Note: F_{IO_2}, fraction of inspired oxygen; PGD, primary graft dysfunction; p-yr, pack-year.

institution demonstrated comparable survival rates regardless of the donor's smoking history,[34] and other previous studies have shown no major adverse outcomes when lungs from smoking donors are used.[35-37] The inconsistencies in donor smoke exposure as a risk for PGD may be due to the inaccuracies inherent in obtaining a smoking history from proxies, and improved methods for determining smoking history (such as biochemical measurement) are warranted.

Recipient risk factors

Recipient variables that have consistently shown an association with the development of PGD include the following: increased body mass index; pretransplant diagnoses of idiopathic pulmonary fibrosis, sarcoidosis, and primary pulmonary hypertension; and increased pulmonary arterial pressure.[1,5,10,18,28,29] The underlying mechanisms of the association between these variables and elevated risk are incompletely understood; however, they are the focus of current studies aimed at improved pathophysiologic understanding of the risk for PGD. Identification of the processes triggered by these specific risk factors for the development of PGD in recipients may lead to therapeutic strategies to reduce such risk. For instance, although changing a patient's diagnosis before transplantation might not be possible, improved understanding of why some individuals are more susceptible to certain diseases (such as sarcoidosis) may allow targeted therapy to decrease patients' risk for the development of PGD before they undergo transplantation.

Operative risk factors

Surgery-related risk factors that have been identified as independent risk factors for PGD include single-lung transplant, donor-recipient size mismatch, large-volume transfusion of packed red blood cells, use of cardiopulmonary bypass, and higher FIO_2 during reperfusion.[1,5,17,18,28,29,38] Establishing the causality of therapeutic variables, such as blood product transfusion and FIO_2 delivery, is notoriously difficult in observational studies because the indication for the therapy may simply mask the many uncaptured factors that define a more complex surgery. Nonetheless, the hypothesis that both transfusion of red blood cells and hypoxia may augment lung injury has reasonable biologic plausibility.[39-42] Several of the aforementioned operative risk factors for PGD, such as higher FIO_2 at reperfusion, are potentially modifiable; therefore, the effect of such factors on the risk for PGD may be amenable to modification by intraoperative management.

SHORT- AND LONG-TERM OUTCOMES

Before the 2005 ISHLT consensus statement, the absence of a standardized definition, in conjunction with a broad spectrum of severity, led to widely divergent reported rates of PGD. Studies based on definitions of PGD similar to that of ARDS (grade 3 PGD) reported rates of PGD between 10% and 25% and 30-day mortality rates near 50%.[3,5,12,43,44]

A recent study in which the consensus definition was used demonstrated that grade 3 PGD at 48 or 72 hours after transplantation is associated with absolute 90-day and 1-year increases in mortality of 18% and 23%, respectively.[28] Additionally, decreased long-term survival is associated with the severity of the PGD syndrome, even among 1-year survivors of PGD.[4]

In addition to being linked to higher mortality, PGD has also been shown to be significantly correlated with adverse short-term outcomes, including prolonged course of ventilatory support, increased length of intensive care unit and hospital stay, and increased health care cost.[2] The long-term outcomes of early PGD survivors include decreased lung function and increased risk for the development of bronchiolitis obliterans syndrome (BOS), which is a barrier to long-term graft survival and a major cause of mortality after the first year following transplantation.[45,46] Initially, the studies examining the link between PGD and BOS yielded conflicting results.[47-51] However, more recent studies have demonstrated that a higher risk for BOS exists even with intermediate grades of PGD and that this risk increases directly with the severity of PGD.[46,52-54] In a retrospective cohort study of 334 lung transplant recipients, Daud and colleagues demonstrated an increased risk for the development of BOS (relative risk = 1.73 to 2.53) in those in whom PGD develops within 24 to 48 hours after transplantation.[54] Furthermore, this association existed independently of acute rejection, lymphocytic bronchiolitis, and community-acquired respiratory viral infections.[54] Later studies showed the existence at all time points of a direct correlation between the severity of PGD and the probability of BOS developing; this correlation is also independent of other potential risk factors for BOS.[46] The potential mechanisms linking PGD to BOS have yet to be elucidated and require further investigation; however, subsequent studies by this group implicated autoimmunity to lung-specific antigens[55,56] after showing that early posttransplant inflammation was associated with PGD and promoted the development of alloimmunity and BOS.[57] The level of proinflammatory mediators released after transplantation may thus have a role in the innate and adaptive immune responses that promote donor-specific alloimmunity and predispose recipients to chronic human lung allograft rejection. Therefore, methods for preventing PGD may have an impact not only on early posttransplant complications but also on long-term outcomes.

PATHOGENESIS

Most aspects of the lung transplant procedure, including the baseline conditions of the donor and recipient at the time of offer, changes in donor homeostasis following brain death, explantation, cold ischemia time during organ transit, intraoperative organ reperfusion, and perhaps, genetic determinants that may alter the donor lung's injury response and repair mechanisms after transplantation, probably contribute to the development of PGD.[1,14] What is eventually manifested in the recipient as PGD probably begins in the donor. Both direct (pneumonia, aspiration, contusion) and indirect (trauma, sepsis, transfusion, brain death) lung injury may occur in donors,[58,59] and it may contribute to an organ's unsuitability for transplantation.[60] In organs with such exposure that are used for transplantation, PGD may reflect organ injury that might have progressed to clinical ARDS had the donor lungs not been explanted.[60]

In vivo experiments on animals indicate the existence of a biphasic response to ischemia-reperfusion injury: an early-phase and a later-phase response. Cells resident in the donor mediate the early phase, whereas the influx of host response cells (including monocytes, T cells, and neutrophils) that occurs in the recipient mediates the later phase.[61,62] Following ischemia, the return of flow across the donor pulmonary endothelium results in shear stress, which can trigger a shift in endothelial cell phenotype and which in turn leads to the generation of reactive oxygen species, inflammatory cell adhesion and migration, coagulation, and vascular permeability.[63] Likewise, the neutrophil-independent[62,68] alveolar macrophages and lymphocytes that are resident in the donor lung play a role in the initial pathogenesis of lung ischemia-reperfusion injury within 1 to 2 hours.[14,61,64-67] Subsequent recruitment and activation of recipient monocytes, neutrophils, and lymphocytes to the sites of lung injury amplify the injury process.[14,69,70] Additional studies suggest that the downstream effects include activation of the complement pathway,[71,72] generation of neutrophil extracellular traps,[73] and release of platelet-activating factors by activated neutrophils.[74-77]

In recent years, both bench and human research studies have highlighted the importance of the innate immune system in the development of PGD.[78,79] Sterile inflammation resulting from tissue damage during donor brain death, ischemia, and reperfusion may lead to inflammasome formation. Danger- and pathogen-associated molecular pattern (DAMP and PAMP) recognition[80] of bacterial and viral pathogens in the donor lung,[81] mitochondrial dysfunction and damage,[82,83] and products of cell apoptosis[83,84] could lead to amplification of the inflammatory response via production of interleukin-1β (IL-1β). Recently, as part of the National Institute of Allergy and Infectious Diseases (NIAID) Clinical Trials in Organ Transplantation Study, the nucleotide-binding oligomerization domain–like receptor inflammasome pathway and toll-like receptor pathways were both found to be upregulated in lung lavage fluid during clinical PGD within 1 hour of lung implantation.[85]

In some individuals, a preexisting humoral immune response to lung antigens may also be important. A study of 142 lung transplant recipients showed that recipients with pretransplant antibodies to specific self-antigens (K-α1-tubulin, collagen type V, and collagen type I) are at higher risk for PGD (relative risk = 3.09) than recipients with no antibodies.[55] Furthermore, those in the antibody-positive group were found to have elevated levels of proinflammatory mediators, de novo production of anti-human leukocyte antigen type II alloantibodies, and a higher incidence of BOS than did patients in the antibody-negative group,

thus indicating a possible link between PGD and BOS in these individuals.[55,57,86,87]

INSIGHT FROM MOLECULAR BIOMARKERS IN HUMAN STUDIES

Several biomarkers and genetic variants in clinical PGD have been examined. Investigators have drawn on previous knowledge of pathophysiologic mechanisms that was gained through basic cell and animal studies[1] aimed at identification of such biomarkers. Currently, potential markers for PGD include the following: markers of alveolar epithelial and endothelial injury, adhesion molecules, cytokines and chemokines, adhesion molecules, markers of thrombophilia and impaired fibrinolysis, markers of vascular permeability and cell proliferation, and markers of homeostasis and immunity, as summarized in Table 26.4.[7,8,87-109]

Several plasma biomarkers appear to be the most highly correlated with concurrent PGD, thus suggesting pathophysiologic activation of these pathways. They include, but are not limited to soluble receptors for advanced glycation end products (sRAGE), club (Clara) cell secretory protein (CC16), plasminogen activator inhibitor-1 (PAI-1), protein C, intercellular adhesion molecule 1 (ICAM-1), and long pentraxin 3 (PTX3).[7,6,74,92,110] Recently, combined biomarker assessments have indicated that sRAGE and PAI-1 provide the strongest discrimination of clinical PGD and may thus be useful as quantitative traits.[105] Lung biopsy studies have also proved useful in indicating human involvement of pathogenic pathways, such as in identifying endothelin-1 expression as being associated with recipient PGD development.[104] Conversely, the use of biomarkers for preoperative prediction of PGD has been less fruitful to date. Preoperative levels of CC16 appear to be associated with PGD in patients without a pretransplant diagnosis of idiopathic pulmonary fibrosis,[107] thus suggesting that the degree of certain recipients' response to epithelial injury, as indicated by plasma CC16 levels, may make them more susceptible to the development of PGD before the transplant operation.[107]

PREVENTIVE INTERVENTIONS

Current PGD prevention strategies include improved donor selection and donor-recipient matching, better preoperative management and care of donors and recipients, and improved surgical and reperfusion techniques that are based on established PGD risk factors.[14,17,18,111,112] Optimal organ preservation techniques are needed to increase the ischemic time tolerated by lungs and ensure optimal lung function after transplantation. Oto and colleagues have shown that when compared with Euro-Collins or Papworth preservation solutions, Perfadex is associated with fewer occurrences of grades 2 and 3 PGD at 48 hours after transplantation.[113] Likewise, proper reperfusion technique is also essential to prevent lung injury. One of the main problems with reperfusion after the ischemic period during transplantation, as reviewed by Barr and colleagues, is the activity of neutrophil

Table 26.4 Biomarkers for primary graft dysfunction in human lung transplantation

Biomarker	Role
Il-1β	Inflammatory cytokine[96]
sRAGE	Marker of epithelial cell injury[107]
CC16	Marker of epithelial injury caused by Clara cells[107]
Protein C	Anticoagulant[92]
ICAM-1	Adhesion molecule in lung tissue[74]
IL-6, IL-8, TNF-α	Inflammatory cytokine[97,99,107]
Collagen V	Self-antigen and influences certain IL-17–dependent cellular autoimmunity[87]
Th17	Produces IL-17 and is linked to production of certain autoimmune diseases[87]
SP-D	Hydrophilic polymer that manages lung immunity[58]
PTX3 in patients with IPF	Marker produced during inflammation[7,98,102,103]
Endothelin-1	Vasoconstrictive protein that manages vascular porosity[90,91,104,108]
MCP-1	Cytokine that gathers monocytes, memory T cells, and natural killer cells in response to lung injuries[94,106,109]
P-selectin	Platelet adhesion molecule that acts as a recruiter of neutrophils to the endothelial lining[93,100]
PAI-1	Inhibits fibrinolysis[92,105]
IL-17	Inflammatory cytokine produced by Th17[87]
VEGF-A, VEGF-B	Vascular porosity regulation and angiogenesis[88,101]
IL-10	Anti-inflammatory cytokine[99]
Leptin	Inflammatory cytokine that regulates adipose tissue mass and leads to lung fibrosis[8]
Angiopoietin-2 in patients with IPF	Marker that promotes higher endothelial permeability[95]
Estradiol levels in males	Inflammatory female sex hormone[89]

Source: Adapted from references 7, 8, 87–109.
Note: CC16, serum Clara cell protein 16; ICAM-1, intercellular adhesion molecule 1; IL, interleukin; IPF, idiopathic pulmonary fibrosis; MCP-1, monocyte chemotactic protein-1; PAI-1, plasminogen activator inhibitor 1; PTX3, pentraxin 3; SP-D, surfactant protein D; sRAGE, soluble receptor for advanced glycation end products; Th17, helper T cells; TNF, tumor necrosis factor; VEGF, vascular endothelial growth factor.

migration and capillary plugging.[18] In a study by Schnickel and colleagues at the University of California at Los Angeles (UCLA), an adjusted reperfusion procedure without white blood cells was used in 100 transplant patients; the incidence of severe PGD 48 hours after transplantation was 2%.[114]

Other therapeutic agents to reduce the development of PGD that have been explored include agents relieving endogenous cytoprotective substances (nitric oxide, prostaglandins, surfactant, endothelium-derived relaxing factor, and adenosine), agents constraining proinflammatory mediators (platelet-activating factor of reactive oxygen species), and agents constraining neutrophil-derived mediators (inhibitors of reactive oxygen species, tumor necrosis factor α [TNF-α], IL-1β, proteases, adhesion molecules, complement cascade, and, cytokines, including TNF-α and IL-1β).[1,14,112,115] However, only a few randomized trials have been conducted, and they have generally been limited by small sample size.[1] Additionally, the results of these small trials have not been consistent; accordingly, future research is necessary.[116-122]

TREATMENT

Treatment of PGD is largely supportive, and management of PGD is influenced by the treatment strategies applied to patients with ARDS. Mainstays of therapy include protective ventilation approaches, avoidance of excess fluid administration, use of inhaled nitric oxide (iNO), prostaglandin E1, and extracorporeal membrane oxygenation (ECMO) when needed.[112] Retransplantation is a treatment option that is typically available only to highly selected patients with no other organ damage, and the results have not been very encouraging: 30-day, 1-year, and 5-year survival rates are 52.2%, 34.8%, and 29.0%, respectively.[123]

Several animal studies and clinical series had previously reported encouraging results regarding the effectiveness of iNO in the treatment of postoperative PGD and refractory hypoxemia[124-127]; however, subsequent clinical trials failed to demonstrate that administration of iNO during the reperfusion phase has a significant effect on the development of PGD, improvement of oxygenation, occurrence of pulmonary edema, 30-day mortality, length of intensive care unit stay, or time to extubation.[119,128,129] Although the use of iNO for the prevention and treatment of PGD is still not well established, its use may be acceptable in selected patients with refractory hypoxemia and elevated pulmonary artery pressure.[112] If patients with severe PGD do not respond to conventional treatment, initiation of ECMO support may serve as a lifesaving measure[112,130-132] that maintains adequate oxygenation and gas exchange and also avoids the harmful effects of aggressive ventilation while lung function recovers.[133-135] A study of 28 patients who were treated with ECMO for severe PGD between 2001 and 2009 reported 30-day, 1-year, and 5-year survival rates of 82%, 64%, and 49%, respectively.[133] Although overall survival for patients with PGD managed with ECMO has improved thanks to advances in venoarterial and venovenous ECMO techniques, future studies examining the use of ECMO in recipients before transplantation and throughout the procedure may suggest changes in its use with the highest-risk recipients.

PRIMARY GRAFT DYSFUNCTION IN THE CONTEXT OF EXPANDING THE DONOR POOL

The success of lung transplantation in patients with advanced lung disease has been tempered by the limited organ supply. The large disparity between the number of suitable lung donors and the number of patients on the waiting list has resulted in many potential recipients dying while on the waiting list or being removed from the list because of clinical decline.[136] In the recent era, the number of lung donors has remained relatively unchanged whereas the number of patients on the lung transplant waiting list has continued to trend upward.[137] As lung transplant technique and patient selection criteria have matured, transplant groups have increasingly relaxed their donor selection criteria and begun using extended criteria donors in an effort to expand the door lung pool. Most studies examining the use of extended criteria donors suggest rates of PGD, BOS, early morbidity, and mortality equivalent to those when standard criteria donors are used.[35-37,111,138-145]

As lung transplant centers continue their efforts to expand the donor lung pool by liberalizing the strict donor selection criteria, the extent to which the guidelines can be loosened without increasing the risk for and severity of PGD remains unclear.

Additional strategies to increase the lung utilization rate and expand the donor lung pool include the use of donation after cardiocirculatory death (DCD) and EVLP.[137] Currently, most lung grafts come from brain-dead donors; however, only 20% of such donors in the United States provide lungs that are satisfactory for transplantation.[143] Despite studies reporting equivalent clinical outcomes when using lungs from brain-dead donors and lungs from DCD donors,[146-149] DCD lung transplantation is still limited to only a few transplant programs. Many previous reports examining outcomes of DCD have been limited by small sample size.[150-153] Levvey and associates recently published a multicenter collaborative study of 174 controlled DCD lung transplants. The overall incidence of severe PGD at 24 hours after transplantation was 8.5%, and the 1- and 5-year actuarial survival rates were 97% and 90%, respectively.[154] In addition, these DCD donors represented an extra 28% increase in lungs suitable for transplantation.[154] Enthusiasm for increasing the donor pool through the use of DCD donors has been tempered because of increased risk for hypotension,[155] warm ischemia time,[156-158] aspiration, and inability to predict a lung's usability for transplantation. However, ex vivo assessment and reconditioning of lungs may allow an additional opportunity to examine lungs from heart-beating donors before transplantation and thus may prove critical to expanding the donor lung pool and including the use of DCD donors (see also Chapter 8).

SUMMARY

PGD continues to have a significant impact on short- and long-term outcomes following lung transplantation; it is responsible for nearly one third of all deaths in the first 90 days after lung transplantation.[159] Survivors continue to have a higher risk for mortality and development of BOS in the long-term. Better understanding of the clinical and molecular risk factors for PGD and the underlying pathophysiologic mechanisms of PGD will enhance our ability to develop potential therapeutic agents and better methods for matching donors and recipients. Future research and understanding of the PGD syndrome may require further refinement of the definition of and criteria for grading PGD to improve the reliability and accuracy of research findings. Finally, strategies to expand the donor lung pool have increased the use of DCD donors and EVLP methods, thus necessitating that their impact on PGD be continually reassessed.

REFERENCES

1. Lee JC, Christie JD. Primary graft dysfunction. Clin Chest Med 2011;32:279-293.
2. Arcasoy SM, Fisher A, Hachem RR, et al. Report of the ISHLT Working Group on Primary Lung Graft Dysfunction part V: Predictors and outcomes. J Heart Lung Transplant 2005;24:1483-1488.
3. Christie JD, Bavaria JE, Palevsky HI, et al. Primary graft failure following lung transplantation. Chest 1998;114:51-60.
4. Christie JD, Kotloff RM, Ahya VN, et al. The effect of primary graft dysfunction on survival after lung transplantation. Am J Respir Crit Care Med 2005;171:1312-1316.
5. Christie JD, Kotloff RM, Pochettino A, et al. Clinical risk factors for primary graft failure following lung transplantation. Chest 2003;124:1232-1241.
6. Diamond JM, Kawut SM, Lederer DJ, et al. Elevated plasma Clara cell secretory protein concentration is associated with high-grade primary graft dysfunction. Am J Transplant 2011;11:561-567.
7. Diamond JM, Lederer DJ, Kawut SM, et al. Elevated plasma long pentraxin-3 levels and primary graft dysfunction after lung transplantation for idiopathic pulmonary fibrosis. Am J Transplant 2011;11:2517-2522.

8. Lederer DJ, Kawut SM, Wickersham N, et al. Obesity and primary graft dysfunction after lung transplantation: The Lung Transplant Outcomes Group Obesity Study. Am J Respir Crit Care Med 2011;184:1055-1061.

9. Lee JC, Christie JD. Primary graft dysfunction. Proc Am Thorac Soc 2009;6:39-46.

10. Diamond JM, Lee JC, Kawut SM, et al. Clinical risk factors for primary graft dysfunction after lung transplantation. Am J Respir Crit Care Med 2013;187:527-534.

11. Lee JC, Christie JD, Keshavjee S. Primary graft dysfunction: Definition, risk factors, short- and long-term outcomes. Semin Respir Crit Care Med 2010;31:161-171.

12. Christie JD, Van Raemdonck D, de Perrot M, et al. Report of the ISHLT Working Group on Primary Lung Graft Dysfunction part I: Introduction and methods. J Heart Lung Transplant 2005;24:1451-1453.

13. Christie JD, Carby M, Bag R, et al. Report of the ISHLT Working Group on Primary Lung Graft Dysfunction part II: Definition. A consensus statement of the International Society for Heart and Lung Transplantation. J Heart Lung Transplant 2005;24:1454-1459.

14. de Perrot M, Liu M, Waddell TK, et al. Ischemia-reperfusion–induced lung injury. Am J Respir Crit Care Med 2003;167:490-511.

15. Trulock EP. Lung transplantation. Am J Respir Crit Care Med 1997;155:789-818.

16. de Perrot M LM, Waddell TK, Keshavjee S. Ischemia-reperfusion–induced lung injury. Am J Respir Crit Care Med 2003;167:490-511.

17. de Perrot M, Bonser RS, Dark J, et al. Report of the ISHLT Working Group on Primary Lung Graft Dysfunction part III: Donor-related risk factors and markers. J Heart Lung Transplant 2005;24:1460-1467.

18. Barr ML, Kawut SM, Whelan TP, et al. Report of the ISHLT Working Group on Primary Lung Graft Dysfunction part IV: Recipient-related risk factors and markers. J Heart Lung Transplant 2005;24:1468-1482.

19. Christie JD, Bellamy S, Ware LB, et al. Construct validity of the definition of primary graft dysfunction after lung transplantation. J Heart Lung Transplant 2010;29:1231-1239.

20. Prekker ME, Nath DS, Walker AR, et al. Validation of the proposed International Society for Heart and Lung Transplantation grading system for primary graft dysfunction after lung transplantation. J Heart Lung Transplant 2006;25:371-378.

21. Christie J, Keshavjee S, Orens J, et al. Potential refinements of the International Society for Heart and Lung Transplantation primary graft dysfunction grading system. J Heart Lung Transplant 2008;27:138.

22. Meade MO, Cook RJ, Guyatt GH, et al. Interobserver variation in interpreting chest radiographs for the diagnosis of acute respiratory distress syndrome. Am J Respir Crit Care Med 2000;161:85-90.

23. Oto T, Griffiths AP, Levvey BJ, et al. Definitions of primary graft dysfunction after lung transplantation: Differences between bilateral and single lung transplantation. J Thorac Cardiovasc Surg 2006;132:140-147.

24. Oto T, Griffiths AP, Levvey BJ, et al. Unilateral radiographic abnormalities after bilateral lung transplantation: Exclusion from the definition of primary graft dysfunction? J Thorac Cardiovasc Surg 2006;132:1441-1446.

25. Oto T, Levvey BJ, Snell GI. Potential refinements of the International Society for Heart and Lung Transplantation primary graft dysfunction grading system. J Heart Lung Transplant 2007;26:431-436.

26. Prekker ME, Herrington CS, Hertz MI, et al. Early Trends in PaO_2/fraction of inspired oxygen ratio predict outcome in lung transplant recipients with severe primary graft dysfunction. Chest 2007;132:991-997.

27. Shah RJ, Diamond JM, Cantu E, et al. Latent class analysis identifies distinct phenotypes of primary graft dysfunction after lung transplantation. Chest 2013;144:616-622.

28. Diamond JM, Lee JC, Kawut SM, et al. Clinical risk factors for primary graft dysfunction after lung transplantation. Am J Respir Crit Care Med 2013;187:527-534.

29. Kuntz CL, Hadjiliadis D, Ahya VN, et al. Risk factors for early primary graft dysfunction after lung transplantation: A registry study. Clin Transplant 2009;23:819-830.

30. Oto T, Excell L, Griffiths AP, et al. The implications of pulmonary embolism in a multiorgan donor for subsequent pulmonary, renal, and cardiac transplantation. J Heart Lung Transplant 2008;27:78-85.

31. Cystic fibrosis woman died with smoker's donor lungs. BBC News. December 18, 2012.

32. Bonser RS, Taylor R, Collett D, et al. Effect of donor smoking on survival after lung transplantation: A cohort study of a prospective registry. Lancet 2012;380:747-755.

33. Cypel M, Keshavjee S. Expansion of the donor lung pool: Use of lungs from smokers. Lancet 2012;380:709-711.

34. Sabashnikov A, Patil NP, Mohite PN, et al. Influence of donor smoking on midterm outcomes after lung transplantation. Ann Thorac Surg 2014;97:1015-1021.

35. Bhorade SM, Vigneswaran W, McCabe MA, et al. Liberalization of donor criteria may expand the donor pool without adverse consequence in lung transplantation. J Heart Lung Transplant 2000;19:1199-1204.

36. Gabbay E, Williams TJ, Griffiths AP, et al. Maximizing the utilization of donor organs offered for lung transplantation. Am J Respir Crit Care Med 1999;160:265-271.

37. Sundaresan S, Semenkovich J, Ochoa L, et al. Successful outcome of lung transplantation is not compromised by the use of marginal donor lungs. J Thorac Cardiovasc Surg 1995;109:1075-1079; discussion 1079-1080.

38. Eberlein M, Reed RM, Bolukbas S, et al. Lung size mismatch and primary graft dysfunction after bilateral lung transplantation. J Heart Lung Transplant 2015;34:233-240.

39. Bhandari V, Choo-Wing R, Lee CG, et al. Hyperoxia causes angiopoietin 2–mediated acute lung injury and necrotic cell death. Nat Med 2006;12:1286-1293.

40. Kozower BD, Christofidou-Solomidou M, Sweitzer TD, et al. Immunotargeting of catalase to the pulmonary endothelium alleviates oxidative stress and reduces acute lung transplantation injury. Nat Biotechnol 2003;21:392-398.

41. Christie JD, Shah CV, Kawut SM, et al. Plasma levels of receptor for advanced glycation end products, blood transfusion, and risk of primary graft dysfunction. Am J Respir Crit Care Med 2009;180:1010-1015.

42. Qing DY, Conegliano D, Shashaty MG, et al. Red blood cells induce necroptosis of lung endothelial cells and increase susceptibility to lung inflammation. Am J Respir Crit Care Med 2014;190:1243-1254.

43. Fiser SM, Cope JT, Kron IL, et al. Aerosolized prostacyclin (epoprostenol) as an alternative to inhaled nitric oxide for patients with reperfusion injury after lung transplantation. J Thorac Cardiovasc Surg 2001;121:981-982.

44. King RC, Binns OA, Rodriguez F, et al. Reperfusion injury significantly impacts clinical outcome after pulmonary transplantation. Ann Thorac Surg 2000;69:1681-1685.

45. Christie JD, Edwards LB, Kucheryavaya AY, et al. The Registry of the International Society for Heart and Lung Transplantation: Twenty-ninth adult lung and heart-lung transplant report—2012. J Heart Lung Transplant 2012;31:1073-1086.

46. Huang HJ, Yusen RD, Meyers BF, et al. Late primary graft dysfunction after lung transplantation and bronchiolitis obliterans syndrome. Am J Transplant 2008;8:2454-2462.

47. Khalifah AP, Hachem RR, Chakinala MM, et al. Minimal acute rejection after lung transplantation: A risk for bronchiolitis obliterans syndrome. Am J Transplant 2005;5:2022-2030.

48. Hachem RR, Khalifah AP, Chakinala MM, et al. The significance of a single episode of minimal acute rejection after lung transplantation. Transplantation 2005;80:1406-1413.

49. Fisher AJ, Wardle J, Dark JH, et al. Non-immune acute graft injury after lung transplantation and the risk of subsequent bronchiolitis obliterans syndrome (BOS). J Heart Lung Transplant 2002;21:1206-1212.

50. Fiser SM, Tribble CG, Long SM, et al. Ischemia-reperfusion injury after lung transplantation increases risk of late bronchiolitis obliterans syndrome. Ann Thorac Surg 2002;73:1041-1047; discussion 1047-1048.

51. Girgis RE, Tu I, Berry GJ, et al. Risk factors for the development of obliterative bronchiolitis after lung transplantation. J Heart Lung Transplant 1996;15:1200-1208.

52. Kreisel D, Krupnick AS, Puri V, et al. Short- and long-term outcomes of 1000 adult lung transplant recipients at a single center. J Thorac Cardiovasc Surg 2011;141:215-222.

53. Whitson BA, Prekker ME, Herrington CS, et al. Primary graft dysfunction and long-term pulmonary function after lung transplantation. J Heart Lung Transplant 2007;26:1004-1011.

54. Daud SA, Yusen RD, Meyers BF, et al. Impact of immediate primary lung allograft dysfunction on bronchiolitis obliterans syndrome. Am J Respir Crit Care Med 2007;175:507-513.

55. Bharat A, Saini D, Steward N, et al. Antibodies to self-antigens predispose to primary lung allograft dysfunction and chronic rejection. Ann Thorac Surg 2010;90:1094-1101.

56. Hachem RR, Tiriveedhi V, Patterson GA, et al. Antibodies to K-alpha 1 tubulin and collagen V are associated with chronic rejection after lung transplantation. Am J Transplant 2012;12:2164-2171.

57. Bharat A, Narayanan K, Street T, et al. Early post-transplant inflammation promotes the development of alloimmunity and chronic human lung allograft rejection. Transplantation 2007;83:150-158.

58. Matute-Bello G, Frevert CW, Martin TR. Animal models of acute lung injury. Am J Physiol Lung Cell Mol Physiol 2008;295:L379-L399.

59. Ware LB. Pathophysiology of acute lung injury and the acute respiratory distress syndrome. Semin Respir Crit Care Med 2006;27:337-349.

60. Wilkes DS, Egan TM, Reynolds HY. Lung transplantation: Opportunities for research and clinical advancement. Am J Respir Crit Care Med 2005;172:944-955.

61. Fiser SM, Tribble CG, Long SM, et al. Lung transplant reperfusion injury involves pulmonary macrophages and circulating leukocytes in a biphasic response. J Thorac Cardiovasc Surg 2001;121:1069-1075.

62. Eppinger MJ, Jones ML, Deeb GM, et al. Pattern of injury and the role of neutrophils in reperfusion injury of rat lung. J Surg Res 1995;58:713-718.

63. Chatterjee S, Nieman GF, Christie JD, et al. Shear stress–related mechanosignaling with lung ischemia: Lessons from basic research can inform lung

transplantation. Am J Physiol Lung Cell Mol Physiol 2014;307:L668-L680.

64. Naidu BV, Krishnadasan B, Farivar AS, et al. Early activation of the alveolar macrophage is critical to the development of lung ischemia-reperfusion injury. J Thorac Cardiovasc Surg 2003;126:200-207.

65. Yang Z, Sharma AK, Linden J, et al. CD4+ T lymphocytes mediate acute pulmonary ischemia-reperfusion injury. J Thorac Cardiovasc Surg 2009;137:695-702; discussion 702.

66. van der Kaaij NP, Kluin J, Haitsma JJ, et al. Ischemia of the lung causes extensive long-term pulmonary injury: An experimental study. Respir Res 2008;9:28.

67. Sharma AK, LaPar DJ, Zhao Y, et al. Natural killer T cell–derived IL-17 mediates lung ischemia-reperfusion injury. Am J Respir Crit Care Med 2012;183:1539-1549.

68. Johnston LK, Rims CR, Gill SE, et al. Pulmonary macrophage subpopulations in the induction and resolution of acute lung injury. Am J Respir Cell Mol Biol 2012;47:417-426.

69. Kreisel D, Nava RG, Li W, et al. In vivo two-photon imaging reveals monocyte-dependent neutrophil extravasation during pulmonary inflammation. Proc Natl Acad Sci U S A 2010;107:18073-18078.

70. Spahn JH, Kreisel D. Monocytes in sterile inflammation: Recruitment and functional consequences. Arch Immunol Ther Exp (Warsz) 2014;62:187-194.

71. Frank MM. Complement in the pathophysiology of human disease. N Engl J Med 1987;316:1525-1530.

72. Shah RJ, Emtiazjoo AM, Diamond JM, et al. Plasma complement levels are associated with primary graft dysfunction and mortality after lung transplantation. Am J Respir Crit Care Med 2014;189:1564-1567.

73. Sayah DM, Mallavia B, Liu F, et al. Neutrophil extracellular traps are pathogenic in primary graft dysfunction after lung transplantation. Am J Respir Crit Care Med 2015;191;455-463.

74. Covarrubias M, Ware LB, Kawut SM, et al. Plasma intercellular adhesion molecule-1 and von Willebrand factor in primary graft dysfunction after lung transplantation. Am J Transplant 2007;7:2573-2578.

75. Miotla JM, Jeffery PK, Hellewell PG. Platelet-activating factor plays a pivotal role in the induction of experimental lung injury. Am J Respir Crit Care Mol Biol 1998;18:197-204.

76. Moreno I, Vicente R, Ramos F, et al. Determination of interleukin-6 in lung transplantation: Association with primary graft dysfunction. Transplant Proc 2007;39:2425-2426.

77. Serrick C, Adoumie R, Giaid A, et al. The early release of interleukin-2, tumor necrosis factor-alpha and interferon-gamma after ischemia reperfusion injury in the lung allograft. Transplantation 1994;58:1158-1162.

78. Kreisel D, Goldstein DR. Innate immunity and organ transplantation: Focus on lung transplantation. Transpl Int 2013;26:2-10.

79. Spahn JH, Li W, Kreisel D. Innate immune cells in transplantation. Curr Opin Organ Transplant 2014;19:14-19.

80. Dowling JK, O'Neill LA. Biochemical regulation of the inflammasome. Crit Rev Biochem Mol Bio 2012;47:424-443.

81. Lamkanfi M, Dixit VM. Modulation of inflammasome pathways by bacterial and viral pathogens. J Immunol 2011;187:597-602.

82. Zhou R, Tardivel A, Thorens B, et al. Thioredoxin-interacting protein links oxidative stress to inflammasome activation. Nat Immunol 2010;11:136-140.

83. Nakahira K, Haspel JA, Rathinam VA, et al. Autophagy proteins regulate innate immune responses by inhibiting the release of mitochondrial DNA mediated by the NALP3 inflammasome. Nat Immunol 2011;12:222-230.

84. Iyer SS, Pulskens WP, Sadler JJ, et al. Necrotic cells trigger a sterile inflammatory response through the Nlrp3 inflammasome. Proc Natl Acad Sci U S A 2009;106:20388-20393.

85. Cantu E, Lederer DJ, Meyer K, et al. Gene set enrichment analysis identifies key innate immune pathways in primary graft dysfunction after lung transplantation. Am J Transplant 2013;13:1898-1904.

86. Bharat A, Kuo E, Steward N, et al. Immunological link between primary graft dysfunction and chronic lung allograft rejection. Ann Thorac Surg 2008;86:189-195; discussion 196-197.

87. Burlingham WJ, Love RB, Jankowska-Gan E, et al. IL-17-dependent cellular immunity to collagen type V predisposes to obliterative bronchiolitis in human lung transplants. J Clin Invest 2007;117:3498-3506.

88. Abraham D, Taghavi S, Riml P, et al. VEGF-A and -C but not -B mediate increased vascular permeability in preserved lung grafts. Transplantation 2002;73:1703-1706.

89. Bastarache JA, Diamond JM, Kawut SM, et al. Postoperative estradiol levels associate with development of primary graft dysfunction in lung transplantation patients. Gend Med 2012;9:154-165.

90. Chalmers GW, Little SA, Patel KR, et al. Endothelin-1–induced bronchoconstriction in asthma. Am J Respir Crit Care Med 1997;156:382-388.

91. Chalmers GW, MacLeod KJ, Thomson LJ, et al. Sputum cellular and cytokine responses to inhaled endothelin-1 in asthma. Clin Exp Allergy 1999;29:1526-1531.

92. Christie JD, Robinson N, Ware LB, et al. Association of protein C and type 1 plasminogen activator inhibitor with primary graft dysfunction. Am J Respir Crit Care Med 2007;175:69-74.

93. Colombat M, Castier Y, Leseche G, et al. Early expression of adhesion molecules after lung transplantation: Evidence for a role of aggregated P-selectin–positive platelets in human primary graft failure. J Heart Lung Transpl 2004;23:1087-1092.

94. Deshmane SL, Kremlev S, Amini S, et al. Monocyte chemoattractant protein-1 (MCP-1): An overview. J Interferon Cytokine Res 2009;29:313-326.

95. Diamond JM, Porteous MK, Cantu E, et al. Elevated plasma angiopoietin-2 levels and primary graft dysfunction after lung transplantation. PloS One 2012;7:e51932.

96. Dolinay T, Kim YS, Howrylak J, et al. Inflammasome-regulated cytokines are critical mediators of acute lung injury. Am J Respir Crit Care Med 2012;185:1225-1234.

97. Fisher AJ, Donnelly SC, Hirani N, et al. Elevated levels of interleukin-8 in donor lungs is associated with early graft failure after lung transplantation. Am J Respir Crit Care Med 2001;163:259-265.

98. Han B, Haitsma JJ, Zhang Y, et al. Long pentraxin PTX3 deficiency worsens LPS-induced acute lung injury. Intensive Care Med 2011;37:334-342.

99. Kaneda H, Waddell TK, de Perrot M, et al. Pre-implantation multiple cytokine mRNA expression analysis of donor lung grafts predicts survival after lung transplantation in humans. Am J Transplant 2006;6:544-551.

100. Kawut SM, Okun J, Shimbo D, et al. Soluble P-selectin and the risk of primary graft dysfunction after lung transplantation. Chest 2009;136:237-244.

101. Krenn K, Klepetko W, Taghavi S, et al. Recipient vascular endothelial growth factor serum levels predict primary lung graft dysfunction. Am J Transplant 2007;7:700-706.

102. Mauri T, Coppadoro A, Bellani G, et al. Pentraxin 3 in acute respiratory distress syndrome: An early marker of severity. Crit Care Med 2008;36:2302-2308.

103. Peri G, Introna M, Corradi D, et al. PTX3, a prototypical long pentraxin, is an early indicator of acute myocardial infarction in humans. Circulation 2000;102:636-641.

104. Salama M, Andrukhova O, Hoda MA, et al. Concomitant endothelin-1 overexpression in lung transplant donors and recipients predicts primary graft dysfunction. Am J Transplant 2010;10:628-636.

105. Shah RJ, Bellamy SL, Localio AR, et al. A panel of lung injury biomarkers enhances the definition of primary graft dysfunction (PGD) after lung transplantation. J Heart Lung Transplant. 2012;31:942-949.

106. Shah RJ, Diamond JM, Lederer DJ, et al. Plasma monocyte chemotactic protein-1 levels at 24 hours are a biomarker of primary graft dysfunction after lung transplantation. Transl Res 2012;160:435-442.

107. Shah RJ, Wickersham N, Lederer DJ, et al. Preoperative plasma club (Clara) cell secretory protein levels are associated with primary graft dysfunction after lung transplantation. Am J Transplant 2014;14:446-452.

108. Sirois MG, Filep JG, Rousseau A, et al. Endothelin-1 enhances vascular permeability in conscious rats: Role of thromboxane A_2. Eur J Pharmacol 1992;214:119-125.

109. Yoshimura T, Yuhki N, Moore SK, et al. Human monocyte chemoattractant protein-1 (MCP-1). Full-length cDNA cloning, expression in mitogen-stimulated blood mononuclear leukocytes, and sequence similarity to mouse competence gene JE. FEBS Let 1989;244:487-493.

110. Christie JD, Shah CV, Kawut SM, et al. Plasma levels of receptor for advanced glycation end products, blood transfusion, and risk of primary graft dysfunction. Am J Respir Crit Care Med 2009;180:1010-1015.

111. Van Raemdonck D, Neyrinck A, Verleden GM, et al. Lung donor selection and management. Proc Am Thorac Soc 2009;6:28-38.

112. Shargall Y, Guenther G, Ahya VN, et al. Report of the ISHLT Working Group on Primary Lung Graft Dysfunction part VI: Treatment. J Heart Lung Transplant 2005;24:1489-1500.

113. Oto T, Griffiths AP, Rosenfeldt F, et al. Early outcomes comparing Perfadex, Euro-Collins, and Papworth solutions in lung transplantation. Ann Thorac Surg 2006;82:1842-1848.

114. Schnickel GT, Ross DJ, Beygui R, et al. Modified reperfusion in clinical lung transplantation: The results of 100 consecutive cases. J Thorac Cardiovasc Surg 2006;131:218-223.

115. de Perrot M, Keshavjee S. Lung preservation. Semin Thorac Cardiovasc Surg 2004;16:300-308.

116. Herrington CS, Prekker ME, Arrington AK, et al. A randomized, placebo-controlled trial of aprotinin to reduce primary graft dysfunction following lung transplantation. Clin Transplant 2011;25:90-96.

117. Moreno I, Vicente R, Mir A, et al. Effects of inhaled nitric oxide on primary graft dysfunction in lung transplantation. Transplant Proc 2009;41:2210-2212.

118. Struber M, Fischer S, Niedermeyer J, et al. Effects of exogenous surfactant instillation in clinical lung transplantation: A prospective, randomized trial. J Thorac Cardiovasc Surg 2007;133:1620-1625.

119. Botha P, Jeyakanthan M, Rao JN, et al. Inhaled nitric oxide for modulation of ischemia-reperfusion injury in lung transplantation. J Heart Lung Transplant 2007;26:1199-1205.

120. Keshavjee S, Davis RD, Zamora MR, et al. A randomized, placebo-controlled trial of complement inhibition in ischemia-reperfusion injury after lung transplantation in human beings. J Thorac Cardiovasc Surg 2005;129:423-428.

121. Meade MO, Granton JT, Matte-Martyn A, et al. A randomized trial of inhaled nitric oxide to prevent ischemia-reperfusion injury after lung transplantation. Am J Respir Crit Care Med 2003;167:1483-1489.

122. Wittwer T, Grote M, Oppelt P, et al. Impact of PAF antagonist BN 52021 (Ginkolide B) on post-ischemic graft function in clinical lung transplantation. J Heart Lung Transplant 2001;20:358-363.

123. Aigner C, Jaksch P, Taghavi S, et al. Pulmonary retransplantation: Is it worth the effort? A long-term analysis of 46 cases. J Heart Lung Transplant 2008;27:60-65.

124. Struber M, Harringer W, Ernst M, et al. Inhaled nitric oxide as a prophylactic treatment against reperfusion injury of the lung. Thorac Cardiov Surg 1999;47:179-182.

125. Date H, Triantafillou AN, Trulock EP, et al. Inhaled nitric oxide reduces human lung allograft dysfunction. J Thorac Cardiovasc Sururg 1996;111:913-919.

126. Macdonald P, Mundy J, Rogers P, et al. Successful treatment of life-threatening acute reperfusion injury after lung transplantation with inhaled nitric oxide. J Thorac Cardiovasc Surg 1995;110:861-863.

127. Adatia I, Lillehei C, Arnold JH, et al. Inhaled nitric oxide in the treatment of postoperative graft dysfunction after lung transplantation. Ann Thorac Surg 1994;57:1311-1318.

128. Perrin G, Roch A, Michelet P, et al. Inhaled nitric oxide does not prevent pulmonary edema after lung transplantation measured by lung water content: A randomized clinical study. Chest 2006;129:1024-1030.

129. Meade M, Granton JT, Matte-Martyn A, et al. A randomized trial of inhaled nitric oxide to prevent reperfusion injury following lung transplantation. J Heart Lung Transplant 2001;20:254-255.

130. Bermudez CA, Adusumilli PS, McCurry KR, et al. Extracorporeal membrane oxygenation for primary graft dysfunction after lung transplantation: Long-term survival. Ann Thorac Surg 2009;87:854-860.

131. Fischer S, Bohn D, Rycus P, et al. Extracorporeal membrane oxygenation for primary graft dysfunction after lung transplantation: Analysis of the Extracorporeal Life Support Organization (ELSO) registry. J Heart Lung Transplant 2007;26:472-477.

132. Dahlberg PS, Prekker ME, Herrington CS, et al. Medium-term results of extracorporeal membrane oxygenation for severe acute lung injury after lung transplantation. J Heart Lung Transplant 2004;23:979-984.

133. Hartwig MG, Walczak R, Lin SS, et al. Improved survival but marginal allograft function in patients treated with extracorporeal membrane oxygenation after lung transplantation. Ann Thorac Surg 2012;93:366-371.

134. Fiser SM, Kron IL, Long SM, et al. Early intervention after severe oxygenation index elevation improves survival following lung transplantation. J Heart Lung Transplant 2001;20:631-636.

135. Meyers BF, Sundt TM, Henry S, et al. Selective use of extracorporeal membrane oxygenation is warranted after lung transplantation. J Thorac Cardiovasc Surg 2000;120:20-28.

136. Naik PM, Angel LF. Special issues in the management and selection of the donor for lung transplantation. Semin Immunopathol 2011;33:201-210.

137. Cypel M, Keshavjee S. Strategies for safe donor expansion: Donor management, donations after cardiac death, ex-vivo lung perfusion. Curr Opin Organ Transplant 2013;18:513-517.

138. Aigner C, Winkler G, Jaksch P, et al. Extended donor criteria for lung transplantation—a clinical reality. Eur J Cardiothorac Surg 2005;27:757-761.

139. Botha P, Trivedi D, Weir CJ, et al. Extended donor criteria in lung transplantation: Impact on organ allocation. J Thorac Cardiovasc Surg 2006;131:1154-1160.

140. Kron IL, Tribble CG, Kern JA, et al. Successful transplantation of marginally acceptable thoracic organs. Ann Surg 1993;217:518-522; discussion 522-524.

141. Lardinois D, Banysch M, Korom S, et al. Extended donor lungs: Eleven years experience in a consecutive series. Eur J Cardiothorac Surg 2005;27:762-767.

142. Meers C, Van Raemdonck D, Verleden GM, et al. The number of lung transplants can be safely doubled using extended criteria donors; a single-center review. Transpl Int 2010;23:628-635.

143. Moreno P, Alvarez A, Santos F, et al. Extended recipients but not extended donors are associated with poor outcomes following lung transplantation. Eur J Cardiothorac Surg 2014;45:1040-1047.

144. Pierre AF, Sekine Y, Hutcheon MA, et al. Marginal donor lungs: A reassessment. J Thorac Cardiovasc Surg 2002;123:421-427; discussion, 427-428.

145. Straznicka M, Follette DM, Eisner MD, et al. Aggressive management of lung donors classified as unacceptable: Excellent recipient survival one year after transplantation. J Thorac Cardiovasc Surg 2002;124:250-258.

146. Love RB. Perspectives on lung transplantation and donation-after-determination-of-cardiac-death donors. Am J Transplant 2012;12:2271-2272.

147. Wigfield CH, Love RB. Donation after cardiac death lung transplantation outcomes. Curr Opin Organ Transplant 2011;16:462-468.

148. De Oliveira NC, Osaki S, Maloney JD, et al. Lung transplantation with donation after cardiac death donors: Long-term follow-up in a single center. J Thorac Cardiovasc Surg 2010;139:1306-1315.

149. Mason DP, Thuita L, Alster JM, et al. Should lung transplantation be performed using donation after cardiac death? The United States experience. J Thorac Cardiovasc Surg 2008;136:1061-1066.

150. Snell GI, Levvey BJ, Oto T, et al. Early lung transplantation success utilizing controlled donation after cardiac death donors. Am J Transplant 2008;8:1282-1289.

151. Mason DP, Murthy SC, Gonzalez-Stawinski GV, et al. Early experience with lung transplantation using donors after cardiac death. J Heart Lung Transplant 2008;27:561-563.

152. Oto T, Levvey B, McEgan R, et al. A practical approach to clinical lung transplantation from a Maastricht Category III donor with cardiac death. J Heart Lung Transplant 2007;26:196-199.

153. de Antonio DG, Marcos R, Laporta R, et al. Results of clinical lung transplant from uncontrolled non–heart-beating donors. J Heart Lung Transplant 2007;26:529-534.

154. Levvey BJ, Harkess M, Hopkins P, et al. Excellent clinical outcomes from a national donation-after-determination-of-cardiac-death lung transplant collaborative. Am J Transplant 2012;12:2406-2413.

155. Mauney MC, Cope JT, Binns OA, et al. Non–heart-beating donors: A model of thoracic allograft injury. Ann Thorac Surg 1996;62:54-61; discussion 61-62.

156. Snell GI, Oto T, Levvey B, et al. Evaluation of techniques for lung transplantation following donation after cardiac death. Ann Thorac Surg 2006;81:2014-2019.

157. Van Raemdonck DE, Rega FR, Neyrinck AP, et al. Non–heart-beating donors. Semin Thorac Cardiovasc Surg 2004;16:309-321.

158. Egan TM. Non–heart-beating donors in thoracic transplantation. J Heart Lung Transplant 2004;23:3-10.

159. Christie JD, Edwards LB, Kucheryavaya AY, et al. The Registry of the International Society for Heart and Lung Transplantation: Twenty-seventh official adult lung and heart-lung transplant report—2010. J Heart Lung Transplant 2010;29:1104-1118.

27

Management of surgical complications

MATHEW THOMAS AND JOHN A. ODELL

INTRODUCTION

Lung transplantation involves multiple complex steps from procurement to implantation, each of which can potentially result in a complication. Such complications may develop at any time from the intraoperative phase to weeks or months after transplantation (Table 27.1).

Posttransplantation complications can be broadly classified into two major groups: surgical and nonsurgical. The latter include medical and immunologic complications such as side effects of immunosuppressive drugs. This chapter focuses on the prevention and management of surgical complications.

The International Society of Heart and Lung Transplantation Registry annual report for 2013 identified technical complications as the cause of death in 11% of 43,428 lung transplant recipients within the first month after surgery, with the rate decreasing to 3.4% between 30 days and 1 year after transplantation and to 0.9% after the first year.[1]

VASCULAR COMPLICATIONS

During implantation of each lung, the bronchial anastomosis is performed first, followed by the two major vascular anastomoses. The pulmonary vein anastomosis is commonly created between the donor left atrial cuff and the confluence of the recipient's pulmonary veins. The donor main pulmonary artery is anastomosed either to the ipsilateral main pulmonary artery or to an equally sized large branch. Both the venous and arterial anastomoses are susceptible to complications, almost of all of which can be prevented by proper surgical technique.

Vascular complications can be broadly classified as follows:

1. Anastomotic leakage.
2. Anastomotic stenosis.
3. Nonanastomotic obstruction (e.g., intravascular thrombus, redundancy, kinking, extraluminal obstruction).

Anastomotic leakage

Anastomotic leakage (bleeding) is usually identified intraoperatively and can often be managed by reinforcing the incompetent area with horizontal mattress or figure-of-eight sutures. As a result of chronic disease and the frequent use of steroids in lung transplant recipients, the vascular tissue (especially the pulmonary arteries) is quite fragile, and rough handling can affect anastomotic integrity. We routinely preserve a portion of the donor pericardium to be used for pledgets during reinforcement of the anastomosis, thereby avoiding the use of nonbiologic (e.g., felt) pledgets and the associated risk for contamination and foreign body infection in an immunocompromised host. Placing the repair sutures with the clamps released and vessel distended reduces the risk of incorporating the back wall and creating an obstruction. However, when significant bleeding impairs proper visualization, reapplication of the vascular clamps to improve exposure may be required. In our experience,

Table 27.1 Surgical complications after lung transplantation

I. Vascular complications
- Anastomotic bleeding
- Anastomotic stenosis
- Nonanastomotic obstruction
  - Kinking
  - Thrombosis and pulmonary embolism
  - Extraluminal compression
II. Airway complications
- Dehiscence
- Stenosis
- Fistula
- Endobronchial granuloma
- Bronchial infection
- Bronchomalacia
III. Air leaks
IV. Phrenic nerve injury and diaphragm paralysis
V. Postoperative hemorrhage
- Hemothorax
- Hemomediastinum, including hemopericardium
- Chest wall hematoma
VI. Pleural space complications
- Pneumothorax
- Pleural effusion
- Empyema
- Chylothorax
VII. Donor-recipient lung size mismatch
VIII. Complications occurring in the nontransplanted lung
IX. Others
- Primary graft dysfunction
- Lung hernia
- Surgical site infection
- Wound dehiscence
- Complications related to cardiopulmonary bypass

complete revision of the entire anastomosis to manage bleeding is rarely necessary.

Anastomotic bleeding may not be immediately obvious; its appearance may be delayed and accompanied by a large amount of sanguineous chest tube drainage and, often, signs of hemorrhagic shock. Chest radiographs may show worsening opacification of one or both hemithoraces. When available, bedside ultrasound can be a valuable tool for real-time assessment of the pleural cavity.[2,3]

Management of postoperative hemorrhage is based on the amount of bleeding, the patient's hemodynamic status and response to resuscitation, coagulation profiles, and degree of lung compression. In patients with significant bleeding or hemodynamic instability, emergency reexploration to control the source of bleeding and evacuate the hemothorax is necessary to ensure both their survival and survival of the graft. In cases of subtler or intermittent bleeding, deciding whether to reoperate can be challenging

because reexploration is not without its own risks. Lung isolation with a double-lumen tube is optimal during reexploration but may not always be feasible because of respiratory or hemodynamic instability, as a result of which, identifying or repairing the source of bleeding is quite difficult. Intermittent apnea is a ventilation strategy that we often use in such situations. Occasionally, cardiopulmonary bypass may be necessary to facilitate surgical exploration and repair.

Anastomotic stenosis

Anastomotic stenosis is a rare complication that occurs in less than 5% of lung transplant procedures.[4,5] Although stenosis may occur in either the pulmonary vein or artery, the findings are often more pronounced and the results more devastating when the vein is involved.

Close attention to detail can significantly reduce the risk for vascular stenosis because it is nearly always a technical problem.[6] Careful size matching of the donor and recipient vascular lumina when performing the anastomosis is important. Some techniques that may be used to deal with a significant severe size mismatch include excising any excess edges on the larger vessel and enlarging the smaller vessel by spatulation, pericardial patch angioplasty, or division of the common wall between two small vessels to create a common orifice.[6-9] Trimming the donor vessels close to the lobar branch origins creates a risk that the orifices will be narrowed during suturing.[6] To avoid a purse-string effect, the sutures should not be pulled or cinched too tightly when a single continuous suturing technique is used. In most cases, a purse-string effect is not significant enough to cause any vascular compromise; however, it may become relevant if the lumen has already been narrowed because of a size mismatch or improperly placed sutures.

Severe venous stenosis may appear as pulmonary congestion and edema soon after the transplanted lung has been reperfused, thus leading to cardiopulmonary instability. The transplanted lung may appear dusky and lose its elasticity, becoming heavy and firm to the touch. In cases of moderate to mild stenosis, findings may be delayed for a few hours or days and often include persistent radiographic opacification of the affected lobe or lung and clinical signs of pulmonary edema.[6] In addition to frothy secretions, an excessive amount of clear chest tube drainage (>1000 mL/ day) was noted in a patient of ours with severe venous stenosis (Figure 27.1). Pulmonary artery stenosis may be associated with persistent pulmonary hypertension, hypoxia, or unsuccessful weaning from the ventilator. Anastomotic stenosis can result in a predisposition to thrombus formation in response to turbulent flow patterns (Figure 27.2).

Because the clinical picture of primary graft dysfunction may be similar to that of venous stenosis,[10] any doubt about the patency of an anastomosis should be investigated by transesophageal echocardiography (TEE).[11] The degree of stenosis can also be assessed with TEE by measuring the pressure gradients across the anastomosis.[11,12] When

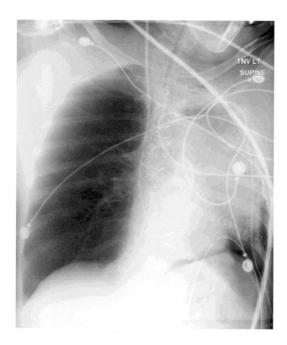

Figure 27.1 Edema and consolidation of the left lung because of severe venous stenosis following a single–left lung transplant.

combined with direct visual assessment of the lung, TEE is an excellent tool for intraoperative assessment of a vascular anastomosis, except for one involving the left lower pulmonary vein, which may not be well visualized.[12] Noninvasive computed tomography (CT) pulmonary angiography is now being used very commonly for the diagnosis of vascular obstructions.[4] Traditional pulmonary angiography can be both diagnostic and therapeutic but is considered an invasive procedure.[5] Ventilation-perfusion scans may show perfusion defects in the affected areas of the lung (see Figure 27.2).[5,6,13]

Survival of the graft and, ultimately, that of the patient depends on expeditious management of vascular stenoses,[4,11] which includes maintaining a low threshold for revision when such stenoses are detected intraoperatively. Postoperatively detected arterial stenoses can often be corrected with percutaneous angioplasty and stenting.[14-16] Venous stenoses are more difficult to treat without surgery and frequently require urgent surgical revision of the anastomosis.[11] When obstructed venous outflow is suspected intraoperatively, the following steps should be undertaken immediately: administer systemic heparin, reapply the pulmonary arterial clamp to stop inflow, and stop ventilation to the affected lung. After the lung has been well drained, the vein is clamped before revision of the anastomosis. Some case reports have described percutaneous treatment of venous stenosis with varying degrees of success.[5,17-19]

Nonanastomotic obstructions

Nonanastomotic obstructions may occur as a result of kinking of a redundant pulmonary vessel, extraluminal

compression, or intraluminal thrombus.[6] Because the vessels are collapsed and the lung is deflated when the anastomosis is being created, determining a vessel's length adequate to allow optimal flow without excessive tension or redundancy requires good judgment. Ensuring that the vessels are not kinked following reperfusion and reinflation of the lung is important. The adjacent vessel could potentially be compressed by large extraluminal clots; by hemostatic material, such as the cellulose-based gauze (e.g., Nuknit, Surgicel) used to stop anastomotic bleeding; or even by soft tissue, such as excessive pericardial fat wrapped around the bronchus (Figure 27.3).[20,21] Any suspicion of inadequate blood flow should be thoroughly investigated and managed as already described.

Intraluminal thrombus formation can also lead to abnormal pulmonary blood flow. Residual thrombi resulting from inadequate perfusion or flushing techniques during procurement can be dislodged later when the transplanted lung is reperfused. Although quite rare, pulmonary arterial embolism from such retained thrombi can occur and cause varying degrees of lung infarction or even loss of the entire transplanted lung.[22] In addition to standardization of the perfusion and flushing techniques, careful examination of the lumina of the donor pulmonary vein and artery for thrombi should be performed during the back-table preparation. If the inspection reveals a clot, it can be removed by extraction with Fogarty[23] or suction catheters[24] and repetition of antegrade and retrograde flushing of the lung with pulmonary protective perfusate.[22,25]

A prospective TEE study showed that pulmonary venous thrombi develop in up to 15% of patients during the early postoperative period, thus leading to a mortality rate of 38% in the first 90 days.[12] Other similar studies have reported an incidence of venous anastomotic thrombi ranging from 9% to 29% and associated mortality rates of up to 67%.[26,27] Allograft failure and stroke resulting from

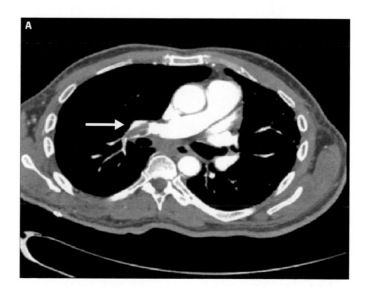

Figure 27.2 (A) Pulmonary arterial thrombus (arrow) distal to a stenotic anastomosis. (Continued)

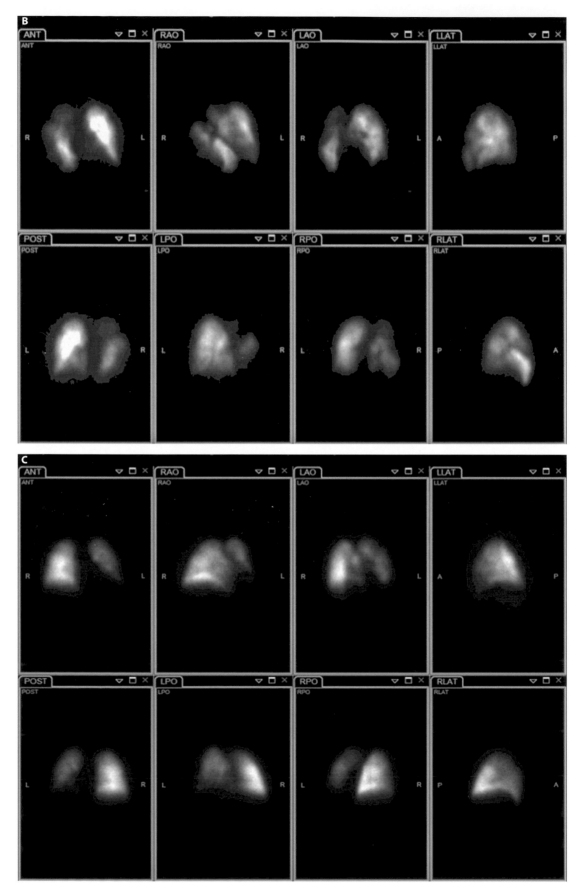

Figure 27.2 (*Continued*) **(B)** Initial perfusion scan showing a significant defect in flow to the right lung. **(C)** Perfusion scan 4 months after treatment with heparin and then warfarin showing reestablishment of normal perfusion to the right lung.

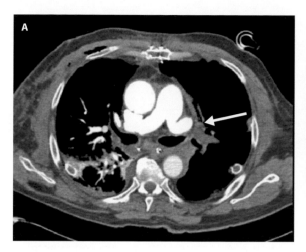
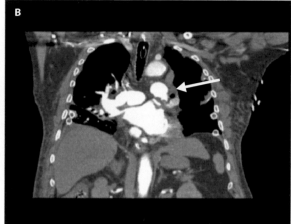

Figure 27.3 Axial **(A)** and coronal **(B)** views of a computed tomography pulmonary angiogram showing abrupt cutoff (arrows) of the left pulmonary artery after a bilateral lung transplant. Surgical reexploration revealed that an engorged piece of hemostatic cellulose-based gauze placed between the artery and the bronchus had caused compression of the vessel.

systemic embolization are well-known consequences of pulmonary venous thrombosis. Systemic antithrombotic therapy should be initiated for moderate or large thrombi with evidence of narrowing on TEE.[12] Because of the high risk for bleeding associated with systemic anticoagulants, observation may be sufficient for small thrombi with minimal elevation of peak pulmonary venous velocity.[12] For thrombi requiring initial therapy, treatment with an anticoagulant such as warfarin is usually lifelong. Severe venous obstruction from thrombi may occasionally require surgery to extract the clot and revise the anastomosis, but it may be associated with very high mortality rates.[11]

AIRWAY COMPLICATIONS

Blood flow to the normal lung has two main sources: the pulmonary and systemic blood circulation. Pulmonary transplantation is unique among all other types of organ transplantation in that the systemic arterial blood supply (i.e., bronchial artery) is not usually restored during engraftment. As a result, the viability of the donor bronchus is initially dependent on retrograde low-pressure collaterals (derived from the pulmonary artery), which supply poorly oxygenated blood.[28] Ischemia of the donor bronchus is universally present after transplantation but is often not severe enough to be clinically significant. Full-thickness ischemia can lead to early (e.g., anastomotic dehiscence) or late (e.g., stenosis) postoperative airway complications. As with many other surgical complications, the lack of a proper definition precludes true understanding of the incidence of airway complications. More recent publications have reported rates of anastomotic complications that require intervention of approximately 7% to 18%.[28-30]

Six main types of airway complications exist: bronchial dehiscence, fistulas, stenosis (the most common type), endobronchial granulomas, bronchomalacia, and endobronchial infections.[28] The first two types appear early in the postoperative period, whereas the others usually become evident after the first month. Different classifications have been proposed for posttransplantation airway complications but have failed to gain universal acceptance.[31-34] The most recent classification, which was proposed by a French group of experts, is based on endoscopic appearance of the airway.[35]

Multiple preoperative and postoperative factors that decrease bronchial healing and increase the risk for airway complications have been identified, although not without controversy. Preoperative risk factors include pulmonary infections, donor-recipient size mismatch involving a taller recipient, and prolonged ventilation of the donor before procurement.[28,29] Rejection, intense immunosuppression therapy, invasive infections, inadequate organ preservation, severe reperfusion edema, prolonged mechanical ventilation (longer than 7 days), and early rejection episodes affect bronchial healing after transplantation.[29,36,37] The incidence of airway complications has decreased in recent years, with the decrease being attributed to better patient selection, lung preservation and surgical techniques, postoperative care, and immunosuppression.[28]

In addition to proper patient selection and matching, meticulous surgical technique is essential to reduce the degree of anastomotic ischemia.[6] Extensive trimming of peribronchial tissue during preparation of the donor lung should be avoided. Similarly, unlike the case in an oncologic operation, lymph nodes around the bronchus and hilum do not require large-scale resection during the recipient pneumonectomy. Because these lymph nodes are highly vascularized, extensive lymphadenectomy may not only compromise the peribronchial blood supply but also increase the risk for perioperative bleeding. It is our practice to avoid denuding the donor *and* recipient bronchi as much as possible and to expose only the cartilage necessary to perform the anastomosis. We routinely resect the donor bronchus to approximately one or two rings above the secondary (lobar) carina because such resection reduces the length of the bronchial segment at risk for ischemia.[38]

In an attempt to improve bronchial healing, different anastomotic techniques have been tried. The two most commonly used techniques for bronchial reconstruction are the telescoping and direct end-to-end anastomoses, which are sometimes performed with modifications. Multiple studies have shown that the telescoping anastomosis is associated with a higher incidence of airway complications,[39-41] which has led many surgical groups to abandon the technique over time.[6,41]

Because of high rates of bronchial necrosis and breakdown (>80%) during the early years of lung transplantation, various techniques were advocated to increase the blood supply to the anastomosis. They included wrapping a pedicled omental flap around the bronchus and bronchial arterial revascularization; however, they are no longer used routinely because of their technical complexity and also because of a decrease in the rates of airway complications over the years.[6,42-44] Some institutions still favor using some type of vascularized flap, such as intercostal muscle or pericardium, to wrap around the anastomosis.[45] We do not consider this step critical during the initial anastomosis,[46] but if an in situ lappet of donor pericardium is readily available, we loosely wrap it around the anastomosis and anchor it to the peribronchial tissue with 3-0 absorbable suture.

Dehiscence

Perianastomotic mucosal necrosis is almost always seen on posttransplantation bronchoscopy but is usually partial-thickness necrosis and often resolves spontaneously.[30,40] Full-thickness necrosis occurs in 1.5% to 10% of anastomoses and leads to varying degrees of dehiscence, which significantly increases the risk for pleural space contamination and, subsequently, empyema, sepsis, and death.[39-41] The delayed radiographic appearance of pneumothorax or air leak in chest tubes should lead to suspicion of dehiscence and be promptly investigated with bronchoscopy. High-resolution CT of the chest is quite sensitive from the standpoint of detection of dehiscence and may show peribronchial or hilar extraluminal air, air-fluid collections, or loss of continuity of the bronchial wall (Figure 27.4).[47,48] Small (≤4 mm) bronchial wall defects have exhibited extremely good spontaneous healing, whereas a larger dehiscence has unpredictable outcomes.[49] Currently, bronchoscopic stenting with self-expandable metallic or silicone stents, which promote the growth of granulation tissue, is often the treatment of choice for most airway dehiscence.[50-52] Large airway disruptions that are refractory or not amenable to stenting can be difficult to manage because the same risk factors that compromised the blood supply to the original anastomosis will probably persist after resection and reconstruction. The use of a vascularized pedicle flap such as intercostal muscle, pericardial fat, or pericardium to wrap around the bronchus is critical to augment the blood supply and ensure a successful repair.[53] In the rare absence of any of the aforementioned

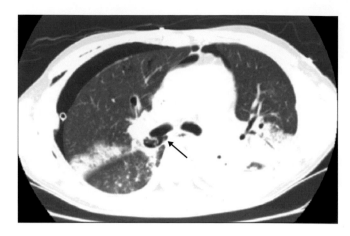

Figure 27.4 High-resolution computed tomography scan showing dehiscence of the right bronchial anastomosis (arrow).

flaps, a pedicled omental flap should be considered as an alternative. Some case reports have described sleeve lobectomies as a successful strategy to manage posttransplant airway dehiscence.[53]

Fistulas

Bronchial dehiscence may lead to fistulas connecting the airway to the pleural space or adjacent structures such as blood vessels, mediastinum, or even the heart.[54-56] Fortunately, these challenging complications are very rare. Bronchovascular fistulas usually appear as sudden massive hemoptysis and may be preceded by smaller amounts of blood-stained sputum, which is known as "herald bleeding." Bronchoatrial fistulas can lead to air embolism.[55] Investigative techniques for intermittent minor hemoptysis include bronchoscopy and pulmonary angiography. Massive hemoptysis is a surgical emergency[57,58] and requires immediate intubation, bronchoscopy, and isolation of the affected lung. Patients should be placed in a lateral decubitus position with the affected side dependent to prevent drowning the opposite lung in blood. Cardiopulmonary bypass may be required to stabilize patients and buy time while fistulas are being exposed.

Management of fistulas to nonvascular structures will depend on fistula size, symptoms, and the patient's clinical condition. The goals of treatment are to stabilize the patient, eradicate ongoing infection, prevent cross-contamination of the contralateral lung, and identify and permanently close the fistula. Treatment options range from more conservative management with endoscopic therapy,[30,59-61] antibiotics, and tube thoracostomy to complex surgical procedures,[62] including the Eloesser window, a modified Clagett procedure, and even lobectomy[54] or pneumonectomy.[57] Small fistulas without significant infection or abscesses can be closed primarily on the bronchial side after resection of the fistula tract; larger fistulas may require more extensive resection and reconstruction, a description of which is outside the scope of this chapter. Regardless of a bronchial fistula's size, surgical repair should include the use of a well-vascularized soft tissue interposition flap.

Strictures

Stenosis is the most common posttransplantation airway complication; it occurs in approximately 8.3% to 32% of anastomoses[33,37,39,50,53] as a delayed consequence of severe ischemia. Preoperative recipient risk factors specific for stenosis include male sex, restrictive lung disease, and the need for hospitalization before transplantation, whereas early rejection appears to be a significant postoperative risk factor.[37] Various patterns of stenosis have been described, with the majority (>85%) involving the anastomosis. In a small number of cases (2.5% to 3%) nonanastomotic segmental stenosis can occur (Figure 27.5),[63] with the bronchus intermedius being the more commonly involved airway.[64,65] The mean time for development of stenosis ranges from 2 to 10 months.[36,63] Reduced predicted forced expiratory volume in the first second of respiration (FEV_1) is a finding associated with stenosis, which is in turn predictive of lower postoperative survival.[34] Airway stenosis is now commonly managed by bronchoscopic dilatation, with or without the use of airway stents.[50,51,61]

PHRENIC NERVE INJURY AND DIAPHRAGM PARALYSIS

The proximity of the phrenic nerve to the pulmonary hilum places it at high risk of being injured during hilar dissection, either directly or by thermal injury.[66] Identification and protection of the phrenic nerve should be a standard part of the lung transplantation operation. In patients with severe intrathoracic adhesions, either from inherent pulmonary pathology or from previous operations, the nerve may not be easily identified and can easily be severed or injured anywhere along its course.

Injury to the phrenic nerve may lead to temporary or permanent paralysis of the diaphragm (Figure 27.6).[66] Determination of the severity of the injury during the initial postoperative period is difficult and often requires more time. Although long-term adverse events may not be significant, paralysis leads to longer mechanical ventilation and intensive care unit stay.[67,68] Suspected phrenic nerve injury can be evaluated by a sniff test with fluoroscopy or ultrasonography, which may demonstrate a paralyzed diaphragm.[68] Surgical plication of the diaphragm can be considered for severe permanent paralysis; however, no data suggest that early repair of the diaphragm leads to better long-term outcomes than observation does.

AIR LEAKS

Air leaks are well-known complications after any lung surgery, including lung transplantation. Possible sources are the bronchial anastomosis or lung parenchyma, particularly if adhesiolysis was required during procurement of the donor lung. At the time of reperfusion of the lung, we routinely test the integrity of the bronchial anastomosis by performing a Valsalva maneuver with the bronchus immersed in normal saline or sterile water to a pressure of 30 cm H_2O. Obvious parenchymal tears on the surface can be repaired with a running 4-0 Prolene suture or by stapled wedge resection of the disrupted area. Even with extreme caution to prevent this complication, varying degrees of air leakage may still be seen after chest closure. Most air leaks can be managed nonoperatively with chest tubes, and they often resolve spontaneously.[69] Delayed appearance of an air leak should raise suspicion for bronchial dehiscence and must be further investigated as described previously. Persistent or

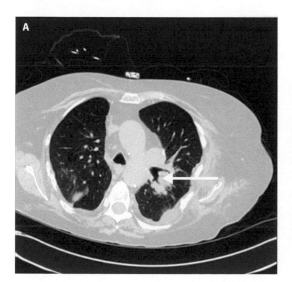 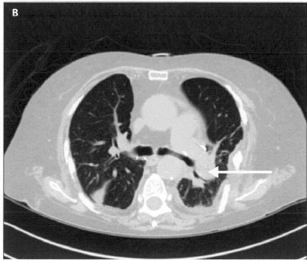

Figure 27.5 **(A)** Computed tomography scan 1 month after bilateral lung transplantation showing nonanastomotic segmental stenosis (arrow) of the left lower lobe and lingular bronchus and lower lobe atelectasis. **(B)** Computed tomography scan of the same patient showing progression of the stenosis (arrow) and atelectasis, which ultimately required a lobectomy.

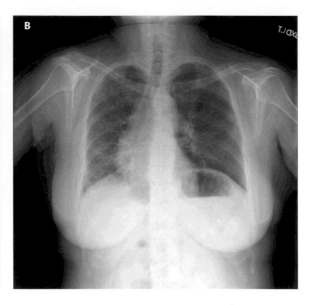

Figure 27.6 Postoperative paralysis of the left hemidiaphragm immediately after transplantation **(A)** and completely resolved after 4 months of observation **(B)**.

large air leaks are associated with increased mortality and may require reexploration and repair.[70,71]

POSTOPERATIVE HEMORRHAGE

Postoperative bleeding has been reported to occur in 9% to 18% of patients after lung transplantation, and multiple studies have shown it to be a major predictor of both morbidity and mortality.[70,72] The studies do not distinguish between anastomotic and other sources of bleeding. Although the pleural space may be the most common site of bleeding, other extrapleural spaces in which blood may collect include the subcutaneous or submuscular planes (Figure 27.7) and the mediastinum. The use of cardiopulmonary bypass and the presence of extensive pleural adhesions in recipients have been associated with an increased risk for postoperative bleeding.[73,74] Thorough examination of the surgical field for hemostasis before the chest is closed may help reduce the incidence of postoperative hematomas. We have found the argon beam coagulator to be a useful tool to stop persistent, diffuse bleeding along the parietal pleural surface after extensive adhesiolysis.

We have a low threshold for early surgical exploration and evacuation of hematomas and hemothoraces. Retained blood clots can easily become infected, thereby leading to wound abscess and empyema. Expansion of the transplanted lung can be severely restricted by a moderate to large hemothorax and result in pulmonary compromise. Pressure necrosis of the skin and wound dehiscence are further complications that may occur because of delay in decompression of chest wall hematomas. In cases in which significant skin ischemia is present, we resect all nonviable skin and do not attempt immediate primary closure, instead opting for intermittent vacuum-assisted dressings

(such as those manufactured by KCI1, San Antonio, Texas) for delayed closure.[75,76]

PLEURAL SPACE COMPLICATIONS

Pleural space conditions that are persistent or require intervention occur after 22% of lung transplant procedures.[69] The well-known pleural space complications of lung transplantation are empyema, pleural effusion, pneumothorax, and less commonly, chylothorax.

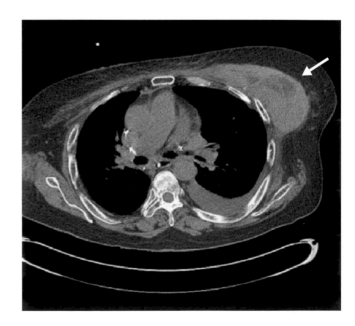

Figure 27.7 Extensive delayed hematoma of the subpectoral chest wall (arrow) after a left single-lung retransplant.

When the donor lung is smaller than the recipient's chest cavity, the transplanted lung may not immediately fill the entire chest, thus giving the appearance of a pneumothorax on a chest radiograph. This possibility must be kept in mind when attempting to treat a postoperative pneumothorax. A small, nonexpanding pneumothorax without any obvious pulmonary compromise can be safely observed. We usually treat symptomatic pneumothoraces or those equal to or more than 5% of the hemithorax volume by percutaneous placement of a 12 French or larger pigtail catheter under ultrasound or CT guidance. This catheter is then connected to a water seal chamber and managed with standard protocols for chest tube management.

Preoperative diagnosis has not been shown to predict the risk for empyema.[69] Pleural effusion is managed according to the size and complexity of the fluid collections. Small pleural effusions without evidence of infection or pulmonary compression are often seen after transplants and can be safely observed.[69] Large nonloculated effusions are often amenable to drainage with percutaneous catheters or chest tubes. In the case of loculated effusions, we frequently administer tissue plasminogen activator in combination with deoxyribonuclease (dornase alfa) as a solution through a chest tube or pigtail catheter to help break down the loculations.[77,78] This regimen can also be used for suspected empyema without evidence of sepsis, although in such cases we have a lower threshold for surgical management. Thoracoscopy is often used during exploration and washout, but thoracotomy may be required for dense and more complex collections. The pleural space may appear abnormal in more than 80% of patients after 1 year, but this finding does not require intervention in asymptomatic patients.[70]

DONOR-RECIPIENT SIZE MISMATCH

Donor-recipient size mismatch is commonly encountered in lung transplantation. In many such instances, the donor lungs are larger than the recipient's chest cavity. Such situations include a female recipient and male donor; small chest cavities in patients with fibrotic lung disease; previous lobectomy in the recipient; and lobes or lungs that are shrunken because of intrinsic pathology, such as idiopathic pulmonary fibrosis or cystic fibrosis.[79] Occasionally, the donor lung is smaller than the recipient's, as in the case of a recipient with long-standing emphysema. Some studies have associated an undersized graft with more complications after transplantation than after transplantation of an oversized graft,[80,81] whereas another large study found that size mismatch has a minimal effect on survival or lung function.[82]

When dealing with a donor-recipient size mismatch, one may be faced with removing a portion of healthy functional lung in an operation in which success depends on keeping as much functional lung as possible. In most instances in which a larger lung needs downsizing, resection of the donor right middle lobe, lingula, or both is usually sufficient.[83,84]

Such resections are generally easily performed, and air leakage usually resolves because of the apposition of pleural surfaces. Some surgeons may use wedge excision of the upper lobes in a procedure similar to lung reduction surgery or even anatomic lobectomy during the back-table preparation of the donor lung.[84,85]

Despite the aforementioned measures to deal with a large lung, primary closure of the chest may occasionally be impossible. Other scenarios in which this situation may be encountered include prolonged use of cardiopulmonary bypass, lung edema secondary to massive resuscitation, and severe primary graft dysfunction.[86,87] Attempts to close the chest in such circumstances may result in hemodynamic and pulmonary compromise because of increased intrathoracic pressure. Leaving the chest open with or without the use of chest retractors, but with an airtight sterile dressing and adequate drains, can help deal with this problem. Final closure can usually be undertaken a few days later.[86,87]

COMPLICATIONS OCCURRING IN THE NONTRANSPLANTED LUNG

Although very little difference in function, survival, and complications exists between patients receiving single-lung versus bilateral lung transplants for noninfective lung conditions, specific complications of which the transplant physician needs to be aware occasionally occur in the nontransplanted lung. In emphysematous patients, cancers related to previous smoking may occur in the nontransplanted lung.[88]

Another infrequently noted problem in an emphysematous contralateral nontransplanted lung is preferential ventilation and consequent overexpansion, mediastinal shift, and compression of the graft. Conversely, the attenuated capillary bed of a diseased lung would lead to preferential perfusion of the graft. Such circumstances may necessitate lung volume reduction surgery or even lobectomy of the remaining lung.[89]

In some long-term survivors of single-lung transplantation for idiopathic pulmonary fibrosis, we have noted marked shrinkage of the nontransplanted lung and the development of persistent, intolerable cough necessitating pneumonectomy of that lung.[90]

MISCELLANEOUS COMPLICATIONS

Other complications that have been described with lung transplantation include surgical site infections, wound dehiscence, sternal dehiscence,[91] lung hernias,[92,93] and complications related to the use of cardiopulmonary bypass.[74,94]

Surgical site infections, including empyema, occur in approximately 5% of patients and thus are not as common with lung transplantation as one would expect given patients' comorbid conditions and use of immunosuppressive therapy.[95] Once present, however, these infections increase length of stay and in-hospital mortality and result in lower long-term survival, with 1-year reported mortality rates of 35% (even when empyema is excluded).[95]

Early in our transplant experience, lung herniation and wide separation of the ribs at the thoracotomy site were noted. These conditions were presumably the result of delayed wound healing and the use of absorbable suture to close the thoracotomy incision, but they are no longer an issue because we now use permanent paracostal sutures for rib reapproximation.

SUMMARY

Despite the significant advances that have been made in the area of lung transplantation during the past decade, surgical complications still play a decisive role in graft and patient survival. Most transplant-related surgical complications can be prevented by awareness of the risk factors, careful patient selection, and use of a standardized surgical technique during each step of the operation.

REFERENCES

1. Yusen RD, Christie JD, Edwards LB, et al. The Registry of the International Society for Heart and Lung Transplantation: Thirtieth adult lung and heart-lung transplant report—2013; focus theme: Age. J Heart Lung Transplant 2013;32:965-978.
2. McEwan K, Thompson P. Ultrasound to detect haemothorax after chest injury. Emerg Med J 2007;24:581-582.
3. Saranteas T, Santaitidis E, Valtzoglou V, Kostopanagiotou G. Emergency lung ultrasound examination for the diagnosis of massive-clotted haemothorax in two cardiac surgery patients. Anaesth Intensive Care 2012;40:564-565.
4. Siddique A, Bose AK, Ozalp F, et al. Vascular anastomotic complications in lung transplantation: A single institution's experience. Interact Cardiovasc Thorac Surg 2013;17:625-631.
5. Clark SC, Levine AJ, Hasan A, et al. Vascular complications of lung transplantation. Ann Thorac Surg 1996;61:1079-1082.
6. Griffith BP, Magee MJ, Gonzalez IF, et al. Anastomotic pitfalls in lung transplantation. J Thorac Cardiovasc Surg 1994;107:743-753; discussion 753-754.
7. Belli EV, Landolfo K, Thomas M, Odell J. Partial anomalous pulmonary venous return in a lung transplant recipient. Ann Thorac Surg 2013;95:1104-1106.
8. Oto T, Rabinov M, Negri J, et al. Techniques of reconstruction for inadequate donor left atrial cuff in lung transplantation. Ann Thorac Surg 2006;81:1199-1204.
9. Bhama JK, Bansal A, Shigemura N, Toyoda Y. Reconstruction technique for a short recipient left atrial cuff during lung transplantation. Eur J Cardiothorac Surg 2014;45:1106-1107.
10. Liguori C, Schulman LL, Weslow RG, et al. Late pulmonary venous complications after lung transplantation. J Am Soc Echocardiogr 1997;10:763-767.
11. Gonzalez-Fernandez C, Gonzalez-Castro A, Rodriguez-Borregan JC, et al. Pulmonary venous obstruction after lung transplantation. Diagnostic advantages of transesophageal echocardiography. Clin Transplant 2009;23:975-980.
12. Schulman LL, Anandarangam T, Leibowitz DW, et al. Four-year prospective study of pulmonary venous thrombosis after lung transplantation. J Am Soc Echocardiogr 2001;14:806-812.
13. Kroshus TJ, Kshettry VR, Hertz MI, Bolman RM 3rd. Deep venous thrombosis and pulmonary embolism after lung transplantation. J Thorac Cardiovasc Surg 1995;110:540-544.
14. Grubstein A, Atar E, Litvin S, et al. Angioplasty using covered stents in five patients with symptomatic pulmonary artery stenosis after single-lung transplantation. Cardiovasc Intervent Radiol 2014;37:686-690.
15. Berger H, Steiner W, Schmidt D, et al. Stent-angioplasty of an anastomotic stenosis of the pulmonary artery after lung transplantation. Eur J Cardiothorac Surg 1994;8:103-105.
16. Chen F, Tazaki J, Shibata T, et al. Stent angioplasty for a kink in the pulmonary artery anastomosis soon after living-donor lobar lung transplantation. Ann Thorac Surg 2011;92:e105-106.
17. Loyalka P, Cevik C, Nathan S, et al. Percutaneous stenting to treat pulmonary vein stenosis after single-lung transplantation. Tex Heart Inst J 2012;39:560-564.
18. Mohamed Mydin MI, Calvert PA, Jenkins DP, Parmar J. Percutaneous dilatation of right inferior pulmonary vein stenosis following single-lung transplant. Interact Cardiovasc Thorac Surg 2012;15:314-316.
19. Pazos-Lopez P, Pineiro-Portela M, Bouzas-Mosquera A, et al. Images in cardiovascular disease. Pulmonary vein stenosis after lung transplantation successfully treated with stent implantation. Circulation 2010;122:2745-2747.
20. Teis A, Camara ML, Ferrer E, Romero-Ferrer B. Critical stenosis of pulmonary homograft induced by Surgicel in Ross procedure. Asian Cardiovasc Thorac Ann 2010;18:382-383.
21. Eto K, Matsumoto M, Kubo Y, Kemmochi R. Superior vena cava syndrome caused by a swollen absorbable haemostat after repair of ischaemic mitral regurgitation. J Cardiothorac Surg 2014;9:1.
22. Oto T, Rabinov M, Griffiths AP, et al. Unexpected donor pulmonary embolism affects early outcomes after lung transplantation: A major mechanism of primary graft failure? J Thorac Cardiovasc Surg 2005;130:1446.
23. Nguyen DQ, Salerno CT, Bolman M 3rd, Park SJ. Pulmonary thromboembolectomy of donor lungs prior to lung transplantation. Ann Thorac Surg 1999;67:1787-1789.

24. Shihata M, Ghorpade N, Lien D, Modry D. Ex vivo bilateral pulmonary embolectomy for donor lungs prior to transplantation. Ann Thorac Surg 2008;85:2110-2112.

25. de Perrot M, Keshavjee S. Lung preservation. Semin Thorac Cardiovasc Surg 2004;16:300-308.

26. Leibowitz DW, Smith CR, Michler RE, et al. Incidence of pulmonary vein complications after lung transplantation: A prospective transesophageal echocardiographic study. J Am Coll Cardiol 1994;24:671-675.

27. McIlroy DR, Sesto AC, Buckland MR. Pulmonary vein thrombosis, lung transplantation, and intraoperative transesophageal echocardiography. J Cardiothorac Vasc Anesth 2006;20:712-715.

28. Santacruz JF, Mehta AC. Airway complications and management after lung transplantation: Ischemia, dehiscence, and stenosis. Proc Am Thorac Soc 2009;6:79-93.

29. Van De Wauwer C, Van Raemdonck D, Verleden GM, et al. Risk factors for airway complications within the first year after lung transplantation. Eur J Cardiothorac Surg 2007;31:703-710.

30. Alvarez A, Algar J, Santos F, et al. Airway complications after lung transplantation: A review of 151 anastomoses. Eur J Cardiothorac Surg 2001;19:381-387.

31. Shennib H, Massard G. Airway complications in lung transplantation. Ann Thorac Surg 1994;57:506-511.

32. Couraud L, Nashef SA, Nicolini P, Jougon J. Classification of airway anastomotic healing. Eur J Cardiothorac Surg 1992;6:496-497.

33. Thistlethwaite PA, Yung G, Kemp A, et al. Airway stenoses after lung transplantation: Incidence, management, and outcome. J Thorac Cardiovasc Surg 2008;136:1569-1575.

34. Chhajed PN, Tamm M, Glanville AR. Role of flexible bronchoscopy in lung transplantation. Semin Respir Crit Care Med 2004;25:413-423.

35. Dutau H, Vandemoortele T, Laroumagne S, et al. A new endoscopic standardized grading system for macroscopic central airway complications following lung transplantation: The MDS classification. Eur J Cardiothorac Surg 2014;45:e33-e38.

36. Kshettry VR, Kroshus TJ, Hertz MI, et al. Early and late airway complications after lung transplantation: Incidence and management. Ann Thorac Surg 1997;63:1576-1583.

37. Castleberry AW, Worni M, Kuchibhatla M, et al. A comparative analysis of bronchial stricture after lung transplantation in recipients with and without early acute rejection. Ann Thorac Surg 2013;96:1008-1017; discussion 1017-1018.

38. Mulligan MS. Endoscopic management of airway complications after lung transplantation. Chest Surg Clin N Am 2001;11:907-915.

39. Garfein ES, McGregor CC, Galantowicz ME, Schulman LL. Deleterious effects of telescoped bronchial anastomosis in single and bilateral lung transplantation. Ann Transplant 2000;5:5-11.

40. Murthy SC, Blackstone EH, Gildea TR, et al. Impact of anastomotic airway complications after lung transplantation. Ann Thorac Surg 2007;84:401-409, 409 e401-e404.

41. Garfein ES, Ginsberg ME, Gorenstein L, et al. Superiority of end-to-end versus telescoped bronchial anastomosis in single lung transplantation for pulmonary emphysema. J Thorac Cardiovasc Surg 2001;121:149-154.

42. Calhoon JH, Grover FL, Gibbons WJ, et al. Single lung transplantation. Alternative indications and technique. J Thorac Cardiovasc Surg 1991;101:816-824; discussion 824-825.

43. Miller JD, DeHoyos A. An evaluation of the role of omentopexy and of early perioperative corticosteroid administration in clinical lung transplantation. The University of Toronto and Washington University Lung Transplant Programs. J Thorac Cardiovasc Surg 1993;105:247-252.

44. Inci I, Weder W. Airway complications after lung transplantation can be avoided without bronchial artery revascularization. Curr Opin Organ Transplant 2010;15:578-581.

45. Emery RW, Arom KV, Von Rueden T, Copeland JG. Use of the pericardial fat pad in pulmonary transplantation. J Card Surg 1990;5:145-148.

46. Khaghani A, Tadjkarimi S, al-Kattan K, et al. Wrapping the anastomosis with omentum or an internal mammary artery pedicle does not improve bronchial healing after single lung transplantation: Results of a randomized clinical trial. J Heart Lung Transplant 1994;13:767-773.

47. Garg K, Zamora MR, Tuder R, et al. Lung transplantation: Indications, donor and recipient selection, and imaging of complications. Radiographics 1996;16:355-367.

48. Semenkovich JW, Glazer HS, Anderson DC, et al. Bronchial dehiscence in lung transplantation: CT evaluation. Radiology 1995;194:205-208.

49. Schlueter FJ, Semenkovich JW, Glazer HS, et al. Bronchial dehiscence after lung transplantation: Correlation of CT findings with clinical outcome. Radiology 1996;199:849-854.

50. Saad CP, Ghamande SA, Minai OA, et al. The role of self-expandable metallic stents for the treatment of airway complications after lung transplantation. Transplantation 2003;75:1532-1538.

51. Kapoor BS, May B, Panu N, et al. Endobronchial stent placement for the management of airway complications after lung transplantation. J Vasc Interv Radiol 2007;18:629-632.

52. Sundset A, Lund MB, Hansen G, et al. Airway complications after lung transplantation: Long-term outcome of silicone stenting. Respiration 2012;83:245-252.

53. Camargo Jde J, Camargo SM, Machuca TN, et al. Surgical maneuvers for the management of bronchial complications in lung transplantation. Eur J Cardiothorac Surg 2008;34:1206-1209.

54. Samano MN, Minamoto H, Junqueira JJ, et al. Bronchial complications following lung transplantation. Transplant Proc 2009;41:921-926.

55. Karmy-Jones R, Vallieres E, Culver B, et al. Bronchial-atrial fistula after lung transplant resulting in fatal air embolism. Ann Thorac Surg 1999;67:550-551.

56. Hoff SJ, Johnson JE, Frist WH. Aortobronchial fistula after unilateral lung transplantation. Ann Thorac Surg 1993;56:1402-1403.

57. Rea F, Marulli G, Loy M, et al. Salvage right pneumonectomy in a patient with bronchial-pulmonary artery fistula after bilateral sequential lung transplantation. J Heart Lung Transplant 2006;25:1383-1386.

58. Guth S, Mayer E, Fischer B, et al. Bilobectomy for massive hemoptysis after bilateral lung transplantation. J Thorac Cardiovasc Surg 2001;121:1194-1195.

59. Lois M, Noppen M. Bronchopleural fistulas: An overview of the problem with special focus on endoscopic management. Chest 2005;128:3955-3965.

60. Chang CC, Hsu HH, Kuo SW, Lee YC. Bronchoscopic gluing for post–lung-transplant bronchopleural fistula. Eur J Cardiothorac Surg 2007;31:328-330.

61. Abdel-Rahman N, Kramer MR, Saute M, et al. Metallic stents for airway complications after lung transplantation: Long-term follow-up. Eur J Cardiothorac Surg 2014;45:854-858.

62. McGiffin D, Wille K, Young K, Leon K. Salvaging the dehisced lung transplant bronchial anastomosis with homograft aorta. Interact Cardiovasc Thorac Surg 2011;13:666-668.

63. Hasegawa T, Iacono AT, Orons PD, Yousem SA. Segmental nonanastomotic bronchial stenosis after lung transplantation. Ann Thorac Surg 2000;69:1020-1024.

64. Lari SM, Gonin F, Colchen A. The management of bronchus intermedius complications after lung transplantation: A retrospective study. J Cardiothorac Surg 2012;7:8.

65. Orons PD, Amesur NB, Dauber JH, et al. Balloon dilation and endobronchial stent placement for bronchial strictures after lung transplantation. J Vasc Interv Radiol 2000;11:89-99.

66. Sheridan PH Jr, Cheriyan A, Doud J, et al. Incidence of phrenic neuropathy after isolated lung transplantation. The Loyola University Lung Transplant Group. J Heart Lung Transplant 1995;14:684-691.

67. Ferdinande P, Bruyninckx F, Van Raemdonck D, et al. Phrenic nerve dysfunction after heart-lung and lung transplantation. J Heart Lung Transplant 2004;23:105-109.

68. Maziak DE, Maurer JR, Kesten S. Diaphragmatic paralysis: A complication of lung transplantation. Ann Thorac Surg 1996;61:170-173.

69. Herridge MS, de Hoyos AL, Chaparro C, et al. Pleural complications in lung transplant recipients. J Thorac Cardiovasc Surg 1995;110:22-26.

70. Ferrer J, Roldan J, Roman A, et al. Acute and chronic pleural complications in lung transplantation. J Heart Lung Transplant 2003;22:1217-1225.

71. Backhus LM, Sievers EM, Schenkel FA, et al. Pleural space problems after living lobar transplantation. J Heart Lung Transplant 2005;24:2086-2090.

72. Ceron Navarro J, de Aguiar Quevedo K, Mancheno Franch N, et al. [Complications after lung transplantation in chronic obstructive pulmonary disease.] Med Clin (Barc) 2013;140:385-389.

73. Shigemura N, Bhama J, Gries CJ, et al. Lung transplantation in patients with prior cardiothoracic surgical procedures. Am J Transplant 2012;12:1249-1255.

74. Burdett C, Butt T, Lordan J, Dark JH, Clark SC. Comparison of single lung transplant with and without the use of cardiopulmonary bypass. Interact Cardiovasc Thorac Surg 2012;15:432-436; discussion 436.

75. O'Connor J, Kells A, Henry S, Scalea T. Vacuum-assisted closure for the treatment of complex chest wounds. Ann Thorac Surg 2005;79:1196-1200.

76. Welvaart WN, Oosterhuis JW, Paul MA. Negative pressure dressing for radiation-associated wound dehiscence after posterolateral thoracotomy. Interact Cardiovasc Thorac Surg 2009;8:558-559.

77. Ahmed AE, Yacoub TE. Empyema thoracis. Clin Med Insights Circ Respir Pulm Med 2010;4:1-8.

78. Wagener JS, Kupfer O. Dornase alfa (Pulmozyme). Curr Opin Pulm Med 2012;18:609-614.

79. Barnard JB, Davies O, Curry P, et al. Size matching in lung transplantation: An evidence-based review. J Heart Lung Transplant 2013;32:849-860.

80. Eberlein M, Arnaoutakis GJ, Yarmus L, et al. The effect of lung size mismatch on complications and resource utilization after bilateral lung transplantation. J Heart Lung Transplant 2012;31:492-500.

81. Eberlein M, Reed RM, Bolukbas S, et al. Lung size mismatch and survival after single and bilateral lung transplantation. Ann Thorac Surg 2013;96:457-463.

82. Mason DP, Batizy LH, Wu J, et al. Matching donor to recipient in lung transplantation: How much does size matter? J Thorac Cardiovasc Surg 2009;137:1234-1240.

83. Slama A, Ghanim B, Klikovits T, et al. Lobar lung transplantation—is it comparable with standard lung transplantation? Transpl Int 2014;27:909-916.

84. Aigner C, Winkler G, Jaksch P, et al. Size-reduced lung transplantation: An advanced operative strategy to alleviate donor organ shortage. Transplant Proc 2004;36:2801-2805.

85. Raja S, Murthy SC, Pettersson GB, Mason DP. Managing extreme airway size mismatch in lung transplantation: The "upper lobectomy" technique. Semin Thorac Cardiovasc Surg 2011;23:336-338.

86. Force SD, Miller DL, Pelaez A, et al. Outcomes of delayed chest closure after bilateral lung transplantation. Ann Thorac Surg 2006;81:2020-2024; discussion 2024-2025.

87. Shigemura N, Orhan Y, Bhama JK, et al. Delayed chest closure after lung transplantation: Techniques, outcomes, and strategies. J Heart Lung Transplant 2014;33:741-748.

88. Belli EV, Landolfo K, Keller C, et al. Lung cancer following lung transplant: Single institution 10 year experience. Lung Cancer 2013;81: 451-454.

89. Anderson MB, Kriett JM, Kapelanski DP, et al. Volume reduction surgery in the native lung after single lung transplantation for emphysema. J Heart Lung Transplant 1997;16:752-757.

90. Elicker BM, Golden JA, Ordovas KG, et al. Progression of native lung fibrosis in lung transplant recipients with idiopathic pulmonary fibrosis. Respir Med 2010;104:426-433.

91. Orsini B, D'Journo XB, Reynaud-Gaubert M, Thomas PA. Sternal dehiscence after clamshell incision in lung transplantation treated with the STR Asbourg Thoracic Osteosyntheses System (STRATOS). Ann Thorac Surg 2014;97:e55-e57.

92. Gomez-Arnau J, Novoa N, Isidro MG, et al. Ruptured hemidiaphragm after bilateral lung transplantation. Eur J Anaesthesiol 1999;16:259-262.

93. Jougon J, Duffy J, Delaisement C, Velly JF. Lobar exclusion after transpericardial herniation in a heart-lung transplantation. Eur J Cardiothorac Surg 1997;12:919-921.

94. Nagendran M, Maruthappu M, Sugand K. Should double lung transplant be performed with or without cardiopulmonary bypass? Interact Cardiovasc Thorac Surg 2011;12:799-804.

95. Shields RK, Clancy CJ, Minces LR, et al. Epidemiology and outcomes of deep surgical site infections following lung transplantation. Am J Transplant 2013;13:2137-2145.

28

Immunosuppression strategies in lung transplantation

MIRANDA A. PARASKEVA, GLEN P. WESTALL, AND GREG I. SNELL

INTRODUCTION

Careful pharmacologic manipulation of the host immune system to prevent rejection of the lung allograft remains the cornerstone of management following lung transplantation. This immunologic imperative must in turn be balanced with the need to avoid significant infection. The immunosuppressive regimens used and extent of immunosuppression achieved have a critical effect on the infection and rejection profiles of individuals undergoing lung transplantation, which in turn affects their long-term survival.

As our understanding of the immune system has matured, our ability to manipulate it pharmacologically has evolved. This evolution has in turn provided us with an arsenal of drugs aimed at keeping the host immune system quiescent in an attempt to prevent activation of the immune pathways that ultimately lead to rejection of the lung allograft. The discovery of the first selective immunosuppressive drug, cyclosporine, in 1976 revolutionized solid-organ transplantation (SOT) and heralded the progression toward longer-term survival that would allow lung transplantation to evolve from a technically possible procedure with poor long-term outcomes to the established treatment of end-stage lung disease that it is today.

Current practices in immunosuppressive regimens vary from institution to institution. This variation is reflected in the International Society of Heart and Lung Transplantation (ISHLT) registry data, which describe the broad diversity of induction and maintenance strategies currently in use.[1] Most randomized controlled trials in lung transplantation have involved only small numbers of patients; as a result, practice has also been aided by retrospective case series and expert consensus. In essence, the information from these sources, coupled with local expertise and past experience, is what tends to serve as the basis for the immunosuppressive practices of individual institutions, thus leading to the variations in practices reported to the registry.

The pharmacologic management of lung transplant recipients varies according to the time from transplantation and is influenced by the infection-rejection profile of the individual recipient. In general, immunosuppressive regimens during the posttransplant period can be divided as follows:

1. The induction phase: Induction encompasses the augmentation of immunosuppression in the perioperative or early postoperative period by using agents such as polyclonal antilymphocyte preparations, anti-CD52 antibodies, or interleukin-2 receptor (IL-2R) antagonists in an attempt to reduce the initial robust T-cell response against the lung allograft and minimize the incidence of acute cellular rejection with the aim of improving long-term outcomes.
2. The maintenance phase: Maintenance therapy involves a combination of agents (usually three) aimed at keeping the host immune system quiescent and preventing

rejection while simultaneously avoiding the excessive immune depletion that would make mounting responses to infection impossible.

3. Management of rejection: The precise regimens and algorithms involved in the management of rejection are dependent on the pattern and immunologic pathway underlying the process. They range from augmentation of immunosuppression with pulse methylprednisolone therapy to plasmapheresis and immunoglobulin treatment of antibody-mediated rejection (AMR).

INDUCTION PHASE

Long-term outcomes following lung transplantation are influenced by the development of chronic lung allograft dysfunction (CLAD), including the obstructive phenotype, and bronchiolitis obliterans syndrome (BOS). A factor implicated in the development of BOS is acute cellular rejection, which is a predominantly T-cell–mediated process.[2] Immune reactivity is highest in the first 6 months after graft implantation; therefore, this early posttransplantation period is the time of highest risk for the development of acute cellular rejection. Many institutions use induction therapy during this period in an attempt to decrease the incidence of acute rejection and influence long-term outcomes.

The two categories of induction agents in wide use are lymphocyte-depleting agents and IL-2 receptor antagonists. They are used to augment immunosuppression by inducing profound T-cell inhibition via interruption of T-cell activation and proliferation. Because the perioperative period confers a high risk for renal insufficiency, a secondary benefit of induction therapy is the ability to delay the initiation of calcineurin inhibitors (CNIs) and thereby allow a longer period for renal recovery from the operative stress of hypovolemia and cardiopulmonary bypass.

Use of induction agents was initially encouraged by evidence from other groups undergoing SOT, which suggested that such agents were associated with a reduced incidence of acute rejection of renal, cardiac, and liver allografts.[3-5] The evidence in lung transplantation, however, has not been definitively established.

Interleukin-2 receptor antagonists (daclizumab and basiliximab)

IL-2 is crucial to T-cell activation and proliferation. It acts as a signaling molecule that binds to the T-cell receptor, thereby leading to activation, proliferation, and differentiation of the T cell into an effector cell. The IL-2R antagonists basiliximab and daclizumab are chimeric (murine-human) monoclonal antibodies directed at CD25, the IL-2R α chain. By high-affinity binding to CD25, these agents selectively block activated T cells and thereby inhibit cell proliferation and differentiation. Because CD25 expression is dependent on T-cell activation, these agents affect only activated T cells and thus do not lead to T-cell depletion.

Humanized antibodies are generally well tolerated and do not tend to lead to the cytokine release syndromes that are more commonly seen with the lymphocyte-depleting agents. These agents are traditionally given before or for a number of hours after implantation. One retrospective study has shown that induction with basiliximab before rather than after implantation leads to overall lower acute rejection scores but no significant differences in rates of BOS and survival.[6]

An overall increase in the use of IL-2R antagonists over the last decade has been reported.[1] A prospective study comparing daclizumab induction with the use of OKT3 and antithymocyte globulin (ATG) found no difference between the groups in terms of rates of acute rejection, BOS, or mortality.[7] However, other smaller retrospective studies have provided conflicting results, with several showing the superiority of daclizumab or basiliximab over alternative induction agents and others suggesting poorer outcomes associated with IL-2R antagonists than with ATG.[8-11] ISHLT registry data suggest that the use of IL-2R antagonists confers a lower reported incidence of acute rejection in the first year than other induction strategies do.[1] This finding is supported by a recent study by Whitson and colleagues, which showed that although all induction agents conferred a mortality benefit, basiliximab appeared to confer greater improvement than ATG, antilymphocyte globulin (ALG), or thymoglobulin did.[12]

Lymphocyte-depleting agents

Lymphocyte-depleting agents are monoclonal or polyclonal antibodies that react against one or more lymphocyte surface antigens and thereby lead to profound depletion of cytotoxic T cells.

POLYCLONAL ANTIBODIES

ALG and ATG are polyclonal immunoglobulin preparations that lead to cytotoxic T-cell depletion indirectly through complement- and cell-mediated antibody-related cell lysis and macrophage-mediated opsonization and phagocytosis.[13] Their use commonly leads to an acute reaction at initial administration because of a cytokine release syndrome that results in fevers, rigors, myalgia, and rash.[14] Other reported complications are leukopenia, thrombocytopenia, immune complex glomerulonephritis, and serum sickness, which can be minimized through the use of therapeutic drug monitoring (TDM) targeting CD3 levels of 50 to 100 cells/μL.[15]

A prospective randomized controlled trial comparing ATG with no induction demonstrated an early reduction in acute rejection. The 8-year follow-up study, however, confirmed the reduction in early rejection but did not show a reduction in the overall incidence of acute rejection or a sustained improvement in survival.[16,17] More recently, a large randomized controlled multicenter study examining the efficacy of a single dose of 5 or 9 mg/kg of ATG-Fresenius as opposed to a placebo showed no significant reduction in acute rejection, graft loss, or death in the first year following lung transplantation.[18]

MONOCLONAL ANTIBODIES

Monomurab-CD3 (OKT3) and alemtuzumab are monoclonal antibodies that have been used for lung transplantation. OKT3 is a murine-derived monoclonal antibody that targets the CD3 complex of the T-cell receptor; it was previously used for the management of acute rejection and induction in other types of SOT.[19] Binding of OKT3 to the CD3 complex of the T cell triggers initial T-cell activation and a massive cytokine release syndrome before leading to depletion of circulating T cells. Its use has decreased in all organ transplants because of the availability of newer small-molecule immunosuppressive drugs. In lung transplantation, however, its use has been further limited because of a high associated incidence of infection[20] and a link between prolonged use and posttransplant lymphoproliferative disorder.[21]

Alemtuzumab (Campath) is a monoclonal antibody against CD52, which is a receptor present on the surface of B cells, T cells, macrophages, monocytes, and natural killer cells. It leads to T-cell depletion through complement-mediated cytolysis and direct antibody-mediated cytotoxicity,[22] which depresses CD4 and CD8 cell counts for up to 3 years. Use of alemtuzumab was reported in only 6% of lung transplant recipients from June 2002 to 2012[1] and has been described by the Pittsburgh group,[23] which showed that at 5 years, survival was comparable to that following ATG induction and better than that with daclizumab or no therapy.[24]

ISHLT registry data suggest improved outcomes with the use of induction.[1] This position is supported by a recent study that analyzed United Network for Organ Sharing (UNOS) data and showed that use of any induction agent was associated with improvements in survival and acute rejection rates in the first year following transplantation.[12] However, other case series and randomized controlled trials have not confirmed these results, and whether induction has a proven overall benefit as part of lung transplant management remains unclear.

MAINTENANCE PHASE

The high risk for allograft rejection after single-lung transplantation versus after other types of SOT confers a greater requirement for immunosuppression and, therefore, higher baseline immunosuppression levels over the course of the transplant process. This increased risk for rejection is probably multifactorial and reflects the unique nature of the lung allograft. First, the lung allograft contains a large number of donor-derived dendritic cells that are capable of stimulating T-cell responses.[25] Second, the lung allograft is exposed to the outside environment and hence to exogenous pathogens that are capable of stimulating immune responses. Third, the processes of donor brain death and ischemic reperfusion lead to a proinflammatory state that can in turn result in allograft injury and further T-cell stimulation.[26]

The maintenance phase of immunosuppression typically consists of a triple-drug regimen. This multidrug combination provides more effective immunosuppression by targeting multiple T-cell pathways and simultaneously minimizing side effects by allowing lower target drug levels. The ISHLT registry indicates that although no clear consensus regarding the optimal drug combination exists, the most commonly used combination consists of a CNI, nucleotide-blocking agent, and glucocorticoid.[1] Other agents, such as mammalian target of rapamycin (mTOR) inhibitors, are increasingly being used as part of routine immunosuppression but still only constitute a minority of the immunosuppression used worldwide.

Calcineurin inhibitors: cyclosporine and tacrolimus

The CNIs cyclosporine and tacrolimus form the cornerstone of the immunosuppressive regimen following lung transplantation. They act to block T-cell activation and, consequently, IL-2 production through the inhibition of calcineurin. According to ISHLT registry data, CNIs are invariably given with an antimetabolite and corticosteroid. Since the development of newer agents, however, the combinations have varied. Notably, tacrolimus use has increased globally over the last decade: it is now being administered to 70% of all lung transplant recipients.[1]

CYCLOSPORINE

Cyclosporine is a fungal polypeptide that forms complexes with cytophilin, an intracytoplasmic protein found in most cells, thereby leading to inhibition of calcineurin and hence T-cell activation. As a highly lipophilic compound, cyclosporine is dependent on the presence of bile acids for absorption; consequently, its absorption varies widely within and between individual patients. Such variation is particularly true in patients who have cystic fibrosis (CF) with pancreatic insufficiency and may therefore require larger and more frequent dosing to achieve therapeutic levels.[27] The original commercial preparations were characterized by poor and unpredictable absorption because of their highly lipophilic nature; however, the newer microemulsion (Neoral) features improved bioavailability, more consistent oral absorption, and more reproducible pharmacokinetic behavior.

Because of the narrow therapeutic window, it is essential that TDM be performed. Low systemic exposure to cyclosporine is associated with acute rejection, whereas high systemic exposure can lead to toxicity.[28] TDM has traditionally used the trough level (C_0) and 2-hour postdose level (C_2) for dose adjustment, with C_0 and C_2 target levels dependent on the time from transplantation. Although C_0 remains the more convenient level to measure, studies of other SOT groups have suggested that C_2 correlates better with systemic exposure, a fact that is supported by studies in lung transplantation.[29,30] Cyclosporine is metabolized by the enzyme cytochrome-P450 3A4 (CYP3A4), and substantial drug interactions with other medications metabolized by this pathway occur. This fact is particularly important in the case of azole antifungals, which have been reported to increase immunosuppressant levels by up to four times.[31] Cyclosporine is associated with nephrotoxicity, hypertension, hyperlipidemia, thrombotic microangiopathy, and neurotoxicity, including tremors and posterior reversible encephalopathy syndrome.[32-34]

TACROLIMUS

Tacrolimus is structurally unrelated to cyclosporine. It is a macrolide antibiotic that binds to the immunophillin FK506 binding protein, thereby leading to inactivation of calcineurin, which in turn inhibits T-cell activation and IL-2 production. It is 10 to 100 times more potent than cyclosporine in inhibiting T-cell activation. It has a narrow therapeutic window; its absorption is hindered by food and unaffected by the presence of bile.[35] TDM uses a C_0 value, but strategies for its postdose monitoring have yet to be developed.[36] Like cyclosporine, tacrolimus is also metabolized by the CYP3A4 pathway and its levels are influenced by many drug-drug interactions. Its toxicities are comparable to those of cyclosporine and include nephrotoxicity, hypertension, hyperlipidemia, diabetes mellitus, and neurotoxicity. Of note, the distribution of their toxicities tends to differ. Although all CNIs can lead to nephrotoxicity, tacrolimus is more likely to lead to new-onset diabetes mellitus whereas cyclosporine is more likely to cause hypertension.[37]

Tacrolimus versus cyclosporine

A number of prospective randomized trials have compared the use of tacrolimus with cyclosporine in lung transplant recipients.[38-40] All the studies have shown tacrolimus to be at least as effective as cyclosporine, and a number have supported the ISHLT registry data suggesting that rates of acute rejection in the first year following transplantation are lower in the tacrolimus-based regimens and higher in the cyclosporine-based regimens.[1] Of note, no study has shown a mortality benefit associated with tacrolimus. Most studies have compared tacrolimus and cyclosporine in combination with either azathioprine or mycophenolate mofetil (MMF) and a corticosteroid, thus reflecting the most common triple-drug regimens used. Keenan and colleagues randomly assigned 133 lung transplant recipients to treatment with tacrolimus or cyclosporine in conjunction with azathioprine and prednisolone. They showed reductions in acute rejection episodes and incidence of BOS in the tacrolimus group with a nonsignificant trend toward improved survival at 2 years.[38] Treede and coworkers evaluated tacrolimus and cyclosporine in combination with MMF and prednisolone.[39] Their cohort additionally received induction therapy with ATG. They demonstrated a reduction in treated acute rejection and a decreased incidence of BOS at 3 years but no difference in survival at 6 months, 1 year, or 3 years.[40] A more recent large prospective randomized controlled trial involving more than 200 patients compared tacrolimus with cyclosporine in combination with MMF

and prednisolone; it showed no significant difference in the incidence of acute rejection or survival but did demonstrate a reduced incidence of BOS in the tacrolimus group.[41] Overall, the literature currently suggests that tacrolimus is slightly superior to cyclosporine.

Alternative calcineurin inhibitor strategies

A number of factors can lead to variable or inadequate absorption during the posttransplant period; they range from patient-specific considerations, such as the gastrointestinal abnormalities that accompany CF, to postoperative complications such as gastroparesis.[42] The requirement for safe and efficacious delivery of immunosuppression has led to the evolution of alternative delivery methods.

INTRAVENOUS CALCINEURIN INHIBITOR ADMINISTRATION

The use of intravenous CNI administration strategies had previously been limited by the manufacturers' recommendations for administration as a continuous 24-hour infusion.[43,44] Such an administration method results in the loss of normal predose trough and postdose peak levels, thus making monitoring of drug levels uninterpretable and contributing to higher rates of neurotoxicity and nephrotoxicity.[45]

Our experience with intravenous cyclosporine and tacrolimus has recently been reported.[46] Cyclosporine can be given as a twice-daily 6-hour bolus infusion that is initiated at a dose of 25 mg and titrated according to C_0 at 25-mg increments. After initially administering cyclosporine intravenously, we switch to oral cyclosporine with a conversion ratio of 1:4. More recently we have used tacrolimus as a twice-daily 4-hour bolus infusion that is initiated at a dose of 0.3 to 0.5 mg. Conversion to the oral formulation occurs at a 1:10 conversion ratio. Twice-daily intravenous bolus administration of cyclosporine and tacrolimus is a practical approach that appears to be efficacious in attaining therapeutic levels and minimizing toxicity.[44,47] Furthermore, in contrast to 24-hour infusion, the bolus approach provides an interpretable C_0.

SUBLINGUAL TACROLIMUS

The early posttransplant period is a time of variable or inadequate gastrointestinal absorption, which is more pronounced in patients with CF, who are at risk for a number of gastrointestinal problems, including gastroesophageal reflux disease, gastric stasis, and pancreatic malabsorption, all of which contribute to significant pharmacokinetic variations in immunosuppression.[48] The sublingual formulation of tacrolimus offers the advantages of not requiring an invasive administration method and facilitating direct systemic uptake, as a result of which variable gastrointestinal absorption is avoided.[48] Use of sublingual tacrolimus requires a 2:1 conversion from oral tacrolimus.[49] Sublingual tacrolimus achieves a C_0 and clinical efficacy that are broadly equivalent to those of the oral formulation.[48-50] Despite the theoretical benefits of the sublingual method of drug delivery, we have found it to be difficult and believe that a significant proportion of the absorption is probably attributable to the swallowed drug rather than to direct sublingual absorption. The sublingual formulation will probably serve as an additional therapeutic option to enable converting a stable cooperative patient from initial intravenous or oral tacrolimus, which might be required during long intensive care unit stays or during periods of variable gut function.

EXTENDED-RELEASE TACROLIMUS

Tacrolimus in a twice-daily formulation has been used in SOT for a number of decades. More recently, a once-daily or extended-release formulation has become available. Although it has been used with other SOT groups,[51-53] the new formulation has only recently been incorporated into routine lung transplant regimens. Tacrolimus XL is a modified galenic formulation that allows once-daily administration. It was designed to provide an area under the concentration-time curve from 0 to 24 hours (AUC_{0-24}) similar to that of the twice-daily formulation and with equivalent efficacy and safety.[53]

The rationale for using tacrolimus XL is to simplify medication regimens with the aim of increasing medication adherence and the additional benefit of potentially providing a better safety profile by avoiding toxic peak concentrations. In patients with impaired gastric motility the formulation's stability may improve total drug exposure. A recent pharmacokinetic study suggested a conversion of 1:1 mg/mg total daily dose and confirmed the existence of a good correlation and similar relationship between AUC_{0-12} and the minimum concentration (C_{min}) after conversion from the twice-daily to once-daily formulation.[54] Unfortunately, this study excluded patients with CF, who are known to have irregular intestinal absorption and thus constitute the group to which such a formulation might offer the most benefits.

We have reported our experience in switching 91 lung transplant recipients to this preparation at a median of 465 days after transplantation.[55] The most common indication for the change in formulation was the concomitant use of an azole requiring significant dose reduction because the once-daily preparation provides the advantage of allowing the administration of 0.5 mg daily (i.e., half the traditional lowest dose of the immediate-release tacrolimus). Other indications were gastrointestinal and renal impairment leading to highly variable tacrolimus levels and suspected or proven nonadherence. Few individuals experienced adverse effects, and no episodes of acute rejection were documented. Although formal longitudinal studies in lung transplantation are lacking, at this point, the extended-release tacrolimus formulation seems to be a useful and efficacious addition to immunosuppression in lung transplantation.

Variance in calcineurin inhibitor levels

Variability in CNI level has been associated with higher rates of acute rejection, graft loss, and other adverse effects

that lead to increased health care costs after SOT.[56-58] Additionally, in liver transplantation, a tacrolimus standard deviation (SD) of greater than 2 is predictive of late rejection.[58] The variation in CNI level has been attributed to nonadherence, intercurrent illness, concomitant medications, and poor absorption.

We recently described the impact of tacrolimus variability on posttransplantation outcomes.[59] The SD for tacrolimus was calculated for 108 lung transplant recipients. Most importantly, the risk for acute rejection increased by 23% for each unit increase in SD. Of note, the mean tacrolimus level of the "rejecters" was higher than that of the "nonrejecters." The proportion of patients with CF was significantly higher in the rejecter group, which suggests that poor absorption may contribute to this variability. A secondary study undertaken by our group examined lung transplant recipients with CF and found that increased variability in tacrolimus levels was associated with poor long-term outcomes, including CLAD and death. We found that recipients with a higher tacrolimus SD were more likely to be nonadherent to their medication regimens, thus suggesting that poor absorption does not explain all the variability seen in this population.[60]

Variability in CNI level has also been used to compare different drug formulations. A comparative examination of bioequivalent generic and branded cyclosporine found evidence that individuals receiving generic cyclosporine have an increased variance in C_0.[61] Similarly, comparison of the standard twice-daily and once-daily extended-release formulations of tacrolimus has shown 50% less variance with the extended-release formulation.[62] Given the simplicity of calculating variability, we believe that it should be the subject of further research in lung transplantation.

Inhaled immunosuppression strategies

The concept of localized therapy in the form of inhaled immunosuppressive agents as an opportunity to reduce systemic immunosuppression is appealing. Although a number of groups have described using inhaled corticosteroids,[63] cyclosporine,[64,65] and tacrolimus[66] in the setting of lung transplantation, few have shown positive outcomes of doing so. A small randomized controlled trial of inhaled fluticasone propionate did not show the drug's efficacy,[63] and although the initial trials of inhaled cyclosporine suggested that it provides a survival benefit when compared with placebo,[65] confirmatory studies have been difficult to initiate and no results are available.[67] Inhaled tacrolimus has been shown to be safe and potentially efficacious in rat models, but no data on humans have been published.[66]

Cell cycle inhibitors

AZATHIOPRINE

Azathioprine is a prodrug for 6-mercaptopurine; it acts to suppress purine synthesis, thereby interrupting DNA and RNA synthesis and inhibiting the proliferation of T and B lymphocytes. Its effect on de novo purine synthesis leads to nonspecific inhibition of proliferating cells and is responsible for its major side effects, in particular myelosuppression. Azathioprine is partly metabolized by thiopurine methyltransferase (TPMT). Ten percent of individuals have a TPMT genetic polymorphism that leads to decreased enzyme activity and increases the probability of myelosuppression[68]; consequently, some units undertake TPMT genotyping to predict risk. The other major adverse effect associated with azathioprine is hepatotoxicity. With the introduction of MMF, use of azathioprine in the management of lung transplantation has declined.

MYCOPHENOLATE MOFETIL

MMF is a prodrug that is converted to its active compound mycophenolic acid (MPA). MPA acts by inhibiting inosine monophosphate dehydrogenase, which is the rate-limiting enzyme in the synthesis of de novo purines and thus inhibits lymphocyte proliferation. MMF is rapidly absorbed in the upper gastrointestinal tract and hydrolyzed to MPA and an inactive metabolite in the liver. The inactive metabolite is reconverted to MPA in the gut and reenters the enterohepatic circulation, thereby leading to a secondary drug peak at 6 to 12 hours after the dose.[69] Large interpatient and intrapatient variations in MPA pharmacokinetics exist. The concentration of MMF is affected by concurrent CNI use, with lower exposure levels achieved when it is coadministered with cyclosporine than with tacrolimus (possibly because of inhibition of enterohepatic circulation). Doses of MMF for patients who are receiving cyclosporine should be higher (3 g/day) than those for patients who are taking tacrolimus (2 g/day). Despite the suggestion that systemic exposure may be correlated with clinical events, the C_0 of MPA is not correlated with its AUC_{12}, as a result of which TDM is not routinely used. MMF can result in significant myelosuppression; consequently, blood counts should be monitored. Its other major side effects are gastrointestinal (nausea, vomiting, and diarrhea). An enteric-coated formula of MPA has been developed and is associated with fewer gastrointestinal side effects.

Azathioprine versus mycophenolate

Large prospective randomized controlled trials in renal and heart transplantation have suggested that MMF is superior to azathioprine in terms of acute rejection rates and survival.[70,71] On the basis of this suggestion, a number of studies have examined the use of MMF following lung transplantation.[72-76] Two prospective multicenter randomized trials compared azathioprine and MMF in conjunction with cyclosporine and prednisolone. The initial study randomly assigned 81 patients and found no differences in acute rejection rates or survival at 6 months[74]; the larger trial investigated 315 patients and supported the initial study's finding, with 3-year follow-up data showing no difference in rates of acute rejection, incidence of BOS, or survival.[72] Nonrandomized data from the ISHLT registry suggest that

the highest rates of acute rejection in the first 12-months following transplantation occur in those who are receiving a combination of azathioprine and cyclosporine.[1] The advantage of MMF over azathioprine may depend on the CNI used because the difference between them when used in combination with a CNI is not as evident as when each is combined with tacrolimus. Irrespective of the findings for other SOT groups, no evidence of the superiority of MMF over azathioprine in lung transplantation currently exists, despite its increasing use.

MTOR INHIBITORS

mTOR is a serine threonine kinase that is downstream of IL-2 in the T-cell activation pathway. It is blocked by both everolimus and sirolimus through their binding to FK506 binding protein-12 (FKBP-12). Blocking of mTOR inhibits the proliferation of lymphocytes and mesenchymal cells. Both everolimus and sirolimus additionally impair fibroblast proliferation, thereby resulting in impaired wound healing. The use of mTOR inhibitors increases with time following transplantation: ISHLT registry data show that they are used twice as frequently at 5 years (16%) as at 1 year (8%) after transplantation.[1]

Everolimus is a derivative of sirolimus; it is a macrolide antibiotic with an improved side effect profile and better bioavailability. Everolimus has been shown to be effective with other types of SOT[77-79]; however, its use in lung transplantation remains hindered by few trials. Early use of an everolimus-based regimen has shown no benefit in terms of the incidence of BOS and survival.[78,80]

Because of their different mechanism of action, mTOR inhibitors can be used in combination with CNIs. Snell and coworkers randomly assigned 213 BOS-free lung transplant recipients to receive cyclosporine and prednisolone with either everolimus or azathioprine.[78] Efficacy failure was defined as a decline in forced expiratory volume in the first second of respiration (FEV_1) greater than 15%, graft loss, death, or loss to follow-up. At 12 months after transplantation, the rate of efficacy failure was significantly lower in the everolimus group, which showed a reduced incidence of greater than a 15% change in FEV_1 with BOS, thus suggesting that the drug may slow the typical loss of lung function. Discontinuation of treatment was more frequent in the everolimus group, and the data at 36 months' follow-up were less encouraging. The incidence of acute rejection remained significantly lower in the everolimus group, but overall rates of efficacy failure were similar.

A multicenter trial randomly assigned 181 patients to receive sirolimus or azathioprine in a tacrolimus-based regimen following lung transplantation. No significant difference between the two groups in terms of acute rejection, BOS, or graft survival was evident at 1 year after transplantation; however, a greater proportion of patients in the sirolimus group withdrew because of a high incidence of adverse effects.[81]

As mentioned, sirolimus and everolimus impair fibroblast proliferation. Early use of sirolimus is associated with impairment of wound healing following renal, liver, heart, and intestinal transplantation, and following lung transplantation, it has been associated with bronchial anastomotic dehiscence.[82] Despite the nonexistence of published data regarding de novo use of everolimus, the assumption has been that this potential for anastomotic dehiscence and impaired wound healing is an effect inherent to the entire class of mTOR inhibitors. As a result, everolimus is not recommended in the first 3 months following lung transplantation. Additionally, sirolimus has been associated with interstitial pneumonitis, which is an idiosyncratic effect that has affected its use following lung transplantation.[83]

mTOR inhibitors are also metabolized by the CYP3A4 pathway and have interactions similar to those of CNIs. Of note, the use of sirolimus in conjunction with an azole antifungal is contraindicated because of a reported increase in sirolimus levels by up to 70 times.[84] The interaction with everolimus is not as pronounced and dose reduction is required. TDM uses a predose C_0 to maintain efficacy while minimizing side effects.

Use of mTOR inhibitors for renal failure

Prolonged exposure to a CNI often leads to nephrotoxicity. The evidence in other types of SOT indicates that replacing the CNI with an mTOR inhibitor improves creatinine clearance.[85,86] Small studies in lung transplantation have shown that introduction of everolimus or sirolimus has resulted in significant improvement in renal function with no changes in acute rejection rates[87] or significant changes in FEV_1.[88,89] However, the evidence supporting long-term use of CNI-free regimens is limited.

Use of mTOR inhibitors in special situations

Increasing evidence suggests that mTOR inhibitors are associated with a decreased incidence of cytomegalovirus (CMV) infection. Intracellular viruses such as CMV rely on a cellular protein synthesis pathway to support genomic replication and viral synthesis. mTOR inhibitors are believed to interrupt this pathway. A recent randomized controlled trial comparing sirolimus with azathioprine in a tacrolimus-based regimen showed a significant decrease in CMV infection at 1 year after adjustment for serostatus and prophylaxis.[90] Larger trials and meta-analyses involving other SOT groups have support this finding that rates of CMV infection with immunosuppressive regimens combining a CNI and an mTOR inhibitor are lower than those with regimens that include a CNI and an antimetabolite.[91,92] Although the evidence is insufficient to generalize advice regarding the use of mTOR inhibitors, the emerging evidence shows that use of an mTOR inhibitor in the presence of persistent or recurrent CMV infection is promising and should at least be considered.

Additionally, a 2006 study of renal transplant recipients with squamous cell skin cancer showed that switching from a CNI to sirolimus provided an antitumor effect,[93] thus suggesting a role for mTOR inhibitors in managing the difficult situation of recurrent nonmelanoma skin cancer.

Generic substitution of immunosuppressants

The introduction of generic immunosuppressive agents into lung transplantation has been understudied. Approval of a generic medication requires that manufacturers demonstrate their products' bioequivalence to the original proprietary formulation[94-96] by comparing the mean pharmacokinetic parameters of the branded and generic drugs from the standpoints of AUC and maximal concentration (C_{max}).[97] In most jurisdictions a drug is regarded as bioequivalent if the 90% confidence interval of the mean AUC is between 80% and 125%.[97,98] Although this issue is not significant in drug-naïve patients, in which case current practice includes empirical dosing based on weight with dose adjustment by TDM targeting a therapeutic range, it may become a problem in cases in which stable patients are switched to the generic formulation. Given the differences in absorption and drug variation that have been reported with different formulations, unchecked alterations in the mean blood level of a critical drug that could potentially lead to increased mortality and morbidity as a result of decreased efficacy or increased toxicity are a possibility.[98,99]

Bioequivalence studies are usually performed on normal healthy subjects who receive a single dose of each product[97] rather than on the target population. At this time, no study demonstrating bioequivalence of any immunosuppressant has been performed in a lung transplant population. This raises many potential issues because lung transplant recipients are particularly susceptible to the adverse effects of significant alterations in immunosuppression, with the possibility of drug interactions and gastrointestinal factors influencing absorption profiles.

Other practical concerns should be considered when planning a change to a generic formulation. The implementation of strategies to avoid "doubling up" of medication, repeated switching between different generic brands, and inadvertent switching are particularly concerning[99]; each of these actions adds an increased burden of care, and their cost must be considered in any discussions of cost savings associated with the use of generics.[98,99]

Our experience with the introduction of Mycophenolate Sandoz (Sandoz, Sydney, Australia) to replace Cellcept (Roche, Sydney, Australia) in 2012 illustrated the aforementioned issues and was noted in a 4-month short-term observational study. Although the initiation of Mycophenolate Sandoz in de novo patients caused few problems, of the 109 stable patients who were switched to the generic formulation, 7% were switched back because of adverse effects (neutropenia, diarrhea, or both) and 5% experienced a greater than 10% decrease in graft function. Although significant medication cost savings were achieved, staff workload increased significantly, as did patient morbidity and anxiety.

MANAGEMENT OF REJECTION

Acute cellular rejection

Acute cellular rejection following lung transplantation is common: it affects 34% of adult lung transplant recipients in the first year,[1] and despite the use of maintenance immunosuppression, it occurs as a result of immune system activation. Acute cellular rejection is more likely to develop in the setting of nonadherence to medication regimens and is associated with CNI variance.[59] T cells play a central role in its pathogenesis, with T-cell infiltration into the allograft resulting in direct cytotoxic effects on lung parenchymal cells, which in turn leads to allograft injury and loss of function.

The clinical features associated with acute rejection are nonspecific and can range from no symptoms to cough and dyspnea or, in its most severe manifestation, to acute respiratory failure. The main differential diagnosis remains infection, and investigation and ultimate diagnosis rely on transbronchial biopsy and histologic examination of the lung parenchyma. Histologically acute rejection is characterized by a perivascular mononuclear infiltrate.[100] The magnitude of this infiltrate forms the basis of the rejection grading system (A0 to A4) that is used in monitoring lung allograft function.

TREATMENT OF ACUTE CELLULAR REJECTION

ISHLT registry data show that 89% of acute rejection episodes are treated with a short course of high-dose intravenous corticosteroids.[1] Although the direct effects of acute rejection are usually controlled and reversed following treatment, the indirect effects remain problematic, with episodes of acute rejection being strongly associated with the later development of BOS.[2]

Most centers treat acute rejection with a grade of A2 or higher. Because recent studies have suggested that a lower grade of acute rejection (A1) is associated with CLAD,[101] many centers have instituted treatment of this pathologic finding. Despite the lack of an evidence base, the standard treatment of acute rejection is a 3-day course of high-dose intravenous corticosteroids (10 to 15 mg/kg/day) with bronchoscopy repeated to confirm resolution of changes 2 weeks after treatment.

For persistent or recurrent acute rejection episodes, the baseline immunosuppression is changed.[102,103] Although other therapies, including ATG, alemtuzumab,[104] total lymphoid irradiation,[105] photophoresis,[106] and inhaled cyclosporine,[107] have been used, they have not been evaluated in large randomized controlled trials.

Antibody-mediated rejection

Emerging data suggest that humoral immunity plays an important role in allograft dysfunction and the development of chronic rejection. Although AMR following renal and heart transplantation is well recognized and has clear diagnostic criteria, its diagnosis after lung transplantation remains difficult. A number of nonspecific pathologic findings, including acute lung injury and neutrophilic capillary infiltration in association with donor-specific antibodies (DSAs), have been associated with AMR; however, a clear diagnostic algorithm has yet to be developed.[108] Part of the reason for this lack is that the diagnostic criteria used in other SOT groups, including circulating DSAs, C4d deposition, and classic histologic abnormalities, have reduced sensitivity and specificity with respect to the diagnosis of AMR in a lung allograft. In particular, circulating DSAs are not always associated with AMR because not all anti-HLA antibodies are complement fixing.[109] Second, C4d staining as a surrogate marker for complement activity is not reproducible in lung tissue and the histologic features associated with AMR are not specific for the condition.[108] Third, the symptoms and signs associated with AMR are not specific to the condition and may also be associated with infection, acute cellular rejection, and other forms of T-cell–mediated chronic rejection. Currently, the diagnosis of AMR requires multidisciplinary input and is ultimately determined by the clinical picture, the presence or absence of DSAs, and histopathologic interpretation.

The evidence base on the treatment of AMR following lung transplantation is limited. Treatment tends to be reserved for those with DSAs and otherwise unexplained graft dysfunction. In principle, therapy is aimed at removing the potentially allograft-damaging antibodies from the circulation and involves the use of plasmapheresis, intravenous immunoglobulin (IVIG), and rituximab. Of note, the authors of a recent systematic review of treatment of AMR following renal transplantation concluded that despite its large size, their evidence base was insufficient to guide treatment recommendations in that group of SOT recipients.[110]

Plasmapheresis is used by most institutions as their first-line strategy for removing DSAs from the circulation. Our protocol includes six exchanges over a 2-week period. Although we have noted a reduction in the amount of measurable anti-HLA DSAs following treatment, plasmapheresis does not completely remove such antibodies from circulation. A number of retrospective studies have suggested that the overall clinical response may depend on the magnitude of DSA reduction.[111] Use of immunoadsorption columns in place of plasmapheresis to selectively remove antibodies has also been reported.[112]

IVIG is derived from pooled human plasma and has broad immunomodulatory effects: it regulates innate and adaptive cellular immune responses and modifies complement activation. Its additional anti-infective effects makes it an attractive treatment option in an immunosuppressed population.[113] Although the evidence in renal transplantation suggests that IVIG lowers DSAs,[114] randomized trials showing its efficacy are lacking.

Rituximab, which is a monoclonal antibody against the CD20 molecule expressed on B cells, has been used by a number of institutions for the treatment of AMR with variable results. Much of the evidence regarding its efficacy comes from renal transplant studies,[110] and its value in the treatment of AMR following lung transplantation remains to be convincingly shown. Through its action against CD20, rituximab results in prolonged and significant depletion of B cells and is used to impair antibody production. A recent retrospective study showed that whereas 62% of patients cleared DSAs following therapy with IVIG, no additional clearance occurred in patients who received rituximab in addition to IVIG.[115]

Bortezomib is a proteasome inhibitor that is widely used for the treatment of multiple myeloma. By acting on the 26S proteasome it selectively targets the antibody-producing plasma cell; theoretically, it should be more efficacious than rituximab, which targets B cells. Experience in treating AMR following lung transplantation is limited to case reports.[116,117]

Eculizumab is a humanized monoclonal antibody that targets the C5 complement protein and prevents formation of the C5b-C9 membrane complex. Its therapeutic effects are thought to occur through its inhibition of complement activation. Its use in lung transplantation is limited to a single case report.[118]

Management of chronic lung allograft dysfunction

CLAD encompasses all phenotypes of chronic rejection. Although chronic rejection has traditionally been characterized histopathologically by obliterative bronchiolitis and its clinical correlate BOS,[2] other phenotypes, including restrictive allograft syndrome (RAS)[119] and acute fibrinous and organizing pneumonia, have been described more recently.[120] There is no universally agreed definition of CLAD and no consensus regarding the optimal treatment regimens.

THERAPEUTIC APPROACHES IN THE MANAGEMENT OF CHRONIC LUNG ALLOGRAFT DYSFUNCTION

Modification of the immunosuppressant regimen

A number of studies have examined augmenting immunosuppression (e.g., with ATG) or switching between similar maintenance agents (i.e., substituting CNIs, MMF, or everolimus for azathioprine) as strategies for managing established BOS.[121,122] Despite studies showing slowing of allograft deterioration or stabilization of allograft function, no single proven strategy exists. In general, alteration of immunosuppression is thought to possibly lead to apparent stabilization. Because no convincing evidence of the absolute efficacy of these approaches exists, avoiding excessive immunosuppression is important because of the significant risk for infection that it poses.

Use of azithromycin

Macrolide use for the treatment and prevention of BOS has been assessed extensively.[37,123-125] Evidence from a number of studies suggests that azithromycin attenuates inflammatory responses and can lead to improvements in FEV_1 and BOS. Despite the uncertainty regarding the optimal time to initiate treatment, therapy that is commenced early appears to be the most successful.[125] The effect of macrolides on RAS remains unclear.

Possible mechanisms of macrolides' effectiveness include the following: alteration of sensitivity to the epithelial-to-mesenchymal transition,[126] prevention of oxidative damage,[127] enhancement of esophageal motility,[128] and reduction of airway epithelial matrix metalloproteinase activity.[129] Treatment tends to be provided in doses of 250 to 500 mg three times per week. Of note, azithromycin can effect QT interval and has been associated with arrhythmia and cardiovascular death in other populations.[130] Care should be taken when azithromycin is used concurrently with other drugs that lead to QTc prolongation, including azoles and tacrolimus.

Other medication-based approaches

Small case series have suggested potential efficacy of a number of other agents and therapies. Some evidence indicates that patients receiving statin therapy to manage hypercholesterolemia have an improved survival rate and decreased incidence of BOS.[131] The role of statins in the prevention and treatment of CLAD and RAS remains unclear, however.

Extracorporeal photopheresis,[132] total lymphoid irradiation,[133] and montelukast[134] have been studied in small nonrandomized trials, and extension of the preliminary work with antifibrotics (i.e., pirfenidone),[135] IL-7 antagonists,[136] and stem cells[126,137] may be fruitful.

CONCLUSION

The modern era of SOT was heralded by the development of cyclosporine in the 1970s. More than 3 decades later, CNIs remain the cornerstone of the immunosuppressive regimen of lung transplant recipients. Although the last decade has not brought any new classes of drugs to the armory, new methods of administration and a stronger focus on TDM have broadened the tools available to manipulate the immune system, which hopefully will in turn translate into better long-term outcomes.

REFERENCES

1. Christie JD, Edwards LB, Kucheryavaya AY, et al. Registry of the International Society for Heart and Lung Transplantation: Twenty-ninth adult lung and heart-lung transplant report—2012. J Heart Lung Transplant 2012;31:1073-1086.
2. Estenne M, Maurer JR, Boehler A, et al. Bronchiolitis obliterans syndrome 2001: An update of the diagnostic criteria. J Heart Lung Transplant 2002;21:297-310.
3. Mehra MR, Zucker MJ, Wagoner L, et al. A multicenter, prospective, randomized, double-blind trial of basiliximab in heart transplantation. J Heart Lung Transplant 2005;24:1297-1304.

4. Szczech LA, Berlin JA, Aradhye S, et al. Effect of anti-lymphocyte induction therapy on renal allograft survival: A meta-analysis. J Am Soc Nephrol 1997;8:1771-1777.

5. Vincenti F, Kirkman R, Light S, et al. Interleukin-2-receptor blockade with daclizumab to prevent acute rejection in renal transplantation. Daclizumab triple therapy study group. N Engl J Med 1998;338:161-165.

6. Swarup R, Allenspach LL, Nemeh HW, et al. Timing of basiliximab induction and development of acute rejection in lung transplant patients. J Heart Lung Transplant 2011;30:1228-1235.

7. Brock MV, Borja MC, Ferber L, et al. Induction therapy in lung transplantation: A prospective, controlled clinical trial comparing OKT3, anti-thymocyte globulin, and daclizumab. J Heart Lung Transplant 2001;20:1282-1290.

8. Garrity ER Jr, Villanueva J, Bhorade SM, et al. Low rate of acute lung allograft rejection after the use of daclizumab, an interleukin 2 receptor antibody. Transplantation 2001;71:773-777.

9. Burton CM, Andersen CB, Jensen AS, et al. The incidence of acute cellular rejection after lung transplantation: A comparative study of anti-thymocyte globulin and daclizumab. J Heart Lung Transplant 2006;25:638-647.

10. Ailawadi G, Smith PW, Oka T, et al. Effects of induction immunosuppression regimen on acute rejection, bronchiolitis obliterans, and survival after lung transplantation. J Thorac Cardiovasc Surg 2008;135:594-602.

11. Hachem RR, Chakinala MM, Yusen RD, et al. A comparison of basiliximab and anti-thymocyte globulin as induction agents after lung transplantation. J Heart Lung Transplant 2005;24:1320-1326.

12. Whitson BA, Lehman A, Wehr A, et al. To induce or not to induce: A 21st century evaluation of lung transplant immunosuppression's effect on survival. Clin Transplant 2014;28:450-461.

13. Taniguchi Y, Frickhofen N, Raghavachar A, et al. Antilymphocyte immunoglobulins stimulate peripheral blood lymphocytes to proliferate and release lymphokines. Eur J Haematol 1990;44:244-251.

14. Halloran PF. Immunosuppressive drugs for kidney transplantation. N Engl J Med 2004;351:2715-2729.

15. Krasinskas AM, Kreisel D, Acker MA, et al. CD3 monitoring of antithymocyte globulin therapy in thoracic organ transplantation. Transplantation 2002;73:1339-1341.

16. Hartwig MG, Snyder LD, Appel JZ 3rd, et al. Rabbit anti-thymocyte globulin induction therapy does not prolong survival after lung transplantation. J Heart Lung Transplant 2008;27:547-553.

17. Palmer SM, Miralles AP, Lawrence CM, et al. Rabbit antithymocyte globulin decreases acute rejection after lung transplantation: Results of a randomized, prospective study. Chest 1999;116:127-133.

18. Snell GI, Westall GP, Levvey BJ, et al. A randomized, double-blind, placebo-controlled, multicenter study of rabbit ATG in the prophylaxis of acute rejection in lung transplantation. Am J Transplant 2014;14:1191-1198.

19. A randomized clinical trial of OKT3 monoclonal antibody for acute rejection of cadaveric renal transplants. Ortho multicenter transplant study group. N Engl J Med 1985;313:337-342.

20. Sweet SC. Induction therapy in lung transplantation. Transpl Int 2013;26:696-703.

21. Swinnen LJ, Costanzo-Nordin MR, Fisher SG, et al. Increased incidence of lymphoproliferative disorder after immunosuppression with the monoclonal antibody OKT3 in cardiac-transplant recipients. N Engl J Med 1990;323:1723-1728.

22. Ciancio G, Burke GW 3rd. Alemtuzumab (campath-1h) in kidney transplantation. Am J Transplant 2008;8:15-20.

23. van Loenhout KC, Groves SC, Galazka M, et al. Early outcomes using alemtuzumab induction in lung transplantation. Interact Cardiovasc Thorac Surg 2010;10:190-194.

24. Shyu S, Dew MA, Pilewski JM, et al. Five-year outcomes with alemtuzumab induction after lung transplantation. J Heart Lung Transplant 2011;30:743-754.

25. Game DS, Lechler RI. Pathways of allorecognition: Implications for transplantation tolerance. Transpl Immunol 2002;10:101-108.

26. Avlonitis VS, Fisher AJ, Kirby JA, Dark JH. Pulmonary transplantation: The role of brain death in donor lung injury. Transplantation 2003;75:1928-1933.

27. Reynaud-Gaubert M, Viard L, Girault D, et al. Improved absorption and bioavailability of cyclosporine A from a microemulsion formulation in lung transplant recipients affected with cystic fibrosis. Transplant Proc 1997;29:2450-2453.

28. Lindholm A, Kahan BD. Influence of cyclosporine pharmacokinetics, trough concentrations, and AUC monitoring on outcome after kidney transplantation. Clin Pharmacol Ther 1993;54:205-218.

29. Glanville AR, Aboyoun CL, Morton JM, et al. Cyclosporine C_2 target levels and acute cellular rejection after lung transplantation. J Heart Lung Transplant 2006;25:928-934.

30. Levy GA. Neoral C_2 monitoring in solid organ transplantation. Transplant Proc 2004;36:392S-395S.

31. Capone D, Tarantino G, Gentile A, et al. Effects of voriconazole on tacrolimus metabolism in a kidney transplant recipient. J Clin Pharm Ther 2010;35:121-124.

32. Bechstein WO. Neurotoxicity of calcineurin inhibitors: Impact and clinical management. Transpl Int 2000;13:313-326.

33. Burdmann EA, Andoh TF, Yu L, Bennett WM. Cyclosporine nephrotoxicity. Semin Nephrol 2003;23:465-476.

34. Curtis JJ. Hypertensinogenic mechanism of the calcineurin inhibitors. Curr Hypertens Rep 2002;4:377-380.

35. Knoop C, Haverich A, Fischer S. Immunosuppressive therapy after human lung transplantation. Eur Respir J 2004;23:159-171.

36. Knoop C, Thiry P, Saint-Marcoux F, et al. Tacrolimus pharmacokinetics and dose monitoring after lung transplantation for cystic fibrosis and other conditions. Am J Transplant 2005;5:1477-1482.

37. Zuckermann A, Reichenspurner H, Birsan T, et al. Cyclosporine A versus tacrolimus in combination with mycophenolate mofetil and steroids as primary immunosuppression after lung transplantation: One-year results of a 2-center prospective randomized trial. J Thorac Cardiovasc Surg 2003;125:891-900.

38. Keenan RJ, Konishi H, Kawai A, et al. Clinical trial of tacrolimus versus cyclosporine in lung transplantation. Ann Thorac Surg 1995;60:580-584; discussion 584-585.

39. Treede H, Klepetko W, Reichenspurner H, et al. Tacrolimus versus cyclosporine after lung transplantation: A prospective, open, randomized two-center trial comparing two different immunosuppressive protocols. J Heart Lung Transplant 2001;20:511-517.

40. Zuckermann A, Reichenspurner H, Jaksch P, et al. Long term follow-up of a prospective randomized trial comparing tacrolimus versus cyclosporine in combination with MMF after lung transplantation. J Heart Lung Transplant 2003;22:S76-S77.

41. Treede H, Glanville AR, Klepetko W, et al. Tacrolimus and cyclosporine have differential effects on the risk of development of bronchiolitis obliterans syndrome: Results of a prospective, randomized international trial in lung transplantation. J Heart Lung Transplant 2012;31:797-804.

42. Raviv Y, D'Ovidio F, Pierre A, et al. Prevalence of gastroparesis before and after lung transplantation and its association with lung allograft outcomes. Clin Transplant 2012;26:133-142.

43. Garrity ER Jr, Hertz MI, Trulock EP, et al. Suggested guidelines for the use of tacrolimus in lung-transplant recipients. J Heart Lung Transplant 1999;18:175-176.

44. Abu-Elmagd KM, Fung J, Draviam R, et al. Four-hour versus 24-hour intravenous infusion of FK 506 in liver transplantation. Transplant Proc 1991;23:2767-2770.

45. Snell GI, Westall GP. Immunosuppression for lung transplantation: Evidence to date. Drugs 2007;67:1531-1539.

46. Snell GI, Ivulich S, Mitchell L, et al. Evolution to twice daily bolus intravenous tacrolimus: Optimizing efficacy and safety of calcineurin inhibitor delivery early post lung transplant. Ann Transplant 2013;18:399-407.

47. Hibi T, Tanabe M, Hoshino K, et al. Cyclosporine A–based immunotherapy in adult living donor liver transplantation: Accurate and improved therapeutic drug monitoring by 4-hr intravenous infusion. Transplantation 2011;92:100-105.

48. Reams BD, Palmer SM. Sublingual tacrolimus for immunosuppression in lung transplantation: A potentially important therapeutic option in cystic fibrosis. Am J Respir Med 2002;1:91-98.

49. Watkins KD, Boettger RF, Hanger KM, et al. Use of sublingual tacrolimus in lung transplant recipients. J Heart Lung Transplant 2012;31:127-132.

50. Romero I, Jimenez C, Gil F, et al. Sublingual administration of tacrolimus in a renal transplant patient. J Clin Phar Ther 2008;33:87-89.

51. Abecassis MM, Seifeldin R, Riordan ME. Patient outcomes and economics of once-daily tacrolimus in renal transplant patients: Results of a modeling analysis. Transplant Proc 2008;40:1443-1445.

52. Beckebaum S, Iacob S, Sweid D, et al. Efficacy, safety, and immunosuppressant adherence in stable liver transplant patients converted from a twice-daily tacrolimus-based regimen to once-daily tacrolimus extended-release formulation. Transpl Int 2011;24:666-675.

53. Marzoa-Rivas R, Paniagua-Martin MJ, Barge-Caballero E, et al. Conversion of heart transplant patients from standard to sustained-release tacrolimus requires a dosage increase. Transplant Proc 2010;42:2994-2996.

54. Mendez A, Berastegui C, Lopez-Meseguer M, et al. Pharmacokinetic study of conversion from tacrolimus twice-daily to tacrolimus once-daily in stable lung transplantation. Transplantation 2014;97:358-362.

55. Levvey B, Cunningham A, Ivulich S, et al. Once-daily tacrolimus: A valuable option post lung transplantation. J Heart Lung Transplant 2014;33:S187-S188.

56. Pollock-Barziv SM, Finkelstein Y, Manlhiot C, et al. Variability in tacrolimus blood levels increases the risk of late rejection and graft loss after solid organ transplantation in older children. Pediatr Transplant 2010;14:968-975.

57. Shemesh E, Fine RN. Is calculating the standard deviation of tacrolimus blood levels the new gold standard for evaluating non-adherence to medications in transplant recipients? Pediatr Transplant 2010;14:940-943.

58. Venkat VL, Nick TG, Wang Y, Bucuvalas JC. An objective measure to identify pediatric liver transplant recipients at risk for late allograft rejection related to non-adherence. Pediatr Transplant 2008;12:67-72.

59. Chiang CY, Schneider HG, Levvey B, et al. Tacrolimus level variability is a novel measure associated with increased acute rejection in lung transplant (LTx) recipients. J Heart Lung Transplant 2013;32:S170.

60. Paraskeva M, Paul E, Ivulich S, et al. Non-adherence is associated with mortality in adolescent lung transplant recipients. J Heart Lung Transplant 2014;33:S223.

61. Taber DJ, Baillie GM, Ashcraft EE, et al. Does bioequivalence between modified cyclosporine formulations translate into equal outcomes? Transplantation 2005;80:1633-1635.

62. Kurnatowska I, Krawczyk J, Oleksik T, Nowicki M. Tacrolimus dose and blood concentration variability in kidney transplant recipients undergoing conversion from twice daily to once daily modified release tacrolimus. Transplant Proc 2011;43:2954-2956.

63. Whitford H, Walters EH, Levvey B, et al. Addition of inhaled corticosteroids to systemic immunosuppression after lung transplantation: A double-blind, placebo-controlled trial. Transplantation 2002;73:1793-1799.

64. Iacono AT, Johnson BA, Grgurich WF, et al. A randomized trial of inhaled cyclosporine in lung-transplant recipients. N Engl J Med 2006;354:141-150.

65. Verleden GM, Dupont LJ. Inhaled cyclosporine in lung transplantation. N Engl J Med 2006;354:1752-1753; author reply 1752-1753.

66. Deuse T, Blankenberg F, Haddad M, et al. Mechanisms behind local immunosuppression using inhaled tacrolimus in preclinical models of lung transplantation. Am J Respir Cell Mol Biol 2010;43:403-412.

67. Johnson BA, Rolfe M, Johnson C, et al.: Inhaled cyclosporine is well tolerated in the CYCLIST clinical trial [Abstract 194]. J Heart Lung Transplant 2010;29:S68.

68. Nguyen CM, Mendes MA, Ma JD. Thiopurine methyltransferase (TPMT) genotyping to predict myelosuppression risk. PLoS Curr 2011;3:RRN1236.

69. Van Gelder T, Klupp J, Barten MJ, et al. Co-administration of tacrolimus and mycophenolate mofetil does not increase mycophenolic acid (MPA) exposure, but co-administration of cyclosporine inhibits the enterohepatic recirculation of MPA, thereby decreasing its exposure. J Heart Lung Transplant 2001;20:160-161.

70. Halloran P, Mathew T, Tomlanovich S, et al. Mycophenolate mofetil in renal allograft recipients: A pooled efficacy analysis of three randomized, double-blind, clinical studies in prevention of rejection. The International Mycophenolate Mofetil Renal Transplant Study Groups. Transplantation 1997;63:39-47.

71. Kobashigawa J, Miller L, Renlund D, et al. A randomized active-controlled trial of mycophenolate mofetil in heart transplant recipients. Mycophenolate mofetil investigators. Transplantation 1998;66:507-515.

72. Glanville AR, Corris PA, McNeil KD, Wahlers T. Mycophenolate mofetil (MMF) vs azathioprine (AZA) in lung transplantation for the prevention of bronchiolitis obliterans syndrome (BOS): Results of a 3 year international randomised trial. J Heart Lung Transplant 2003;22:S207.

73. O'Hair DP, Cantu E, McGregor C, et al. Preliminary experience with mycophenolate mofetil used after lung transplantation. J Heart Lung Transplant 1998;17:864-868.

74. Palmer SM, Baz MA, Sanders L, et al. Results of a randomized, prospective, multicenter trial of mycophenolate mofetil versus azathioprine in the prevention of acute lung allograft rejection. Transplantation 2001;71:1772-1776.

75. Ross DJ, Waters PF, Levine M, et al. Mycophenolate mofetil versus azathioprine immunosuppressive regimens after lung transplantation: Preliminary experience. J Heart Lung Transplant 1998;17:768-774.

76. Zuckermann A, Birsan T, Thaghavi S, et al. Mycophenolate mofetil in lung transplantation. Transplant Proc 1998;30:1514-1516.

77. Dantal J, Berthoux F, Moal MC, et al. Efficacy and safety of de novo or early everolimus with low cyclosporine in deceased-donor kidney transplant recipients at specified risk of delayed graft function: 12-month results of a randomized, multicenter trial. Transpl Int 2010;23:1084-1093.

78. Snell GI, Valentine VG, Vitulo P, et al. Everolimus versus azathioprine in maintenance lung transplant recipients: An international, randomized, double-blind clinical trial. Am J Transplant 2006;6:169-177.

79. Vigano M, Tuzcu M, Benza R, et al. Prevention of acute rejection and allograft vasculopathy by everolimus in cardiac transplants recipients: A 24-month analysis. J Heart Lung Transplant 2007;26:584-592.

80. Glanville AR, Aboyoun C, Klepetko W, et al. 3-year results of the CeMyLungs study, a 3-year randomised, open label, multi-centre investigator driven study comparing de novo enteric coated mycophenolate sodium with delayed onset everolimus, both arms in combination with cyclosporin (using C_2 monitoring) and corticosteroids for the prevention of bronchiolitis obliterans syndrome in heart-lung, bilateral lung and single lung transplant recipients [Abstract 171]. J Heart Lung Transplant 2012;31:S66.

81. Bhorade S, Ahya VN, Baz MA, et al. Comparison of sirolimus with azathioprine in a tacrolimus-based immunosuppressive regimen in lung transplantation. Am J Respir Crit Care Med 2011;183:379-387.

82. King-Biggs MB, Dunitz JM, Park SJ, et al. Airway anastomotic dehiscence associated with use of sirolimus immediately after lung transplantation. Transplantation 2003;75:1437-1443.

83. McWilliams TJ, Levvey BJ, Russell PA, et al. Interstitial pneumonitis associated with sirolimus: A dilemma for lung transplantation. J Heart Lung Transplant 2003;22:210-213.

84. Vfend (Voriconazole) [product information]. Kirkland, Quebec, CN: Pfizer, 2005.

85. Hunt J, Lerman M, Magee MJ, et al. Improvement of renal dysfunction by conversion from calcineurin

inhibitors to sirolimus after heart transplantation. J Heart Lung Transplant 2005;24:1863-1867.

86. Mulay AV, Cockfield S, Stryker R, et al. Conversion from calcineurin inhibitors to sirolimus for chronic renal allograft dysfunction: A systematic review of the evidence. Transplantation 2006;82:1153-1162.

87. Gullestad L, Iversen M, Mortensen SA, et al. Everolimus with reduced calcineurin inhibitor in thoracic transplant recipients with renal dysfunction: A multicenter, randomized trial. Transplantation 2010;89:864-872.

88. Villanueva J, Boukhamseen A, Bhorade SM. Successful use in lung transplantation of an immunosuppressive regimen aimed at reducing target blood levels of sirolimus and tacrolimus. J Heart Lung Transplant 2005;24:421-425.

89. Shitrit D, Rahamimov R, Gidon S, et al. Use of sirolimus and low-dose calcineurin inhibitor in lung transplant recipients with renal impairment: Results of a controlled pilot study. Kidney Int 2005;67:1471-1475.

90. Ghassemieh B, Ahya VN, Baz MA, et al. Decreased incidence of cytomegalovirus infection with sirolimus in a post hoc randomized, multicenter study in lung transplantation. J Heart Lung Transplant 2013;32:701-706.

91. Brennan DC, Legendre C, Patel D, et al. Cytomegalovirus incidence between everolimus versus mycophenolate in de novo renal transplants: Pooled analysis of three clinical trials. Am J Transplant 2011;11:2453-2462.

92. Vigano M, Dengler T, Mattei MF, et al. Lower incidence of cytomegalovirus infection with everolimus versus mycophenolate mofetil in de novo cardiac transplant recipients: A randomized, multicenter study. Transpl Infect Dis 2010;12:23-30.

93. Campistol JM, Eris J, Oberbauer R, et al. Sirolimus therapy after early cyclosporine withdrawal reduces the risk for cancer in adult renal transplantation. J Am Soc Nephrol 2006;17:581-589.

94. Medicines and Healthcare Products Regulatory Agency. Oral tacrolimus products: Measures to reduce risk of medication errors. Drug Saf Update 2010;3:5-7.

95. Generic medicines: Dealing with multiple brands. NPS News 2007;55:25-26.

96. Therapeutic Goods Administration. Biopharmaceutics studies. Australian Regulatory Guidelines for Prescriptions Medicines 2004; appendix 15:91-116.

97. Christians U, Klawitter J, Clavijo CF. Bioequivalence testing of immunosuppressants: Concepts and misconceptions. Kidney Int Suppl 2010;115:S1-S7.

98. Uber PA, Ross HJ, Zuckermann AO, et al. Generic drug immunosuppression in thoracic transplantation: An ISHLT educational advisory. J Heart Lung Transplant 2009;28:655-660.

99. Ensor CR, Trofe-Clark J, Gabardi S, et al. Generic maintenance immunosuppression in solid organ transplant recipients. Pharmacotherapy 2011; 31:1111-1129.

100. Stewart S, Fishbein MC, Snell GI, et al. Revision of the 1996 working formulation for the standardization of nomenclature in the diagnosis of lung rejection. J Heart Lung Transplant 2007;26:1229-1242.

101. Hopkins PM, Aboyoun CL, Chhajed PN, et al. Association of minimal rejection in lung transplant recipients with obliterative bronchiolitis. Am J Respir Crit Care Med 2004;170:1022-1026.

102. Horning NR, Lynch JP, Sundaresan SR, et al. Tacrolimus therapy for persistent or recurrent acute rejection after lung transplantation. J Heart Lung Transplant 1998;17:761-767.

103. Onsager DR, Canver CC, Jahania MS, et al. Efficacy of tacrolimus in the treatment of refractory rejection in heart and lung transplant recipients. J Heart Lung Transplant 1999;18:448-455.

104. Reams BD, Musselwhite LW, Zaas DW, et al. Alemtuzumab in the treatment of refractory acute rejection and bronchiolitis obliterans syndrome after human lung transplantation. Am J Transplant 2007;7:2802-2808.

105. Valentine VG, Robbins RC, Wehner JH, et al. Total lymphoid irradiation for refractory acute rejection in heart-lung and lung allografts. Chest 1996;109:1184-1189.

106. Dall'Amico R, Messina C. Extracorporeal photochemotherapy for the treatment of graft-versus-host disease. Ther Apher 2002;6:296-304.

107. Keenan RJ, Zeevi A, Iacono AT, et al. Efficacy of inhaled cyclosporine in lung transplant recipients with refractory rejection: Correlation of intragraft cytokine gene expression with pulmonary function and histologic characteristics. Surgery 1995;118:385-391.

108. Berry G, Burke M, Andersen C, et al. Pathology of pulmonary antibody-mediated rejection: 2012 update from the pathology council of the ISHLT. J Heart Lung Transplant 2013;32:14-21.

109. Roberts JA, Barrios R, Cagle PT, et al. The presence of anti-HLA donor-specific antibodies in lung allograft recipients does not correlate with C4d immunofluorescence in transbronchial biopsy specimens. Arch Pathol Lab Med 2014;138:1053-1058.

110. Roberts DM, Jiang SH, Chadban SJ. The treatment of acute antibody-mediated rejection in kidney transplant recipients—a systematic review. Transplantation 2012;94:775-783.

111. Jackups R Jr, Canter C, Sweet SC, et al. Measurement of donor-specific HLA antibodies following plasma exchange therapy predicts clinical outcome in pediatric heart and lung transplant recipients with antibody-mediated rejection. J Clin Apher 2013;28:301-308.

112. Appel JZ 3rd, Hartwig MG, Davis RD, Reinsmoen NL. Utility of peritransplant and rescue intravenous immunoglobulin and extracorporeal immunoadsorption in lung transplant recipients sensitized to HLA antigens. Hum Immunol 2005;66:378-386.

113. Jordan SC, Toyoda M, Kahwaji J, Vo AA. Clinical aspects of intravenous immunoglobulin use in solid organ transplant recipients. Am J Transplant 2011;11:196-202.

114. Shehata N, Palda VA, Meyer RM, et al. The use of immunoglobulin therapy for patients undergoing solid organ transplantation: An evidence-based practice guideline. Transfus Med Rev 2010;24(Suppl 1):S7-S27.

115. Hachem RR, Yusen RD, Meyers BF, et al. Anti-human leukocyte antigen antibodies and preemptive antibody-directed therapy after lung transplantation. J Heart Lung Transplant 2010;29:973-980.

116. Neumann J, Schio S, Tarrasconi H, et al. Bortezomib in lung transplantation: A promising start. Clin Transplant 2009:421-424.

117. Neumann J, Tarrasconi H, Bortolotto A, et al. Acute humoral rejection in a lung recipient: Reversion with bortezomib. Transplantation 2010;89:125-126.

118. Dawson KL, Parulekar A, Seethamraju H. Treatment of hyperacute antibody-mediated lung allograft rejection with eculizumab. J Heart Lung Transplant 2012;31:1325-1326.

119. Sato M, Waddell TK, Wagnetz U, et al. Restrictive allograft syndrome (RAS): A novel form of chronic lung allograft dysfunction. J Heart Lung Transplant 2011;30:735-742.

120. Paraskeva M, McLean C, Ellis S, et al. Acute fibrinoid organizing pneumonia after lung transplantation. Am J Respir Crit Care Med 2013;187:1360-1368.

121. Knoop C, Estenne M. Acute and chronic rejection after lung transplantation. Semin Respir Crit Care Med 2006;27:521-533.

122. Zamora MR. Updates in lung transplantation. Clin Transplant 2012:185-192.

123. Gerhardt SG, McDyer JF, Girgis RE, et al. Maintenance azithromycin therapy for bronchiolitis obliterans syndrome: Results of a pilot study. Am J Respir Crit Care Med 2003;168:121-125.

124. Vos R, Vanaudenaerde BM, Ottevaere A, et al. Long-term azithromycin therapy for bronchiolitis obliterans syndrome: Divide and conquer? J Heart Lung Transplant 2010;29:1358-1368.

125. Vos R, Vanaudenaerde BM, Verleden SE, et al. A randomised controlled trial of azithromycin to prevent chronic rejection after lung transplantation. Eur Respir J 2011;37:164-172.

126. Banerjee B, Musk M, Sutanto EN, et al. Regional differences in susceptibiity of bronchial epithelium to mesenchymal transition and inhibition by the macrolide antibiotic azithromycin. PLoS 2012;7:e52309.

127. Persson HL, Vainikka LK, Sege M, et al. Leaky lysosomes in lung transplant macrophages: Azithromycin prevents oxidative damage. Respir Res 2012;13:83.

128. Mertens V, Blondeau K, Pauwels A, et al. Azithromycin reduces gastroesophageal reflux and aspiration in lung transplant recipients. Dig Dis Sci 2009;54:972-979.

129. Verleden SE, Vandooren J, Vos R, et al. Azithromycin decreases MMP-9 expression in the airways of lung transplant recipients. Transpl Immunol 2011;25:159-162.

130. Ray WA, Murray KT, Hall K, et al. Azithromycin and the risk of cardiovascular death. N Engl J Med 2012;366:1881-1890.

131. Johnson BA, Iacono AT, Zeevi A, et al. Statin use is associated with improved function and survival of lung allografts. Am J Respir Crit Care Med 2003;167:1271-1278.

132. Morrell MR, Despotis GJ, Lublin DM, et al. The efficacy of photopheresis for bronchiolitis obliterans syndrome after lung transplantation. J Heart Lung Transplant 2010;29:424-431.

133. Verleden GM, Lievens Y, Dupont LJ, et al. Efficacy of total lymphoid irradiation in azithromycin nonresponsive chronic allograft rejection after lung transplantation. Transplant Proc 2009;41:1816-1820.

134. Verleden GM, Verleden SE, Vos R, et al. Montelukast for bronchiolitis obliterans syndrome after lung transplantation: A pilot study. Transpl Int 2011;24:651-656.

135. Bizargity P, Liu K, Wang L, et al. Inhibitory effects of pirfenidone on dendritic cells and lung allograft rejection. Transplantation 2012;94:114-122.

136. Vanaudenaerde BM, De Vleeschauwer SI, Vos R, et al. The role of the IL23/IL17 axis in bronchiolitis obliterans syndrome after lung transplantation. Am J Transplant 2008;8:1911-1920.

137. Sinclair K, Yerkovich ST, Chambers DC. Mesenchymal stem cells and the lung. Respirology 2013;18:397-411.

29

Viral infections in lung transplantation

LARA DANZIGER-ISAKOV, ERIK VERSCHUUREN, AND ORIOL MANUEL

INTRODUCTION

Viral infection causes specific morbidity and mortality after lung transplantation. In addition, several viral infections have been associated with long-term morbidity such as chronic lung allograft dysfunction (CLAD), which was previously identified as bronchiolitis obliterans syndrome (BOS). This chapter reviews common viral infections that have a significant impact on lung transplantation.

RESPIRATORY VIRUSES

Infection with community-acquired respiratory virus (CARV) can develop after lung transplantation. The viral pathogens commonly reported include long-standing members of the families Orthomyxoviridae (influenza A and B) and Paramyxoviridae (respiratory syncytial virus [RSV], parainfluenza virus [PIV], and human metapneumovirus), picornaviruses (rhinovirus and enteroviruses), and adenoviruses. Other emerging viruses have been reported in lung transplantation with limited data on specifically associated symptoms; they include human coronaviruses (HCoV-229E, NL63, HKU1, and OC43), polyomaviruses (WU and KI), and a parvovirus (human bocavirus).[1-3]

Epidemiology and risk factors

The epidemiology of CARV infection in lung transplant recipients has been described in retrospective and prospective studies. Acquisition of virus can occur at any time after a transplant; cases of donor-derived influenza and adenovirus infection have been reported and caused significant morbidity in some cases.[4,5] In lung transplant recipients CARV infection occurs with seasonal variability patterns similar to those of the virus circulating in the broader community.[1,6] The individual episodes recorded in the literature range from cases involving asymptomatic recovery during surveillance studies to mild rhinorrhea and nasal congestion to severe lower respiratory tract symptoms resulting in respiratory failure. Although most studies have focused on single episodes, cases of persistent infection with rhinovirus lasting for up to 15 months have been reported.[7]

Recovery of CARV is highly dependent on the presence of respiratory symptoms. Virus is recovered from only 3% to 5% of asymptomatic adult lung transplant recipients,[8] whereas 34% to 66% of symptomatic lung transplant recipients have virus recovered during an episode.[8-12] In a single-center prospective single-season study, episodes of suspected CARV infection developed in two thirds of lung transplant recipients, with a virus recovered in 34% of those cases.[10] In a year-long study from Switzerland, investigators recovered a virus in the bronchoalveolar lavage (BAL) fluid of 55% of subjects,[8] whereas in Canada 66% of subjects with clinical symptoms of CARV infection had a virus identified.[11] However, only 21 of 80 CARV episodes in a recent cohort of lung transplant recipients were symptomatic when respiratory viral testing was included in surveillance bronchoscopy.[1] In pediatrics, a multinational retrospective study revealed that only 13.8% of 576 subjects had a reported CARV infection within the first year after their transplant.[6] The viruses recovered in these studies included rhinovirus, influenza, parainfluenza, RSV, human metapneumovirus, and adenovirus. Differences in the recovery rates may be related to diagnostic techniques used.

Risk factor assessment for CARV reveals that younger age is associated with symptomatic CARV infection in pediatric lung transplant recipients.[6] However, age, type of transplant, and underlying diagnoses are not specific risk factors for CARV infection in adult lung transplant recipients.[1,10,13] Although hypogammaglobulinemia has been associated with increased risk for bacterial, fungal, and cytomegalovirus (CMV) infection after lung transplantation,[14] serum immunoglobulin levels lower than 700 mg/dL were not associated with increased risk for CARV infection in one retrospective review.[15]

Associated outcomes

Outcomes associated with CARV infection, including acute cellular rejection (ACR) and BOS, have been explored in the literature. A recent study did show CARV to be associated with a higher incidence of ACR than in the noninfected control group.[1] In contrast, several pediatric and adult studies in lung transplantation have failed to show an association between ACR and CARV[6,12,13,16]; in most of these studies, however, transbronchial biopsy was not systematically performed to assess for ACR in each episode, and one study enrolled patients who had been treated preemptively with corticosteroids, which may have resulted in underestimation of an association between CARV and ACR.[17,18] Finally, a systematic review of the literature and pooled analysis of clinical studies failed to show an association between CARV and ACR.[19]

Conversely, an epidemiologic link between CARV episodes and the development of BOS appears in multiple studies of adult lung transplant recipients. Retrospective evaluations reported the subsequent development of BOS in 32% to 60% of subjects with a diagnosis of previous CARV infection.[4,13,20] A case-control study of recipients with and without CARV revealed an association between CARV and the subsequent development of BOS, with BOS developing in 18% of the symptomatic subjects but in none of the controls.[11] Early infection within the first year after transplantation has additionally been associated with increased long-term risk for the development of BOS as long as 10 years following transplantation.[21] However, a single pediatric study of nearly 600 recipients did not reveal an association between CARV and BOS (although patients were monitored for only 1 year after transplantation),[6] and a prospective single-season study by Milstone and colleagues found no association between CARV and BOS.[10] The aforementioned pooled analysis of clinical studies was limited by the number of BOS cases reported and the variable duration of follow-up, which led its authors to suggest that more specific prospective assessment of a relationship between CARV and BOS is required.[19]

The impact of CARV on BOS has been hypothesized as being related to the type of CARV infection. Recently, nonrhinovirus infection was associated with a higher rate of allograft dysfunction (as measured by forced expiratory volume in the first second after respiration [FEV_1] 1 to 3 months after CARV infection) than is rhinovirus infection.[18] Additionally, a significant incidence of BOS 6 months after episodes of CARV involving RSV infection but not after cases involving human metapneumovirus has been reported.[9]

The potential immunologic mechanisms underlying this epidemiologic association are currently being investigated. Weigt and colleagues reported that increased concentrations of the chemokine receptor CXCR3 ligands CXCL10 and CXCL11 in BAL fluid during CARV infection were associated with greater declines in FEV_1 at 6 months after infection.[22] With the improvement in molecular diagnostics for respiratory virus,[23] increased surveillance, and increased insight into the potential mechanisms of inflammatory injury with CARV, the association between CARV and BOS can be further delineated and measures for novel treatment strategies developed.

Treatment

Interventions for CARV infection vary depending on the virus recovered and the currently available therapeutic agents. In the case of influenza infection, therapy is generally dictated by the susceptibility of the circulating virus and can vary over time. Because influenza virus is a well-evaluated pathogen, its optimal therapy should be assessed yearly on the basis of local, national, and international evaluation of circulating virus; therefore, treatment should follow national and international guidelines based on the most recent reports. The spectrum of available antiviral agents against influenza continues to expand, and early initiation of antiviral therapy for influenza has been associated with improved outcomes in pediatric and adult solid-organ transplant (SOT) recipients.[24]

Therapeutic interventions for RSV that include ribavirin (aerosolized, intravenous [IV], or oral) with or without a concomitant steroid and IV immunoglobulin have been described in several case series.[25,26] Similar response rates have been reported with all modes of ribavirin administration in lung transplant recipients.[25,27] Reports of a newer agent, ALN-RSV01, which is a small interfering RNA that can enter the cell to target RSV-specific viral mRNA, have appeared in the literature. In two randomized placebo-controlled trials involving more than 100 lung transplant recipients who received aerosolized ALN-RSV01 for 3 to 5 days, lower rates of new or progressive BOS were reported in the subjects who received ALN-RSV01 regardless of whether ribavirin had been coadministered.[28,29] Additionally, several antivirals targeting RSV are under development; they include polyclonal high-titer anti-RSV immunoglobulin and two fusion inhibitors that target the F protein of RSV, thus allowing attachment but blocking fusion of the virus to the host cell. These antivirals have not been evaluated in lung transplant recipients to date.

Successful treatment of other cases of paramyxoviral infection with ribavirin has been reported in the literature. Raza and colleagues reported a single case of human metapneumovirus and McCurdy and coworkers reported treating PIV infection in five subjects with ribavirin.[29a] In addition, case reports describe successful treatment of PIV type 3 lower respiratory tract infection in two lung transplant recipients with the novel agent DAS-181. Both patients showed a reduction in viral load and mild side effects that resolved after completion of therapy.[30,31]

Adenoviral infections were treated effectively with cidofovir and IV immunoglobulin in three of four pediatric lung transplant recipients identified by Doan and colleagues.[32] The use of a lipid-conjugated oral form of cidofovir, brincidofovir (Chimerix, Durham, North Carolina), to treat adenovirus in hematopoietic stem cell transplant recipients and other immunocompromised hosts has been reported in the literature; however, the treated patients did not included any lung transplant recipients.

Finally, although rhinovirus has become the virus most commonly recovered in the era of molecular diagnostic use, no approved antiviral treatment options for this infection currently exist. Several potential therapeutic agents are being evaluated in patients with asthma, including the new oral drug vapendavir or BTA793 (Biota Pharmaceuticals, Inc., Melbourne, Australia), which binds to the viral capsid to inhibit or interfere with receptor binding and subsequently prevent further infection, and the inhaled interferon beta SNG001 (Synairgen PLC, Southampton, England), which is being evaluated as an agent to prevent progression from upper to lower respiratory tract infection. Additional investigation in immunocompromised hosts, including lung transplant recipients, is needed.

Prevention strategies

Even before treatment strategies are used, prevention methods aimed at avoiding CARV have the capacity to eliminate any potential downstream effects of respiratory viral infections. For all viruses, standard precautions, including avoidance of sick contacts and appropriate hand hygiene, are essential. Additional virus-specific precautions include yearly influenza vaccination for all lung transplant recipients and their close contacts[33,34] and influenza prophylaxis in cases of known exposure. During the 2009 H1N1 pandemic, adjuvant influenza vaccination was well tolerated and appeared to have clinical efficacy, with influenza infection developing in only 2 of 148 vaccinated individuals in a Swiss cohort as compared with 5 of 20 unvaccinated individuals.[35] However, additional data from another Swiss group revealed that seroprotection is significantly less likely to develop in lung transplant recipients (43.5%) than in other SOT recipients (72% to 85%) and healthy controls (87%).[36] Additionally, intradermal vaccination boosters did not appear to increase vaccine seroresponse in another cohort of lung transplant recipients.[37] Although vaccination has elicited a lower rate of seroresponse in lung transplant recipients than in other SOT recipients, it has been shown to reduce the incidence of influenza-associated pneumonia[38] and has therefore been recommended as an effective prevention strategy after lung transplantation.

In addition, the importance of infection control in hospitalized patients with CARV cannot be underestimated as a way of preventing spread within the hospital setting. Standard, contact, and droplet infection control precautions should be implemented with suspected CARV infection and can be narrowed to target the virus identified in accordance with local and national guidelines.

HERPESVIRUS INFECTIONS

Viruses belonging to the Herpesviridae family remain the pathogens most commonly responsible for infectious complications occurring after lung transplantation.[39] Depending on its seroprevalence in the general population and the age of the recipient at the time of transplantation, herpesvirus infection may be a consequence of reactivation of a previous infection, transmission from the donor allograft, or development of a natural infection after transplantation. For example, the majority of adult transplant recipients are seropositive for herpes simplex virus (HSV) and varicella-zoster virus (VZV), and consequently, most cases of clinical manifestation of HSV and VZV are reactivations of previous latent infection.[40] On the other hand, patients who are seronegative for CMV and Epstein-Barr virus (EBV) and receive an organ from a seropositive donor (the D+/R- constellation) are at higher risk for the development of symptomatic disease than seropositive recipients are.[41] Therefore, assessment of the serologic status of the donor and the recipient for each virus at the time of transplantation is of major importance to determine the risk for posttransplantation viral replication and to individualize antiviral preventive strategies accordingly.[42]

Cytomegalovirus

CMV belongs to the β-herpesvirus family and has historically been the number one pathogen occurring after organ transplantation. CMV disease has been associated with morbidity and even mortality in lung transplant recipients,[43] but because of a significant improvement in CMV prevention and treatment strategies, direct mortality resulting from CMV is rarely seen today.[44] However, concern remains regarding the potential association between CMV infection and the development of CLAD, which is the most significant complication impairing graft and patient survival after lung transplantation.

Current accepted definitions of CMV events in lung transplant recipients include active CMV infection, which refers to the identification of CMV replication (by either nucleic acid testing or antigenemia) irrespective of symptoms, and CMV disease, which refers to active CMV infection with attributable symptoms. The main risk factors for the development of CMV disease after lung transplantation include the high-risk D+/R- CMV serostatus,[45] use of lymphocyte-depleting antibodies as induction or antirejection therapy,[46] and previous occurrence of acute rejection with subsequent enhanced immunosuppression.[47] Some studies have correlated the presence of certain genetic polymorphisms in innate immune genes with a higher incidence of CMV replication after transplantation.[47] Of note, the incidence of CMV disease is higher in lung transplant recipients than in other transplant recipients, which is potentially due to a higher state of immunosuppression and higher CMV viral load within the lung allograft. The current incidence of CMV disease in lung transplant recipients varies from 5% to 40% and depends mainly on CMV serostatus and the duration of antiviral prophylaxis.[44,48,49]

Clinical manifestations of CMV disease include a viral syndrome characterized by malaise, myalgia, low-grade fever, and an end-organ disease such as colitis, esophagitis, or hepatitis. Of note, despite frequent reactivation of CMV in allografts (CMV in BAL fluid), the incidence of CMV pneumonitis in lung transplant recipients in the current era is relatively low. Data from two different prospective cohorts of lung transplant recipients showed that CMV replication in the allograft, as measured by polymerase chain reaction (PCR), was 41% to 44% at 1 year after transplantation, whereas CMV pneumonitis occurred in only 5.3% to 8% of these patients.[50,51]

The relationship between CMV infection and its indirect effects in lung transplant recipients is controversial. CMV replication after transplantation is driven by a lack of control of the specific cell-mediated immunity induced by immunosuppressive drugs, which is in turn associated with a proinflammatory and immunomodulatory state that may affect transplant recipients' alloimmune response and, eventually, allograft function and survival.[52] In early studies involving no prevention or a short duration of prophylaxis, CMV was associated with impaired allograft function and survival after lung transplantation.[53] Since the introduction of universal preventive strategies, particularly those involving the use of extended antiviral prophylaxis, this association has become less clear.[54,55] In a study published in 1995, CMV disease was associated with CLAD only before the introduction of prophylaxis with IV ganciclovir.[56] More recently, CMV infection was identified as a significant risk factor for the development of CLAD in a study from Australia (hazard ratio [HR] = 2.1, P = .003)[51] but not in another study from Canada (HR = 1.04, P = .89).[50] In both studies, all patients received at least 3 months of antiviral prophylaxis with ganciclovir, valganciclovir, or both. Another study involving a cohort of lung transplant recipients in Sweden who underwent antiviral prophylaxis for 3 months found that both CMV disease and asymptomatic CMV replication remained associated with a lower CLAD-free survival rate (32% and 36%, respectively, as opposed to 69% in patients without CMV infection).[57] Taken together, these data suggest that antiviral prophylaxis has the potential to reduce, but not completely eliminate the indirect effects of CMV on the lung allograft.

Prevention of CMV disease (Table 29.1) in organ transplantation consists of administering an antiviral drug for a specified time after transplantation (universal prophylaxis), monitoring CMV viral load by PCR, or administering an antiviral drug to patients with active CMV replication (a preemptive approach).[58] In lung transplantation, most centers use antiviral prophylaxis for prevention of CMV and it is the preferred strategy recommended in published guidelines.[59] The optimal duration of prophylaxis has not been established, but most studies have shown that prophylaxis lasting less than 6 months is associated with a higher incidence of CMV disease.[60] A randomized controlled trial comparing 3 and 12 months of valganciclovir prophylaxis in lung transplant recipients showed a significantly lower incidence of CMV disease in the 12-month group (4% versus 32% in the 3-month group, P < .001).[44] However, in intermediate-risk groups (particularly in D⁻/R⁺ patients), 6 months of prophylaxis appears to be appropriate for preventing late-onset CMV disease.[61] Some centers use CMV-specific immunoglobulin in combination with antiviral drugs for prevention of CMV disease, but the benefit of this approach has not been completely established. Recently, the role of CMV-specific cell-mediated immunity assays in stratifying the risk for CMV disease in individual patients has been investigated; observational studies found that patients with detectable cellular immunity are at lower risk for the development of CMV disease.[62-64] The value of incorporating CMV immune monitoring into the routine management of lung transplant recipients requires validation in interventional trials.[58]

Therapy for established CMV disease (see Table 29.1) usually consists of the administration of IV ganciclovir.[48] In other SOT recipients valganciclovir has been shown to be as efficacious as IV ganciclovir in treating CMV disease[65]; however, the published experience in lung transplant recipients is limited. Given the enhanced bioavailability of oral valganciclovir,[66] oral therapy should be expected to be appropriate for the treatment of mild to moderate cases of CMV disease, but IV therapy should be preferred for severe cases with end-organ involvement. In patients with a favorable response to therapy, a switch from IV to oral therapy can be safely proposed. Duration of therapy is determined by the time until clinical and virologic response; 3 to 4 weeks of antiviral therapy is usually needed, although severe cases with a slow reduction in CMV viral load may require longer therapy. Secondary prophylaxis for 4 to 8 weeks after completion of a full-dose course of ganciclovir or valganciclovir may be recommended in high-risk patients to avoid early relapse.[58] Lung transplant recipients are at higher risk for the development of antiviral-resistant CMV infection than other transplant recipients are, with the incidence ranging from 5% to 15%, particularly in D⁺/R⁻ patients.[67] Most mutations responsible for antiviral resistance are located in the UL97 kinase and UL54 polymerase. UL97 mutations can usually be treated with high doses of ganciclovir, whereas UL54 mutations require alternative antiviral drugs such as foscarnet. The role of new antiviral drugs such as letermovir or brincidofovir in therapy for resistant CMV infection must be evaluated in lung transplant recipients.[68]

Table 29.1 Antiviral strategies for herpesvirus in lung transplant recipients

Virus	Prevention	Therapy	Comments
HSV-1 and HSV-2	Ganciclovir and valganciclovir for CMV prophylaxis are effective for prevention of HSV Acyclovir, valaciclovir, and famciclovir for 8 to 12 weeks are recommended in CMV D-/R- lung transplant recipients or in patients followed by using the preemptive approach	Mucocutaneous disease: acyclovir, valaciclovir, and famciclovir Disseminated or severe disease: IV acyclovir Infection with acyclovir-resistant HSV: foscarnet	
VZV	Ganciclovir and valganciclovir for CMV prophylaxis are effective for prevention of VZV infection Acyclovir, valaciclovir, and famciclovir for 8 to 12 weeks are recommended for CMV D-/R- lung transplant recipients or for patients monitored by the preemptive approach	Localized HZ: Acyclovir, valaciclovir, and famciclovir Disseminated HZ or primary varicella: IV acyclovir	Acyclovir seems to be less effective than the other drugs in reducing PHN
CMV	For D+/R- lung transplant recipients: prophylaxis with valganciclovir for 6 to 12 months For R+ lung transplant recipients: prophylaxis with valganciclovir for 6 to 12 months. Alternatively, a strict preemptive approach may be used in these patients. For D-/R- lung transplant recipients: HSV and VZV prophylaxis	End-organ disease: IV ganciclovir Viral syndrome: IV ganciclovir or valganciclovir In case of initial use of IV ganciclovir, a switch to valganciclovir can be made after clinical and virologic improvement once absorption is ensured	In highly immunosuppressed patients, CMVIg or IVIG can be used as additional prevention or therapy
EBV	For D+/R- lung transplant recipients: prophylaxis with valganciclovir for 6 months may be considered specifically for prevention of EBV	Antiviral therapy for persistent EBV viremia or as adjunctive therapy for PTLD is not recommended	
HHV-6 and HHV-7	No specific antiviral preventive strategy is recommended	End-organ HHV-6 disease: foscarnet	
HHV-8	No specific antiviral preventive strategy is recommended	No specific antiviral therapy is recommended	Some cases of HHV-8–associated disease have improved after valganciclovir therapy, although the role of antivirals in this setting is controversial

Note: CMV, cytomegalovirus; CMVIg, specific CMV immunoglobulin; D, donor; EBV, Epstein-Barr virus; HHV, human herpes virus; HSV, herpes simplex virus; HZ, herpes zoster; IV, intravenous; IVIG, intravenous immunoglobulin; PHN, postherpetic neuralgia; PTLD, posttransplant lymphoproliferative disorder; R, recipient; VZV, varicella-zoster virus.

Epstein-Barr virus

Epstein-Barr virus (EBV) is a γ-herpesvirus that infects more than 95% of the world population. Primary infection occurs in children and young adults; it is usually asymptomatic but can appear as a viral syndrome with fever and adenopathy that is known as infectious mononucleosis. In transplant recipients, EBV is responsible for a variety of clinical manifestations ranging from an infectious mononucleosis–like syndrome (in pediatric transplant recipients with EBV primary infection) to proliferation of monoclonal lymphocytes leading to high-grade lymphoma.[69] Such clinical entities associated with EBV infection after transplantation are known as posttransplant lymphoproliferative disorder (PTLD) and are mainly the consequence of the lack of cell-mediated immune surveillance of EBV-infected lymphocytes as a result of immunosuppression.[70]

The main risk factor for the development of EBV-associated PTLD in lung transplant recipients is the EBV serostatus of the donor and the recipient.[71] EBV D+/R- patients are at particular risk for the development of primary EBV infection, which may lead to PTLD. Because most seronegative recipients are children, PTLD is a particular problem in pediatric lung transplantation. The incidence of PTLD in lung transplant recipients at the age of 5 years ranges from 1.5% to 16%, depending on the recipient's age.[69,71] Although the net state of immunosuppression clearly influences risk for the development of PTLD, the role of each specific immunosuppressive drug in increasing the risk for EBV replication and the development of PTLD is not well described. Induction therapy with lymphocyte-depleting antibodies appears to be associated with a higher incidence of PTLD in large nationwide registries,[72] but no particular maintenance antirejection drug seems to influence the risk for PTLD. In particular, despite some promising in vitro data showing a role for mammalian target of rapamycin (mTOR) inhibitors in inhibiting the proliferation of EBV-infected cells in PTLD mouse models,[73] its role in protecting against the development PTLD in transplant recipients has not been proved in terms of a reduction in incidence.[72]

Prevention of EBV-associated PTLD is a major issue in lung transplant recipients (see Table 29.1). D+/R- patients at high risk for EBV infection are generally managed with reduced immunosuppressive regimens, particularly regimens in which the use of lymphocyte-depleting antibodies is avoided. Acyclovir and ganciclovir have exhibited in vitro antiviral activity against EBV; therefore, antiviral prophylaxis with these drugs to prevent (or delay) the development of primary EBV infection is frequently given to EBV D+/R- patients.[69] However, antiviral drugs act only against lytic virus and not against latently EBV-infected B cells. Hence, whether antiviral drugs have a beneficial effect in preventing EBV DNAemia and PTLD is not clear. Of note, no randomized controlled trials have addressed the benefits of antiviral prophylaxis and the data from observational studies are inconclusive. Monitoring the blood for EBV DNAemia may identify patients with persistent EBV replication. Because such patients are at highest risk for EBV-associated PTLD, they are candidates to receive some intervention to reduce the level of EBV DNAemia, such as a reduction of immunosuppression or the administration of antiviral or anti–lymphocyte B cytotoxic therapy. However, very few prospective studies have addressed such a preemptive approach in SOT recipients. In a study of pediatric liver transplant recipients, EBV DNAemia was monitored by PCR testing of blood samples every 1 to 2 weeks after transplantation, and immunosuppression was actively reduced in patients with two consecutive positive assays. This preemptive approach resulted in a significantly lower incidence of PTLD than in the a historical cohort (2% versus 16%, respectively).[74] On the other hand, the use of acyclovir or ganciclovir as preemptive therapy for persistent EBV DNAemia does not appear to be effective in this setting, and data on the long-term safety of administration of the anti-CD20 monoclonal antibody rituximab for preemptive treatment require further validation.[75] Some groups have used infusion of autologous or allogeneic (third-party) EBV-specific cytotoxic T cells for restoring cell-mediated immunity to

EBV in patients in whom reduction of immunosuppression did not successfully eradicate EBV DNAemia; however, this strategy appears to be less efficacious in SOT recipients than in stem cell transplant recipients.[76]

Management of established EBV-related PTLD requires a reduction in immunosuppression as a first step. Some cases of polyclonal proliferation may respond to this single measure, but more aggressive PTLD requires additional therapy with rituximab with or without chemotherapy.[69] Nonresponsive cases may benefit from EBV-specific cytotoxic T-cell infusion.

Other herpesvirus

HERPES SIMPLEX VIRUS TYPES 1 AND 2

HSV reactivation is one of the most common forms of viral infection after organ transplantation.[40] HSV-1 is generally responsible for oropharyngeal manifestations, whereas HSV-2 is most commonly associated with genital disease; however, both viruses can be found in either location. In adults the seroprevalence of HSV-1 is estimated to be 70% to 90% and that of HSV-2 is estimated to be 20%.[77] The clinical manifestations of HSV infection are usually similar to those observed in immunocompetent patients and include oral and genital mucocutaneous vesicular rash. In highly immunosuppressed patients, more extensive lesions with necrotic ulcers can be observed. In addition, cases of disseminated HSV disease, including HSV hepatitis and pneumonitis, have been reported in SOT recipients.[78] Diagnosis of HSV infection is usually clinical and can be confirmed by PCR. The use of antiviral prophylaxis with acyclovir or valacyclovir during the first weeks after transplantation can effectively prevent HSV infection (see Table 29.1). Because the drugs used for CMV prophylaxis are also active against HSV, specific herpes prophylaxis is needed only in low-risk CMV D-/R- patients who are not receiving CMV prophylaxis or in patients who are being monitored by the preemptive approach.[40] Therapy for HSV consists of the administration of oral acyclovir, valacyclovir, or famciclovir for nonsevere cutaneous lesions. For HSV infection that is severe, disseminated, or both, high-dose IV acyclovir is recommended.

VARICELLA-ZOSTER VIRUS

VZV is transmitted from person to person through aerosolized secretions; after primary infection (chickenpox), VZV latently infects the sensory ganglia. If immune surveillance is reduced, VZV can reactivate and appear as vesicular lesions (herpes zoster [HZ]) in the vicinity of the affected nerve. Because the seroprevalence of VZV infection in adults in Europe and North America is close to 100%, HZ is the most common clinical manifestation of VZV infection in adult transplant recipients. In the pediatric transplant population, however, primary VZV infection may occur after transplantation and be associated with significant mortality. Lung transplant recipients appear to be at the highest risk for the development of HZ of all organ transplants, with an estimated incidence of 15% to 20% at 5 years after transplantation.[79,80] In patients receiving CMV prophylaxis, episodes of HZ appear after use of the antiviral drug has been discontinued.[80] The clinical manifestations of VZV infection in lung transplant recipients are usually similar to those in the general population. In a cohort of 239 lung transplant recipients, rates of disseminated cutaneous and visceral involvement were only 6% and 0%, respectively,[80] although some cases of fatal disseminated HZ after lung transplantation have been reported.[81] Importantly, a significant number of lung transplant recipients (up to 20%) may develop postherpetic neuralgia.[80] As for HSV infection, diagnosis of VZV infection is usually clinical, although in some cases microbiologic confirmation by PCR can be useful to differentiate between HSV and VZV infection (see Table 29.1). Therapy for VZV infection consists of administration of oral acyclovir, valacyclovir, or famciclovir in nonsevere cases of HZ. IV acyclovir is the drug of choice in cases involving primary infection or disseminated reactivation. Screening for VZV infection and administration of the live attenuated Oka vaccine to seronegative transplant candidates is an essential strategy to reduce the burden of VZV infection after transplantation.[33] Posttransplantation vaccination of seronegative patients has recently been shown to be safe and immunogenic in a selected cohort of pediatric liver transplant recipients, although no data about the safety of this approach in lung transplant recipients exist.[82] A live attenuated zoster vaccine has been approved for use in the elderly, but the impact of pretransplantation vaccination on the incidence of posttransplantation IIZ has not yet been investigated.[33] A heat-inactivated zoster vaccine has been tested in different immunocompromised populations but not in SOT recipients.

HUMAN HERPESVIRUS 6 AND HUMAN HERPESVIRUS 7

The human herpesviruses HHV-6 and HHV-7 are closely related β-herpesviruses that latently infect most of the adult population.[83] In immunocompetent children, HHV-6 and HHV-7 are the cause of exanthema subitum (roseola). In SOT recipients (lung transplant recipients in particular), the clinical significance of HHV-6 and HHV-7 infection has not yet been well established. HHV-6 and HHV-7 reactivation after transplantation is common; some series have shown that HHV-6 and HHV-7 may replicate in the allografts of 20% to 50% of lung transplant recipients during the first year after transplantation.[50,84] However, very few cases of symptomatic HHV-6 disease have been reported, and HHV-7 appears to not be associated with clinical disease.[85] The clinical manifestations of HHV-6 infection are similar to those observed with CMV infection, including a viral syndrome, pneumonitis, and gastrointestinal disease.[86] Additionally, some cases of HHV-6 encephalitis after organ transplantation have been reported. Some series have associated the presence of HHV-6 in BAL with a higher incidence of CLAD,[87] but this association has not been confirmed in all studies.[50] A unique feature of HHV-6 is

that it may integrate into the host chromosome in approximately 1% of the population and be transmitted vertically or through the donor (a condition that has been named chromosomally integrated HHV-6).[88] Because HHV-6 DNA is present in each of their cells, patients with chromosomally integrated HHV-6 have high viral loads of HHV-6 in their blood samples without clinical significance, which may complicate diagnosing active HHV-6 infection on the basis of PCR results. Whether HHV-6 infection may be reactivated in transplant recipients with chromosomally integrated HHV-6 and be manifested as clinical HHV-6 disease is not known.[88] Universal CMV prophylaxis may reduce the occurrence of HHV-6 and HHV-7 replication, although the impact of prevention of HHV-6 infection on patient and allograft outcomes has not been assessed (see Table 29.1).[85] Foscarnet demonstrates better antiviral activity against HHV-6 than ganciclovir does, and it is the preferred drug for treating symptomatic HHV-6 disease.

HUMAN HERPESVIRUS-8

HHV-8 belongs to the γ-herpesvirus family, and as an oncogenic virus, it shares many characteristics with EBV. The seroprevalence of HHV-8 infection varies greatly between geographic regions, with a high prevalence in Africa (50%) and Mediterranean Europe (10% to 30%) and a low prevalence in northern Europe and North America (<10%).[89] Therefore, the incidence of HHV-8–associated disease after lung transplantation depends on the origin of the donor and the recipient. However, screening for HHV-8 in the donor and recipient at the time of transplantation is not routinely performed in most countries because of the limited specificity of the HHV-8 serology, which leads to false-positive results. In a French cohort of kidney transplant recipients in which HHV-8 serology was systematically performed, 3.2% of recipients were seropositive for HHV-8 and 1.3% of patients had a D+/R- serostatus.[90] The most common clinical manifestation of HHV-8 infection in lung transplant recipients is Kaposi sarcoma (KS), which is estimated to be 100 to 1000 times more frequent in SOT recipients than in the general population. The incidence of KS in lung transplant recipients has been reported to be 6.67 per 1000 patient-years (2.8- and 428-fold higher than in kidney transplant recipients and the general population, respectively).[91] Although KS is limited to the skin in most patients, disseminated KS with visceral involvement may develop in lung transplant recipients . Localization of KS within the lung allograft has been described in several case reports.[92] SOT recipients may have more severe manifestations of HHV-8–associated disease, including multicentric Castleman disease (MCD), primary effusion lymphoma, and a sepsis-like syndrome with hemophagocytosis.[93] Of note, most of these cases occurred in HHV-8–seronegative patients who received an organ from a seropositive donor, and they were associated with high mortality.[93] The first strategy to treat KS in lung transplant recipients is reduction of immunosuppression. mTOR inhibitors have antiproliferative effects, and switching from calcineurin inhibitors to mTOR inhibitors has been associated with resolution of the KS lesions in most cases,[94] although experience in lung transplant recipients is limited. Cases of disseminated KS, MCD, and sepsis-like syndrome require aggressive therapy, including reduction of immunosuppressive therapy, rituximab, and chemotherapy. The role of antiviral drugs in preventing or treating HHV-8–associated disease has not been well established (see Table 29.1).[83]

HEPATITIS VIRUS INFECTIONS

Some viruses cause specific issues after lung transplantation. Hepatitis B virus (HBV) and hepatitis C virus (HCV) are the most important and best-known viruses that cause both acute and chronic hepatitis after transplantation.[95] Hepatitis E virus (HEV) was recently identified as a pathogen associated with chronic hepatitis in lung transplant patients.[96,97]

Hepatitis B virus

HBV is a DNA virus, a member of the Hepadnaviridae family, and the major cause of acute and chronic hepatitis, cirrhosis, and hepatocellular carcinoma. HBV is a worldwide health problem that affects more than 350 million individuals.[98] Thanks to effective vaccination programs, HBV's prevalence and associated mortality have decreased during the last decade; however, it remains a major health issue and results in more than 600,000 deaths worldwide annually.[99]

Candidates for lung transplantation should be screened for HBV and categorized on the basis of serologic test results (Table 29.2). Group 1 is the largest group in developed countries and includes patients who are HBV negative or have been vaccinated for HBV (anti-HBV+). The second group consists of previously infected patients who have cleared the virus (anti-HBVc+ and anti-HBVs+). Members of both these groups are candidates for lung transplantation; however, because HBV can be reactivated under immunosuppression, patients with cleared HBV (i.e., those in the second group) should be monitored regularly after transplantation. The third group consists of those with only anti-HBVc; they may be clearing the virus but anti-HBVs has not developed. HBV DNA testing should be performed on these patients, and they should be considered infectious unless their HBV DNA test result is negative. Finally, until recently, chronic HBV infection (HBV surface antigen–positive individuals) was an absolute contraindication to lung transplantation.[100] Emerging guidelines from the International Society of Heart and Lung Transplantation (ISHLT) now describe chronic HBV infection as a relative contraindication to lung transplantation, thus indicating that transplantation can be considered in selected HBV-positive candidates in the absence of cirrhosis and hepatocellular carcinoma.[101]

The use of HBV-positive donors has also been reported in the literature. Dhillon and colleagues explored the United Network for Organ Sharing (UNOS) data comparing the outcomes of 13,233 recipients of organs from anti-HBc–negative donors with those of 333 recipients of anti-HBc–positive organs for lung and heart-lung transplantation. Their analysis indicated an increase in the overall percentage of anti-HBc–positive lung donors from 2.8% to 4.8% between 1994 and 2004.[102] Additionally, 5-year mortality was not significantly different between the groups, and anti-HBc–positive donor status was not an independent risk factor for 1- or 5-year mortality in multivariate analysis. Additional studies have assessed pretransplant vaccination as well as posttransplant prophylaxis with lamivudine.[103] Vaccination appears to be successful, with no reports of HBV transmission and similar 1-year survival rates in the 29 fully vaccinated recipients of anti-HBc–positive donor lungs despite the lack of documentation about seroconversion. In addition, none of the seven patients who underwent 12 months of lamivudine prophylaxis after receiving an anti-HBc–positive organ exhibited evidence of de novo hepatitis.[103] These data highlight the importance of appropriate vaccination against HBV in the pretransplant period. No data on the use of hepatitis B surface antigen–positive donors in lung transplantation exist. Further information on the impact of HBV in lung transplantation is needed.

HEPATITIS C VIRUS

HCV is a single-stranded RNA virus belonging to the family Flaviviridae.[104] Several HCV genotypes are recognized, with genotypes 1, 2, and 3 being the most common in developed countries. Chronic HCV infection affects approximately 170 million people worldwide and may result in liver cirrhosis and hepatocellular carcinoma.[105] Transmission by blood products and transplantation has been nearly eliminated by blood screening, but HCV remains a common cause of chronic hepatitis, with more than 4 million cases in the United States alone.[106]

Table 29.2 Hepatitis B serology patterns

Status	HBs–Ag	Anti–HBs	Anti–HBc	Group
No infection	−	−	−	1
Vaccinated	−	+	−	1
Cleared infection	−	+	+	2
Resolving infection	−	−	+	3
Active infection (chronic hepatitis B)	+	−	±	4

Note: Anti-HBc, anti–hepatitis B core antibodies; anti-HBs, anti–hepatitis B surface antibodies; HBs-Ag, hepatitis B surface antigen.

Until recently, chronic HCV was also listed as an absolute contraindication to lung transplantation in guidelines from the ISHLT.[100] Two small series that examined a combined total of 20 lung transplant patients showed that the patient and graft survival rates of those with HCV were similar to those of controls.[107,108] In addition, analysis of the Organ Procurement and Transplantation Network (OPTN)/UNOS database showed similar 5-year survival for HCV-seropositive and HCV-seronegative recipients.[109]

The current standard therapy for HCV is a combination of pegylated interferon (PEG-INF) and ribavirin, with its efficacy dependent on HCV genotype. The current treatment leads to a sustained viral response in approximately 80% of non–transplant recipients with HCV genotype 2 or 3 and in approximately 45% with genotype 1. However, many new classes and combinations of anti-HCV therapy are currently under evaluation with encouraging results. Medication regimens that include agents such as sofosbuvir and daclatasvir are expected to increase the response rates considerably.[110] It is anticipated that with these emerging treatment algorithms, more patients with HCV will achieve a sustained viral response. In the absence of cirrhosis and hepatocellular carcinoma, patients with chronic HCV infection may be considered candidates for lung transplantation.

HEPATITIS E VIRUS

In developed countries HEV is known as a major cause of hepatitis transmitted via the fecal-oral route.[111] HEV is a single-stranded RNA virus belonging to the Hepeviridae family, and in developed countries it is known as a traveler's disease. Travel-related HEV infection is caused by hepatitis E genotype 1 or 2.[112] Genotype 3 has recently been identified as a cause of chronic hepatitis in lung transplant patients and is now recognized as a zoonotic pathogen.[113,114]

In lung transplant recipients HEV infection may lead to chronic hepatitis and cirrhosis.[115,116] Its mode of transmission to transplant recipients is unclear, although its high prevalence in the swine population supports the view that it is a porcine zoonosis.[117] Transmission by blood transfusion is rare, and donor-derived infection via lung transplantation has not been described.[118]

The clinical features of HEV infection range from asymptomatic mild hepatitis to subacute liver failure.[114,119,120] Chronic HEV infection has been established in up to 2% to 3% of lung transplant recipients in some European populations.[96] Serologic tests are usually negative; real-time PCR for HEV RNA is the test of choice.[113,121] HEV RNA can remain detectable in stool after it is no longer detectable in serum.

Therapeutic options are reduction of immunosuppression, PEG-INF, and ribavirin. For transplant recipients, ribavirin monotherapy for 3 to 4 months is currently suggested as the treatment of choice to avoid the risk for rejection associated with either reduction of immunosuppression or initiation of PEG-INF.[122] The end points for HEV treatment remain unclear, with either duration (3 to 5 months) and undetectable viral load in serum or absence of HEV RNA in stool being the leading markers to date.[96,97,122] Relapses after treatment do occur, even in patients whose serum and stool samples become HEV RNA negative during treatment.[122,123] Additional studies of HEV infection in lung transplant recipients are needed to define its epidemiology in different groups and to identify its outcomes and appropriate strategies for its treatment.

HUMAN IMMUNODEFICIENCY VIRUS

In the past, human immunodeficiency virus (HIV) was considered an absolute contraindication to lung transplantation.[100] However, with the availability of highly active antiretroviral therapy, the prognosis for patients infected with HIV has improved dramatically. In addition, prospective research on kidney and liver transplantation in HIV-positive patients has shown survival rates similar to those of noninfected recipients.[124] Therefore, an increasing number of centers are now offering SOT to HIV-positive patients with undetectable viral loads.[125,126]

Pulmonary arterial hypertension is a recognized complication of HIV infection,[127-130] as well as an established indication for lung transplantation.[100] As survival of HIV-positive patients improves, the prevalence of PAH in transplant recipients in the HIV-positive population will increase; thus far, however, many such patients have been refused as transplant candidates. To date, only one HIV-positive lung transplant recipient has been reported in the literature. The patient, who received a transplant for cystic fibrosis at an Italian center, was alive with a functioning graft 1 year after transplantation.[131] With the emerging early data on successful lung transplantation at selected centers and successful liver and kidney transplantation in HIV-positive patients, the arguments for exclusion of HIV positive patients from lung transplantation are abating. An increase in the number of requests for lung transplantation in HIV-positive patients can be expected. Stable patients with undetectable HIV RNA viral loads who fulfill the criteria for lung transplantation are expected to be increasingly referred and accepted for lung transplantation. The substantive posttransplant issue will be the numerous interactions between antiretroviral and immunosuppressive drugs.[132,133] Lung transplantation in HIV-infected individuals should therefore be performed only in centers with combined expertise in HIV and lung transplantation.

REFERENCES

1. Kumar D, Husain S, Chen MH, et al. A prospective molecular surveillance study evaluating the clinical impact of community-acquired respiratory viruses in lung transplant recipients. Transplantation 2010;89:1028-1033.
2. Gottlieb J, Schulz TF, Welte T, et al. Community-acquired respiratory viral infections in lung transplant recipients: A single season cohort study. Transplantation 2009;87:1530-1537.

3. Astegiano S, Bergallo M, Solidoro P, et al. Prevalence and clinical impact of polyomaviruses KI and WU in lung transplant recipients. Transplant Proc 2010;42:1275-1278.

4. Bridges ND, Spray TL, Collins MH, et al. Adenovirus infection in the lung results in graft failure after lung transplantation. J Thorac Cardiovasc Surg 1998;116:617-623.

5. Meylan PR, Aubert JD, Kaiser L. Influenza transmission to recipient through lung transplantation. Transpl Infect Dis 2007;9:55-57.

6. Liu M, Worley S, Arrigain S, et al. Respiratory viral infections within one year after pediatric lung transplant. Transpl Infect Dis 2009;11:304-312.

7. Kaiser L, Aubert JD, Pache JC, et al. Chronic rhinoviral infection in lung transplant recipients. Am J Respir Crit Care Med 2006;174:1392-1399.

8. Garbino J, Gerbase MW, Wunderli W, et al. Lower respiratory viral illnesses: Improved diagnosis by molecular methods and clinical impact. Am J Respir Crit Care Med 2004;170:1197-1203.

9. Hopkins P, McNeil K, Kermeen F, et al. Human metapneumovirus in lung transplant recipients and comparison to respiratory syncytial virus. Am J Respir Crit Care Med 2008;178:876-881.

10. Milstone AP, Brumble LM, Barnes LM, et al. A single-season prospective study of respiratory viral infections in lung transplant recipients. Eur Respir J 2006;28:131-137.

11. Kumar D, Erdman D, Keshavjee D, et al. Clinical impact of community-acquired respiratory viruses on bronchiolitis obliterans after lung transplant. Am J Transplant 2005;5:2031-2036.

12. Bridevaux PO, Aubert JD, Soccal PM, et al. Incidence and outcomes of respiratory viral infections in lung transplant recipients: A prospective study. Thorax 2014;69:32-38.

13. Khalifah AP, Hachem RR, Chakinala MM, et al. Respiratory viral infections are a distinct risk for bronchiolitis obliterans syndrome and death. Am J Respir Crit Care Med 2004;170:181-187.

14. Goldfarb NS, Avery RK, Goormastic M, et al. Hypogammaglobulinemia in lung transplant recipients. Transplantation 2001;71:242-246.

15. Noell BC, Dawson KL, Seethamraju H. Effect of hypogammaglobulinemia on the incidence of community-acquired respiratory viral infections after lung transplantation. Transplant Proc 2013;45:2371-2374.

16. Soccal PM, Aubert JD, Bridevaux PO, et al. Upper and lower respiratory tract viral infections and acute graft rejection in lung transplant recipients. Clin Infect Dis 2010;51:163-170.

17. Glanville AR, Community-acquired respiratory viruses after lung transplantation: Common, sometimes silent, potentially lethal. Thorax 2014;69:1-2.

18. Sayah DM, Koff JL, Leard LE, et al. Rhinovirus and other respiratory viruses exert different effects on lung allograft function that are not mediated through acute rejection. Clin Transplant 2013;27:E64-E71.

19. Vu DL, Bridevaus PO, Aubert PO, et al. Respiratory viruses in lung transplant recipients: A critical review and pooled analysis of clinical studies. Am J Transplant 2011;11:1071-1078.

20. Billings JL, Hertz MI, Savik K, et al. Respiratory viruses and chronic rejection in lung transplant recipients. J Heart Lung Transplant 2002;21:559-566.

21. Magnusson J, Westin J, Andersson LM, et al. The impact of viral respiratory tract infections on long-term morbidity and mortality following lung transplantation: A retrospective cohort study using a multiplex PCR panel. Transplantation 2013;95:383-388.

22. Weigt SS, Derhovanessian A, Liao E, et al. CXCR3 chemokine ligands during respiratory viral infections predict lung allograft dysfunction. Am J Transplant 2012;12:477-484.

23. Weinberg A, Zamora MR, Li A, et al. The value of polymerase chain reaction for the diagnosis of viral respiratory tract infections in lung transplant recipients. J Clin Virol 2002;25:171-175.

24. Kumar D, Michaels MG, Morris MI, et al. Outcomes from pandemic influenza A H1N1 infection in recipients of solid-organ transplants: A multicentre cohort study. Lancet Infect Dis 2010;10:521-526.

25. Glanville AR, Scott AI, Morton JM, et al. Intravenous ribavirin is a safe and cost-effective treatment for respiratory syncytial virus infection after lung transplantation. J Heart Lung Transplant 2005;24:2114-2119.

26. Pelaez A, Lyon GM, Force SD, et al. Efficacy of oral ribavirin in lung transplant patients with respiratory syncytial virus lower respiratory tract infection. J Heart Lung Transplant 2009;28:67-71.

27. Li L, Avery R, Budev M, et al. Oral versus inhaled ribavirin therapy for respiratory syncytial virus infection after lung transplantation. J Heart Lung Transplant 2012;31:839-844.

28. Simon A, Karsten V, Cehelsky J, et al. Results of a phase 2b multi-center trial of ALN-RSV01 in respiratory syncytial virus (RSV)-infected lung transplant patients. Eur Resp J 1 Sept 2012.

29. Zamora MR, Budev M, Rolfe M, et al. RNA interference therapy in lung transplant patients infected with respiratory syncytial virus. Am J Respir Crit Care Med 2011;183:531-538.

29a. McCurdy LH, Milstone A, Dummer S. Clinical features and outcomes of paramyxoviral infection in lung transplant recipients treated with ribavirin. J Heart Lung Transplant 2003;22:745-753.

30. Drozd DR, Limaye AP Moss RB, et al. DAS181 treatment of severe parainfluenza type 3 pneumonia

in a lung transplant recipient. Transpl Infect Dis 2013;15:E28-E32.

31. Guzman-Suarez BB, Buckley MW, Gilmore ET, et al. Clinical potential of DAS181 for treatment of parainfluenza-3 infections in transplant recipients. Transpl Infect Dis 2012;14:427-433.

32. Doan ML, Mallory GB, Kaplan SL, et al. Treatment of adenovirus pneumonia with cidofovir in pediatric lung transplant recipients. J Heart Lung Transplant 2007;26:883-889.

33. Danziger-Isakov L, Kumar D, AST Infectious Diseases Community of Practice. Vaccination in solid organ transplantation. Am J Transplant 2013;13(Suppl 4):311-317.

34. Rubin LG, Levin MJ Ljungman P, et al. 2013 IDSA clinical practice guideline for vaccination of the immunocompromised host. Clin Infect Dis 2014;58:e44-e100.

35. Schuurmans MM, Tini GM, Dalar L, et al. Pandemic 2009 H1N1 influenza virus vaccination in lung transplant recipients: Coverage, safety and clinical effectiveness in the Zurich cohort. J Heart Lung Transplant 2011;30:685-690.

36. Siegrist CA, Ambrosioni J, Bel M, et al. Responses of solid organ transplant recipients to the AS03-adjuvanted pandemic influenza vaccine. Antivir Ther 2012;17:893-903.

37. Manuel O, Humar A, Chen MH, et al. Immunogenicity and safety of an intradermal boosting strategy for vaccination against influenza in lung transplant recipients. Am J Transplant 2007;7:2567-2572.

38. Perez-Romero P, Aydillo TA, Perez-Ordoñez A, et al. Reduced incidence of pneumonia in influenza-vaccinated solid organ transplant recipients with influenza disease. Clin Microbiol Infect 2012;18:E533-E540.

39. Fishman JA. Overview: Cytomegalovirus and the herpesviruses in transplantation. Am J Transplant 2013;13(Suppl 3):1-8; quiz 8.

40. Zuckerman RA, Limaye AP. Varicella zoster virus (VZV) and herpes simplex virus (HSV) in solid organ transplant patients. Am J Transplant 2013;13(Suppl 3):55-66; quiz 66.

41. Manuel O, Kralidis G, Mueller NJ, et al. Impact of antiviral preventive strategies on the incidence and outcomes of cytomegalovirus disease in solid organ transplant recipients. Am J Transplant 2013;13:2402-2410.

42. Fischer SA, Lu K. AST Infectious Diseases Community of Practice. Screening of donor and recipient in solid organ transplantation. Am J Transplant 2013;13(Suppl 4):9-21.

43. Duncan AJ, Dummer JS, Paradis IL, et al. Cytomegalovirus infection and survival in lung transplant recipients. J Heart Lung Transplant 1991;10:638-644; discussion 645-646.

44. Palmer SM, Limaye AP, Banks M, et al. Extended valganciclovir prophylaxis to prevent cytomegalovirus after lung transplantation: A randomized, controlled trial. Ann Intern Med 2010;152:761-769.

45. Hammond SP, Martin ST, Roberts K, et al. Cytomegalovirus disease in lung transplantation: Impact of recipient seropositivity and duration of antiviral prophylaxis. Transpl Infect Dis 2013;15:163-170.

46. Boland GJ, Hene RJ, Ververs C, et al. Factors influencing the occurrence of active cytomegalovirus (CMV) infections after organ transplantation. Clin Exp Immunol 1993;94:306-312.

47. Mitsani D, Nguyen MH, Girnita DM, et al. A polymorphism linked to elevated levels of interferon-gamma is associated with an increased risk of cytomegalovirus disease among Caucasian lung transplant recipients at a single center. J Heart Lung Transplant 2011;30:523-529.

48. Humar A, Kumar D, Preiksaitis J, et al. A trial of valganciclovir prophylaxis for cytomegalovirus prevention in lung transplant recipients. Am J Transplant 2005;5:1462-1468.

49. Mitsani D, Nguyen MH, Kwak EJ, et al. Cytomegalovirus disease among donor-positive/recipient-negative lung transplant recipients in the era of valganciclovir prophylaxis. J Heart Lung Transplant 2010;29:1014-1020.

50. Manuel O, Kumar D, Moussa G, et al. Lack of association between beta-herpesvirus infection and bronchiolitis obliterans syndrome in lung transplant recipients in the era of antiviral prophylaxis. Transplantation 2009;87:719-725.

51. Paraskeva M, Bailey M, Levvey BJ, et al. Cytomegalovirus replication within the lung allograft is associated with bronchiolitis obliterans syndrome. Am J Transplant 2011;11:2190-2196.

52. Smith C, Khanna R. Immune regulation of human herpesviruses and its implications for human transplantation. Am J Transplant 2013;13(Suppl 3):9-23; quiz 23.

53. Chaparro C, Maurer JR, Chamberlain D, et al. Causes of death in lung transplant recipients. J Heart Lung Transplant 1994;13:758-766.

54. Chmiel C, Speich R, Hofer M, et al. Ganciclovir/valganciclovir prophylaxis decreases cytomegalovirus-related events and bronchiolitis obliterans syndrome after lung transplantation. Clin Infect Dis 2008;46:831-839.

55. Tamm M, Aboyoun CL, Chhajed PN, et al. Treated cytomegalovirus pneumonia is not associated with bronchiolitis obliterans syndrome. Am J Respir Crit Care Med 2004;170:1120-1123.

56. Bando K, Paradis IL, Similo S, et al. Obliterative bronchiolitis after lung and heart-lung transplantation. An analysis of risk factors and management. J Thorac Cardiovasc Surg, 1995;110:4-13; discussion 13-14.

57. Johansson I, Mårtensson G, Nyström U, et al. Lower incidence of CMV infection and acute rejections with valganciclovir prophylaxis in lung transplant recipients. BMC Infect Dis 2013;13:582.

58. Kotton CN, Kumat D, Caliendo AM, et al. Updated international consensus guidelines on the management of cytomegalovirus in solid-organ transplantation. Transplantation 2013;96:333-360.

59. Zuk DM, Humar A, Weinkauf JG, et al. An international survey of cytomegalovirus management practices in lung transplantation. Transplantation 2010;90:672-676.

60. Zamora MR, Nicolls MR, Hodges TN, et al. Following universal prophylaxis with intravenous ganciclovir and cytomegalovirus immune globulin, valganciclovir is safe and effective for prevention of CMV infection following lung transplantation. Am J Transplant 2004;4:1635-1642.

61. Schoeppler KE, Lyu DM, Grazia TJ, et al. Late-onset cytomegalovirus (CMV) in lung transplant recipients: Can CMV serostatus guide the duration of prophylaxis? Am J Transplant 2013;13:376-382.

62. Manuel O, Husain S, Kumar D, et al. Assessment of cytomegalovirus-specific cell-mediated immunity for the prediction of cytomegalovirus disease in high-risk solid-organ transplant recipients: A multicenter cohort study. Clin Infect Dis 2013;56:817-824.

63. Weseslindtner L, Kerschner H, Steinacher D, et al. Prospective analysis of human cytomegalovirus DNAemia and specific CD8+ T cell responses in lung transplant recipients. Am J Transplant 2012;12:2172-2180.

64. Westall GP, Mifsud NA, Kotsimbos T. Linking CMV serostatus to episodes of CMV reactivation following lung transplantation by measuring CMV-specific CD8+ T-cell immunity. Am J Transplant 2008;8:1749-1754.

65. Asberg A, Humar A, Rollag H, et al. Oral valganciclovir is noninferior to intravenous ganciclovir for the treatment of cytomegalovirus disease in solid organ transplant recipients. Am J Transplant 2007;7:2106-2013.

66. Kiser TH, Fish DN, Zamora MR. Evaluation of valganciclovir pharmacokinetics in lung transplant recipients. J Heart Lung Transplant 2012;31:159-166.

67. Minces LR, Nguyen MN, Mitsani D, et al. Ganciclovir-resistant cytomegalovirus infections among lung transplant recipients are associated with poor outcomes despite treatment with foscarnet-containing regimens. Antimicrob Agents Chemother 2014;58:128-135.

68. Marty FM, Winston DJ, Rowley SD, et al. CMX001 to prevent cytomegalovirus disease in hematopoietic-cell transplantation. N Engl J Med 2013;369:1227-1236.

69. Green M, Michaels MG. Epstein-Barr virus infection and posttransplant lymphoproliferative disorder. Am J Transplant 2013;13(Suppl 3):41-54; quiz 54.

70. Bollard CM, Rooney CM, Heslop HE. T-cell therapy in the treatment of post-transplant lymphoproliferative disease. Nat Rev Clin Oncol 2012;9:510-519.

71. Sampaio MS, Cho YW, Qazi Y, et al. Posttransplant malignancies in solid organ adult recipients: An analysis of the U.S. National Transplant Database. Transplantation 2012;94:990-998.

72. Kirk AD, Cherikh WS, Ring M, et al. Dissociation of depletional induction and posttransplant lymphoproliferative disease in kidney recipients treated with alemtuzumab. Am J Transplant 2007;7:2619-2625.

73. Cen O, Longnecker R. Rapamycin reverses splenomegaly and inhibits tumor development in a transgenic model of Epstein-Barr virus–related Burkitt's lymphoma. Mol Cancer Ther 2011;10:679-686.

74. Lee TC, Savoldo B, Rooney CM, et al. Quantitative EBV viral loads and immunosuppression alterations can decrease PTLD incidence in pediatric liver transplant recipients. Am J Transplant 2005; 5:2222-2228.

75. Martin SI, Dodson B, Wheeler B, et al. Monitoring infection with Epstein-Barr virus among sero-mismatch adult renal transplant recipients. Am J Transplant 2011;11:1058-1063.

76. Haque T, Wilkie GM, Jones MM, et al. Allogeneic cytotoxic T-cell therapy for EBV-positive post-transplantation lymphoproliferative disease: Results of a phase 2 multicenter clinical trial. Blood 2007;110:1123-1131.

77. Xu F, Sternberg MR, Kottiri BJ, et al. Trends in herpes simplex virus type 1 and type 2 seroprevalence in the United States. JAMA 2006;296:964-973.

78. Basse G, Mengelle C, Kamar N, et al. Disseminated herpes simplex type-2 (HSV-2) infection after solid-organ transplantation. Infection 2008;36:62-64.

79. Gourishankar S, McDermid JC, Jhangri GS, et al. Herpes zoster infection following solid organ transplantation: Incidence, risk factors and outcomes in the current immunosuppressive era. Am J Transplant 2004;4:108-115.

80. Manuel O, Kumar D, Singer LG, et al. Incidence and clinical characteristics of herpes zoster after lung transplantation. J Heart Lung Transplant 2008;27:11-16.

81. Carby M, Jones A, Burke M, et al. Varicella infection after heart and lung transplantation: A single-center experience. J Heart Lung Transplant 2007;26:399-402.

82. Posfay-Barbe KM, Pittet LF, Scottas C, et al. Varicella-zoster immunization in pediatric liver transplant recipients: Safe and immunogenic. Am J Transplant 2012;12:2974-2985.

83. Razonable RR, Human herpesviruses 6, 7 and 8 in solid organ transplant recipients. Am J Transplant 2013;13(Suppl 3):67-77; quiz 77-78.

84. Costa C, Delsedime L, Solidoro P, et al. Herpesviruses detection by quantitative real-time polymerase chain reaction in bronchoalveolar

lavage and transbronchial biopsy in lung transplant: Viral infections and histopathological correlation. Transplant Proc 2010;42:1270-1274.

85. Lehto JT, Halme M, Tukiainen P, et al. Human herpesvirus-6 and -7 after lung and heart-lung transplantation. J Heart Lung Transplant 2007;26:41-47.

86. Lamoth F, Jayet PY, Aubert JD, et al. Case report: Human herpesvirus 6 reactivation associated with colitis in a lung transplant recipient. J Med Virol 2008;80:1804-1807.

87. Neurohr C, Huppmann P, Leuchte H, et al. Human herpesvirus 6 in bronchalveolar lavage fluid after lung transplantation: A risk factor for bronchiolitis obliterans syndrome? Am J Transplant 2005;5:2982-2991.

88. Pellett PE, Ablashi DV, Ambros PF, et al. Chromosomally integrated human herpesvirus 6: Questions and answers. Rev Med Virol 2012;22:144-155.

89. Mesri EA, Cesarman E, Boshoff C. Kaposi's sarcoma and its associated herpesvirus. Nat Rev Cancer 2010;10:707-719.

90. Frances C, Marcelin AG, Legendre Ch, et al. The impact of preexisting or acquired Kaposi sarcoma herpesvirus infection in kidney transplant recipients on morbidity and survival. Am J Transplant 2009;9:2580-2586.

91. Piselli P, Busnach G, Citterio F, et al. Risk of Kaposi sarcoma after solid-organ transplantation: Multicenter study in 4,767 recipients in Italy, 1970-2006. Transplant Proc 2009;41:1227-1230.

92. Sathy SJ, Martinu T, Youens K, et al. Symptomatic pulmonary allograft Kaposi's sarcoma in two lung transplant recipients. Am J Transplant 2008;8:1951-1956.

93. Pietrosi G, Vizzini G, Pipitone L, et al. Primary and reactivated HHV8 infection and disease after liver transplantation: A prospective study. Am J Transplant 2011;11:2715-2723.

94. Stallone G, Schena A, Infante B, et al. Sirolimus for Kaposi's sarcoma in renal-transplant recipients. N Engl J Med 2005;352:1317-1323.

95. Levitsky J, Doucette K, AST Infectious Diseases Community of Practice. Viral hepatitis in solid organ transplantation. Am J Transplant 2013;13(Suppl 4):147-168.

96. Riezebos-Brilman A, Puchhammer-Stöckl E, van der Weide HY, et al. Chronic hepatitis E infection in lung transplant recipients. J Heart Lung Transplant 2013;32:341-346.

97. Riezebos-Brilman A, Verschuuren EA, van Son WJ, et al. The clinical course of hepatitis E virus infection in patients of a tertiary Dutch hospital over a 5-year period. J Clin Virol 2013;58:509-514.

98. Lee WM. Hepatitis B virus infection. N Engl J Med 1997;337:1733-1745.

99. Poland GA, Jacobson RM. Clinical practice: Prevention of hepatitis B with the hepatitis B vaccine. N Engl J Med 2004;351:2832-2838.

100. Orens JB, Estenne M, Arcasoy S, et al. International guidelines for the selection of lung transplant candidates: 2006 update—a consensus report from the Pulmonary Scientific Council of the International Society for Heart and Lung Transplantation. J Heart Lung Transplant 2006;25:745-755.

101. Weill D, Bendon C, Ciorris PA, et al. A consensus document for the selection of lung transplant candidates: 2014—an update from the Pulmonary Transplantation Council of the International Society for Heart and Lung Transplantation. J Heart Lung Transplant 2015;34:1-15.

102. Dhillon GS, Levitt J, Mallidi H, et al. Impact of hepatitis B core antibody positive donors in lung and heart-lung transplantation: An analysis of the United Network for Organ Sharing Database. Transplantation 2009;88:842-846.

103. Shitrit AB, Kramer MR, Bakal I, Morali G, et al. Lamivudine prophylaxis for hepatitis B virus infection after lung transplantation. Ann Thorac Surg 2006;81:1851-1852.

104. Robertson B, Myers G, Howard C, et al. Classification, nomenclature, and database development for hepatitis C virus (HCV) and related viruses: Proposals for standardization. International Committee on Virus Taxonomy. Arch Virol 1998;143:2493-2503.

105. Dienstag JL, McHutchison JG. American Gastroenterological Association technical review on the management of hepatitis C. Gastroenterology 2006;130:231-264; quiz 214-217.

106. Lauer GM, Walker BD. Hepatitis C virus infection. N Engl J Med 2001;345:41-52.

107. Doucette K, Weinkauf J, Jackson K, Lein D. Survival following lung transplantation is not impacted by hepatitis C infection [abstract]. Am J Transplant 2012;12:472.

108. Sahi H, Zein NN, Mehta AC, et al. Outcomes after lung transplantation in patients with chronic hepatitis C virus infection. J Heart Lung Transplant 2007;26:466-471.

109. Fong TL, Cho YW, Hou L, et al. Outcomes after lung transplantation and practices of lung transplant programs in the United States regarding hepatitis C seropositive recipients. Transplantation 2011;91:1293-1296.

110. Ghany MG, Nelson DR, Strader DB, et al. An update on treatment of genotype 1 chronic hepatitis C virus infection: 2011 practice guideline by the American Association for the Study of Liver Diseases. Hepatology 2011;54:1433-1444.

111. Aggarwal R, Jameel S. Hepatitis E. Hepatology 2011;54:2218-2226.

112. Stoszek SK, Engle RE, Abdel-Hamid M, et al. Hepatitis E antibody seroconversion without disease in highly endemic rural Egyptian communities. Trans R Soc Trop Med Hyg 2006;100:89-94.

113. Haagsma EB, Niesters HG, van den Berg AP, et al. Prevalence of hepatitis E virus infection in liver transplant recipients. Liver Transpl 2009;15:1225-1228.

114. Pischke S, Suneetha PV, Baechlein C, et al. Hepatitis E virus infection as a cause of graft hepatitis in liver transplant recipients. Liver Transpl 2010;16:74-82.

115. Kamar N, Mansuy JM, Cointault O, et al. Hepatitis E virus–related cirrhosis in kidney- and kidney-pancreas-transplant recipients. Am J Transplant 2008;8:1744-1748.

116. Pischke S, Greer M, Hardtke S, et al. Course and treatment of chronic hepatitis E virus infection in lung transplant recipients. Transpl Infect Dis 2014;16:333-339.

117. van der Poel WH, Verschoor R, van der Heide R, et al. Hepatitis E virus sequences in swine related to sequences in humans, The Netherlands. Emerg Infect Dis 2001;7:970-976.

118. Dalton HR, Stableforth W, Thurairajah P, et al. Autochthonous hepatitis E in Southwest England: Natural history, complications and seasonal variation, and hepatitis E virus IgG seroprevalence in blood donors, the elderly and patients with chronic liver disease. Eur J Gastroenterol Hepatol 2008;20:784-790.

119. Gerolami R, Moal V, Picard C, et al. Hepatitis E virus as an emerging cause of chronic liver disease in organ transplant recipients. J Hepatol 2009;50:622-624.

120. Kamar N, Abravanel F, Garrouste C, et al. Three-month pegylated interferon-alpha-2a therapy for chronic hepatitis E virus infection in a haemodialysis patient. Nephrol Dial Transplant 2010;25:2792-2795.

121. Kamar N, Rostaing L, Izopet J. Hepatitis E virus infection in immunosuppressed patients: Natural history and therapy. Semin Liver Dis 2013;33:62-70.

122. Kamar N, Izopet J, Tripon S, et al. Ribavirin for chronic hepatitis E virus infection in transplant recipients. N Engl J Med 2014;370:1111-1120.

123. Pischke S, Hardtke S, Bode U, et al. Ribavirin treatment of acute and chronic hepatitis E: A single-centre experience. Liver Int 2013;33:722-726.

124. Ragni MV, Belle SH, Im K, et al. Survival of human immunodeficiency virus–infected liver transplant recipients. J Infect Dis 2003;188:1412-1420.

125. Stock PG, Roland ME. Evolving clinical strategies for transplantation in the HIV-positive recipient. Transplantation 2007;84:563-571.

126. Blumberg EA, Rogers CC, AST Infectious Diseases Community of Practice. Human immunodeficiency virus in solid organ transplantation. Am J Transplant 2013;13(Suppl 4):169-178.

127. Kim KK, Factor SM. Membranoproliferative glomerulonephritis and plexogenic pulmonary arteriopathy in a homosexual man with acquired immunodeficiency syndrome. Hum Pathol 1987;18:1293-1296.

128. Mehta NJ, Khan IA, Mehta RN, et al. HIV-related pulmonary hypertension: Analytic review of 131 cases. Chest 2000;118:1133-1141.

129. Humbert M, Sitbon O, Chaouat A, et al. Pulmonary arterial hypertension in France: Results from a national registry. Am J Respir Crit Care Med 2006;173:1023-1030.

130. Petrosillo N, Chinello P, Cicalini S. Pulmonary hypertension in individuals with HIV infection. AIDS 2006;20:2128-2129.

131. Bertani A, Grossi P, Vitulo P, et al. Successful lung transplantation in an HIV- and HBV-positive patient with cystic fibrosis. Am J Transplant 2009;9:2190-2196.

132. Frassetto LA, Browne M, Cheng A, et al. Immunosuppressant pharmacokinetics and dosing modifications in HIV-1 infected liver and kidney transplant recipients. Am J Transplant 2007;7:2816-2820.

133. Trofe-Clark J, Lemonovich TL, AST Infectious Diseases Community of Practice. Interactions between anti-infective agents and immunosuppressants in solid organ transplantation. Am J Transplant 2013;13(Suppl 4):318-326.

30

Fungal infections in lung transplantation

MELISSA GITMAN AND ME-LINH LUONG

INTRODUCTION

Invasive fungal infection (IFI) is a serious complication of lung transplantation and is associated with significant morbidity and mortality. When compared with other solid-organ transplant (SOT) recipients, lung transplant recipients are more susceptible to fungal infection. This increased susceptibility to fungal infection stems from continuous and direct contact with the environment, profound immunosuppression, and impaired clearance mechanisms caused by allograft denervation and colonization of the airways by organisms from the upper respiratory tract or native lung in the case of single-lung transplantation.[1] In this setting, infection can occur as a result of contamination from the allograft or the recipient's airway flora and reactivation of a previously acquired latent infection and primary posttransplant infection. The cumulative incidence of IFI in the first year after lung transplantation is approximately 8.6%.[2] Molds account for 70% of IFI after lung transplantation, with *Aspergillus* being the most frequent pathogen.[3] Although observed less frequently, non-*Aspergillus* molds such as *Scedosporium* and *Fusarium*, dematiaceous fungi, fungi of the class Zygomycetes, and various fungi responsible for endemic mycoses are increasingly recognized as emerging pathogens in this population. Yeast infection occurs less frequently than mold infection and mainly involves *Candida* and *Cryptococcus* species.

MOLD

Aspergillus

EPIDEMIOLOGY

Aspergillus infection is the most frequent fungal infection after lung transplantation; it accounts for 73% of all cases of mold infection.[3,4] The 12-month cumulative incidence of invasive aspergillosis (IA) is 4.13%.[3] *Aspergillus fumigatus* is the most common species followed by *Aspergillus flavus*, *Aspergillus niger*, *Aspergillus terreus*, *Aspergillus versicolor*, and others.[3] *Aspergillus* infection generally occurs within the first year after a transplant: however, widespread use of antifungal prophylaxis has caused a shift in the time of onset of IA. Current data suggest that IA occurs later after transplantation, with a median time of occurrence of 10.5 months.[3] Although IA is more frequent within the first year after lung transplantation, reports of infection occurring up to 13 years after lung transplantation exist.[5]

RISK FACTORS

Many factors increase the risk for IA in lung transplant recipients (Table 30.1).

Environmental exposure

Aspergillus is a ubiquitous organism that is found in decaying organic matter. In particular, exposure to airborne fungal conidia can occur during construction or renovation,

Table 30.1 Risk factors for invasive aspergillosis in lung transplant recipients

Environmental and recreational exposure
- Construction or renovation
- Gardening
- Composting
- Farming
- Marijuana use (smoking)

Net state of immunosuppression
- High-dose steroids
- Antilymphocytic therapy
- OKT3
- Cytomegalovirus infection
- Hypogammaglobulemia

Risk factors unique to lung transplantation
- Continuous and direct contact with the environment
- Impaired clearance mechanisms caused by allograft denervation
- Airway colonization before transplantation
- Airway colonization after transplantation
- Single-lung transplantation
- Prolonged ischemia
- Donor-derived infection

gardening, composting, and farming activities. Additionally, tobacco and marijuana can be contaminated with fungi, and recreational and medical marijuana use has been associated with IA.[6] Therefore, lung transplant recipients should be advised to avoid such environmental exposure or wear a mask to minimize inhalation of airborne fungal conidia.

Net state of immunosuppression

The net state of immunosuppression is an important determinant for the subsequent development of IA. High-dose steroids, antilymphocytic therapy, and OKT3 have been associated with increased risk for IA.[7] Hypogammaglobulinemia, which is commonly observed after lung transplantation, increases risk for IA. In a recent study by Florescu and colleagues, patients with severe hypogammaglobulinemia (immunoglobulin G <400 mg/dL) had an 8.19-fold higher risk for IA than did those without hypogammaglobulinemia.[8] Cytomegalovirus (CMV) infection increases the risk for IA, although whether this association is caused by an immunomodulatory effect of CMV itself or CMV is a surrogate marker of severe immunosuppression remains unclear.[9]

Risk factors unique to lung transplant recipients

Lung transplant recipients have several unique risk factors that heighten their risk for IA, including transplantation of a single lung,[10] prolonged anastomotic ischemia,[5] *Aspergillus* colonization (before and after transplantation),[11-13] and infection derived from the donor.[14] *Aspergillus* colonization before transplantation is an important risk factor for the development of IA after transplantation.[11-13] Pretransplant

Aspergillus colonization occurs primarily in patients with cystic fibrosis (CF) and can be observed in up to 60% of lung transplant recipients with CF.[12] Whether transient or remote *Aspergillus* colonization before transplantation increases the risk for posttransplant development of invasive disease is unclear. What is clear, however, is that the presence of *Aspergillus* in the airways at the time of transplantation (as determined by intraoperative culture) is associated with a fourfold increased risk for the posttransplant development of IA.[11]

CLINICAL MANIFESTATION

Four main clinical manifestations of *Aspergillus* infection in lung transplant recipients are recognized: colonization, tracheobronchitis or bronchial anastomotic site infections, pulmonary disease, and disseminated disease.[15]

Aspergillus colonization may occur in up to 46% of lung transplant recipients.[16] In most patients colonization develops within the first 3 months after transplantation.[10] Colonized patients are asymptomatic and the diagnosis is established by culture without evidence of tissue invasion (see the section on diagnosis for details). Although colonization itself is benign, it may lead to complications such as invasive disease[16] or bronchiolitis obliterans syndrome (BOS).[17,18] Posttransplant *Aspergillus* colonization is associated with an 11-fold risk for progression to IA in the absence of prophylaxis.[16] It is also associated with an increased risk for the development of BOS and appears to be associated mainly with small (<3.5 μm) conidia-producing *Aspergillus* species (A. fumigatus, Aspergillus nidulans, A. terreus, and Aspergillus flavipes).[17,18]

Tracheobronchitis aspergillosis (TBA) is an uncommon form of IA that accounts for less than 10% of IA cases. TBA occurs most commonly during the first year after lung transplantation, with a median time of onset of 2.7 months.[10,12] TBA is characterized by local tissue invasion of the trachea, bronchi, or both and endobronchial lesions (such as erythema, ulceration, necrosis, or pseudomembrane formation) along with compatible microbiologic test results.[10,19] Patients are usually asymptomatic but may exhibit increased sputum production, cough, dyspnea, or fever.[10,20] TBA at the site of the bronchial anastomosis is a clinical entity that is unique to lung transplantation and characterized by local infection at the suture line of the bronchial anastomosis (Figure 30.1). The anastomosis is particularly vulnerable to fungal infection in the immediate posttransplant period because of devascularization, which may result in sloughing of necrotic epithelial tissue in the airway lumen, thus creating an environment favorable for fungal growth and local tissue invasion. Diagnosis is difficult because of the lack of symptoms in the early course of the disease. Routine bronchoscopic examination performed early after transplantation may allow detection of asymptomatic anastomotic infection. Overall, TBA is associated with a favorable outcome, although serious complications such as bronchial stenosis, dehiscence, bronchopleural fistula, and fatal hemorrhage have been reported.[10]

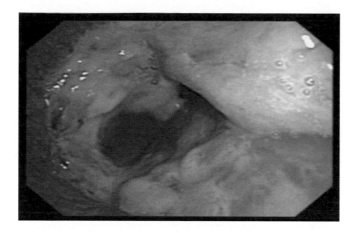

Figure 30.1 Tracheobronchial anastomotic site infection showing ischemic appearance of the tissue.

Invasive pulmonary aspergillosis (IPA) is the most common manifestation and accounts for up to 93% of cases of IA.[3] The median time of onset of IA after lung transplantation is 10.5 months. Patients usually exhibit dyspnea (65%), cough (58%), and sputum production (42%); fever is present in less than one third of patients.[3] Patients with vascular invasion secondary to *Aspergillus* infection may have pleuritic chest pain or hemoptysis secondary to infarction of lung tissue. Historically, IPA in lung transplant recipients was associated with a high mortality rate of 60% to 75%; however, more recent studies have reported a lower mortality rate (22%).[3,21]

If not diagnosed early, *Aspergillus* can spread to other organs. Disseminated disease accounts for 4% of all cases of IA.[3] Extrapulmonary disease can involve any organ, but the central nervous system (CNS) is a site of predilection. CNS aspergillosis is considered the most severe form of IA and is associated with a poor prognosis.[22] Other forms of disseminated disease include skin lesions, gastrointestinal tract infection, osteomyelitis, endocarditis, and endovascular infection.

DIAGNOSIS

Diagnosis of IA is particularly challenging because of the nonspecific symptoms, insensitive and slow conventional diagnostic modalities, and necessity for an invasive procedure to obtain adequate histopathologic specimens.

To standardize the definitions of IFI used in research and clinical trials, the European Organization for Research and Treatment of Cancer/Mycoses Study Group (EORTC/MSG) proposed three levels of probability of IFI: "proven," "probable," and "possible."[23] Proven IFI requires demonstration of fungal invasion identified by histopathologic testing or fungal culture from a normally sterile site. Probable IFI requires that host factors be present and the radiologic and mycologic criteria be met. Patients not meeting the mycologic criteria are considered to have "possible IFI." Radiologic criteria associated with IA include dense, well-circumscribed lesions with or without a halo sign, air-crescent sign, or cavity on a chest computed tomography scan. However, these radiologic criteria are based largely on data

from neutropenic patients[24] and thus may not be applicable to lung transplant recipients. The International Society of Heart and Lung Transplantation (ISHLT) published distinct definitions of IFI in lung transplant recipients that take the unique features of this patient population into account.[19] The guidelines also provide definitions of tracheobronchitis, anastomotic infection, and colonization.

Radiology

Plain chest radiography is neither sensitive nor specific enough to detect pulmonary fungal infection.[10] Chest computed tomography is the modality of choice for assessment of the pulmonary parenchyma. Classically, the presence of IA is heralded by the halo sign (Figure 30.2), which is characterized by a nodular mass lesion surrounded by ground-glass opacity that gives the appearance of a halo sign.[24] The nodular area represents a focus of pulmonary infarction, and the surrounding ground-glass opacity is caused by alveolar hemorrhage. Although this finding is commonly observed in neutropenic patients, it is rarely present in nonneutropenic SOT recipients.[25] In a study assessing radiologic findings in lung transplant recipients with either proven or probable IA, bilateral bronchial wall thickening and centrilobular opacities with a tree-in-bud pattern (Figure 30.3) were the most common findings, whereas nodules (Figure 30.4) or the halo sign were rarely observed.[26] Accordingly, neutropenic patients are more susceptible to angioinvasive disease, whereas nonneutropenic patients (including lung transplant recipients) are less susceptible to angioinvasive disease and more susceptible to the development of airway-invasive disease. Finally, in the setting of suspected nonpulmonary IA, appropriate imaging of the involved organ should be obtained to assess the extent of disease.

Microbiology

Fungal culture is limited by its slow turnaround time and low sensitivity. Obtaining a positive culture may take up to

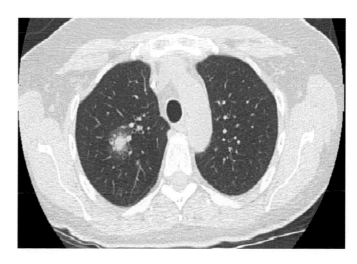

Figure 30.2 Thoracic computed tomography showing a right side nodule surrounded by ground-glass opacity giving the appearance of a "halo."

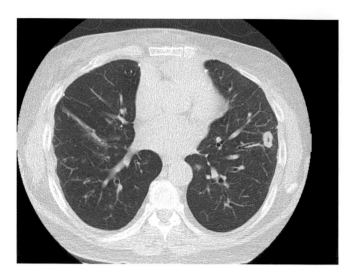

Figure 30.3 Thoracic computed tomography showing bilateral bronchial wall thickening.

14 days. The sensitivity of sputum culture ranges between 8% and 34% and that of bronchoalveolar lavage (BAL) culture is moderately higher (45% to 62%).[27] In an effort to improve the diagnosis of IA, several non–culture-based tests have been developed: galactomannan (GM) tests, the $(1\rightarrow3)$-β-D-glucan (BDG) test, and *Aspergillus* nucleic acid–based assays such as polymerase chain reaction (PCR).

GM is a component of the *Aspergillus* cell wall that is released during fungus growth. Detection of GM by enzyme-linked immunoassay (EIA) in serum precedes the appearance of clinical symptoms and radiologic abnormality by 7 to 8 days.[28] The serum GM assay has proved useful for the diagnosis of IA, particularly in immunocompromised individuals.[29] Although testing based on serum GM is sensitive when used for neutropenic patients with IA (detection rate = 72% to 80%), its performance in nonneutropenic SOT recipients is disappointing.[29] Serum GM has unacceptably low sensitivity for IA in lung transplant recipients (range = 30% to 55%).[30] The rate of detection of GM in BAL fluid is higher than the

rate of detection in serum (82% to 86% with a positivity threshold of 0.5).[31,32] In fact, detection of GM in BAL fluid is deemed more suitable for diagnosis of IA in lung transplant recipients because the sensitivity of the assay in this specific population ranges between 77% and 100% (a positivity threshold of 0.5).[33-35] One drawback of the GM assay is the occurrence of false-positive results caused by fungus genetically similar to *Aspergillus* (such as *Penicillium*, *Paecilomyces*, and *Alternaria*), which lowers its specificity. Increasing the cutoff value from 0.5 to 1.0 or higher improves the test's specificity without compromising its sensitivity.[34-36] However, one study reported significantly decreased sensitivity when a higher cutoff value is used.[33] Hence, the optimal positivity threshold value for GM in BAL fluid remains uncertain. Additionally, administration of antifungals before testing is associated with an increased risk for false-negative results because it lowers the fungal burden.[33]

BDG is another polysaccharide that is present in the fungal cell wall and released as the fungus grows. BDG is present in the cell wall of many fungal organisms, including *Candida* species, other molds (with the exception of Zygomycetes, *Blastomyces dermatitidis*, and *Cryptococcus* species), and *Pneumocystis* species; therefore, BDG is not specific to IA. Detection of BDG in serum by EIA has been used for the diagnosis of IFI with moderate accuracy.[37] Serial monitoring of serum BDG in lung transplant recipients has been demonstrated to provide marginal accuracy, with a sensitivity and specificity of 71% and 59%, respectively.[38]

Nucleic acid–based testing (*Aspergillus* PCR protocols) is also available for the diagnosis of IA. Until recently, however, PCR testing suffered from a lack of standardization that resulted in extensive interlaboratory variability of test performance.[39] Thus, nucleic acid–based assays are not included in the EORTC/MSG microbiologic criteria.[23] Recently, two standardized PCR assays targeting the *18S RNA* gene have been introduced: the mycAssay (Mycanostica, Manchester, United Kingdom) and the *Aspergillus* PCR Panel (Viracor-IBT Laboratories, Lee's Summit, Missouri). The use of the Viracor *Aspergillus* PCR in BAL samples for the diagnosis of IA among lung transplant recipients was found to be highly sensitive (100%) in one study.[33] Overall, nucleic acid–based tests appear promising but need further validation before they can be incorporated into routine clinical use.

TREATMENT

Management of IA requires a twofold approach: reduction of immunosuppression and selection of an appropriate antifungal agent. The choice of antifungal drug should be based on efficacy as well as toxicity, with consideration for the patient's comorbid conditions. Attention should be paid to special circumstances. For instance, tracheobronchitis requires bronchoscopic débridement and inhaled antifungal therapy in addition to systemic therapy. If dehiscence of the anastomosis occurs, such patients may need surgical intervention with stent placement. Although no evidence supports its use, combination inhaled and systemic antifungal therapy has been proposed.

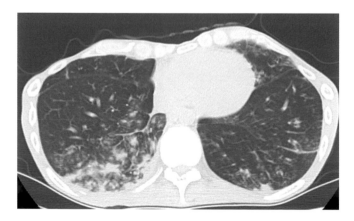

Figure 30.4 Thoracic computed tomography showing multiple pulmonary nodules (predominant on the right side) surrounded by ground-glass opacities (halo sign).

Voriconazole

Voriconazole is the recommended treatment of IA.[40] Voriconazole results in a better clinical response than conventional amphotericin B does.[41] It is available in intravenous and oral formulations, which facilitates continuation of treatment in the outpatient setting. Voriconazole is metabolized by hepatic cytochrome P-450 2C19 (CYP2C19), CYP2C9, and CYP3A4 and is notoriously associated with drug-drug interactions. Specifically, voriconazole inhibits the metabolism of calcineurin inhibitors (CNIs), and if the latter is not adjusted, high potentially toxic CNI serum levels will occur. Hence, a 50% reduction in the CNI dose is required at the start of voriconazole therapy. Common side effects include visual disturbances (20%), hepatic enzyme abnormalities (12% to 20%), and photosensitivity (8% to 10%).[42] High rates of voriconazole-associated hepatotoxicity have been reported in lung transplant recipients, with the incidence ranging between 34% and 60%[43-45]; therefore, careful monitoring of liver enzymes throughout therapy should be ensured. Periostitis is an infrequent adverse effect associated with prolonged voriconazole exposure.[46] It is characterized by inflammation of the cortical layer of the bones and diffuse pain associated with elevated alkaline phosphatase. Periostitis is thought to be caused by accumulation of fluoride (contained in voriconazole) and deposition in the bone cortex, thus resulting in inflammation of the periosteum. Diagnosis is made by demonstration of a periosteal reaction on a plain bone radiograph or bone scan. Resolution of symptoms occurs with discontinuation of voriconazole. Finally, recent studies have linked voriconazole to increased risk for cutaneous malignancies, particularly squamous cell carcinoma.[47-49] In these studies, prolonged voriconazole exposure, residence in a sun-exposed area, age, and history of skin cancer increased the risk for skin malignancies.

Voriconazole metabolism is subject to significant variability because of drug-drug interactions, underlying liver disease, and pharmacogenetic variations in CYP2C19, which in turn leads to variations in levels of the drug. Low serum levels of voriconazole have been associated with poor outcomes in patients with IA, whereas high levels have been associated with neurotoxicity.[50,51] Some experts recommend therapeutic drug monitoring (TDM) of voriconazole, with target serum levels between 1.0 and 5.5 mg/L to optimize clinical response and minimize toxicity.[50] Although a number of studies have examined the role of TDM in patients with hematologic malignancy, few studies have addressed the role of TDM in lung transplant recipients. To date, one study has assessed the efficacy of voriconazole prophylaxis in lung transplant recipients and found that a serum level of voriconazole greater than 1.0 mg/L is associated with fewer occurrences of breakthrough IFI and fewer instances of fungal colonization during prophylaxis.[52] No study has assessed the utility of TDM of voriconazole for treatment of IA in lung transplant recipients.

Posaconazole

Posaconazole, a new-generation azole, has demonstrated excellent in vitro activity against *Aspergillus*.[53] Because it is a newer agent, it is less well studied than voriconazole. To date, posaconazole has been used as salvage therapy for patients who are intolerant or unresponsive to first-line therapy. Posaconazole salvage therapy is associated with a response rate of 42% (versus 26% in the control group).[54] Overall, posaconazole has a favorable safety profile, with the main side effects being headache (17%), dry mouth (9%), and dizziness (6%).[55] Posaconazole is a CYP3A4 inhibitor and can thus induce drug interactions with CNIs. Its main limitations are lack of an intravenous formulation, reduced absorption with antacid drugs, and dietary restrictions (including the requirement of a fatty meal for adequate absorption).

Amphotericin B

Conventional amphotericin B and its lipid formulations are considered alternative therapies for IA. Its use is limited by significant adverse effects, including infusion-related reactions and nephrotoxicity (32.5% with the conventional formulation and 14.5% with lipid formulations).[56] The risk for nephrotoxicity is increased by concurrent use of other nephrotoxic drugs, which is usually the case with lung transplant recipients who are receiving CNIs.

Echinocandins

Echinocandins (which include caspofungin, anidulafungin, and micafungin) also demonstrate activity against *Aspergillus*. In general, these compounds have good safety and tolerability profiles. Side effects include headaches (3% to 15%), fever (35%), and elevated liver enzymes (2% to 16%).[57] To date, only one study has assessed the use of caspofungin as primary therapy for IA in heart or lung transplant recipients; it reported a positive response rate of 67%.[58] Because of the limited data on their use as primary therapy for IA, echinocandins are not recommended for this indication but may be used for salvage therapy.[59,60]

Combination therapy

Increasing data support the use of combination antifungal therapy for the treatment of IA. The combination of voriconazole and caspofungin for primary treatment of IA has resulted in a trend toward better survival than with liposomal amphotericin B.[59] The combination of voriconazole and caspofungin for IA in lung transplant recipients has yielded good response, although the retrospective and noncomparative design of this study limits interpretation of its results.[61] Finally, in a recent randomized controlled trial, the combination of voriconazole and anidulafungin as primary therapy for IA in patients with hematologic malignancies did not provide any survival benefit when compared with voriconazole monotherapy.[62] However, combination therapy was associated with a trend toward better clinical outcomes, particularly in patients who tested positive for GM in their serum.

PROPHYLAXIS

Given the risk for the development of IA following lung transplantation and the significant morbidity associated with it, many lung transplant centers implement preventive measures. Two strategies exist: universal or preemptive prophylaxis. The preemptive prophylaxis strategy targets therapy toward patients deemed at high risk for the development of IA. A recent worldwide survey reported that 58.6% of lung transplant centers use universal prophylaxis within the first 6 months after transplantation whereas 36.2% opt for preemptive prophylaxis.[63] Voriconazole, either alone or in combination with inhaled amphotericin, is the most commonly administered agent. Only 5.2% of centers do not provide any form of antifungal prophylaxis. The efficacy of antifungal prophylaxis following lung transplantation has been evaluated in several small single-center studies. Unfortunately, these studies are limited by their small sample size, retrospective design, different antifungal regimens, local practices, and epidemiologic bias. A recent meta-analysis assessed the efficacy of antifungal prophylaxis for prevention of IA after lung transplantation and found no significant reduction in IA when prophylaxis is used.[64] Consequently, the efficacy of antifungal prophylaxis to prevent IA in lung transplant recipients remains uncertain.

Non-*Aspergillus* mold

SCEDOSPORIUM

The genus *Scedosporium* consists of four medically important species: *Scedosporium apiospermum*, *Scedosporium boydii*, *Scedosporium aurantiacum*, and *Scedosporium prolificans*. *Scedosporium* is a ubiquitous saprophytic mold that can be recovered from polluted water, soil, and decaying vegetation. Like *Aspergillus*, *Scedosporium* can colonize or infect the sinus or respiratory airways of individuals with underlying lung disease such as bronchiectasis, sarcoidosis, tuberculosis, and CF. *Scedosporium* can be found in cultures of sputum obtained from up to 8% of patients with CF, thus putting them at greater risk for invasive disease after lung transplantation.[65,66]

Overall, *Scedosporium* infection accounts for 27% of cases of mold infection in lung transplant recipients and occurs at a median of 12 months after lung transplantation.[3] *Scedosporium* is associated with various conditions, such as colonization, mycetoma, sinopulmonary disease, and disseminated disease with CNS involvement.[67] Approximately 50% of cases of scedosporiosis in SOT recipients are disseminated.[68] The clinical symptoms, radiologic findings, and histopathologic features of *Scedosporium* infection are indistinguishable from those characterizing *Aspergillus*, but unlike *Aspergillus*, *Scedosporium* is resistant to many antifungal agents and is thus associated with high rates of therapeutic failure and relapses.[67]

Scedosporium species are inherently resistant to amphotericin and flucytosine but display variable susceptibility to itraconazole, voriconazole, posaconazole, and micafungin. Voriconazole is the agent most active against *Scedosporium* species and is frequently used alone or in combination with other antifungal agents.[69] *Scedosporium prolificans* is particularly resistant to most antifungal agents; however, the combination of voriconazole and terbinafine appears to be synergistic in vitro, and good clinical outcomes have been reported with its use.[70,71] Reduction of immunosuppression and surgical excision of localized disease should be considered whenever possible. Overall, the prognosis of *Scedosporium* infection is poor, with the mortality rate ranging from 54% to 78% or even higher in cases of dissemination.[68]

FUSARIUM

Fusarium is another ubiquitous saprophytic fungus; it is found in soil and decaying vegetation but can also be pathogenic in certain plants. More than 50 *Fusarium* species have been identified but only 12 have been associated with human disease. Most *Fusarium* species associated with infection in humans are classified within two species complexes that are typically referred to as single species, *Fusarium solani* (50% of cases) and *Fusarium oxysporum* (20% of cases).[72]

Fusariosis is emerging as a serious opportunistic infection in patients with neutropenia or after hematopoietic stem cell transplantation but is rarely seen in SOT recipients.[3,73] Infection is acquired by direct inoculation or inhalation. Clinical symptoms depend largely on the host's immune status and portal of entry. *Fusarium* causes a wide variety of clinical disease ranging from superficial infection to locally invasive infection to deep-seated infection.[74] In immunocompetent individuals, *Fusarium* can cause onychomycosis and keratitis. Semi-invasive infection can lead to breakdown of the skin or mucosal barrier and appears as contact lens–associated keratitis or wound infection following a burn injury or local penetrating trauma. In immunocompromised individuals, *Fusarium* can cause invasive disseminated disease. Neutropenic patients are particularly susceptible to disseminated disease with fungemia and pulmonary and skin involvement. To date, only nine cases of *Fusarium* infection in lung transplant recipients have been reported[75]; they all exhibited pulmonary involvement, and disseminated disease developed in two. *Fusarium* fungemia is reported in 40% to 50% of cases of disseminated infection.[76] The clinical symptoms and radiologic and histopathologic findings are indistinguishable from those of infection caused by other hyalohyphomycosis. Thus, identification must be performed by fungal culture or molecular-based assays. The presence of banana-shaped multicellular macroconidia on fungal culture provides a diagnosis of *Fusarium* infection, but identification to the species level requires molecular-based assays.

Locally invasive disease should be treated by surgical débridement and antifungal therapy. Invasive disease requires antifungal therapy, although the optimal agent remains uncertain. Typically, *Fusarium* species demonstrate relative resistance to most antifungal agents. Different species have different susceptibility patterns: *F. solani* complex and *Fusarium verticilloides* are resistant to all azoles and display high minimum inhibitory concentrations to amphotericin; *F. oxysporum* and *Fusarium moniliforme* appear to be susceptible to voriconazole and posaconazole.[74] Thus, identification to the species level and antifungal susceptibility testing should be performed to guide antifungal therapy. Voriconazole and amphotericin B are the agents of choice.[71] The prognosis of fusariosis is directly related to the host's immune status, with high mortality in patients with profound neutropenia. In lung transplant recipients, fusariosis is associated with a high mortality rate (67%).[75]

Dematiaceous molds

Dematiaceous molds contain melanin pigment in the fungal cell wall, which confers a darker color to fungal cultures. This heterogeneous group contains a wide variety of organisms, including *Cladosporium, Dactylaria, Cladophialophora, Phialophora, Exserohilum, Scopulariopsis, Alternaria, Curvularia, Bipolaris, Ochroconis,* and *Exophiala.* These organisms can cause opportunistic infection in immunocompromised hosts and tend to occur later after transplantation than other opportunistic mold infection does.[77]

Like other molds, dematiaceous molds can cause semiinvasive skin and soft tissue disease (mycetoma and chromoblastomycosis), deep tissue disease with sinopulmonary involvement, or disseminated disease with CNS involvement. Case reports of disease caused by *Cladophialophora, Ochroconis, Exophiala,* and other organisms have been reported in SOT recipients.[78] As with other molds, diagnosis is obtained through a combination of direct microscopy, culture, and histology.

Treatment involves a combination of surgical débridement and systemic antifungal therapy. No standardized therapies exist, but voriconazole, posaconazole, and itraconazole are the agents most active against this group of fungi.[79] Itraconazole is the drug of choice because of the extensive clinical experience with it. Voriconazole may presumably be superior for CNS infection because of its better penetration of cerebrospinal fluid (CSF).

Zygomycosis

Zygomycosis (previously called mucormycosis) is a rare but very aggressive infection. The class Zygomycetes encompasses more than 20 genera, including the following medically important genera: *Rhizopus, Rhizomucor, Mucor, Cunninghamella,* and *Lichtheimia* (previously classified as *Absidia*). Zygomycosis accounts for 2.1% of cases of mold infection in lung transplant recipients and occurs with a median time of onset of 26 months after transplantation.[3] Risk factors for zygomycosis include diabetes, renal failure, malnutrition, iron overload, corticosteroids use, previous rejection, use of thymoglobulin, extremes of age, and

prophylaxis with voriconazole or caspofungin (which are not active against these fungi).[80]

Classically, fungi of the class Zygomycetes cause severe invasive rhinocerebral and sinocerebral disease. Pulmonary involvement is frequent in lung transplant recipients.[81,82] Diagnosis is established by histopathologic examination or fungal culture demonstrating broad, aseptate, ribbon-like hyphae. Of note, fungi of the class Zygomycetes do not possess BDG or GM in their cell wall; consequently, negative BDG and GM test results do not preclude zygomycosis.[83]

Because zygomycosis is a highly aggressive disease, adequate therapy should be initiated as soon as the diagnosis is suspected. Delayed therapy is associated with a fivefold increase in mortality in patients with hematologic diseases.[84] Liposomal amphotericin B (5 mg/kg/day) is the drug of choice for the treatment of zygomycosis.[85] Posazonazole demonstrates good activity against this pathogen and can be used as a step-down therapy once a clinical response has been well documented. Posaconazole can also be used as salvage therapy.[86] Echinocandins are not active against fungi of the class Zygomycetes; however, synergistic activity with polyenes has been demonstrated in an animal model.[87] The combination of a lipid formulation of amphotericin B and caspofungin was associated with better survival than was polyene monotherapy in one retrospective study.[88] Adjunctive therapy with iron depletion chelators may be of benefit, although their efficacy remains uncertain.[85,89] Surgical débridement is a key component in the management of zygomycosis and should be performed whenever feasible. Overall, zygomycosis portends a poor prognosis, with a mortality rate approaching 50% in SOT recipients.[90]

Endemic mycosis

Histoplasmosis, blastomycosis, and coccidioidomycosis are endemic mycoses that are prevalent in restricted geographic areas. Infection can occur in immunocompetent and immunocompromised individuals. Endemic mycoses infrequently occur after transplantation, with a low incidence of only 0.2% in SOT recipients.[91] The disease may occur as primary infection, reactivation of latent infection, or donor-derived infection.

HISTOPLASMOSIS

Histoplasmosis is caused by two human pathogenic strains: *Histoplasma capsulatum* var. *capsulatum,* which is found in the Ohio and Mississippi river valleys in North America as well as in South America, and *Histoplasma capsulatum* var. *duboisii,* which is found in Africa.[92] *H. capsulatum* is found in soil and is often associated with bat guano or bird droppings. Disruption of soil as a result of excavation or construction can release infectious elements that are subsequently inhaled. Posttransplant histoplasmosis in SOT recipients is rare, with a reported incidence of 0.10%.[91] The median time to diagnosis is 27 months after transplantation.[93] In immunocompetent individuals, histoplasmosis is asymptomatic or characterized by symptoms of mild pulmonary disease.

In contrast, in SOT recipients, histoplasmosis causes moderate to severe pneumonia and progression to disseminated disease in 81% of cases.[93] The overall rate of histoplasmosis mortality in SOT recipients is 19%, but it may be higher with disseminated disease. Diagnosis can be achieved by several diagnostic methods: histopathologic examination, fungal culture, antigen detection (in urine or in serum), and serologic testing. Identification of small (2 to 6 μm) narrow-necked budding yeasts by histopathologic examination confirms the diagnosis. Histoplasmosis is fastidious and grows slowly in fungal culture (up to 6 weeks may be required). Detection of histoplasmosis antigen (in urine or serum) by EIA is a rapid and highly sensitive method for diagnosing disseminated disease; the assay is most sensitive (93%) with urine samples.[93] Antigen detection assays have a specificity of 99%; however cross-reactivity commonly occurs with other endemic mycoses.[94,95] Serologic testing is not useful for the diagnosis of acute infection, but seroconversion or a fourfold rise in titer is indicative of recent infection.[95] Lipid formulations of amphotericin B (3 to 5 mg/kg/day) are recommended for the treatment of severe disease; they should be continued for at least 2 weeks or until clinical improvement and followed by oral itraconazole therapy for at least 12 months.[96] Patients with mild to moderate disease can be treated with itraconazole for 6 to 12 weeks. TDM of itraconazole (aiming for serum levels >1 mg/L) is recommended to ensure adequate drug exposure. Relapse occurs in 6% of cases and usually within the first 2 years.[93] The concentration of *Histoplasma* antigen should be less than 2 ng/mL before therapy is stopped, and it should be monitored for at least 12 months after treatment has been discontinued.[96] The effectiveness of prophylaxis in SOT recipients with a history of histoplasmosis is not well established. Current guidelines recommend itraconazole prophylaxis for patients who have recovered from active histoplasmosis infection during the 2 years before initiation of immunosuppression.[95] Routine pretransplant screening is not recommended.

BLASTOMYCOSIS

Blastomycosis is the clinical syndrome caused by *Blastomyces dermatitidis,* which is distributed in the Upper Midwest, Great Lakes region, South Central states and St. Lawrence River area in North America.[97] Blastomycosis in SOT recipients is rare, with an incidence of only 0.14%.[95] Like histoplasmosis, blastomycosis typically involves a spectrum of illness ranging from mild acute pneumonia to severe pneumonia, which may progress to fulminant infection with multiorgan failure. Extrapulmonary involvement is reported in 25% to 40% of those infected and can be manifested as cutaneous, osteoarticular, genitourinary, or CNS disease.[98] Immunocompromised individuals often have severe pneumonia or disseminated disease.[91,99] To date, the largest series of blastomycosis in SOT recipients has included 11 patients (1 lung transplant recipient).[97] Most patients had severe pneumonia, and disseminated disease with cutaneous involvement developed in one third of them. The overall mortality rate in SOT recipients is 36%.

Diagnostic modalities are similar to those for histoplasmosis and include histopathologic analysis, fungal culture, antigen detection (in urine and in serum), and serologic testing. Identification of large (8 to 15 μm) broad-based budding yeasts by histopathologic analysis confirms the diagnosis. Like fungal culture for histoplasmosis, that for blastomycosis is very fastidious and up to 6 weeks may be required for a positive result. Detection of blastomycosis antigen in serum or urine is also possible and may be useful for providing a rapid diagnosis. The sensitivity and specificity of detection of blastomycosis antigen in urine are 90% and 99%, respectively.[100] However, cross-reactivity with histoplasmosis is common.[101] The recommended treatment of immunocompromised individuals with blastomycosis is a lipid formulation of amphotericin (3 to 5 mg/kg/day for 1 to 2 weeks or until clinical improvement, with longer duration in cases involving CNS disease).[95,98] Once a clinical response has been achieved, step-down therapy can be continued with oral itraconazole (200 mg three times per day for 3 days followed by 200 mg twice daily for at least 12 months). The effectiveness of monitoring of blastomycosis antigen as a guide to the duration of therapy has not been established.[95] Relapse is rare.[97,99] Pretransplant screening and antifungal prophylaxis after transplantation are not recommended.

COCCIDIOIDOMYCOSIS

Coccidioides is found in the soil of arid desert areas of the southwestern United States, including California, Arizona, New Mexico, Texas, Utah, and northern Mexico. Coccidioidomycosis is caused by two species, *Coccidioides immitis,* which is endemic to California, and *Coccidioides posadasii,* which is found in Arizona and New Mexico. Infection is acquired through inhalation of dust-borne infectious arthroconidia. In SOT recipients, the incidence of posttransplant coccidioidomycosis ranges from 1.4% to 6.9%.[95] The majority of cases (70%) occur within the first year after transplantation, thus suggesting that most cases of infection result from reactivation of previous infection.[102] Primary infection can occur in patients who have traveled, even briefly, to an endemic area.[103] Albeit rare, donor-derived infection has been reported.[104] Risk factors for posttransplant coccidioidomycosis include a history of infection, serologic test results positive for positive *Coccidioides* before transplantation, and treatment for acute rejection.[105] In immunocompetent individuals, coccidioidomycosis is asymptomatic or self-limited in 60% of cases.[106] Symptomatic disease includes pneumonia and may be associated with myalgia, maculopapular rash, or arthralgia. Atypical manifestations and disseminated disease occur in 1% to 5% of infected individuals. The clinical symptoms of coccidioidomycosis in immunocompromised hosts are similar to those in immunocompetent individuals; however, atypical symptoms and disseminated disease involving the skin, skeleton, and meninges are encountered more frequently (in 30% to 75% of cases).[105] The overall mortality rate in SOT recipients is 30%. The diagnosis can be made by histopathologic analysis, fungal culture, serologic testing, or antigen detection by EIA. Identification of characteristic spherules by histopathologic analysis or positive fungal culture (with intercalated arthroconidia) is diagnostic for coccidioidomycosis. Unfortunately, such diagnostic modalities perform poorly in SOT recipients (sensitivity of 75% and 33%, respectively).[107] Serologic testing is a highly sensitive method for diagnosis of coccidioidomycosis in immunocompetent individuals; however, its sensitivity is significantly lower in SOT recipients and ranges from 10% to 45%.[107,108] A meticulous search for extrapulmonary involvement (with lumbar puncture to exclude meningeal involvement) should be performed even in patients with presumed localized disease. Fungal culture of CSF is insensitive: only 15% of patients with coccidioidomycosis meningitis have a positive culture.[109] Serologic testing by complement fixation should be performed on CSF to increase sensitivity. The recommended treatment of severe or disseminated infection is a lipid formulation of amphotericin B (1.5 to 5 mg/kg/day) or high-dose fluconazole (800 mg daily) until improvement occurs. Step-down therapy with fluconazole should be continued for at least 12 months or until the infection has resolved, whichever takes longer.[110] Mild to moderate infection can be treated with fluconazole. Lifelong fluconazole prophylaxis is recommended for all SOT recipients with coccidioidomycosis to prevent relapse.[95] Transplant candidates with previous exposure to coccidioidomycosis (either by travel history, medical history, or positive serologic test results) are at risk for reactivation after transplantation and should receive fluconazole prophylaxis (400 mg daily for 6 to 12 months or for life) to reduce the risk for reactivation.[95]

YEAST

Candida

Candida species are responsible for 23% of all IFI in lung transplant recipients.[4] Many Candida species can cause human disease, but most infection is caused by Candida albicans (66%), followed by Candida glabrata, Candida parapsilosis, Candida tropicalis, and Candida krusei. Risk factors for invasive candidiasis (IC) include the use of broad-spectrum antibiotics, lengthy antibiotic therapy, presence of central venous catheters, and necessity of renal replacement therapy. Colonization with Candida is a risk factor for anastomotic infection and candidemia.

Candidiasis is usually a nosocomial infection that occurs early after transplantation (median time of onset, 25 days).[111] Clinical manifestations range from mucocutaneous involvement to deep organ (eye, spleen, and heart valves) seeding. In lung transplant recipients, bronchial anastomotic involvement is the most common manifestation (38%), followed by bloodstream infection (28%) and disseminated disease (13%).[1,111] Recovery of Candida from a respiratory tract culture usually indicates colonization and does not require therapy. Candida pneumonia is extremely rare, and its diagnosis

requires demonstration of tissue invasion by histopathologic examination. The overall mortality rate associated with IC is 40%.[112] The diagnosis of IC is usually established by a positive culture of blood or sterile body fluid. Although earlier studies highlighted the limited sensitivity (50%) of blood culture for detection of IC, new and improved blood culture systems have higher sensitivity (93%) for detection of IC.[113] Serum BDG antigen may be useful for the diagnosis of IC; as mentioned earlier, however, its overall accuracy in lung transplant recipients is marginal.[38]

Patients with IC should receive treatment with an echinocandin until species and antifungal susceptibility have been determined. Once these results become available and clinical improvement has been achieved, therapy can be modified according to the aforementioned tests results.[114] Candida albicans and C. parapsilosis are usually susceptible to fluconazole; C. glabrata demonstrates elevated minimum inhibitory concentrations with fluconazole and requires high-dose fluconazole or an alternative antifungal agent; C. krusei is intrinsically resistant to fluconazole and should be treated with another agent. Alternative agents include echinocandin, amphotericin, and other azoles. Fungemia should be treated for at least 14 days after the first negative blood culture. Disseminated disease requires prolonged therapy until infection is cured.

Cryptococcus

Cryptococcus is an encapsulated yeast that is often found in soil contaminated with bird droppings. Of the 37 species included in the genus, only 2 cause human disease: Cryptococcus neoformans which is distributed worldwide, and Cryptococcus gattii, which can be acquired in the Pacific Northwest in both Canada and the United States, as well as in some parts of Africa and Australia.[115]

The incidence of cryptococcosis in SOT recipients is 2.8%.[116] Cryptococcosis after lung transplantation may be acquired as a result of primary infection, reactivation of latent infection, or donor-derived infection. Disease onset is late, usually beyond 3 years after transplantation.[2] Early onset of disease, particularly within 30 days after transplantation, should raise suspicion for donor-derived infection.[117] Cryptococcosis is usually manifested as CNS disease or pneumonia. Pulmonary disease ranges from asymptomatic colonization to severe pneumonia. Other clinical manifestations of cryptococcosis include skin infection, osteoarticular infection, prostatitis, liver disease, kidney disease, or disseminated disease with or without CNS involvement.[116] Approximately 50% to 75% of SOT recipients with pneumonia have concomitant CNS disease that may or may not be asymptomatic. Overall, cryptococcosis in SOT recipients is associated with a mortality rate between 15% and 49%, depending on the extent of disease.[116]

Determining the site and extent of disease is essential when evaluating patients with suspected cryptococcosis. Brain imaging should be performed before lumbar puncture to determine the presence of mass lesions or hydrocephalus.

Disseminated disease should always be excluded with a lumbar puncture and blood and urine cultures. The diagnosis of cryptococcosis can be obtained by histopathologic analysis, direct microscopic examination of specimens stained with India ink, fungal culture, or detection of cryptococcal antigen in the serum or CSF. Identification of oval narrow-based budding yeast cells of variable size (2 to 15 μm) in tissue subjected to histopathologic examination is suggestive of cryptococcosis. In patients with cryptococcal meningitis, direct microscopy of samples stained with India ink, fungal culture, and detection of cryptococcal antigen in serum and CSF have a sensitivity of 59%, 92%, 93%, and 94%, respectively.[118] Serum cryptococcal antigen assay is highly sensitive in patients with cryptococcal meningitis; however, its sensitivity is much lower in those with localized pulmonary disease.[119] Lung transplant recipients with isolated pulmonary disease tend to have lower levels of cryptococcal antigen or none at all.[119]

Patients with CNS involvement and disseminated or severe pulmonary infection should be treated with liposomal amphotericin (3 to 4 mg/kg/day) and flucytosine (100 mg/kg/day divided into four doses) for at least 2 weeks or until clinical improvement. Once the patient improves, therapy can be stepped down to fluconazole (400 to 800 mg daily for 6 to 12 months). Patients with mild pulmonary infection may be treated with fluconazole (400 to 800 mg daily for 6 to 12 months).[120] Relapse is uncommon. Whenever possible, reduction of immunosuppression should be attempted. However, rapid reduction of immunosuppression may cause rejection or lead to immune reconstitution inflammatory syndrome (IRIS).[121] IRIS is manifested as worsening of disease despite adequate therapy in the absence of microbiologic resistance, and it usually occurs 4 to 6 weeks after initiation of therapy. IRIS develops in approximately 5% to 11% of SOT recipients with cryptococcosis. No laboratory marker for IRIS exists. Antifungal therapy should be continued in conjunction with additional anti-inflammatory therapy with a corticosteroid.[122]

CONCLUSION

Despite advances in understanding of the biology and epidemiology of fungal pathogens, improvement in diagnostic modalities, and introduction of new more efficacious therapeutic agents, IFI remains an important cause of morbidity and mortality after lung transplantation. An in-depth understanding of the epidemiology of the fungal pathogen, careful assessment of patient risk factors and clinical symptoms, judicious use of diagnostic tests, and early initiation of appropriate therapy are the key elements to improve outcome associated with IFI in lung transplant recipients.

REFERENCES

1. Husain S. Unique characteristics of fungal infections in lung transplant recipients. Clin Chest Med 2009;30:307-313, vii.
2. Pappas PG, Alexander BD, Andes DR, et al. Invasive fungal infections among organ transplant recipients: Results of the Transplant-Associated Infection Surveillance Network (TRANSNET). Clin Infect Dis 2010;50:1101-1111.
3. Doligalski CT, Benedict K, Cleveland AA, et al. Epidemiology of invasive mold infections in lung transplant recipients. Am J Transplant 2014;14:1328-1333.
4. Neofytos D, Fishman JA, Horn D, et al. Epidemiology and outcome of invasive fungal infections in solid organ transplant recipients. Transpl Infect Dis 2010;12:220-229.
5. Iversen M, Burton CM, Vand S, et al. Aspergillus infection in lung transplant patients: Incidence and prognosis. Eur J Clin Microbiol Infect Dis 2007;26:879-886.
6. Gargani Y, Bishop P, Denning DW. Too many mouldy joints—marijuana and chronic pulmonary aspergillosis. Mediterr J Hematol Infect Dis 2011;3:e2011005.
7. Issa NC, Fishman JA. Infectious complications of antilymphocyte therapies in solid organ transplantation. Clin Infect Dis 2009;48:772-786.
8. Florescu DF, Kalil AC, Qiu F, et al. What is the impact of hypogammaglobulinemia on the rate of infections and survival in solid organ transplantation? A meta-analysis. Am J Transplant 2013;13:2601-2610.
9. Husni RN, Gordon SM, Longworth DL, et al. Cytomegalovirus infection is a risk factor for invasive aspergillosis in lung transplant recipients. Clin Infect Dis 1998;26:753-755.
10. Singh N, Husain S. Aspergillus infections after lung transplantation: Clinical differences in type of transplant and implications for management. J Heart Lung Transplant 2003;22:258-266.
11. Luong ML, Chaparro C, Stephenson A, et al. Pretransplant Aspergillus colonization of cystic fibrosis patients and the incidence of post–lung transplant invasive aspergillosis. Transplantation 2014;97:351-357.
12. Helmi M, Love RB, Welter D, et al. Aspergillus infection in lung transplant recipients with cystic fibrosis: Risk factors and outcomes comparison to other types of transplant recipients. Chest 2003;123:800-808.
13. Nunley DR, Ohori P, Grgurich WF, et al. Pulmonary aspergillosis in cystic fibrosis lung transplant recipients. Chest 1998;114:1321-1329.
14. Ruiz I, Gavalda J, Monforte V, et al. Donor-to-host transmission of bacterial and fungal infections in lung transplantation. Am J Transplant 2006;6:178-182.
15. Sole A, Salavert M. Fungal infections after lung transplantation. Curr Opin Pulm Med 2009;15:243-253.

16. Cahill BC, Hibbs JR, Savik K, et al. *Aspergillus* airway colonization and invasive disease after lung transplantation. Chest 1997;112:1160-1164.

17. Weigt SS, Elashoff RM, Huang C, et al. *Aspergillus* colonization of the lung allograft is a risk factor for bronchiolitis obliterans syndrome. Am J Transplant 2009;9:1903-1911.

18. Weigt SS, Copeland CA, Derhovanessian A, et al. Colonization with small conidia *Aspergillus* species is associated with bronchiolitis obliterans syndrome: A two-center validation study. Am J Transplant 2013;13:919-927.

19. Husain S, Mooney ML, Danziger-Isakov L, et al. A 2010 working formulation for the standardization of definitions of infections in cardiothoracic transplant recipients. J Heart Lung Transplant 2011;30:361-374.

20. Karnak D, Avery RK, Gildea TR, et al. Endobronchial fungal disease: An under-recognized entity. Respiration 2007;74:88-104.

21. Steinbach WJ, Marr KA, Anaissie EJ, et al. Clinical epidemiology of 960 patients with invasive aspergillosis from the PATH Alliance registry. J Infect 2012;65:453-464.

22. Lin SJ, Schranz J, Teutsch SM. Aspergillosis case-fatality rate: Systematic review of the literature. Clin Infect Dis 2001;32:358-366.

23. De Pauw B, Walsh TJ, Donnelly JP, et al. Revised definitions of invasive fungal disease from the European Organization for Research and Treatment of Cancer/Invasive Fungal Infections Cooperative Group and the National Institute of Allergy and Infectious Diseases Mycoses Study Group (EORTC/MSG) Consensus Group. Clin Infect Dis 2008;46:1813-1821.

24. Greene RE, Schlamm HT, Oestmann JW, et al. Imaging findings in acute invasive pulmonary aspergillosis: Clinical significance of the halo sign. Clin Infect Dis 2007;44:373-379.

25. Park SY, Kim SH, Choi SH, et al. Clinical and radiological features of invasive pulmonary aspergillosis in transplant recipients and neutropenic patients. Transpl Infect Dis 2010;12:309-315.

26. Gazzoni FF, Hochhegger B, Severo LC, et al. High-resolution computed tomographic findings of *Aspergillus* infection in lung transplant patients. Eur J Radiol 2014;83:79-83.

27. Patterson JE. Epidemiology of fungal infections in solid organ transplant patients. Transpl Infect Dis 1999;1:229-236.

28. Sulahian A, Boutboul F, Ribaud P, et al. Value of antigen detection using an enzyme immunoassay in the diagnosis and prediction of invasive aspergillosis in two adult and pediatric hematology units during a 4-year prospective study. Cancer 2001;91:311-318.

29. Pfeiffer CD, Fine JP, Safdar N. Diagnosis of invasive aspergillosis using a galactomannan assay: A meta-analysis. Clin Infect Dis 2006;42:1417-1427.

30. Husain S, Kwak EJ, Obman A, et al. Prospective assessment of Platelia *Aspergillus* galactomannan antigen for the diagnosis of invasive aspergillosis in lung transplant recipients. Am J Transplant 2004;4:796-802.

31. Zou M, Tang L, Zhao S, et al. Systematic review and meta-analysis of detecting galactomannan in bronchoalveolar lavage fluid for diagnosing invasive aspergillosis. PloS One 2012;7:e43347.

32. Heng SC, Morrissey O, Chen SC, et al. Utility of bronchoalveolar lavage fluid galactomannan alone or in combination with PCR for the diagnosis of invasive aspergillosis in adult hematology patients: A systematic review and meta-analysis. Crit Rev Microbiol 2015;41:124-134.

33. Luong ML, Clancy CJ, Vadnerkar A, et al. Comparison of an *Aspergillus* real-time polymerase chain reaction assay with galactomannan testing of bronchoalvelolar lavage fluid for the diagnosis of invasive pulmonary aspergillosis in lung transplant recipients. Clin Infect Dis 2011;52:1218-1226.

34. Pasqualotto AC, Xavier MO, Sanchez LB, et al. Diagnosis of invasive aspergillosis in lung transplant recipients by detection of galactomannan in the bronchoalveolar lavage fluid. Transplantation 2010;90:306-311.

35. Husain S, Clancy CJ, Nguyen MH, et al. Performance characteristics of the Platelia *Aspergillus* enzyme immunoassay for detection of *Aspergillus* galactomannan antigen in bronchoalveolar lavage fluid. Clin Vaccine Immunol 2008;15:1760-1763.

36. Clancy CJ, Jaber RA, Leather HL, et al. Bronchoalveolar lavage galactomannan in diagnosis of invasive pulmonary aspergillosis among solid-organ transplant recipients. J Clin Microbiol 2007;45:1759-1765.

37. Karageorgopoulos DE, Vouloumanou EK, Ntziora F, et al. β-D-Glucan assay for the diagnosis of invasive fungal infections: A meta-analysis. Clin Infect Dis 2011;52:750-770.

38. Alexander BD, Smith PB, Davis RD, et al. The (1,3) {beta}-D-glucan test as an aid to early diagnosis of invasive fungal infections following lung transplantation. J Clin Microbiol 2010;48:4083-4088.

39. White PL, Mengoli C, Bretagne S, et al. Evaluation of *Aspergillus* PCR protocols for testing serum specimens. J Clin Microbiol 2011;49:3842-3848.

40. Walsh TJ, Anaissie EJ, Denning DW, et al. Treatment of aspergillosis: Clinical practice guidelines of the Infectious Diseases Society of America. Clin Infect Dis 2008;46:327-360.

41. Herbrecht R, Denning DW, Patterson TF, et al. Voriconazole versus amphotericin B for primary therapy of invasive aspergillosis. N Engl J Med 2002;347:408-415.

42. Vfend [package insert]. New York: Pfizer, 2015.

43. Cadena J, Levine DJ, Angel LF, et al. Antifungal prophylaxis with voriconazole or itraconazole

in lung transplant recipients: Hepatotoxicity and effectiveness. Am J Transplant 2009;9: 2085-2091.

44. Luong ML, Hosseini-Moghaddam SM, Singer LG, et al. Risk factors for voriconazole hepatotoxicity at 12 weeks in lung transplant recipients. Am J Transplant 2012;12:1929-1935.

45. Husain S, Paterson DL, Studer S, et al. Voriconazole prophylaxis in lung transplant recipients. Am J Transplant 2006;6:3008-3016.

46. Wang TF, Wang T, Altman R, et al. Periostitis secondary to prolonged voriconazole therapy in lung transplant recipients. Am J Transplant 2009;9:2845-2850.

47. Vadnerkar A, Nguyen MH, Mitsani D, et al. Voriconazole exposure and geographic location are independent risk factors for squamous cell carcinoma of the skin among lung transplant recipients. J Heart Lung Transplant 2010;29:1240-1244.

48. Singer JP, Boker A, Metchnikoff C, et al. High cumulative dose exposure to voriconazole is associated with cutaneous squamous cell carcinoma in lung transplant recipients. J Heart Lung Transplant 2012;31:694-699.

49. Feist A, Lee R, Osborne S, et al. Increased incidence of cutaneous squamous cell carcinoma in lung transplant recipients taking long-term voriconazole. J Heart Lung Transplant 2012;31:1177-1181.

50. Pascual A, Calandra T, Bolay S, et al. Voriconazole therapeutic drug monitoring in patients with invasive mycoses improves efficacy and safety outcomes. Clin Infect Dis 2008;46:201-211.

51. Smith J, Safdar N, Knasinski V, et al. Voriconazole therapeutic drug monitoring. Antimicrob Agents Chemother 2006;50:1570-1572.

52. Mitsani D, Nguyen MH, Shields RK, et al. Prospective, observational study of voriconazole therapeutic drug monitoring among lung transplant recipients receiving prophylaxis: Factors impacting levels of and associations between serum troughs, efficacy, and toxicity. Antimicrob Agents Chemother 2012;56:2371-2377.

53. Pfaller MA, Messer SA, Hollis RJ, et al. Antifungal activities of posaconazole, ravuconazole, and voriconazole compared to those of itraconazole and amphotericin B against 239 clinical isolates of Aspergillus spp. and other filamentous fungi: Report from SENTRY Antimicrobial Surveillance Program, 2000. Antimicrob Agents Chemother 2002;46:1032-1037.

54. Walsh TJ, Raad I, Patterson TF, et al. Treatment of invasive aspergillosis with posaconazole in patients who are refractory to or intolerant of conventional therapy: An externally controlled trial. Clin Infect Dis 2007;44:2-12.

55. Posaconazole [package insert]. Merck, White House Station, NJ, 2006.

56. Mistro S, Maciel Ide M, de Menezes RG, et al. Does lipid emulsion reduce amphotericin B nephrotoxicity? A systematic review and meta-analysis. Clin Infect Dis 2012;54:1774-1777.

57. Mora-Duarte J, Betts R, Rotstein C, et al. Comparison of caspofungin and amphotericin B for invasive candidiasis. N Engl J Med 2002;347:2020-2029.

58. Groetzner J, Kaczmarek I, Wittwer T, et al. Caspofungin as first-line therapy for the treatment of invasive aspergillosis after thoracic organ transplantation. J Heart Lung Transplant 2008;27:1-6.

59. Singh N, Limaye AP, Forrest G, et al. Combination of voriconazole and caspofungin as primary therapy for invasive aspergillosis in solid organ transplant recipients: A prospective, multicenter, observational study. Transplantation 2006;81:320-326.

60. Hiemenz JW, Raad, II, Maertens JA, et al. Efficacy of caspofungin as salvage therapy for invasive aspergillosis compared to standard therapy in a historical cohort. Eur J Clin Microbiol Infect Dis 2010;29:1387-1394.

61. Thomas A, Korb V, Guillemain R, et al. Clinical outcomes of lung-transplant recipients treated by voriconazole and caspofungin combination in aspergillosis. J Clin Pharm Ther 2010;35:49-53.

62. Marr KA, Schlamm H, Rottinghaus ST, et al. A randomised, double-blind study of combination antifungal therapy with voriconazole and anidulafungin versus voriconazole monotherapy for primary treatment of invasive aspergillosis. Abstract LB 2812. 22nd European Congress of Clinical Microbiology and Infectious Diseases. London; 2012.

63. Neoh CF, Snell GI, Kotsimbos T, et al. Antifungal prophylaxis in lung transplantation—a world-wide survey. Am J Transplant 2011;11:361-366.

64. Bhaskaran A, Mumtaz K, Husain S. Anti-Aspergillus prophylaxis in lung transplantation: A systematic review and meta-analysis. Curr Infect Dis Rep 2013;15:514-525.

65. Cimon B, Carrere J, Vinatier JF, et al. Clinical significance of Scedosporium apiospermum in patients with cystic fibrosis. Eur J Clin Microbiol Infect Dis 2000;19:53-56.

66. Sahi H, Avery RK, Minai OA, et al. Scedosporium apiospermum (Pseudoallescheria boydii) infection in lung transplant recipients. J Heart Lung Transplant 2007;26:350-356.

67. Cortez KJ, Roilides E, Quiroz-Telles F, et al. Infections caused by Scedosporium spp. Clin Microbiol Rev 2008;21:157-197.

68. Husain S, Munoz P, Forrest G, et al. Infections due to Scedosporium apiospermum and Scedosporium prolificans in transplant recipients: Clinical characteristics and impact of antifungal agent therapy on outcome. Clin Infect Dis 2005;40:89-99.

69. Troke P, Aguirrebengoa K, Arteaga C, et al. Treatment of scedosporiosis with voriconazole: Clinical experience with 107 patients. Antimicrob Agents Chemother 2008;52:1743-1750.

70. Bhat SV, Paterson DL, Rinaldi MG, Veldkamp PJ. *Scedosporium prolificans* brain abscess in a patient with chronic granulomatous disease: Successful combination therapy with voriconazole and terbinafine. Scand J Infect Dis 2007;39:87-90.

71. Tortorano AM, Richardson M, Roilides E, et al. ESCMID and ECMM joint guidelines on diagnosis and management of hyalohyphomycosis: *Fusarium* spp., *Scedosporium* spp. and others. Clin Microbiol Infect 2014;20(Suppl 3):27-46.

72. O'Donnell K, Sutton DA, Rinaldi MG, et al. Genetic diversity of human pathogenic members of the *Fusarium oxysporum* complex inferred from multilocus DNA sequence data and amplified fragment length polymorphism analyses: Evidence for the recent dispersion of a geographically widespread clonal lineage and nosocomial origin. J Clin Microbiol 2004;42:5109-5120.

73. Nucci M, Marr KA, Queiroz-Telles F, et al. *Fusarium* infection in hematopoietic stem cell transplant recipients. Clin Infect Dis 2004;38:1237-1242.

74. Nucci M, Anaissie E. *Fusarium* infections in immunocompromised patients. Clin Microbiol Rev 2007;20:695-704.

75. Carneiro HA, Coleman JJ, Restrepo A, Mylonakis E. *Fusarium* infection in lung transplant patients: Report of 6 cases and review of the literature. Medicine (Baltimore) 2011;90:69-80.

76. Boutati EI, Anaissie EJ. *Fusarium*, a significant emerging pathogen in patients with hematologic malignancy: Ten years' experience at a cancer center and implications for management. Blood 1997;90:999-1008.

77. Virgili A, Zampino MR, Mantovani L. Fungal skin infections in organ transplant recipients. Am J Clin Dermatol 2002;3:19-35.

78. Singh N, Chang FY, Gayowski T, Marino IR. Infections due to dematiaceous fungi in organ transplant recipients: Case report and review. Clin Infect Dis 1997;24:369-374.

79. Chowdhary A, Meis JF, Guarro J, et al. ESCMID and ECMM joint clinical guidelines for the diagnosis and management of systemic phaeohyphomycosis: Diseases caused by black fungi. Clin Microbiol Infect 2014;20(Suppl 3):47-75.

80. Singh N, Aguado JM, Bonatti H, et al. Zygomycosis in solid organ transplant recipients: A prospective, matched case-control study to assess risks for disease and outcome. J Infect Dis 2009;200:1002-1011.

81. Almyroudis NG, Sutton DA, Linden P, et al. Zygomycosis in solid organ transplant recipients in a tertiary transplant center and review of the literature. Am J Transplant 2006;6:2365-2374.

82. Sun HY, Aguado JM, Bonatti H, et al. Pulmonary zygomycosis in solid organ transplant recipients in the current era. Am J Transplant 2009;9:2166-2171.

83. Wingard JR, Hiemenz JW, Jantz MA. How I manage pulmonary nodular lesions and nodular infiltrates in patients with hematologic malignancies or undergoing hematopoietic cell transplantation. Blood 2012;120:1791-1800.

84. Chamilos G, Lewis RE, Kontoyiannis DP. Delaying amphotericin B–based frontline therapy significantly increases mortality among patients with hematologic malignancy who have zygomycosis. Clin Infect Dis 2008;47:503-509.

85. Cornely OA, Cuenca-Estrella M, Meis JF, Ullmann AJ. European Society of Clinical Microbiology and Infectious Diseases (ESCMID) Fungal Infection Study Group (EFISG) and European Confederation of Medical Mycology (ECMM) 2013 joint guidelines on diagnosis and management of rare and emerging fungal diseases. Clin Microbiol Infect 2014;20(Suppl 3):1-4.

86. Alexander BD, Perfect JR, Daly JS, et al. Posaconazole as salvage therapy in patients with invasive fungal infections after solid organ transplant. Transplantation 2008;86:791-796.

87. Ibrahim AS, Gebremariam T, Fu Y, et al. Combination echinocandin-polyene treatment of murine mucormycosis. Antimicrob Agents Chemother 2008;52:1556-1558.

88. Reed C, Bryant R, Ibrahim AS, et al. Combination polyene-caspofungin treatment of rhino-orbital-cerebral mucormycosis. Clin Infect Dis 2008;47:364-371.

89. Spellberg B, Ibrahim AS, Chin-Hong PV, et al. The Deferasirox-AmBisome Therapy for Mucormycosis (DEFEAT Mucor) study. A randomized, double-blinded, placebo-controlled trial. J Antimicrob Chemother 2012;67:715-722.

90. Husain S, Alexander BD, Munoz P, et al. Opportunistic mycelial fungal infections in organ transplant recipients: Emerging importance of non-*Aspergillus* mycelial fungi. Clin Infect Dis 2003;37:221-229.

91. Kauffman CA, Freifeld AG, Andes DR, et al. Endemic fungal infections in solid organ and hematopoietic cell transplant recipients enrolled in the Transplant-Associated Infection Surveillance Network (TRANSNET). Transpl Infect Dis 2014;16:213-224.

92. Kauffman CA. Histoplasmosis: A clinical and laboratory update. Clin Microbiol Rev 2007;20:115-132.

93. Assi M, Martin S, Wheat LJ, et al. Histoplasmosis after solid organ transplant. Clin Infect Dis 2013;57:1542-1549.

94. Hage C, Kleiman MB, Wheat LJ. Histoplasmosis in solid organ transplant recipients. Clin Infect Dis 2010;50:122-123; author reply 123-124.

95. Miller R, Assi M, AST Infectious Diseases Community of Practice. Endemic fungal infections in solid organ transplantation. Am J Transplant 2013;13(Suppl 4):250-261.

96. Wheat LJ, Freifeld AG, Kleiman MB, et al. Clinical practice guidelines for the management of patients with histoplasmosis: 2007 update by the Infectious Diseases Society of America. Clin Infect Dis 2007;45:807-825.

97. Gauthier GM, Safdar N, Klein BS, Andes DR. Blastomycosis in solid organ transplant recipients. Transpl Infect Dis 2007;9:310-317.

98. Chapman SW, Dismukes WE, Proia LA, et al. Clinical practice guidelines for the management of blastomycosis: 2008 update by the Infectious Diseases Society of America. Clin Infect Dis 2008;46:1801-1812.

99. Grim SA, Proia L, Miller R, et al. A multicenter study of histoplasmosis and blastomycosis after solid organ transplantation. Transpl Infect Dis 2012;14:17-23.

100. Connolly P, Hage CA, Bariola JR, et al. *Blastomyces dermatitidis* antigen detection by quantitative enzyme immunoassay. Clini Vaccine Immunol 2012;19:53-56.

101. Durkin M, Witt J, Lemonte A, et al. Antigen assay with the potential to aid in diagnosis of blastomycosis. J Clin Microbiol 2004;42:4873-4875.

102. Blair JE, Logan JL. Coccidioidomycosis in solid organ transplantation. Clin Infect Dis 2001;33:1536-1544.

103. Cha JM, Jung S, Bahng HS, et al. Multi-organ failure caused by reactivated coccidioidomycosis without dissemination in a patient with renal transplantation. Respirology 2000;5:87-90.

104. Wright PW, Pappagianis D, Wilson M, et al. Donor-related coccidioidomycosis in organ transplant recipients. Clin Infect Dis 2003;37:1265-1269.

105. Vikram HR, Dosanjh A, Blair JE. Coccidioidomycosis and lung transplantation. Transplantation 2011;92:717-721.

106. Parish JM, Blair JE. Coccidioidomycosis. Mayo Clin Proc 2008;83:343-348; quiz 348-349.

107. Mendoza N, Blair JE. The utility of diagnostic testing for active coccidioidomycosis in solid organ transplant recipients. Am J Transplant 2013;13:1034-1039.

108. Blair JE, Coakley B, Santelli AC, et al. Serologic testing for symptomatic coccidioidomycosis in immunocompetent and immunosuppressed hosts. Mycopathologia 2006;162:317-324.

109. Johnson RH, Einstein HE. Coccidioidal meningitis. Clin Infect Dis 2006;42:103-107.

110. Galgiani JN, Ampel NM, Blair JE, et al. Coccidioidomycosis. Clin Infect Dis 2005;41:1217-1223.

111. Schaenman JM, Rosso F, Austin JM, et al. Trends in invasive disease due to *Candida* species following heart and lung transplantation. Transpl Infect Dis 2009;11:112-121.

112. Pappas PG, Rex JH, Lee J, et al. A prospective observational study of candidemia: Eidemiology, therapy, and influences on mortality in hospitalized adult and pediatric patients. Clin Infect Dis 2003;37:634-643.

113. Klingspor L, Muhammed SA, Ozenci V. Comparison of the two blood culture systems, Bactec 9240 and BacT/Alert 3D, in the detection of *Candida* spp. and bacteria with polymicrobial sepsis. Eur J Clin Microbiol Infect Dis 2012;31:2983-2987.

114. Pappas PG, Kauffman CA, Andes D, et al. Clinical practice guidelines for the management of candidiasis: 2009 update by the Infectious Diseases Society of America. Clin Infect Dis 2009;48:503-535.

115. Datta K, Bartlett KH, Baer R, et al. Spread of *Cryptococcus gattii* into Pacific Northwest region of the United States. Emerg Infect Dis 2009;15:1185-1191.

116. Husain S, Wagener MM, Singh N. *Cryptococcus neoformans* infection in organ transplant recipients: Variables influencing clinical characteristics and outcome. Emerg Infect Dis 2001;7:375-381.

117. Sun HY, Alexander BD, Lortholary O, et al. Unrecognized pretransplant and donor-derived cryptococcal disease in organ transplant recipients. Clin Infect Dis 2010;51:1062-1069.

118. Antinori S, Radice A, Galimberti L, et al. The role of cryptococcal antigen assay in diagnosis and monitoring of cryptococcal meningitis. J Clin Microbiol 2005;43:5828-5829.

119. Singh N, Alexander BD, Lortholary O, et al. Pulmonary cryptococcosis in solid organ transplant recipients: Clinical relevance of serum cryptococcal antigen. Clin Infect Dis 2008;46:e12-e18.

120. Perfect JR, Dismukes WE, Dromer F, et al. Clinical practice guidelines for the management of cryptococcal disease: 2010 update by the Infectious Diseases Society of America. Clin Infect Dis 2010;50:291-322.

121. Singh N, Perfect JR. Immune reconstitution syndrome associated with opportunistic mycoses. Lancet Infect Dis 2007;7:395-401.

122. Baddley JW, Forrest GN, AST Infectious Diseases Community of Practice. Cryptococcosis in solid organ transplantation. Am J Transplant 2013;13(Suppl 4):242-249.

31

Bacterial infections after lung transplantation

JENNIFER DELACRUZ, JENNIFER L. STEINBECK, KENNETH PURSELL, AND DAVID PITRAK

OVERVIEW AND PATHOPHYSIOLOGY

Lung transplantation survival rates are lower than those for other types of solid-organ transplantation. The reason is higher rates of infection and rejection-related complications.[1,2] Infectious complications are the leading cause of morbidity and mortality at every time point following lung transplantation and the cause of death of at least 50% of lung transplant recipients (LTRs). Bacterial infection is the most frequent infectious complication of lung transplantation and accounts for 35% to 66% of infections. Overall, 50% to 85% of LTRs experience at least one episode of bacterial infection.[3] Most of these episodes occur in the immediate post-transplant period (i.e., 2 weeks after transplantation), with more than 80% of infections occurring in the lung, mediastinum, and pleural space.[2,3] Although such bacterial infection creates a considerable hazard in LTRs, most patients respond to antibiotic therapy and survive. Maurer and colleagues reported that although bacterial infection (more than half of which is pneumonia) is the most common type, it results in a lower mortality rate than either viral or fungal infection does.[4] Another study of early bacterial pneumonia (i.e., occurring within 2 weeks of lung transplantation) reported an overall rate of mortality resulting from bacterial pneumonia of only 3% for the entire cohort, although 1 of 11 patients with bacterial pneumonia did die.[5] In absolute numbers, however, bacterial pneumonia is responsible for the greatest number of early deaths caused by infection.[6] One autopsy study of 131 patients who received transplants between 1986 and 1995 showed that 48% of deaths after lung transplantation were caused by bacterial infections (in most cases by pneumonia).[7] Other causes of death were surgical complications (19%), posttransplant lymphoproliferative disorder (7%), and unrelated causes (7%). Rejection was not a major cause of death during the early posttransplant period or the first year after transplantation.[7] Although pneumonia is common, other serious life-threatening types of infection, such as bacteremia and urinary tract infections, also occur. Pediatric lung transplants pose a significant risk for bacteremia, which does carry significant mortality.[8]

Risk for infection following lung transplantation varies according to time after transplant.[9,10] A large majority of infectious complications (approximately 75%) occur during the first year after transplantation, with most of those cases clustered in the first month. Parada and coworkers reported that the critical period for the development of bacterial infection in lung transplantation is the first 3 months after the transplant.[11] Pneumonia is quite common. Complicated deep surgical site infection, empyema, surgical wound infection, mediastinitis, sternal osteomyelitis, and pericarditis also occur in 5% of patients at a mean of 25 days after transplantation. Such infection is associated with decreased 1-year survival.[11] In another series, early pleural space infection in patients with pleural effusion (occurring in the first 90 days after transplantation) was not uncommon: it occurred in 27% (34 of 124). Interestingly, most of these cases (60%) were fungal, with *Candida albicans* being the predominant species isolated, and 25% were caused by bacterial pathogens.[12]

In patients who have received a transplant within the past month, nosocomial multidrug-resistant (MDR) pathogens, such as vancomycin-resistant *Enterococcus*, methicillin-resistant *Staphylococcus aureus* (MRSA), MDR *Pseudomonas aeruginosa* (PsAR), and other gram-negative organisms predominate. Sources include both donor and recipient lungs, central and peripheral venous catheters, arterial catheters, urinary catheters, wound infections, and anastomotic leaks. *Clostridium difficile* infection (CDI) is also seen. Although infection in most patients is caused by the typical nosocomial pathogens that affect all populations, some LTRs have a particularly difficult time with pathogens unique to the LTR population (for example, pneumonia with *Burkholderia* species in patients with cystic fibrosis [CF]). Between 1 and 6 months after transplantation, anastomotic leaks and CDI remain prevalent. Routine *Pneumocystis jirovecii* prophylaxis with trimethoprim-sulfamethoxazole (TMP-SMX), which does provide some antibacterial protection, is widely implemented by almost all transplant centers. Despite the use of TMP-SMX, breakthrough infection caused by *Nocardia* and *Listeria* species is occasionally seen within this time frame. *Mycobacterium tuberculosis* (MTB) infection does occur rarely during this period as well. Beginning at 6 months after transplantation, community-acquired pathogens that cause pneumonia and urinary tract infections are seen and *Streptococcus pneumoniae* becomes a significant pathogen. Infection caused by *Nocardia* and *Rhodococcus* has also been reported.

Little information exists on the risk factors for late infection that complicate solid-organ transplants (SOTs), including lung transplants. San Juan and colleagues looked at the risk factors for late infection (defined as infection occurring more than 6 months after transplantation) associated with different types of SOTs.[13] Risk factors included acute rejection during the early posttransplant period, relapsing cytomegalovirus (CMV) infection, and previous bacterial infection. In contrast to other types of solid-organ transplantation, lung transplantation was itself a risk factor.[13] Patients could benefit from closer monitoring, prolonged prophylactic measures, or both.

Chronic rejection, which is characterized histologically by obliterative bronchiolitis, remains the major impediment to successful long-term outcomes in lung transplantation. Obliterative bronchiolitis afflicts two thirds of patients. Infection increases the risk for bronchiolitis obliterans syndrome (BOS), with BOS subsequently becoming the major predisposing factor for cumulative increased infection.[14]

Risk is determined by a combination of exposure and the effect of immunosuppression. Patients are at risk for infection with typical nosocomial pathogens and also for the development of infection with organisms with which they have previously been colonized or infected. Twenty-three percent of patients with deep surgical site involvement had infection involving organisms that had colonized their native lungs before transplantation.[15] Patients with CF and previous infection with MDR organisms, PsAR, or other gram-negative bacilli were at risk for infection with these organisms.[16] The currently available data regarding whether patients with CF and a pretransplant history of infection with MDR organisms have worse outcomes after lung transplantation are conflicting.

PATHOGENESIS

The determinants of bacterial infection after lung transplantation include altered anatomy, aggressive immunosuppression, recipients' colonizing flora before their transplant, posttransplant changes in flora that occur in connection with constant exposure to the environment, and recipients' own genetic makeup. LTRs possess a unique constellation of anatomic predisposing risk factors, most of which are specific for pneumonia. Such factors include decreased cough reflex, decreased mucociliary clearance, loss of bronchial circulation, and loss of lymphatic drainage, and they all contribute to risk for pneumonia.[17,18]

Immune factors

Etienne and Mornex described lung transplantation as "an immune state characterized by an increase in infection and an alloreactive state."[19] The process of increasing immunosuppression to manage rejection and obliterative bronchiolitis, coupled with markedly impaired lung function and mucus clearance, dramatically raises the predisposition to infection in such patients.

Innate immune effector cells are important in host defense against bacterial pathogens. Immune suppression is associated with a decrease in certain macrophage functions that are part of the innate immune response to infection. Immune suppression to prevent rejection and BOS reduce proinflammatory and Th1 cytokines, which are important in host defense against bacterial infection. Some have proposed monitoring levels of these cytokines to help avoid excessive immunosuppression in stable lung transplant patients. A number of studies of cells collected by bronchoalveolar lavage (BAL) have shown that the T cells of patients with infection demonstrate lower intracellular cytokine production than do those of patients without infection.[20] Interleukin-2 [IL-2] production by CD4[+] T cells and production of tumor necrosis factor α by CD8[+] T cells decreased after stimulation.

Other investigators have demonstrated that other indicators of the degree of immunosuppression can determine the risk for infection. The ImmuKnow Immune Cell Function Assay (Cylex, Inc., Columbia, Maryland), which measures the production of adenosine triphosphate (ATP) by lymphocytes in response to stimulation with a mitogen, was used to study 175 LTRs who had 129 episodes of infection. The ATP levels of patients in whom CMV disease or bacterial infection developed were significantly lower than those of stable patients; ATP levels less than 100 ng/mL were associated with increased risk for infection (odds ratio = 2.8:1).[21] A study of 57 LTRs showed that a low ATP level predicted bacterial infection.[22] Although immune monitoring appears to have the potential for identifying patients at risk for bacterial infection, no particular protocol is currently the standard of care.

Infectious complications are the most common cause of death in patients in whom obliterative bronchiolitis develops. Furthermore, evidence indicates that bacterial infection may play a role in the establishment of obliterative bronchiolitis by amplifying or extending an inflammatory immune response to foreign antigens and providing another form of nonalloimmune lung injury.[23,24] In fact, pilot studies of long-term antimicrobial antibiotic therapy have provided preliminary evidence of a positive influence on the outcome of obliterative bronchiolitis.[25]

Another important mechanism of immune deficiency that can occur after lung transplantation is hypogammaglobulinemia. Goldfarb and colleagues reported that 70% of LTRs had below normal IgG levels; 37% had IgG levels below 400 mg/dL (the level of hypogammaglobulinemia that identifies a population at high risk for bacterial and fungal infection and poor survival).[26] Interestingly, the authors recommended close monitoring of hypogammaglobulinemic patients but did not make any recommendation about replacement therapy with immune globulin. Significant hypogammaglobulinemia also develops frequently in pediatric LTRs and is associated with increased risk for infection and hospital stays in this population as well.[27] Yip and coworkers reported that lower IgG levels before transplantation, which are common with severe chronic obstructive pulmonary disease independent of steroid use, are associated with hypogammaglobulinemia after lung transplantation.[28] Use of mycophenolate mofetil was also associated with hypogammaglobulinemia after transplantation. The development of hypogammaglobulinemia is not unique to lung transplantation; it is a problem that occurs with other SOTs as well[29]: severe hypogammaglobulinemia (IgG <400 mg/dL) occurs in 15% of SOT recipients. A recent meta-analysis of the effect of hypogammaglobulinemia on the risk for infection and mortality after a SOT showed a 21.9-fold higher relative risk for death in patients with severe hypogammaglobulinemia during the first year after a transplant.[29] A recent review advocated routine monitoring for hypogammaglobulinemia in SOT recipients and replacement therapy when indicated.[30]

Microbial flora

The microbiota of LTRs may play an important role in the outcome of bacterial infection. Shteinberg and colleagues reported that patients colonized with fluoroquinolone-resistant gram-negative bacilli have significantly worse outcomes, with a relative risk for mortality of 9.2% even in patients without CF.[31] The risk for colonization by these pathogens is directly related to previous antibiotic exposure. Infection with PsAR, *Stenotrophomonas*, *Burkholderia* species, and mycobacteria plays a major role in patient outcomes and recipient selection; colonization or infection with MDR bacteria may be a contraindication to lung transplantation. Complex bacterial infection following lung transplantation is a particular problem for patients with CF. Certain species of the *Burkholderia cepacia* complex, such as *Burkholderia gladioli* and *Burkholderia cenocepacia*, pose a greater risk for death after transplantation in patients with CF.[32] The effect of the existing microbial flora on outcome has been variable, however. Dobbin and coworkers showed that pretransplant colonization with pan-resistant bacteria was not associated with poor outcome or reduced survival.[33] Aris and associates also demonstrated that the presence of MDR bacteria did not increase the risk for infection or adversely affect survival.[34] Therefore, at this time each center needs to decide whether colonization or infection with MDRgram-negative rods is a contraindication to lung transplantation.

Charlson and colleagues looked at the microbiome of patients following lung transplantation.[35] The organisms present in the lung and upper respiratory tract were determined by bacterial and fungal 16S rDNA sequencing from BAL and oral wash specimens, respectively. The microbiota was compared to that of controls. LTRs had a higher bacterial burden in their BAL fluid, frequent appearance of predominant organisms, greater differences between their lower and upper respiratory tract flora and BAL profile, and decreased respiratory tract diversity. Better understanding of the microbiome of LTRs may be an important focus of interventions in the future.

Genetics

Genetic studies may provide greater insight into the risk for bacterial infection after lung transplantation. Palmer and coworkers reported that polymorphisms in Toll-like receptor 4 (TLR4) that are associated with endotoxin hyporesponsiveness are linked to a significantly lower risk for rejection in the first 3 years after lung transplantation. A trend toward decreased onset of grade 2 or 3 BOS was also discovered.[36] Targeting innate immune signaling could be an important strategy for preventing allograft rejection.

Genetic studies focusing on heart and stem cell transplant patients may also be applicable to the risk for infection in lung transplantation. A recent study of heart transplant recipients showed that late infection (>60 days after transplantation) is common and occurs in 48% of recipients.[37] Late bacterial infection was associated with polymorphisms of the gene *HMOX1* (a gene regulating neutrophil activation), whereas viral infection was related to polymorphisms of *CTLA4* (a regulator of T-cell activation). A recent study of stem cell transplant recipients showed that genetic deficiency of pentraxin 3 (PTX3), which is a soluble pattern recognition receptor, contributes to the risk for invasive aspergillosis by affecting the antifungal capacity of neutrophils; moreover, PTX3 is known to have an effect on tuberculosis and PsAR colonization in patients with CF.[38] Future studies will uncover other genetic differences with an impact on the risk for infection in transplant recipients, including LTRs.

Effects of bacterial infection on lung allografts

Infection can have multiple effects on graft function, including creation of increased risk for rejection. Rat models of lung transplantation have clearly shown that CMV and *Listeria* infection enhance chronic rejection[39]; however, the mechanisms that result in rejection after bacterial infection have not been completely elucidated. Activation of the innate immune system can enhance adaptive immunity and induce lung rejection. Animal studies show that bacterial infection can induce granulocyte colony-stimulating factor–dependent neutrophilia and graft infiltration, which can induce acute rejection. Neutrophil elastase activity increases with bacterial infection, which may cause lung allograft damage.[40] Although this pattern of activity appears to be more pronounced in patients with α_1-antitrypsin deficiency, the same pattern was seen for patients without α_1-antitrypsin deficiency. Increased endothelin-1 is associated with bacterial lung infection and results in increased fibrosis, which plays a major part in the pathogenesis of bronchiolitis obliterans.[41]

Colonization with gram-negative bacteria, including PsAR, may also contribute to risk for the development of BOS. Yamamoto and colleagues demonstrated that PsAR infection could abolish tolerance of a transplanted lung by stimulating B7 expression on neutrophils that infiltrate the lung,[42] which in turn results in activation of CD4+ T cells; production of IL-2, interferon, and IL-17; and subsequent loss of graft tolerance. The same investigators also showed that blocking B7 and still having adequate clearance of PsAR may be possible and a potential strategy for future management of patients.

TYPES OF BACTERIAL INFECTION IN LUNG TRANSPLANT RECIPIENTS

Site-specific disease

In 2012, the Registry of the International Society for Heart and Lung Transplantation reported that bronchiolitis and infection (non-CMV infection) were the leading causes of mortality in LTRs during the first 3 years following lung transplantation. Infection was the leading cause of mortality from day 31 through the first year after lung transplantation and second only to graft failure through day 30.[43] Most infection occurred within the first year, specifically during the first 90 days after transplantation.[1,11] According to an epidemiologic study of early and late transplant infection, bacteria remain the most common source of infection. Bacterial disease (other than mycobacterial disease, which accounted for 4% of cases) was responsible for 48% of

causative infectious organisms after lung transplantation.[11] Infection is nearly twice as frequent in LTRs as in heart transplant recipients, with most cases of infection arising from the respiratory tract.[3] At least half of deaths of LTRs are caused by or complications of infection, and more than one third of LTRs with fatal outcomes also had BOS. This syndrome is one of the highest risk factors for the development of infection in LTRs, which is probably attributable to the amount of immunosuppression they receive and their impaired lung function.[3] Because infection is directly related to mortality in LTRs, prevention, early diagnosis, and initiation of treatment are imperative.

Pneumonia

EARLY-ONSET PNEUMONIA

Bacterial pneumonia is the most common infection after a lung transplant.[1,3,43-45] LTRs are particularly susceptible to respiratory tract infection because of impaired postoperative function of the lung graft, including impaired mucociliary clearance and denervation, which interferes with the cough reflex. Moreover, LTRs are the only SOT recipients whose transplanted organ is itself directly exposed to environmental pathogens.[3,11,45-47] Pneumonia that develops in the first 30 days after a transplant is most frequently health care associated and secondary to nosocomial organisms; PsAR is the causative organism isolated most commonly.[1,11,44-47] A retrospective epidemiologic study reported that PsAR was the pathogen most commonly isolated in LTRs with pneumonia (isolated in 33% of cases), followed by *S. aureus and Acinetobacter* (isolated in 26% and 16% of cases, respectively) and *Aspergillus* (16%).[1,45] Likewise, a more extensive retrospective study analyzed infection in LTRs over a 15-year period and found that 178 of 208 LTRs experienced a total of 859 episodes of infection. Most episodes were respiratory tract infection (559 episodes [65.1%]), followed by mucocutaneous (skin, wound, catheter-related, and oral) infection (88 episodes [10.2%]), and bloodstream infection (85 [9.9%]). Infection in other sites (urine, bowel, eye, and peritoneum) accounted for 127 (14.8%) episodes. Most (83.6%) of the episodes of respiratory tract infection were bacterial; gram-negative organisms were encountered most frequently, and PsAR was the most commonly isolated pathogen.[47]

LATE-ONSET PNEUMONIA

LTRs struggle with respiratory tract infection indefinitely. Because these patients are continuously exposed to the health care setting, they will continue to be at risk for hospital-acquired pneumonia and, frequently, more resistant organisms throughout their lifetime.[1] In addition to nosocomial respiratory infection, community-acquired pneumonia is more commonly observed in the late posttransplant setting (longer than 6 months after transplantation) because patients are commonly no longer hospitalized at that point. Community-acquired pathogens such as *S. pneumoniae, Legionella,* and viral sources of respiratory infection should be considered in LTRs with late-onset pneumonia.[48] De Bryun and colleagues reported the presence of invasive pneumococcal infection in 14 of 220 LTRs (6.4%) at a median of 1.3 years after lung transplantation. All the patients with invasive pneumococcal disease were receiving TMP-SMX prophylaxis at diagnosis, and their disease was associated with TMP-SMX resistance in 71% of cases.[48] Urinary antigen tests exist for both *S. pneumoniae* and *Legionella pneumophila* and are used as a diagnostic tool. In the case of *Legionella*, however, urinary testing can be used only for the diagnosis of *L. pneumophila* serotype 1; therefore, infection with other serotypes or other common species (e.g., *Legionella micdadei*) would need to be diagnosed by culture, typically from BAL fluid. Because of the narrow scope of the *Legionella* urinary antigen, if the pretest probability of legionella is high, empiric treatment should be considered regardless of the results of urinary antigen testing.[44,49-51] The diagnosis of *Legionella* infection can easily be missed and should be considered in patients with progressive disease despite broad-spectrum antibiotic therapy. In addition, *Legionella* can be nosocomial or community acquired; for this reason, it is important that *Legionella* not be overlooked as a potential pathogen in patients in whom pneumonia develops while they are hospitalized.[44,49-51] Tkatch and colleagues reported that SOT recipients with legionellosis were the only patients found to have empyema. SOT recipients were also the only patients to have *Legionella* isolated from nonpulmonary sources, such as blood, fascia, and chest wounds.[49]

Community-acquired respiratory virus is also a potential pathogen that should be considered at any time in the posttransplant setting, especially in patients with a history of exposure and during the appropriate season. Influenza, parainfluenza, and respiratory syncytial viruses are the commonly isolated viral pathogens associated with late-onset viral pneumonia.[1,44,47] Community-acquired respiratory virus is linked to both severe and life-threatening pneumonitis, as well as to the development of death from BOS.[1] Viral respiratory infection can also result in the development of secondary bacterial pneumonia.[1,44]

Secondary bacterial pneumonia after viral lower respiratory tract infection is an important source of morbidity and mortality in both immunocompetent and immunocompromised patients.[44] Secondary bacterial infection is responsible for up to 25% of influenza-associated deaths. *S. pneumoniae*, *S. aureus*, and *Haemophilus influenzae* are the predominant pathogens in normal hosts.[44,52-55] As in the general population, this syndrome should be suspected in patients who initially improve after a viral illness and subsequently experience recrudescence.[44]

DONOR-DERIVED INFECTION

Campos and coworkers did reveal a link between early-onset pneumonia and pretransplant colonization in LTRs with suppuration; however, donor lung organisms did not affect the incidence of pneumonia after lung transplantation.[45] The relationship between positive donor Gram stains and the potential for transmission of infection has also

been reviewed in several studies, one of which reported that donor Gram stain was not predictive of the development of early postoperative pneumonia.[56] Of note, neither study mentioned posttransplantation prophylactic antibiotics in LTRs being directed by the donor lung organisms isolated or duration of prophylaxis. Ruiz and coworkers reported that some microorganisms isolated from bacterial cultures of donor or preservation fluids pose an increased risk for donor-derived infection and consequently result in increased morbidity, death, or graft loss. They determined that *S. aureus*, Enterobacteriaceae, PsAR, and fungi carry a higher risk for the development of donor-derived infection than do *Staphylococcus epidermidis* or diphtheroids.[57] Their conclusion was that donor-to-host transmission of infection is encountered after lung transplantation. To avoid increased mortality and morbidity, a suitable prophylactic antibiotic regimen should be instituted initially and adjusted on the basis of the results of culturing samples from the donor, grafts, preservative fluid, and recipient results.[57] However, LTRs with CF should not be treated solely on the basis of the results of donor cultures because patients with CF frequently have a history of resistant organisms and their prophylactic antibiotics are typically tailored accordingly.[3]

PNEUMONIA IN LUNG TRANSPLANT RECIPIENTS WITH CYSTIC FIBROSIS

LTRs with CF who have airway colonization with pathogens such as PsAR, *S. aureus*, and *Aspergillus* before transplantation are not at greater risk for the development of posttransplantation infectious complications secondary to the presence of these organisms than are LTRs without CF.[3] Nunley and colleagues reported that *Pseudomonas* is isolated from LTRs with CF earlier and more frequently. They also reported that infection with *Pseudomonas* as the causative organism occurs more frequently in LTRs with CF but is not linked to an increase in mortality. The presence of *Pseudomonas* in lung grafts is associated with marked inflammation in the airways of all LTRs.[58] Smith and coworkers found that resistant *Pseudomonas* does not affect the survival of patients with CF who receive heart-lung transplants.[59] One question that remains is whether the higher incidence of PsAR colonization in LTRs with CF, which results in more inflammation (which in turn leads to the development of BOS), is related indirectly to increased morbidity and mortality.

PNEUMONIA AND OTHER INFECTION SECONDARY TO ATYPICAL BACTERIAL PATHOGENS

Mycobacterial infection after lung transplantation is uncommon. Its relative risk in LTRs with MTB infection is greater than that in the general population. LTRs have a higher incidence of MTB infection than other SOT recipients do. Nontuberculosis *Mycobacterium* (NTM) infection is rare, albeit more common than MTB infection.[1,41,60-61] LTRs are at greater risk for pulmonary infection in general because the allograft is in direct contact with the pathogen.[1,41,60] In countries in which tuberculosis is endemic, MTB disease is more prevalent, whereas in countries in which MTB is not endemic, NTM prevails.[41,61] The incidence of NTM seems to be on the rise.[1,61]

Doucette and associates reported a case of *Mycobacterium abscessus* at their institution that involved an LTR with invasive *M. abscessus* infection of the sternum requiring extensive débridement; the LTR did have sputum cultures positive for the organism before transplantation. Another case described is that of a 20-year-old man in whom disseminated *M. abscessus* infection developed shortly after his transplant; the cultures before his transplant were also positive for *M. abscessus*.[61] *Mycobacterium abscessus* is observed in LTRs at a higher rate than in other SOT recipients. It has been reported as causing skin, soft tissue, pulmonary, and disseminated disease in LTRs. The most common manifestation in all SOT recipients is cutaneous lesions. Such infection has been reported throughout the posttransplant period with no increase in incidence at any specific point in that period.[62] Pleuropulmonary disease in LTRs is described most commonly.[61] Increases in both mortality and disseminated disease associated with *M. abscessus* in SOT recipients have been observed. *Mycobacterium avium* complex and other NTM infection is less common, and the impact of such infection on morbidity and mortality is less severe than that of *M. abscessus* infection. If pretransplant clinical and radiographic evidence raises concern for NTM infection, further evaluation and probable treatment should be carefully considered before transplantation.[1]

Nocardia, although encountered less frequently, is associated with an increase in mortality in LTRs. Husain and coworkers retrospectively reviewed the clinical histories and outcomes of 473 LTRs over a 9-year span. In their study *Nocardia* infection was diagnosed in 0.6% to 2.1% of LTRs, the overall mortality rate was 40%, and rate of *Nocardia*-related mortality was 75%, which is much higher than that in previous studies. The researchers attributed this disparity to the fact that the study patient population had lung transplants exclusively, as well as an increased frequency of infection with *Nocardia farcinica*, which is a more virulent strain.[63] LTRs with *Nocardia* pneumonia typically had nonspecific findings on imaging, and recipients of single-lung transplants frequently had native lung involvement, which the researchers presumed to be secondary to native structural and functional lung abnormalities rather than to reactivation of preexisting infection.[63] The LTRs who were receiving Bactrim (TMP-SMX) prophylaxis were among the recipients in whom *Nocardia* developed, which illustrates that Bactrim-resistant strains exist.[1,63] Bactrim prophylaxis should not preclude *Nocardia* as a potential pathogen in LTRs. Cutaneous lesions are the most common form of extrapulmonary disease.[63] Cutaneous lesions have been reported in liver and renal transplant recipients; however, cutaneous lesions were not reported in the LTRs in this study or in other reviewed cases outside their institution. Hussain and coworkers concluded that unlike other transplant recipients, LTRs exhibit nonspecific

symptoms.[63] Like many other atypical pathogens, *Nocardia* is a great mimicker of other infection; therefore, *Nocardia* should be considered as a potential pathogen, especially in LTRs with progressive disease who are not responding to broad-spectrum antibiotics.[1]

Tracheobronchitis

Tracheobronchitis typically arises in the first 6 weeks to 3 months after transplantation. The diagnosis is made by bronchoscopic evaluation, which commonly reveals purulence, ulceration, dehiscence, or necrosis. The organisms most commonly responsible are *Pseudomonas* and *Staphylococcus*, followed by *Aspergillus* and (reportedly) *Candida*.[1]

Bloodstream infections

Valentine and coworkers showed that bacteremia (bloodstream infection) affected 9.4% of lung transplant patients, with *Staphylococcus* species being the predominant pathogens.[44,47] Almost 50% of the organisms causing bacteremia after lung transplantation were MDR organisms (appearing at an average of 172 days after transplantation); pulmonary infection was the most common source of drug-resistant gram-negative bacteremia. The rate of mortality attributable to bacteremia in these patients at day 28 was high (reported as 25%).[44,47]

Mediastinitis

Mediastinitis after sternotomy is associated with high morbidity and mortality, especially in transplant recipients. Abid and coworkers reviewed cardiopulmonary transplant data over a 15-year period and found *S. aureus* to be the most common causative organism in all cardiac transplant recipients with mediastinitis. In LTRs, however, various causative organisms, including *Pseudomonas*, *B. cepacia*, *S. epidermidis*, *Escherichia coli*, and *Klebsiella*, were reported. *Candida albicans* was the causative agent of mediastinitis in three patients, two of whom died. Fungal and polymicrobial mediastinitis was shown to have a 66% mortality rate, whereas *S. aureus* resulted in a mortality rate of 11%. In addition to fungal and polymicrobial infection, delayed diagnosis, bacteremia, shock, and leukopenia also carry a poor prognosis. Surgery in addition to antibiotic therapy, antifungal therapy, or both is the mainstay of treatment.[64]

Empyema

Empyema is not a common complication after lung transplantation; when it does occur, however, it carries high mortality. Nunley and colleagues evaluated 392 LTRs and identified empyema in 14 patients (3.6%), most commonly at 6 weeks after transplantation. Of the 14 LTRs with empyema, 28.6% died as a result of infectious complications related to empyema.[65] Gram-positive, gram-negative, and saprophytic organisms were found to cause empyema in this population. No predominant organism was found to be responsible for transplant-associated empyema.[65] The researchers also compared LTRs who received their transplant for a septic lung disorder with LTRs who received their transplant because of a nonseptic lung disorder; the incidence of empyema did not differ regardless of whether a single-lung, double-lung, or heart-lung transplant was received. Of note, the researchers did report that the LTRs with septic lung disorders received a longer course of perioperative prophylactic antibiotics, which may have resulted in decreased development of empyema in the LTRs with previous septic lung disorders.[65] *Mycobacterium abscessus* causing pneumonia and empyema has been reported in LTRs; however, it is a very rare occurrence.[66]

Other bacterial infection

Other bacterial infection, including urinary tract infection, cutaneous infection, and CDI, is commonly encountered in the post–lung transplant setting. Valentine and colleagues reported that urinary tract infection affected 3.1% of the LTRs in the cases they reviewed, with PsAR being the prevalent pathogen.[44,47] Cutaneous infection affected 5.5% of the patients, with the prevalent pathogens being *Staphylococcus* species.[44,47] Severe and relapsing CDI has also been described in immunocompromised hosts. Past reports showed that CDI affects 7.4% of LTRs, with the main risk factor being antibiotic exposure.[44,67-68] Given that CDI is becoming more prevalent, its incidence is probably greatly underestimated. Diarrhea warrants a workup for non-CDI, especially in patients who have a history of travel to or are from regions with a high incidence of endemic gastrointestinal pathogens.[39,67-68]

ASSOCIATION OF BACTERIAL INFECTION WITH BRONCHIOLITIS OBLITERANS SYNDROME

BOS has been reported to be an indicator of poorer survival after the first year following transplantation and is the main cause of death after the first posttransplant year. Bacterial infection has been associated with the development of BOS and the poorer prognosis of patients with BOS. In view of this association, infectious complications and the resultant mortality in LTRs are probably underestimated.[1,14] *Pseudomonas* has been linked to significant inflammation in airways[58]; some studies suggest a possible relationship between persistent airway colonization with *Pseudomonas* and BOS.[68,70-71] Additionally, aspiration of bile acid as a result of gastroesophageal reflux disease (GERD) and pulmonary colonization with PsAR appear to be linked,[44,72] as do GERD and BOS.[44,73] The relationship between chronic airway colonization, GERD, and BOS is the focus of considerable ongoing research.[44] A link between CDI and BOS, which is thought to be secondary to the inflammatory response, has also been reported; however, the role of CDI in chronic rejection remains unclear.[69]

THERAPY

Therapy for posttransplant bacterial infection should be influenced by time after transplantation and results of culture. Obtaining cultures of blood, urine, and sputum as early in the infectious workup as possible is critical because they are the usual sources. Early removal of central venous catheters, arterial catheters, and urinary catheters is critical. In the first month after a transplant, nosocomial pathogens predominate and empiric therapy should have broad-spectrum coverage. In one study that examined mortality in the first month after transplantation, bacterial infection accounted for most deaths, with death being attributed primarily to pneumonia and catheter-associated bacteremia.[74] Interestingly, MDR pathogens such as *Acinetobacter*, which are classically seen during this period, are increasingly being identified late (>6 months) in the posttransplant course.[75] Overall rates of posttransplant infection decreased; however, more infection involving MDR bacteria and a marked shift toward isolation of more gram-negative bacilli with extensive drug resistance have occurred.[76] Mortality is higher in thoracic transplant recipients who are infected with nosocomial pathogens.[77] LTRs can require extended ventilator support and significant exposure to broad-spectrum antibiotics, which has been associated with the acquisition of extensive drug-resistant gram-negative bacilli. Infection with carbapenem-resistant gram-negative bacilli has been associated with decreases in allograft and patient survival.[76]

Choice of antibiotic

Directed antimicrobial therapy depends on the pathogen causing the disease and review of the results of antimicrobial susceptibility testing. The emergence of MDR pathogens has made this choice particularly challenging, and susceptibility data should always guide therapeutic decisions. MRSA can be treated with vancomycin, linezolid, or daptomycin, although the use of daptomycin as therapy for MRSA lung infection should be avoided because pulmonary surfactant inactivates it. Vancomycin-resistant *Enterococcus* can be treated with daptomycin or linezolid. Gram-negative pathogens that produce extended-spectrum β-lactamases or contain AmpC beta-lactamases (both of which confer resistance to many β-lactam antibiotics) can be treated with carbapenem.[76] *Acinetobacter* isolates are frequently resistant to most antibiotics and are usually treated with carbapenems or colistimethate. Carbapenem-resistant Enterobacteriaceae have limited, nonstandardized treatment options. Polymyxins are commonly used against these isolates; however, they have poor pulmonary penetration when administered intravenously. Adjunctive therapy with aerosolized polymyxins is frequently used for such infection. Consultation with an infectious diseases specialist is recommended. Table 31.1 lists increasingly prevalent MDR pathogens and reasonable empiric antimicrobial coverage.

Table 31.1 Empiric therapy for emerging multidrug-resistant pathogens

Pathogen	Common sites of infection	Empiric therapy
Community-acquired methicillin-resistant *Staphylococcus aureus*	Skin and soft tissue Lung (pneumonia, often postviral) Bacteremia	Vancomycin Linezolid Daptomycin (not for pneumonia)
ESBL or cAMP–producing organisms	Pneumonia Bacteremia Intra-abdominal	Carbapenems (note that ertapenem has no *Pseudomonas* coverage)
Clostridium difficile infection	Gastrointestinal tract	Metronidazole or vancomycin (oral), depending on disease severity
Stenotrophomonas maltophilia	Lung Sinuses Skin Bacteremia	Trimethoprim-sulfamethoxazole
Acinetobacter	Pneumonia Bacteremia	Colestimethate Imipenem and cilastatin
Vancomycin-resistant *Enterococcus*	Bacteremia Pneumonia	Daptomycin Linezolid

Note: cAMP, cyclic adenosine monophosphate; ESBL, extended-spectrum β-lactamase.

As always, local susceptibility data, culture-specific susceptibility results, and infectious disease guidance should be used.[76]

Less prevalent pathogens include *Nocardia* (which affects approximately 1.9% of LTRs), *Listeria*, and *Rhodococcus*. For *Nocardia*, treatment with TMP-SMX is classically administered, although because many patients are receiving this medication when breakthrough infection occurs, combination or alternative therapy (often with carbapenems, cephalosporins, or fluoroquinolones) should be considered.[78,79] *Listeria* is a pathogen that is occasionally encountered after a SOT and is usually treated with ampicillin. The literature includes one report of *Listeria* infection complicating a lung transplant,[80] as well as one report of *Rhodococcus* infection after lung transplantation.[81] Treatment usually consists of multiple agents and should be guided by the results of susceptibility testing and the recommendations of an infectious diseases specialist. Cases of MTB and NTM complicating lung transplantation have been reported.[82,83] Therapy usually consists of three or four antimycobacterial drugs and should be guided by data from susceptibility testing and an infectious diseases specialist's recommendations. Rifampin, which is frequently a component of such regimens, interacts with multiple immunosuppressive agents.

PREVENTION

In view of the significant morbidity and mortality associated with bacterial infection in LTRs, taking all steps possible to prevent the development of infection is of paramount importance. This goal can be accomplished by active immunization, passive immunization, peritransplant chemoprophylaxis, and reduction of exposure to infectious agents.

Vaccination

Vaccination is a powerful tool to prevent the development of infection in all hosts, and it remains important in lung transplant candidates and recipients. Aggressive efforts should be undertaken to ensure that all LTRs are up to date on vaccinations before undergoing transplantation. Because the response to vaccination is often lessened in the setting of organ failure, early vaccination is beneficial. If vaccinations are not completed before transplantation, however, inactivated bacterial vaccinations can be safely administered afterward.[84]

In general, it is recommended that all adults with end-stage lung disease receive all vaccinations that the Centers for Disease Control and Prevention (CDC) guidelines for immunocompetent hosts deem appropriate for individuals of their age and with their exposure history and immune status.[85] The optimal time to initiate vaccination following a transplant is not known. Because the immune response in the immediate posttransplant period in the setting of intense immunosuppression is poor,[85] most centers wait to initiate vaccination until 3 to 6 months after a transplant, at which time baseline immunosuppression has been reached.[84] The Infectious Diseases Society of America guidelines recommend that standard age-appropriate vaccines be given according to the CDC annual schedule 2 to 6 months after a transplant.[85]

Streptococcus pneumoniae infection can result in a variety of invasive diseases, including bacteremia, pneumonia, and meningitis.[60] SOT recipients remain at high risk for invasive disease.[44,48] The previously mentioned retrospective cohort study in which de Bryun and coworkers investigated invasive pneumococcal infection in LTRs established an incidence rate of 22.7 cases per 1000 person-years. All the available isolates were from the 23-valent pneumococcal polysaccharide vaccine (PPSV23)-associated serogroups.[48] Another prospective population-based surveillance study found the incidence of invasive pneumococcal disease in sterile sites in their SOT recipients to be 146 episodes of infection per 100,000 persons per year; for comparison, the incidence in the general population was 11.5 per 100,000 persons per year. Rates of resistance to TMP-SMX and penicillin in SOT recipients were not significantly different from those in the general population. Eighty-five percent of the isolates were strains covered by PPSV23.[60]

It is recommended that all SOT candidates who have not received a dose of PPSV23 within the past 5 years and have not received two lifetime doses be administered this vaccination. Administration of the pneumococcal conjugate vaccine (PCV13) should be completed 8 weeks before giving PPSV23 if both are indicated.[85]

If PCV13 is not provided before the SOT is performed, it should be administered 2 to 6 months following the transplant, depending on the patient's degree of immunosuppression. If the recipient has not received PPSV23 within 5 years and has not received two or more lifetime doses, it should be administered 2 to 6 months following transplantation and at least 8 weeks after PCV13. Some studies have found a seroconversion rate as high as 94% for vaccination with PPSV23.[85] Although SOT recipients can mount an immune response, it is weaker than that achieved by healthy controls.[86]

Despite guidelines, a cross-sectional study of one transplant center found that only 62.4% of patients evaluated for a lung transplant had received the *S. pneumoniae* vaccine.[87] A prime-boost strategy has been found effective for the pneumococcal conjugate vaccine PCV7 followed by PPSV23 in patients with Hodgkin lymphoma and human immunodeficiency virus infection.[88,89] A T-cell–dependent immune response is produced by the conjugate vaccine, which is more effective at producing memory B cells that can then be boosted by the polysaccharide vaccination. The prime-boost strategy was not found to improve immunogenicity in a study of renal transplant patients who received PPSV23 at 1 year following either PCV7 or PPSV23[90] or in a study of liver transplant patients who received PPSV23 8 weeks following PCV7.[91] A retrospective study of 12 LTRs found that PCV7 was immunogenic but that an additional dose of PPSV23 did not provide any additional benefit.[92]

It is recommended that all pediatric transplant patients receive *H. influenzae* type B (Hib) vaccine.[84] A paucity of data regarding this vaccination in SOT patients exists, but one study of renal transplant patients found it to be safe and effective.[93]

Again, the data regarding *Neisseria meningitidis* vaccination in the SOT recipients are limited. Regardless, it is recommended for all patients between the ages of 11 and 18 years and for adults who are in the military, have terminal complement component deficiency, travel to high-risk areas, have functional or anatomic asplenia, or are living on campus while attending college.[84]

If a candidate or recipient has not received a tetanus booster in the past 10 years, the tetanus, diphtheria, and acellular pertussis (Tdap) vaccine should be given. All adults should receive at least one dose of acellular pertussis vaccine.[84]

Protection of LTRs from vaccine-preventable infection is not limited to vaccination of the patients alone but should also include vaccination of their household members and close contacts. Immunocompetent individuals living in the same household as transplant recipients should receive all inactivated vaccinations according to the age-appropriate CDC schedule.[85]

The possibility of vaccinations triggering rejection has been proposed, but study of this issue has been limited to small case series, case reports, and expositions of theoretical beliefs.[85,94-96] Moreover, most of the available reports deal with heart or kidney transplant recipients who received influenza vaccination.[44] A study of 18 heart transplant patients found a nonsignificant increase in the incidence of rejection in those who received the influenza vaccine[96]; however, larger-scale studies found no evidence of or data on increased rejection or allograft dysfunction in association with vaccination. Multiple studies support the absence of risk for rejection and the safety of vaccination of transplant recipients in this regard.[85,88,94,97-101]

Passive immunization

No guidelines currently exist regarding the use of nonspecific intravenous immunoglobulin (IVIG) or pathogen-specific immunoglobulin preparations for the prevention of bacterial infection in LTRs. Uncontrolled trials in heart transplant recipients have shown a benefit of IVIG replacement on morbidity and mortality in patients in whom infection develops.[102] More studies should be pursued to evaluate the role of IVIG replacement therapy for hypogammaglobulinemia after lung transplantation.

Peritransplant prophylaxis

Peritransplant infection can occur as a result of pathogens present in the donor lung or from pretransplant colonization or infection in the recipient. Microbiologic evaluation of samples from donor lungs that have been obtained via bronchoscopy is a key part of posttransplant management of infection. The vast majority of donor lungs will probably have at least one organism identified.[103,104] A review of 28 LTRs at one center over a 1-year period found that infection with the organism originally identified in the donor lung developed in 21% of them.[103] Another study of 197 lung transplants found that donor-to-host transmission of bacterial infection related to donor graft colonization occurred in 10 LTRs (5.1%).[57] Although some isolated organisms, such as coagulase-negative *Staphylococcus* and diphtheroids, may be considered low risk from the standpoint of posttransplant infection, other organisms, such as *S. aureus, S. pneumoniae, H. influenzae,* and PsAR, are considered to be far more pathogenic.[44]

Broad-spectrum antimicrobials are used empirically in the immediate posttransplant setting. At our institution, we then treat posttransplant patients with a 2- week course of antibiotics targeting any pathogens identified in the donor or recipient. Although donor lung colonization is common overall, the risk for subsequent recipient infection is relatively low when proper prophylaxis is used.[104-106]

Patients with CF are known to be colonized with bacteria in both the upper and lower airways. It has been suggested that the sinuses may serve as a reservoir from which bacteria can spread and infect the lung allograft, thereby leading to deleterious effects. Therefore, some centers advocate either pretransplant or posttransplant sinus surgery; however, the data are conflicting and our center does not do so routinely.[107-109] Some lung transplant candidates, such as those with CF, may be colonized or previously infected with resistant and difficult-to-treat pathogens, such as *B. cepacia*, PsAR, *Stenotrophomonas maltophililia*, *Acinetobacter*, or *Alcaligenes xylosoxidans*. Published data suggest decreased graft and patient survival in cases of infection or colonization with extensive drug-resistant *Burkholderia* and *Stenotrophomonas*. Withholding a transplant because of the presence of resistant bacteria is a decision to be made by each individual transplant center.[44]

Minimization of risk

Like all other hospitalized patients, LTRs are at risk for nosocomial infection. Proper precautions, including basic hand hygiene, should always be used. Reports have described outbreaks of infection involving a variety of pathogens and their nosocomial spread among the transplant population.[110-114] Observing proper precautions with all patients to minimize the risk for nosocomial infection and outbreaks is imperative.

REFERENCES

1. Burguete S, Diego M, Levine F, et al. Lung transplant infection. Respirology 2013;18:22-38.
2. Alexander BD, Tapson VF. Infectious complications of lung transplantation. Transpl Infect Dis 2001;3:128-137.
3. Speich R, van der Bij W. Epidemiology and management of infections after lung transplantation. Clin Infect Dis 2001;33(Suppl 1):S58-S65.
4. Maurer JR, Tullis DE, Grossman RF, et al. Infectious complications following isolated lung transplantation. Chest 1992;10:1056-1059.
5. Zander DS, Baz MA, Visner GA, et al. Analysis of early deaths after isolated lung transplantation. Chest 2001;120:225-232.
6. Deusch E, End A, Griomm M, et al. Early bacterial infections in lung transplant recipients. Chest 1993;104:1412-1416.
7. Husain AN, Siddiqui MT, Reddy VB, et al. Postmortem findings in lung transplant recipients. Mod Pathol 1996;9:752-761.
8. Danziger-Isakov L, Sweet S, Delamorena M, et al. Epidemiology of bloodstream infections in the first year after pediatric lung transplantation. Pediatr Infect Dis J 2005;24:324-330.
9. Fishman JA. Infection in solid-organ transplant recipients. N Engl J Med 2007;357:2601-2614.
10. Patel R, Paya CV. Infections in solid-organ transplant recipients. Clin Microbiol Rev 1997;10:86-124.
11. Parada M, Alba A, Sepúlveda C. Early and late infections in lung transplantation patients. Transplant Proc 2010;42:333-335.
12. Wahidi M, Willner DA, Snyder LD, et al. Diagnosis and outcome of early pleural space infection following lung transplantation. Chest 2009;135:484-491.
13. San Juan R, Aguado JM, Diaz-Pedroche C, et al. Incidence, clinical characteristics, and risk factors of late infection in solid organ transplant recipients: Data from the RESITRA study group. Am J Transplant 2007;7:964-971.
14. Parada M, Alba A, Sepúlveda C. Bronchiolitis obliterans syndrome development in lung transplantation patients. Transplant Proc 2010;42:331-332.
15. Shields RK, Clancy CJ, Minces LR, et al. Epidemiology and outcomes of deep surgical site infections following lung transplantation. Am J Transplant 2013;13:2137-2145.
16. Lechtzin N, Majnu J, Merlo C, et al. Outcomes of adults with cystic fibrosis infected with antibiotic-resistant *Pseudomonas aeruginosa*. Respiration 2006;73:27-33.
17. D'Ovidio F, Keshavjee S. Gastroesophageal reflux and lung transplantation. Dis Esophagus 2006;19:315-320.
18. Duarte AG, Terminella L, Smith JT, et al. Restoration of cough reflex in lung transplant recipients. Chest 2008;134:310-316.
19. Etienne B, Mornex JF. Immunological aspects of lung transplantation. Rev Mal Respir 1996;13(Suppl 5):S15-S22.
20. Hodge G, Hodge S, Reynolds PN, et al. Airway infection in stable lung transplant patients is associated with decreased intracellular T-helper type 1 proinflammatory cytokines in bronchoalveolar lavage T-cell subsets. Transpl Infect Dis 2008;10:99-105.
21. Husain S, Raza K, et al. Experience with immune monitoring in lung transplant recipients: Correlation of low immune function with infection. Transplantation 2009;87:1852-1857.
22. Bhorade SM, Janata K, Vigneswaran WT, et al. Cylex ImmuKnow assay levels are lower in lung transplant recipients with infection. J Heart Lung Transplant 2008;27:990-994.
23. Heng D, Sharples LD, McNeil K, et al. Bronchiolitis obliterans syndrome: Incidence, natural history, prognosis, and risk factors. J Heart Lung Transplant 1998;17:1255-1263.

24. Girgis RE, Tu I, Berry GJ, et al. Risk factors for the development of obliterative bronchiolitis after lung transplantation. J Heart Lung Transplant 1996;15:1200-1208.

25. Egan JJ. Obliterative bronchiolitis after lung transplantation: A repetitive multiple injury airway disease. Am J Respir Crit Care Med 2004;170:931-932.

26. Goldfarb NS, Avery RK, Goormastic M, et al. Hypogammaglobulinemia in lung transplant recipients. Transplantation 2001;71:242-246.

27. Robertson J, Eidemir O, Saz EU, et al. Hypogammaglobulinemia: Incidence, risk factors, and outcomes following pediatric lung transplantation. Pediatr Transplant 2009;13:754-759.

28. Yip NH, Lederer DJ, Kawut SM, et al. Immunoglobulin levels before and after lung transplantation. Am J Respir Crit Care Med 2006;173:917-921.

29. Florescu DF, Kalil AC, Qui F, et al. What is the impact of hypogammaglobulinemia on the rate of infections and survival in solid organ transplantation? A meta-analysis. Am J Transplant 2013;13:2601-2610

30. Avery RK, Blumberg EA. Hypogammaglobuloinemia: Time to reevaluate? Am J Transplant 2013;13:2517-2518.

31. Shteinberg M, Raviv Y, Bishara J, et al. The impact of fluoroquinolone resistance of gram-negative bacteria in respiratory secretions on the outcome of lung transplant (non–cystic fibrosis) recipients. Clin Transplant 2012;26:884-890.

32. Hafkin J, Blumberg E. Infections in lung transplantation: New insights. Curr Opin Organ Transplant 2009;14:483-487.

33. Dobbin C, Maley M, Harkness J, et al. The impact of pan-resistant bacterial pathogens on survival after lung transplantation in cystic fibrosis: Results from a single large referral centre. J Hosp Infect 2004;56:277-282.

34. Aris RM, Gilligan PH, Neuringer IP, et al. The effects of panresistant bacteria in cystic fibrosis patients on lung transplant outcome. Am J Respir Crit Care Med 1997;155:1699-1704.

35. Charlson E, Diamond J, Bittinger K, et al. Lung-enriched organisms and aberrant bacterial and fungal respiratory microbiota after lung transplant. Am J Respir Crit Care Med 2012;186:536-545.

36. Palmer S, Burch L, Davis R, et al. The role of innate immunity in acute allograft rejection after lung transplantation. Am J Respir Crit Care Med 2003;168:628-632.

37. Ohmann EL, Brooks MM, Webber SA, et al. Association of genetic polymorphisms and risk of late post-transplantation infection in pediatric heart recipients. J Heart Lung Transplant 2010;29:1342-1351.

38. Cunha C, Aversa F, Lacerda J, et al. Genetic PTX3 deficiency and aspergillosis in stem-cell transplantation. N Engl J Med 2014;370:421-432.

39. Wiebe K, Fraund S, Steinmuller C, et al. Rare cytomegalovirus and *Listeria monocytogenes* infection enhance chronic rejection after allogenic rate lung transplantation. Transpl Int 2005;18:1166-1174.

40. Meyer KC, Nunley DR, Dauber JH, et al. Neutrophils, unopposed neutrophil elastase, and alpha-1 antiprotease defenses following human lung transplantation. Am J Respir Crit Care Med 2001;164:97-102.

41. Charpin JM, Stern M, Lebrun G, et al. Increased endothelin-1 associated with bacterial infection in lung transplant recipients. Transplantation 2001;7:1840-1847.

42. Yamamoto S, Nava RG, Zhu J, et al. Cutting edge: *Pseudomonas aeruginosa* abolishes established lung tolerance by stimulating B7 expression on neutrophils. J Immunol 2012;189:4221-4225.

43. Christie JD, Edwards LB, Kucheryavaya AY, et al The Registry of the International Society for Heart and Lung Transplantation: Twenty-ninth official adult lung and heart-lung transplantation report—2012. J Heart Lung Transplant 2012;31:1073-1086.

44. Ramaprasad C, Pursell K. Bacterial infections after lung transplantation. In Vigneswaran WT, Garrity ER Jr, eds. Lung Transplantation. London: Informa Healthcare; 2010:311-319.

45. Campos S, Caramori M, Teixeira R, et al. Bacterial and fungal pneumonias after lung transplantation. Transplant Proc 2008;40:822-824.

46. Aguilar-Guisado M, Givalda J, Ussetti P, et al. Pneumonia after lung transplantation in the RESITRA Cohort: A multicenter prospective study. Am J Transplant 2007;7:1989-1996.

47. Valentine VG, Bonvillain RW, Gupta MR, et al. Infections in lung allograft recipients: Ganciclovir era. J Heart Lung Transplant 2008;27:528-535.

48. de Bruyn G, Whelan TP, Mulligan MS, et al. Invasive pneumococcal infections in adult lung transplant recipients. Am J Transplant. 2004;4:1366-1371.

49. Tkatch LS, Kusne S, Irish WD, et al. Epidemiology of *Legionella* pneumonia and factors associated with legionella-related mortality at a tertiary care center. Clin Infect Dis 1998;27:1479-1486.

50. Nichols L, Strollo DC, Kusne S. Legionellosis in a lung transplant recipient obscured by cytomegalovirus infection and *Clostridium difficile* colitis. Transpl Infect Dis 2002;4:41-45.

51. Bangsborg JM, Uldum S, Jensen JS, et al. Nosocomial legionellosis in three heart-lung transplant patients: Case reports and environmental observations. Eur J Clin Microbiol Infect Dis 1995;14:99-104.

52. Simonsen L. The global impact of influenza on morbidity and mortality. Vaccine 1999;17(Suppl 1):S3-S10.

53. Peltola VT, Murti KG, McCullers JA. Influenza virus neuraminidase contributes to secondary bacterial pneumonia. J Infect Dis 2005;192:249-257.

54. Schwarzmann SW, Adler JL, Sullivan RJ Jr, et al. Bacterial pneumonia during the Hong Kong influenza epidemic of 1968-1969. Arch Intern Med 1971;127:1037-1041.

55. Hageman JC, Uyeki TM, Francis JS, et al. Severe community-acquired pneumonia due to *Staphylococcus aureus*, 2003-04 influenza season. Emerg Infect Dis 2006;12:894-899.

56. Weill D, Dey G, Hicks A, et al. A positive donor Gram stain does not predict outcome following lung transplantation. J Heart Lung Transplant 2002;21:555-558.

57. Ruiz I, Gavalda J, Monforte V, et al. Donor-to-host transmission of bacterial and fungal infections in lung transplantation. Am J Transplant 2006;6:178-182.

58. Nunley D. Grgurich W, Iacono A, et al. Allograft colonization and infections with *Pseudomonas* in cystic fibrosis lung transplant recipients. Chest 1998;113:1235-1243.

59. Smith S, Foweraker J, Hamilton D, et al. Impact of antibiotic-resistant *Pseudomonas* on the survival of cystic fibrosis (CF) patients following heart-lung transplantation. J Heart Lung Transplant 2001;20:224.

60. Kumar D, Humar A, Plevneshi A, et al. Invasive pneumococcal disease in solid organ transplant recipients—10-year prospective population surveillance. Am J Transplant 2007;7:1209-1214.

61. Doucette K, Fishman J. Nontuberculous mycobacterial infection in hematopoietic stem cell and solid organ transplant recipients. Clin Infect Dis 2004:38:1428-1439.

62. Garrison A, Morris M, Lewis S, et al. *Mycobacterium abscessus* infection in solid organ transplant recipients: Report of three cases and review of the literature. Transpl Infect Dis 2009;11:541-548.

63. Husain S, McCurry K, Dauber J, et al. *Nocardia* infection in lung transplant recipients. J Heart Lung Transplant 2002;21:354-359.

64. Abid Q, Nkere UU, Hasan A, et al. Mediastinitis in heart and lung transplantation: 15 years experience. Ann Thorac Surg 2003;75:1565-1571.

65. Nunley D, Grgurich W, Keenan R, et al. Empyema complicating successful lung transplantation. Chest 1999;115:1312-1315.

66. Fairhurst R, Kubak B, Shpiner R, et al. *Mycobacterium abscessus* empyema in a lung transplant recipient. J Heart Lung Transplant 2002;21:391-394.

67. Zar FA, Bakkanagari SR, Moorthi KM, et al. A comparison of vancomycin and metronidazole for the treatment of *Clostridium difficile*–associated diarrhea, stratified by disease severity. Clin Infect Dis 2007;45:302-307.

68. Gottlieb J, Mattner F, Weissbrodt H, et al. Impact of graft colonization with gram-negative bacteria after lung transplantation on the development of bronchiolitis obliterans syndrome in recipients with cystic fibrosis. Respir Med 2009;103,743-749.

69. Gunderson CC, Gupta MR, Lopez F, et al. *Clostridium difficile* colitis in lung transplantation. Transpl Infect Dis 2008;10:245-251.

70. Vos R, Vanaudenaerde BM, De Vleeschauwer SI, et al. De novo or persistent pseudomonal airway colonization after lung transplantation: Importance for bronchiolitis obliterans syndrome? Transplantation 2008;86:624-625; author reply 635-636.

71. Vos R, Vanaudenaerde BM, Geudens N, et al. Pseudomonal airway colonisation: Risk factor for bronchiolitis obliterans syndrome after lung transplantation? Eur Respir J 2008;31:1037-1045.

72. Vos R, Blondeau K, Vanaudenaerde BM, et al. Airway colonization and gastric aspiration after lung transplantation: Do birds of a feather flock together? J Heart Lung Transplant 2008;27:843-849.

73. Hartwig MG, Appel JZ, Li B, et al. Chronic aspiration of gastric fluid accelerates pulmonary allograft dysfunction in a rat model of lung transplantation. J Thorac Cardiovasc Surg 2006;131:209-217.

74. Zander MS. Safety and efficacy of influenza vaccination in renal transplant recipients. Nat Clin Pract Nephrol 2008;4:358-359.

75. Sopirala MM, Pope-Harman A, Nunley, DR, et al. Multidrug-resistant *Acinetobacter baumannii* pneumonia in lung transplant recipients. J Heart Lung Transplant 2008;27:804-807.

76. Patel G, Perez F, Bonomo RA. Carbapenem-resistant Enterobacteriaceae and *Acinetobacter baumannii*: Assessing their impact on organ transplantation. Curr Opin Organ Transplant 2010;15:676-682.

77. Mattner F, Fischer S, Weissbrodt H, et al. Postoperative nosocomial infections after lung and heart transplantation. J Heart Lung Transplant 2007;26:241-249.

78. Poonyagariyagorn HK, Gershman A, Avery R, et al. Challenges in the diagnosis and management of *Nocardia* infections in lung transplant recipients. Transpl Infect Dis 2008;10:403-408.

79. Khan BA, Duncan M, Reynolds J, et al. *Nocardia* infection in lung transplant recipients. Clin Transplant 2008;22:562-566.

80. Janssens W, Van Raemdonck D, Dupont L, et al. J Heart Lung Transplant 2006;25:734-737.

81. Le Lay G, Martin F, Leroyer C, et al. *Rhodococcus equi* causing bacteraemia and pneumonia in a pulmonary transplant patient. J Infect 1996;33:239-240.

82. Chernenko SM, Humar A, Hutcheon M, et al. *Mycobacterium abscessus* infections in lung transplant recipients: The international experience. J Heart Lung Transplant 2006;25:1447-1455.

83. Malouf MA, Glanville AR. The spectrum of mycobacterial infection after lung transplantation. Am J Respir Crit Care Med 1999;160:1611-1616.

84. Danziger- Isakov L, Kumar D. Vaccination in solid organ transplantation. Am J Transplant 2013;13:311-317.

85. Rubin LG, Levin MJ, Ljungman P, et al. 2013 IDSA clinical practice guideline for vaccination of the immunocompromised host. Clin Infect Dis 2014;58:309-318.

86. Blumberg EA, Brozena SC, Stutman P, et al. Immunogenicity of pneumococcal vaccine in heart transplant recipients. Clin Infect Dis 2001;32:307-310.

87. Gasink LB, Wurcell AG, Kotloff RM, et al. Low prevalence of prior *Streptococcus pneumoniae* vaccination among potential lung transplant candidates. Chest 2006;130:218-221.

88. Chan CY, Molrine DC, George S, et al. Pneumococcal conjugate vaccine primes for antibody responses to polysaccharide pneumococcal vaccine after treatment of Hodgkin's disease. J Infect Dis 1996;173:256-258.

89. Lesprit P, Pedrono G, Molina JM, et al. Immunological efficacy of a prime-boost pneumococcal vaccination in HIV-infected adults. AIDS. 2007;21:2425-2434.

90. Tobudic S, Plunger V, Sunder-Plassmann, et al. Randomized, single blind, controlled trial to evaluate the prime-boost strategy for pneumococcal vaccination in renal transplant recipients. PLoS One 2012;7:e46133.

91. Kumar D, Chen MH, Wong G, et al. A randomized, double-blind, placebo-controlled trial to evaluate the prime-boost strategy for pneumococcal vaccination in adult liver transplant recipients. Clin Infect Dis 2008;47:885-892.

92. Gattringer R, Winkler H, Roedler S, et al. Immunogenicity of a combined schedule of 7-valent pneumococcal conjugate vaccine followed by a 23-valent polysaccharide vaccine in adult recipients of heart or lung transplants. Transpl Infect Dis 2011;3:540-544.

93. Sever MS, Yildiz A, Eraksoy H, et al. Immune response to *Haemophilus influenzae* type B vaccination in renal transplant recipients with well-functioning allografts. Nephron 1999;81:55-59.

94. Avery RK. Influenza vaccines in the setting of solid-organ transplantation: Are they safe? Curr Opin Infect Dis 2012;25:464-468.

95. Vistoli F, Focosi D, De Donno M, et al. Pancreas rejection after pandemic influenza virus A (H1N1) vaccination or infection: A report of two cases. Transpl Int 2011;24:e28-e29.

96. Blumberg EA, Fitzpatrick J, Stutman PC, et al. Safety of influenza vaccine in heart transplant recipients. J Heart Lung Transplant 1998;17:1075-1080.

97. Kimball P, Verbeke S, Flattery M, et al. Influenza vaccination does not promote cellular or humoral activation among heart transplant recipients. Transplantation 2000;69:2449-2451.

98. Magnani G, Falchetti E, Pollini G, et al. Safety and efficacy of two types of influenza vaccination in heart transplant recipients: A prospective randomised controlled study. J Heart Lung Transplant 2005;24:588-592.

99. White-Williams C, Brown R, Kirklin J, et al. Improving clinical practice: Should we give influenza vaccinations to heart transplant patients? J Heart Lung Transplant 2006;25:320-323.

100. Scharpe J, Evenepoel P, Maes B, et al. Influenza vaccination is efficacious and safe in renal transplant recipients. Am J Transplant. 2008;8:332-337.

101. Hurst FP, Lee JJ, Jindal RM, et al. Outcomes associated with influenza vaccination in the first year after kidney transplantation. Clin J Am Soc Nephrol 2011;6:1192-1197.

102. Carbone J, Sarmiento E, Palomo J, et al. The potential impact of substitutive therapy with intravenous immunoglobulin on the outcome of heart transplant recipients with infections. Transpl Proc 2007;39:2385-2388.

103. Low DE, Kaiser LR, Haydock DA, et al. The donor lung: Infectious and pathologic factors affecting outcome in lung transplantation. J Thorac Cardiovasc Surg 1993;106:614-621.

104. Bonde PN, Patel ND, Borja MC, et al. Impact of donor lung organisms on post–lung transplant pneumonia. J Heart Lung Transplant 2006;25:99-105.

105. Mattner F, Kola A, Fischer S, et al. Impact of bacterial and fungal donor organ contamination in lung, heart-lung, heart and liver transplantation. Infection 2008 36:207-212.

106. Len O, Gavalda J, Blanes M, et al. Donor infection and transmission to the recipient of a solid allograft. Am J Transplant 2008;8:2420-2425.

107. Holzmann D, Speich R, Kaufmann T, et al. Effects of sinus surgery in patients with cystic fibrosis after lung transplantation: A 10-year experience. Transplantation 2004;15;77:134-136.

108. Leung MK, Rachakonda L, Weill D, Hwang PH. Effects of sinus surgery on lung transplantation outcomes in cystic fibrosis. *Am J Rhinol* 2008;22:192-196.

109. Vital D, Hofer M, Benden C, et al. Impact of sinus surgery on pseudomonal airway colonization, bronchiolitis obliterans syndrome and survival in cystic fibrosis lung transplant recipients. Respiration 2013;86:25-31.

110. Paterson DL, Singh N, Rihs JD, et al. Control of an outbreak of infection due to extended-spectrum beta-lactamase–producing *Escherichia coli* in a liver transplantation unit. Clin Infect Dis 2001;33:126-128.

111. Huebner ES, Christman B, Dummer S, et al. Hospital-acquired *Bordetella bronchiseptica* infection following hematopoietic stem cell transplantation. J Clin Microbiol 2006;44:2581-2583.

112. Singh N, Squier C, Wannstedt C, et al. Impact of an aggressive infection control strategy on endemic *Staphylococcus aureus* infection in liver transplant recipients. Infect Control Hosp Epidemiol 2006;27:122-126.

113. Iroh Tam PY, Kline S, Wagner JE, Rapidly growing mycobacteria among pediatric hematopoietic cell transplant patients traced to the hospital water supply. Pediatr Infect Dis J 2014;33: 1043-1046.

114. Boszczowski I, do Prado GV, Dalben MF, et al. Polyclonal outbreak of bloodstream infections caused by *Burkholderia cepacia* complex in hematology and bone marrow transplant outpatient units. Rev Inst Med Trop Sao Paulo 2014;56:71-76.

32

Diagnosis of lung rejection and infection: A pathologist's perspective

VIJAYALAKSHMI ANANTHANARAYANAN AND ALIYA N. HUSAIN

INTRODUCTION

Acute rejection contributes to significant morbidity in lung transplant recipients, and repeated episodes predispose them to the development of chronic rejection. The diagnosis of acute rejection is often made on the basis of routine surveillance transbronchial biopsy. Alternatively, the diagnosis can be based on a patient's symptoms and worsening pulmonary function test results. The frequency with which surveillance biopsies are performed varies from institution to institution. A biopsy sample is considered adequate for evaluation of rejection if it includes at least one airway and four or five fragments of well-expanded, alveolated lung (each containing 50 to 100 alveoli). Specimens may require gentle agitation in formalin to promote inflation of the fragments. It is recommended that after specimens have been processed, at least five 5-μm levels be cut. Generally, levels 1, 3, and 5 are stained with hematoxylin and eosin (H&E). The remaining unstained slides can be used for special stains or immunostains as described later.

REJECTION

Rejection is classified as acute or chronic on the basis of the absence or presence of airway fibrosis. The presence of fibrosis is deemed irreversible, thus making it the key distinction between acute and chronic rejection. Acute rejection can be either cellular or antibody mediated. The grading of acute cellular rejection (ACR) is based on the amount of perivascular (grade A) and airway inflammation (grade B).

The morphology and intensity of perivascular cellular infiltrates, including their extent and distribution, are the cornerstones of histologic grading. Either the 1996[1] or 2007[2] International Society for Heart and Lung Transplantation (ISHLT) classification can be used for grading (Table 32.1). The only difference between the two is that in the latter formulation, airway inflammation grades are collapsed into two grades from four. However, because it is becoming evident that airway inflammation significantly increases the risk for chronic rejection, and as more emphasis is being placed on treating mild airway rejection, many centers are either giving both classifications or using just the 1996 version. Both components (i.e., acute perivascular rejection and airway inflammation) need to be incorporated into the final interpretation of the biopsy sample. The grade AX is used to denote no alveoli and BX is used to indicate no airway in the biopsy specimen.

Acute perivascular rejection (grade A)

Acute perivascular rejection is characterized by circumferential inflammatory cell infiltrates around blood vessels, particularly venules and lymphatics. Grade A0 (no acute rejection) indicates that the pulmonary parenchyma is normal without any inflammation (Figure 32.1A). Grade A1 (minimal ACR) is used for scattered but infrequent perivascular mononuclear infiltrates (Figure 32.1B). These infiltrates may or may not be obvious at low magnification, depending on whether the biopsy sample is adequately alveolated and free of artifacts. The inflammatory infiltrate generally

Table 32.1 Comparison of the 1996 and 2007 ISHLT classification schemes for grading pulmonary allograft rejection

Description of rejection	1996 grade	2007 grade
Perivascular		
None	A0	A0
Minimal	A1	A1
Mild	A2	A2
Moderate	A3	A3
Severe	A4	A4
Airway inflammation		
None	B0	B0R
Minimal	B1	B1R
Mild	B2	B1R
Moderate	B3	B2R
Severe	B4	B2R

Note: ISHLT, International Society for Heart and Lung Transplantation.

consists of a two- to three-cell layer-thick, circumferential ring of small plasmacytoid lymphocytes admixed with transformed lymphocytes. Grade A2 (mild ACR) is characterized by easily appreciable, frequent perivascular infiltrates (Figure 32.1C). In addition to lymphocytes and activated lymphocytes, the infiltrate also includes admixed eosinophils and macrophages. Moreover, the mononuclear cells may infiltrate the subendothelial layer and thus result in endothelialitis. The key difference between A2 and A3 rejection is that in the case of grade A3 (moderate ACR), the inflammatory infiltrate extends beyond the confines of the perivascular interstitium into the adjacent air spaces or alveolar septa. Endothelialitis is common in grade A3 rejection (Figure 32.1D). Grade A4 (severe acute rejection) lesions are characterized by pneumocyte damage and prominent endothelialitis, which is generally accompanied by intra-alveolar necrotic debris, hemorrhage, neutrophils, and hyaline membranes (seen rarely). With current immunosuppressive regimens, grade A4 rejection is not commonly encountered in daily practice. There is reason to believe that some

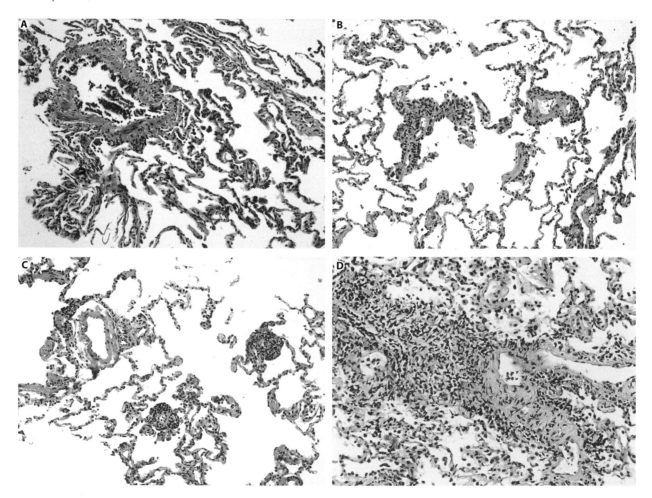

Figure 32.1 Acute cellular vascular rejection. **(A)** Transbronchial lung biopsy specimen showing alveolated lung parenchyma and the associated airway with no cellular rejection (grade A0, B0). **(B)** Minimal acute perivascular rejection with incomplete rimming of vessels by activated lymphocytes (grade A1). **(C)** Mild acute perivascular rejection with more than three layers of perivascular lymphoid infiltrates (grade A2). **(D)** Moderate acute cellular rejection with extensive perivascular lymphoid infiltrates that extend into the alveolar septa (grade A3).

overlap of grade A4 ACR with antibody-mediated rejection (AMR), which is discussed later, might exist.

Airway inflammation and lymphocytic bronchiolitis (grade B acute airway rejection)

According to the ISHLT, grade B was called airway inflammation or lymphocytic bronchiolitis because the pathologists were of the opinion that airway rejection could not be reliably distinguished from infection. On the basis of our experience, however, acute airway rejection is akin to acute cellular perivascular rejection in the sense that it is also characterized by mixed inflammation in the submucosa with activated lymphocytes, eosinophils, and plasma cells. Thus, we recommend that the term *acute airway rejection* be used instead of the nonspecific terms *airway inflammation* and *lymphocytic bronchiolitis*. In cases of predominance of neutrophils (especially intraepithelial neutrophils) in this inflammation, infection is more likely, and this likelihood should be stated in the pathology report (in either the diagnosis or a comment).

In the ISHLT classification of lung rejection[1,2] the designation grade B is assigned to smaller non–cartilage-containing airways (i.e., bronchioles). In our experience, however, both the large and the small airways can show ACR. Airway inflammation was graded from B0 (no inflammation) to B4 (severe airway inflammation) in the 1996 classification (see Table 32.1). However, because of high interobserver and intraobserver variability in the evaluation of airway inflammation, the grading was collapsed into a two-tier (low-grade and high-grade) system in 2007. The previously used terms *B0* and *BX* were retained in the newer classification. At our institution, we still use the 1996 grading system for evaluating airway inflammation because it provides greater information and detail regarding the biopsy sample. Several studies have shown that airway rejection is an independent risk factor for the development of chronic rejection; it may even be more important than perivascular rejection.[3,4]

When no inflammation is present in the airway, the sample is called negative for airway rejection (B0). In cases of minimal acute airway rejection (B1), small and few foci of infiltrates are located between the mucosa and muscle layer (Figure 32.2A). With mild acute airway rejection (B2), a band-like submucosal infiltrate is present (Figure 32.2B). Occasional eosinophils may be seen. In grades B1 and B2 (i.e., B1R according to the new classification) samples, no epithelial damage or intraepithelial lymphocytes are present. The features of moderate acute airway rejection (B3) are similar to those of grade B2 rejection, but with extension into the overlying epithelium (Figure 32.2C). The submucosal mononuclear infiltrates show a greater proportion of larger activated lymphocytes, plasmacytoid cells, and eosinophils. Severe airway rejection (B4) includes ulceration, fibrinopurulent exudate, and epithelial cell necrosis. Having said that, it is important to remember that a disproportionate increase in the number of neutrophils in the epithelium in relation to mononuclear cells in the submucosa probably indicates an underlying infection rather than rejection (Figure 32.2D). It should also be noted that in some patients concurrent rejection and infection may be present because the latter can trigger rejection.

Bronchus-associated lymphoid tissue (BALT) is often hyperplastic in lung transplant recipients and should be considered in the differential diagnosis of ACR. The main histologic features of BALT are nodular infiltrates of mature lymphocytes located eccentrically adjacent to an airway (Figure 32.3A). When doubt exists, immunohistochemical staining for CD21 can be used to demonstrate follicular dendritic cells, which are often present in the center of BALT but are absent in rejection (Figure 32.3B).[5,6]

Chronic airway rejection and obliterative bronchiolitis (grade C)

The incidence of chronic airway rejection is 49% at 5 years and 76% by 10 years after transplantation, and it contributes to significant morbidity and mortality in lung transplant recipients.[7] It can occur anytime from a few weeks to several years after transplantation. The diagnosis of obliterative bronchiolitis (OB) is made clinically; pathologic confirmation is not deemed necessary. In fact, transbronchial biopsy is often considered an insensitive method for detection of OB because of the patchy distribution of the lesions. A wedge biopsy may sometimes be needed to diagnose OB, which is characterized by dense polypoid or eccentric submucosal fibrosis that results in partial or complete luminal obstruction (Figure 32.4). In active OB, intrabronchial and peribronchial mononuclear inflammation is seen in addition to submucosal fibrosis. The distinction between active and inactive OB was included in the 1996 working formulation but subsequently omitted from the 2007 classification, in which a biopsy sample is designated as C1 or C0 depending on the presence of evidence of obliterative bronchiolitis.

The clinical counterpart of OB, bronchiolitis obliterans syndrome, is a subset of the newly introduced clinical diagnosis chronic lung allograft dysfunction, which is defined as dysfunction with any cause that persists for more than 3 weeks.[8]

Chronic vascular rejection (grade D)

Unlike in other types of solid-organ transplantation, chronic vascular rejection is rarely clinically significant in lung transplantation, although it is often seen in patients with OB. Chronic vascular rejection is characterized by fibrointimal thickening of arteries and veins that is similar to the coronary allograft vasculopathy seen in cardiac transplant recipients. Trichrome stain highlights the fibrosis both in airways and in vessels. Chronic vascular rejection can be diagnosed on the basis of wedge biopsies and only rarely by transbronchial biopsies.

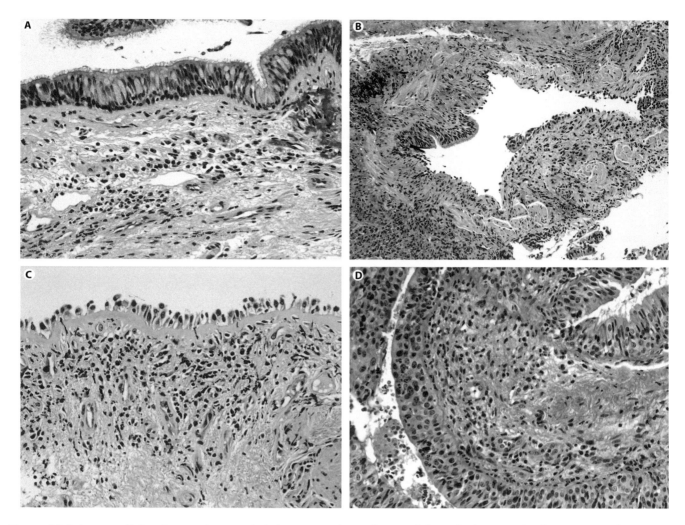

Figure 32.2 Acute cellular airway rejection. **(A)** This airway shows few small foci of submucosal inflammatory infiltrates in minimal rejection (grade B1/B1R). **(B)** A band-like inflammatory infiltrate is present in the submucosa in mild rejection (grade B2/B1R). **(C)** Inflammation extends into the overlying epithelium in moderate acute airway rejection (grade B3/B2R). **(D)** Inflammation with abundant neutrophils is present in both the epithelium and submucosa in this patient with infection.

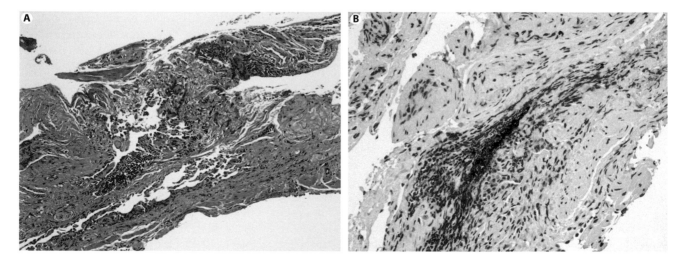

Figure 32.3 Bronchus-associated lymphoid tissue (BALT). **(A)** Rounded focal collections of mature lymphocytes are present in the peribronchial tissue. **(B)** CD21 stain (immunohistochemistry) highlights the dendritic cells in a center of BALT (this stain is negative in rejection).

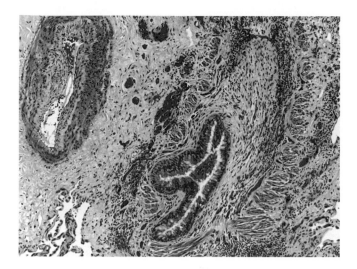

Figure 32.4 Obliterative bronchiolitis. Eccentric submucosal fibrosis and chronic inflammation partially occluding the lumen of this airway (grade C1a) is visible. Also note the pulmonary artery branch in the upper left, which shows intimal fibrosis (chronic vascular rejection, grade D).

Antibody-mediated (humoral) rejection

AMR is caused by interactions between preexisting or de novo donor-specific antibodies (DSAs) that usually react with human leukocyte antigens (HLAs) expressed on endothelial cells.[9] Deposition of the antigen-antibody complex in turn activates the complement cascade, which results in further graft injury.

In 2004, the National Conference to Assess Antibody-Mediated Rejection in Solid Organ Transplantation proposed several stages of humoral rejection in solid organs that can be identified on the basis of the presence of DSAs, deposition of the complement component 4d (C4d), tissue pathology, and clinical allograft dysfunction (Table 32.2).[10] Even though this grading system is very useful in research settings, its use in daily clinical practice is limited.

Although the diagnosis of AMR is well recognized in heart and renal transplantation, in lung transplantation it is fraught with controversies and challenges, and no universally accepted diagnostic criteria exist. AMR remains a diagnosis of exclusion that requires correlation with serologic and microbiologic studies. As in other solid organs, in the lung, AMR can be classified as hyperacute or acute.

HYPERACUTE ANTIBODY-MEDIATED REJECTION

Hyperacute rejection is a rare phenomenon in which preexisting antibodies react with the allograft during or shortly after transplantation. Preexisting antibodies arise from previous antigen exposure as a result of pregnancy, previous transfusions, or transplants. Clinically, acute-onset respiratory failure with pulmonary infiltrates occurs. Pathologic examination reveals neutrophilic margination with vasculitis and fibrinoid necrosis of the vessel walls. Thankfully, the incidence of hyperacute rejection is extremely rare because of better pretransplantation compatibility testing.

ACUTE ANTIBODY-MEDIATED REJECTION

On the basis of extrapolation of the findings seen in kidney and heart allografts with AMR, it has been speculated that capillary dilatation, endothelial swelling, and increased numbers of circulating white blood cells could be features of AMR in the lung. Badesch and colleagues[11] reported the findings of pulmonary capillaritis in patients with graft dysfunction. Pulmonary capillaritis is defined as an increased number of neutrophils along the capillary bed and focal fibrinoid necrosis with or without spillage into the alveolar space.[12,9] Similarly, in 2005, Astor and colleagues reported pulmonary capillaritis in 35 patients with allograft dysfunction.[13] HLA antibody data for these patients were not available; however, it was speculated that the clinical and the pathologic findings were distinct from those seen in typical cases of ACR.

In the 2007 ISHLT classification, no consensus criteria were formulated for the diagnosis of AMR. Instead, the ISHLT coined the term *capillary injury* (in place of *capillaritis*) to describe the pattern of injury in AMR and noted that it represented a nonspecific morphologic spectrum of injury that can also be seen in other conditions, including

Table 32.2 Putative stages of the humoral response to an organ graft

Stage	Features
Stage I: Latent humoral response	Circulating antibody alone (antibodies are directed against HLA or other antigens on donor endothelial cells)
	No C4d deposition
	No tissue pathology
	No clinical evidence of graft dysfunction
Stage II: Silent humoral reaction	Circulating antibody + C4d deposition
	No tissue pathology
	No clinical evidence of graft dysfunction
Stage III: Subclinical humoral rejection*	Circulating antibody + C4d deposition + tissue pathology
	No clinical evidence of graft dysfunction
Stage IV: Humoral rejection	Circulating antibody + C4d deposition + tissue pathology + graft dysfunction

Note: *May differ among organs because the ability to detect mild degrees of graft dysfunction varies.

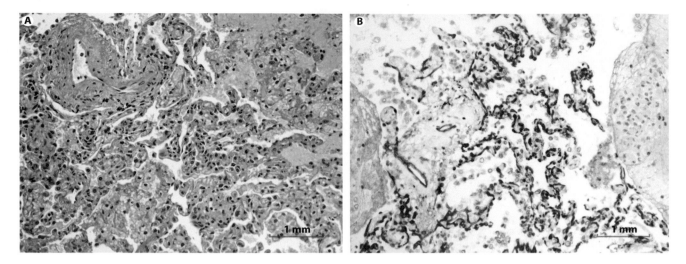

Figure 32.5 Acute antibody-mediated rejection in an HLA-positive patient with severe lung dysfunction 14 days after transplantation. **(A)** Hematoxylin and eosin staining of a transbronchial biopsy sample shows capillary injury. **(B)** Immunohistochemical staining for C4d shows strong diffuse endothelial staining. (Courtesy of M. Angeles Montero M.D, Ph.D, London, England.)

infection, diffuse alveolar damage (DAD), and rejection (Figure 32.5A).[2,13] The 2007 guidelines further suggest that small-vessel intimitis (inflammation within the intima of the vessel) should raise suspicion for AMR.

The ISHLT came to the conclusion that if a reason to suspect AMR on the basis of clinical, morphologic, or serologic grounds exists, immunohistochemistry studies for byproducts of complement activation (C3d and C4d) should be performed. Only strong diffuse endothelial staining should be considered positive (Figure 32.5B). That being said, it is important to remember that there are caveats to interpreting C4d immunostaining in isolation without an appropriate clinical context. C4d immunostaining can also be seen with other causes of complement activation such as infection or DAD (Figure 32.6A).[14,15] At our institution we routinely perform C4d immunostaining on all heart and lung allograft biopsy specimens. Unlike the situation in the heart biopsies, C4d immunostaining of samples from lung transplant recipients (performed prospectively on all biopsy specimens from 100 consecutive patients) was not positive in any case. Furthermore, none of the specimens showed capillaritis or capillary injury. However, almost all the C4d stains demonstrated background staining, especially in the elastic fibers (Figure 32.6B).

In summary, AMR rarely occurs in the lung; it is a diagnosis based on clinical, serologic, and pathologic findings. The biopsy findings have several morphologic overlaps with other causes of graft dysfunction, including infection, ischemia-reperfusion injury, high-grade ACR, aspiration, and drug toxicity.

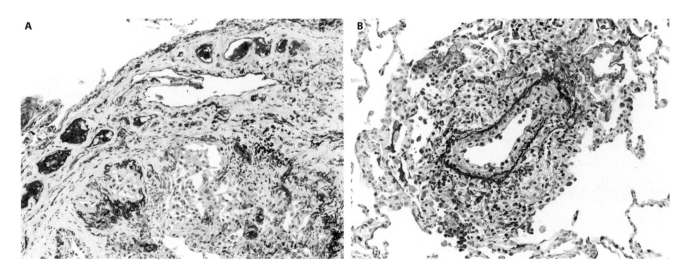

Figure 32.6 Nonspecific C4d staining. **(A)** Posttransplant patient with viral infection showing focal endothelial staining with C4d. **(B)** Patient with cellular rejection and background elastic staining with C4d.

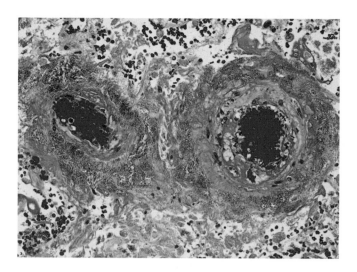

Figure 32.7 Bacterial pneumonia. Numerous bacteria are visible around the blood vessels with no inflammatory response in this severely immunocompromised lung recipient, who died of pneumonia 5 days after transplantation.

INFECTION

The ISHLT has proposed several standardized definitions of bacterial, viral, and fungal infection occurring in cardiothoracic transplant recipients.[16] Of these three types of infection, bacterial infection (respiratory and nonrespiratory) is the major contributor to early and late posttransplant complications. Bacterial infection may originate with the donor or the recipient or it may be nosocomial. Because tissue diagnosis is not used for confirmation of bacterial infection, it is not discussed further here. If infection is present at autopsy, extensive bacterial growth is associated with necrosis but is without a significant inflammatory response in such immunocompromised patients (Figure 32.7).

Approximately 50% to 90% of the North American adult population is infected with and latently harbors cytomegalovirus (CMV) for life within endothelial cells, monocytes, macrophages, neutrophils, and renal and pulmonary epithelial cells. Most CMV infection is inapparent and asymptomatic. The recent explosion in molecular diagnostic techniques has greatly improved the recovery of viral pathogens. CMV remains one of the most common opportunistic viral pathogens in lung transplant recipients. Immunocompromised hosts can exhibit fever, cough, rales, or hypoxemia with radiologic findings of ground-glass opacity, reticular interstitial density, consolidation, or pleural effusion. Dissemination may also occur in immunocompromised hosts and result in hepatitis, thrombocytopenia, or encephalitis.[17] Four main patterns of tissue response exist. The most common is the miliary necroinflammatory form, which consists of small, multicentric nodules of central hemorrhage, necrosis, and fibrin surrounded by necrotic alveolar walls and inflammatory cells. DAD or hemorrhagic pneumonia may also occur. Rarely, CMV infection may assume the form of diffuse interstitial pneumonitis or a solitary nodule with minimal nonspecific inflammation. The cytopathic effects of the virus are very distinct. As the name implies, cytomegaly (i.e., enlargement) of the infected cell, which could be an epithelial cell, an endothelial cell, a macrophage, or tissue fibroblast, is present. Both intranuclear and intracytoplasmic inclusions are present. Intranuclear inclusions are single, large (20 μm), basophilic, round to oval structures with nuclear membrane accentuation and a peripheral halo resulting in an "owl's eye" morphology. Such inclusions are also called Cowdry A inclusions. In contrast, the intracytoplasmic inclusions tend to be approximately 1- to 3-μm multiple, granular, basophilic, or amphophilic bodies (Figure 32.8A).

Immunohistochemistry (Figure 32.8B) can be used to confirm the diagnosis of CMV infection and is considered a very sensitive and specific method for diagnosing the infection at a very early stage.[18] At our institution, CMV immunostaining is routinely performed on the surveillance

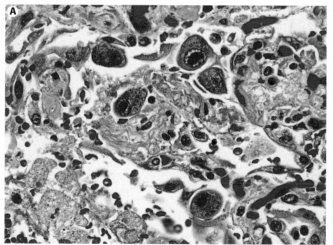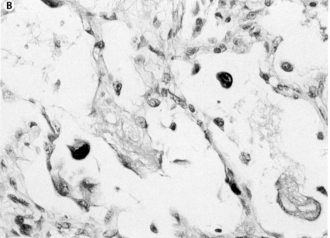

Figure 32.8 Cytomegalovirus (CMV) pneumonia. **(A)** Multiple well-developed inclusions with characteristic features (i.e., enlarged cells, a single intranuclear inclusion, and multiple cytoplasmic inclusions) are visible. **(B)** Immunohistochemical stain for CMV is positive in cells showing little or no cytopathic effect.

biopsies because of the high clinical impact of an early diagnosis. The main differential diagnosis for CMV infection includes other types of viral pneumonia, such as those caused by herpesvirus (which results in eosinophilic ground-glass nuclear inclusions without cytomegaly), adenovirus ("smudgy" nuclear inclusions), and measles virus (intracytoplasmic, eosinophilic inclusions and giant cells). DAD and interstitial pneumonitis of other causes also enter into the differential diagnosis.

Fungal infection likewise remains a serious cause of morbidity and mortality in lung transplant recipients despite the use of antifungal prophylaxis. Although less frequent than either bacterial or viral infection, fungal infection is associated with higher mortality.[19] The cumulative incidence of fungal infection in lung transplant recipients at 1 year is 8%.[20,21] The vast majority of cases of mold infection are caused by *Aspergillus* species, followed by *Scedosporium* species and Zygomycetes.[16] Species of *Candida*, which is a common pathogen in cardiac transplant recipients, are rarely seen in lung transplant recipients in the current era of prophylaxis. In contrast to other solid-organ transplant recipients, lung transplant recipients also show unique clinical syndromes associated with fungal infection, including colonization, tracheobronchitis, and anastomotic site infection.

Of all solid-organ transplant recipients, lung transplant recipients have the highest incidence of invasive aspergillosis (cumulative incidence at 1 year, 3.8%).[20] However, not all patients who have had *Aspergillus* isolated from their respiratory airways have invasive disease. Colonization and anastomotic site infection can also occur, although the incidence of these events has decreased greatly thanks to better surgical techniques. Risk factors for invasive bronchopulmonary aspergillosis include a high level of immunosuppression, single-lung transplantation, environmental exposure, hypogammaglobulinemia, and CMV infection.[19] At initial examination, patients have hemoptysis and pleuritic-type chest pain. Because of angioinvasion and fungal emboli,

lesions appear grossly as targetoid nodules with necrosis and infarction. Microscopically, they are characterized by hemorrhagic infarction with necrotizing pneumonia. Fungal hyphae are septate and show branching at acute angles (Figure 32.9A). The hyphal forms can be demonstrated by using Gomori methenamine silver and periodic acid–Schiff stains (Figure 32.9B). *Aspergillus* species cannot be distinguished from *Fusarium* or *Scedosporium* species on morphologic grounds. The distinction can be made only by culture. On the other hand, Zygomyctes genera (including *Mucor* and *Rhizopus*) can be identified (on most occasions) by the presence of irregular, broad aseptate hyphae that show right-angle branching. The incidence of *Mucor* in transplant recipients is much lower. As mentioned previously, *Candida* is a less common cause of fungal pneumonia but is morphologically distinguishable from other hyphae by the presence of budding yeasts and pseudohyphae, which are secondary to hematogenous dissemination or aspiration from the oral cavity or upper respiratory tract. The other yeast that is not uncommonly encountered in the cardiothoracic transplant setting is *Cryptococcus*, which is differentiated from *Candida* by its round shape and capsule. The capsular material is also stained by mucicarmine, a routine histochemical stain commonly used for making this distinction in daily practice. Another yeast-like fungus causing pneumonia in up to 13% of lung transplant recipients is *Pneumocystis jirovecii* (*Pneumocystis carinii*).[22] Laboratory diagnosis of *Pneumocystis* is usually made by demonstrating the organisms in induced sputum or bronchoalveolar lavage fluid or in a lung biopsy specimen. The classic histologic findings on H&E-stained sections of lung include foamy, acellular exudates within alveolar spaces and chronic interstitial inflammation. The cyst forms of *Pneumocystis* are visualized only by Gomori methenamine silver staining, in which case they appear as crescent-shaped, cup-shaped, or boat-shaped unicellular forms without budding. Rarely, pneumocystis can be associated with a granulomatous inflammation.

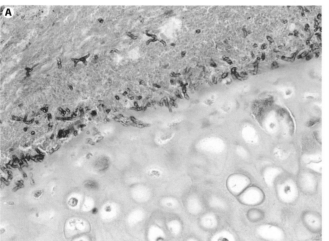 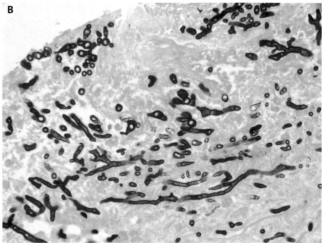

Figure 32.9 Aspergillus infection. **(A)** Fungal hyphae are seen invading soft tissue and necrotic cartilage. **(B)** Gomori methenamine silver stain demonstrating branching septate hyphae.

POSTTRANSPLANT LYMPHOPROLIFERATIVE DISORDER

Posttransplant lymphoproliferative disorder (PTLD) comprises a heterogeneous group of lymphoid or plasmacytic proliferations that occur in solid-organ or bone marrow and stem cell transplant recipients as a consequence of immunosuppression and decreased immunologic surveillance. Most of these proliferations are associated with Epstein-Barr virus (EBV) infection. EBV-negative PTLD is probably caused by human herpesvirus 8, other unknown viruses, or chronic antigenic stimulation. In adult solid-organ allografts, the incidence of PLTD is partially correlated with the intensity of the immunosuppressive regimen, with the lowest frequencies occurring in renal transplant recipients (<1%) and the highest in lung and intestinal transplant recipients (>5%).[23] In stem cell transplant recipients, PTLD is of donor origin, whereas it is of host origin in solid-organ recipients. Furthermore, in lung transplant patients, PTLD frequently involves the allograft, thus resulting in diagnostic challenges. The World Health Organization classifies PTLD into the following types: early lesions, polymorphic PTLD, monomorphic PTLD, and classical Hodgkin lymphoma–type PTLD.[24,25] Lung involvement in PTLD is mostly of the polymorphic or monomorphic type. On the other hand, the early lesions frequently involve the lymph nodes, tonsils, or adenoids and, less frequently, extranodal sites such as the lung. Histologically, they appear as infectious mononucleosis–like lesions or plasmacytic hyperplasia with preservation of lymph node architecture. In situ hybridization reveals EBV-positive cells. In polymorphic PTLD, the infiltrate is more aggressive with necrosis, larger cells with atypical mitosis, and effacement of the tissue architecture. In situ hybridization studies reveal numerous EBV-positive cells.

The early lesions and some of the polymorphic forms of PTLD regress with reduction of immunosuppression. Monomorphic PTLD fulfills the diagnostic criteria for B- and T-cell or natural killer cell neoplasms in immunocompetent patients, and it can demonstrate any of the morphologic patterns of B- and T-cell lymphomas. Classic Hodgkin lymphoma is the least frequent of all forms of PTLD; it is common in renal allografts and almost always EBV positive. Monomorphic, classic Hodgkin-like PTLD does not respond to a reduction in immunosuppression alone and frequently requires systemic chemotherapy. Long-term survival depends on the type of PTLD and other factors such as graft function. As expected, early PTLD lesions tend to have the best prognosis. The main histologic differential diagnosis is ACR, which does not usually appear as a mass lesion. Furthermore, ACR is a mixed mononuclear, perivascular, or peribronchiolar cell infiltrate that tends to be EBV negative.

SUMMARY

The diagnosis of ACR in the lung is not always straightforward. Moreover, the grading of ACR is subject to interobserver variability. Infection remains the key differential diagnosis for ACR. Despite this fact, on most occasions infection can be reliably distinguished from rejection on morphologic grounds alone. Ancillary stains and microbiologic and serologic data can further clarify this diagnostic dilemma. On the other hand, the territory of AMR in the lung continues to remain enigmatic and poses several diagnostic challenges and controversies.

REFERENCES

1. Yousem SA, Berry GJ, Cagle PT, et al. Revision of the 1990 working formulation for the classification of pulmonary allograft rejection: Lung Rejection Study Group. J Heart Lung Transplant 1996;15:1-15.
2. Stewart S, Fishbein MC, Snell GI, et al. Revision of the 1996 working formulation for the standardization of nomenclature in the diagnosis of lung rejection. J Heart Lung Transplant 2007;26:1229-1242.
3. Husain AN, Siddiqui MT, Holmes EW, et al. Analysis of risk factors for the development of bronchiolitis obliterans syndrome. Am J Respir Crit Care Med 1999;159:829-833.
4. Glanville AR, Aboyoun CL, Havryk A, et al. Severity of lymphocytic bronchiolitis predicts long-term outcome after lung transplantation. Am J Respir Crit Care Med 2008;177:1033-1040.
5. Sattar HA, Husain AN, Kim AY, Krausz T. The presence of a CD21+ follicular dendritic cell network distinguishes invasive Quilty lesions from cardiac acute cellular rejection. Am J Surg Pathol 2006;30:1008-1013.
6. Sattar HA, Krausz T, Bhorade S, Husain AN. The presence of a CD21+ follicular dendritic cell (FDC) network is useful in distinguishing bronchus associated lymphoid tissue (BALT) from pulmonary acute cellular rejection. 97th Annual Meeting of the United States and Canadian Academy of Pathology, March 1-7. Mod Pathol 2008;21:1596.
7. Yusen RD, Christie JD, Edwards LB, et al. The Registry of the International Society for Heart and Lung Transplantation: Thirtieth adult lung and heart-lung transplant report—2013; focus theme: Age. J Heart Lung Transplant 2013;32:965-978.
8. Verleden GM, Raghu G, Meyer KC, et al. A new classification system for chronic lung allograft dysfunction. J Heart Lung Transplant 2014;33:127-133.
9. Wallace WD, Weigt SS, Farver CF. Update on pathology of antibody-mediated rejection in the lung allograft. Curr Opin Organ Transplant 2014;19:303-308.
10. Takemoto SK, Zeevi A, Feng S, et al. National conference to assess antibody-mediated rejection in solid organ transplantation. Am J Transplant 2004;4:1033-1041.
11. Badesch DB, Zamora M, Fullerton D, et al. Pulmonary capillaritis: A possible histologic form of acute pulmonary allograft rejection. J Heart Lung Transplant 1998;17:415-422.

12. Daoud AH, Betensley AD. Diagnosis and treatment of antibody mediated rejection in lung transplantation: A retrospective case series. Transpl Immunol 2013;28:1-5.

13. Astor TL, Weill D, Cool C, et al. Pulmonary capillaritis in lung transplant recipients: Treatment and effect on allograft function. J Heart Lung Transplant 2005;24:2091-2097.

14. Wallace WD, Reed EF, Ross D, et al. C4d staining of pulmonary allograft biopsies: An immunoperoxidase study. J Heart Lung Transplant 2005;24:1565-1570.

15. Westall GP, Snell GI, McLean C, et al. C3d and C4d deposition early after lung transplantation. J Heart Lung Transplant 2008;27:722-728.

16. Husain S, Mooney ML, Danziger-Isakov L. A 2010 working formulation for the standardization of definitions of infections in cardiothoracic transplant recipients. J Heart Lung Transplant 2011;30:361-374.

17. Clark NM, Lynch JP 3rd, Sayah D, et al. DNA viral infections complicating lung transplantation. Semin Respir Crit Care Med 2013;34:380-404.

18. Solans EP, Garrity ER Jr, McCabe M, et al. Early diagnosis of cytomegalovirus pneumonitis in lung transplant patients. Arch Pathol Lab Med 1995;119:33-55.

19. Bhaskaran A, Hosseini-Moghaddam SM, Rotstein C, Husain S. Mold infections in lung transplant recipients. Semin Respir Crit Care Med 2013;34:371-379.

20. Pappas PG, Alexander BD, Andes DR, et al. Invasive fungal infections among organ transplant recipients: Results of the Transplant-Associated Infection Surveillance Network (TRANSNET). Clin Infect Dis 2010;50:1101-1111.

21. Kubak BM. Fungal infection in lung transplantation. Transpl Infect Dis 2002;4(Suppl 3):24-31.

22. Sułkowska K, Palczewski P, Gołębiowski M. Radiological spectrum of pulmonary infections in patients post solid organ transplantation. Pol J Radiol 2012;77:64-70.

23. Végso G, Hajdu M, Sebestyén A. Lymphoproliferative disorders after solid organ transplantation—classification, incidence, risk factors, early detection and treatment options. Pathol Oncol Res 2011;17:443-454.

24. Jagadeesh D, Woda BA, Draper J, Evens AM. Post transplant lymphoproliferative disorders: Risk, classification, and therapeutic recommendations. Curr Treat Options Oncol 2012;13:122-136.

25. Al-Mansour Z, Nelson BP, Evens AM. Post-transplant lymphoproliferative disease (PTLD): Risk factors, diagnosis, and current treatment strategies. Curr Hematol Malig Rep 2013;8:173-183.

33

Obliterative bronchiolitis/bronchiolitis obliterans syndrome: Etiology, diagnosis, and management

SUSAN R. RUSSELL AND SANGEETA M. BHORADE

INTRODUCTION

Lung transplantation is a lifesaving option for selected patients with end-stage lung disease. However, long-term outcomes are limited by chronic lung allograft dysfunction (CLAD). Obliterative bronchiolitis (OB) and its clinical counterpart, bronchiolitis obliterans syndrome (BOS), are major causes of allograft dysfunction after lung transplantation.[1] The pathogenesis of the disease is poorly understood and its mortality remains high.[2-4] Once other causes of chronic allograft dysfunction have been excluded and the diagnosis has been confirmed, few available therapies other than repeat transplantation have been proved to positively affect outcomes. This chapter describes the genesis and diagnosis of this disease and the options available for treating it.

DEFINITION OF OBLITERATIVE BRONCHIOLITIS AND BRONCHIOLITIS OBLITERANS SYNDROME

OB, the most recognized subset of CLAD, was initially described in 1984 in a series of 14 patients, 3 of whom had

pathologic confirmation of disease.[5] Histopathologic examination revealed polypoid fibromyxoid granulation tissue with eosinophilic fibrotic scars that were obliterating the lumina of the terminal bronchioles while sparing the surrounding alveoli (Figure 33.1). However, the sensitivity of transbronchial lung biopsy for identification of OB is poor and it cannot be relied on to guide decisions regarding a change in therapy.[6,7]

As a result, in 1993 the International Society of Heart and Lung Transplantation (ISHLT) proposed a clinical definition of the chronic rejection termed *bronchiolitis obliterans syndrome* that was based on a physiologic decline in pulmonary function.[8] *BOS* is the clinical term that has been used to define a progressive and irreversible decline in forced expiratory volume in the first second of respiration (FEV$_1$). The initial consensus document established the threshold for BOS as an irreversible decline in FEV$_1$ of 20% or more in the absence of any confounding factors. To increase the sensitivity of this diagnosis, the classification was updated in 2002 to include potential BOS (BOS-0p). To potentially permit earlier detection of the development of BOS, BOS-0p was defined as a greater than 10%

345

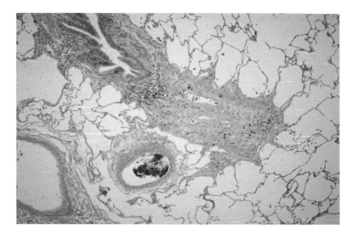

Figure 33.1 Obliterative bronchiolitis.

decline in FEV_1 or a 25% decrease in midexpiratory flow rates ($FEF_{25\%-75\%}$) (Table 33.1). According to the most recent classification of BOS, decrement in lung function and time course of the disease are both essential to the diagnosis.[9] Specifically, to meet the criteria for diagnosis, FEV_1 must decline persistently from the baseline posttransplant value to less than 80% predicted for a minimum of 3 weeks. In addition, the diagnosis cannot be entertained until at least 3 months after patients have received their transplant. BOS is further classified on the basis of severity of decline in FEV_1; this includes "potential BOS" (when a decline in spirometry results is noted but does not cross the 80% threshold [see Table 33.1]). During the clinical evaluation while a diagnosis of OB/BOS is being entertained, it should be remembered that the definition does not include any specific imaging or laboratory testing; possible candidates for addition to the current diagnostic criteria are discussed later in this chapter. This terminology has enabled lung transplant centers worldwide to classify and compare patients with similar physiology. However, whether all patients with clinical BOS have OB as the primary underlying histopathologic process remains unclear because no studies have correlated the two entities.

Table 33.1 Definition and classification of obliterative bronchiolitis/bronchiolitis obliterans syndrome

BOS grade	FEV_1, % of baseline[a]
0	>90% and $FEF_{25\%-75\%}$ > 75%
0p	81% to 90% and $FEF_{25\%-75\%}$ ≤ 75%
1	66% to 80%
2	51% to 65%
3	≤50%

Note: BOS, bronchiolitis obliterans syndrome; FEV_1, forced expiratory volume in first second of respiration; $FEF_{25\%-75\%}$, forced expiratory flow at 25% to 75% of forced vital capacity.

[a] The baseline is the average of the two best FEV_1 values at least 3 weeks apart following lung transplantation. Grade 0p designates "probable" BOS (when a decline in spirometry results is noted but does not meet the criteria for grade 1 disease).

Inadequacies of the current definition of bronchiolitis obliterans syndrome

Given the significance of BOS in lung transplantation, the accuracy of this definition is of utmost importance to identify BOS, determine appropriate therapies, and assess prognosis. A Web-based survey was designed and distributed to members of the pulmonary council of the ISHLT to better understand the accuracy and reliability of the current definition of BOS.[10] The survey included clinical and spirometric data on five patient scenarios from a multicenter lung transplant study. Eighty-seven experienced lung transplant physicians, 95% of whom were pulmonologists and approximately half of whom were medical directors of their respective lung transplant programs, responded to the survey. The survey results showed a 70% level of interobserver agreement regarding the presence or absence of BOS. Of those who agreed on the presence of BOS, 41% agreed on the timing of BOS.

Reliability, objectivity, and ease of performance of spirometry in the clinical setting were identified as positive aspects of the current definition. However, the survey highlighted several potential issues with the current definition, including the variability in the performance of spirometry in individual patients, variability in interpretation of the spirometry results by individual physicians, and difficulties in defining the onset of BOS on the basis of spirometric measurements alone, especially in the presence of an acutely reversible process. As a result, the diagnosis of BOS is often delayed and made in retrospect. Respondents to the survey suggested potential ways to improve the current definition by adding clinical variables, including oxygen saturation, hypercapnia, radiographic findings (inspiratory and expiratory high-resolution computed tomography [HRCT] scans), and exercise tolerance (including the 6-minute walk test), and then adding guidelines defining BOS in the presence of an acute reversible event.

That BOS/OB may be inadequate to define all the conditions associated with a decrease in pulmonary function after lung transplantation has increasingly been recognized. Recently, *chronic lung allograft dysfunction* has been defined as an encompassing term associated with a decline in lung function.[11] The definition of CLAD includes but is not limited to BOS/OB and other elements, such as restrictive physiology, various radiologic findings, and different histopathologic descriptions. The various phenotypes may be associated with different pathogeneses and response to therapies.

EPIDEMIOLOGY

The true incidence and prevalence of OB is unknown—in large part because of inconsistencies in the definition and time periods examined in the studies to date and because of the selection bias of large transplant centers with larger populations of patients. The ISHLT data indicate that whereas the 1-year survival rate has improved consistently to 81%

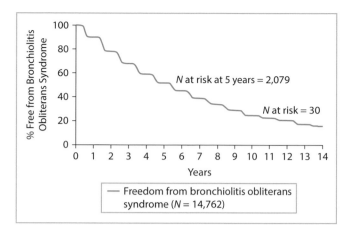

Figure 33.2 Survival of patients with bronchiolitis obliterans syndrome. (Revised from Christie JD, Edwards LB, Kucheryavaya AY, et al. The Registry of the International Society for Heart and Lung Transplantation: Twenty-ninth adult lung and heart-lung transplant report—2012. J Heart Lung Transplant 2012;31:1073-1086.)

in the current era, the overall 5- and 10-year survival rates (53% and 30%, respectively) have stagnated (Figure 33.2). This lack of improvement in the late phase can be attributed to BOS, which is the leading cause of mortality after the first year following transplantation. Twenty-two percent of patients in the ISHLT database reportedly died of bronchiolitis between 3 and 5 years after transplantation; however, this may be an underestimate because another 16% of deaths are listed as having resulted from "graft failure" but may actually have resulted from BOS that was not well defined. The overall prevalence of BOS has been reported to be 48% at 5 years and 76% at 10 years.[12] Diagnosis before transplantation does not affect the incidence of BOS, with the possible exception of the diagnosis of cystic fibrosis versus chronic obstructive pulmonary disease.[13]

Clinical indicators of obliterative bronchiolitis and bronchiolitis obliterans syndrome

Identification of surrogate markers that indicate or herald the development of OB/BOS has been an evolving area of research, with multiple studies focusing on various modalities of imaging and diagnostic testing. None has gained traction to the point of inclusion in currently published guidelines, but each deserves mention as a promising ground for future development.

Using bronchioalveolar lavage (BAL) fluid to look for markers of progression to BOS has been a focus of much research because after lung transplantation recipients undergo routine bronchoscopy as part of surveillance for rejection. Multiple previous studies have indicated that BAL neutrophilia predicts progression toward BOS (see later section on risk factors).[14] Other parameters of BAL fluid that have been linked to BOS are common factors associated

with epithelial injury and a proinflammatory, profibrotic state. One such marker of dysregulated injury and repair is elevation of the proinflammatory cytokine interleukin-8 (IL-8).[15-17] In a cohort of 86 transplant recipients, the IL-8 level was correlated with BAL neutrophilia and established as a driver of neutrophil chemotaxis.[18] The chemokine monocyte chemoattractant protein-1 (MCP-1) may also play a role in inducing a profibrotic state in patients with BOS: it was shown to be elevated in eight patients at an average of approximately 150 days before development of the syndrome in 13 patients without the disease.[16] Markers of innate immunity, particularly α-defensins, have been implicated as well.[19] Matrix metalloproteinase-9 (MMP-9), an enzyme linked to neutrophil migration through the endothelium and remodeling of the extracellular matrix, was shown to be elevated in BAL fluid before the development of BOS in a study that compared 13 patients with 21 controls.[20] Finally, markers of oxidative stress as a surrogate for early epithelial injury, particularly myeloperoxidase and glutathione, have also been implicated in the development of BOS.[21-23]

However, generalizing the results of such studies is difficult because of their small sample size and variations in their collection methods and clinical follow-up.[14,24] The possibility of BOS actually encompassing different entities given the clinically observed phenotypes also confounds these results because patients with more rapidly progressive disease may manifest more markers of inflammation than do patients whose disease is stable. Because most of the aforementioned studies predate the emphasis of the ISHLT guidelines regarding BOS being a separate entity from CLAD, patients with both disease states may have been included in the same data set, thus skewing the results.[1] Further studies are needed to identify the best biomarkers from BAL fluid that could predict the development of BOS and therefore provide a basis for early preventive therapy.

Use of HRCT as a noninvasive method to aid in the diagnosis of BOS has gained support because it can detect findings not seen on chest radiographs and provide useful information in pediatric populations, in which spirometry results are often not reproducible or even obtainable. Findings observed in BOS include air trapping on expiratory images, bronchiectasis, and mosaic perfusion and attenuation.[25,26] One study of 38 heart-lung transplant recipients and 8 healthy controls documented an HRCT sensitivity of 83% and specificity of 89% when air trapping (measured subjectively by a radiologist on the basis of an established scoring system) crossed the threshold of 32%.[27] However, although multiple studies have noted that air trapping is correlated with BOS more than with other features seen on HRCT, this finding was not sufficiently accurate to predict BOS before a decline in spirometry results.[25,28-30]

Exhaled nitric oxide (NO) and carbon monoxide (CO) are alternative measures of lung function that have been investigated as markers of the early development of BOS. Several studies have validated exhaled NO as being reproducible and reflective of NO in the lower airways; hence, they may be correlated with the inflammation in the lower airways that is seen in this syndrome.[31,32] In a study of 64 bilateral transplant recipients and 1 single-lung transplant recipient, the slope of alveolar plateau for helium, the helium slope from a single-breath washout, and chemiluminescence were used to determine NO and CO levels and then compared with spirometric data as a means of assessing the development of BOS. Although the combination of these markers was found to have better sensitivity than any one of them alone, its specificity and positive predictive value remained low.[33] Others have pointed to the usefulness of increases in exhaled NO as an indicator of progression of the disease in patients in whom BOS has been diagnosed or has stabilized (i.e., as a marker of response to a change in therapy).[34,35] To date, however, the use of exhaled NO and CO has not been standardized outside the research setting.

Several caveats regarding the use of these markers for early and definitive diagnosis of BOS exist. In addition to the lack of specificity of many of these markers, none has been validated in a separate cohort of lung transplant recipients, nor have they been validated in patients who receive single-lung transplants. In addition, threshold levels of these markers have not been established. At the current time, none of these markers are used to make the diagnosis of BOS, but they are often used to confirm or support this diagnosis.

Phenotypes of bronchiolitis obliterans syndrome

The existence of several phenotypes of BOS has been increasingly recognized. The rate of decline in FEV_1 was initially described in 1995 by Nathan and colleagues, who noted three primary types of decline: (1) rapid rate of decline in lung function, (2) rapid rate of decline followed by stabilization of lung function, and (3) slow rate of decline.[36] Clinical risk factors for these patterns of decline have subsequently been analyzed further. Lama and colleagues compared the clinical characteristics of 111 lung transplant recipients with BOS who had a rapid decline in FEV_1 with those of recipients who did not.[37] They found that patients with a rapid decline were more likely to be female, have idiopathic pulmonary fibrosis, and have received a single-lung transplant. Such patients had an earlier onset of BOS (within 6 months after their lung transplant) and higher mortality than did patients with a slower decline in FEV_1.

In addition to rate of decline, early onset of a decline in FEV_1 (within 3 years after transplantation) has been associated with a more rapid decline in FEV_1 and decreased survival.[38,39] High-grade BOS (grade 2 or higher) at initial examination has also been associated with a worse outcome. Burton and colleagues have shown that over a 10-year period, progression to higher-grade BOS was linked to increased mortality.[40] Finlen-Copeland found that patients with both a rapid decline in FEV_1 and high-grade BOS (grade 2 or 3) at initial evaluation had higher mortality.[41] Together, all these studies suggest that a rapid decline in FEV_1 along with

a higher grade of BOS when patients are first seen may be indicative of more aggressive phenotypes of BOS that are associated with a disease process characterized by a different pathogenesis and response to alternative therapies.

A separate phenotype of BOS that has recently been identified is azithromycin-responsive airway disease. Characteristics of this disease include the presence of BAL neutrophilia (neutrophil percentage >15%) and HRCT findings of peribronchiolar infiltrates and a "tree-in-bud" appearance.[11] In one study, the decline in FEV_1 was found to be slower in patients who respond to azithromycin. Treatment with azithromycin is discussed in more detail later in this chapter.[42]

RISK FACTORS

Several risk factors predispose lung transplant recipients to BOS. They can be classified as alloimmune (or intrinsically driven) or nonalloimmune (Table 33.2).

Alloimmune risk factors

One of the most important alloimmune risk factors for BOS is acute rejection. The development of OB/BOS is commonly associated with the development and severity of episodes of acute rejection, whether of the perivascular lymphocytic (grade A) or peribronchiolar mononuclear (grade B) form. Grade A2 or higher rejection has been correlated with the subsequent development of BOS in multiple studies.[43-50] An earlier retrospective review of 32 transplant recipients correlated at least three episodes of rejection in a 12-month period with a 100% incidence of BOS.[44] Higher-grade rejection and late diagnosis of acute rejection also increase the risk for the development of BOS.[46,49,50] Links have also been documented between minimal (grade A1) rejection and the development of OB/BOS, although this is an area of

Table 33.2 Risk factors for bronchiolitis obliterans syndrome

Alloimmune
  Acute vascular rejection (grade A)
  Lymphocytic bronchiolitis (grade B)
  Antibody-mediated rejection/donor-specific antibodies
  Autoimmunity: collagen V, K-α_1-tubulin
Nonalloimmune
  Primary graft dysfunction
  Reflux disease
  Infection: CMV, community-acquired viruses,
  PA, *Aspergillus*
Other
  BAL neutrophilia
  Single- versus double-lung transplant
  Medication noncompliance

Note: BAL, bronchoalveolar lavage; CMV, cytomegalovirus, PA, *Pseudomonas aeruginosa.*

evolving research. In a study analyzing surveillance biopsy samples from 184 transplant recipients, the development of grade A1 rejection, even in asymptomatic patients, was correlated with an increased incidence of the development of BOS.[51] Other studies have confirmed that a single episode of grade A1 rejection independently predicts this syndrome.[52] Therefore current guidelines recommend augmenting immunosuppressive therapy in patients with minimal rejection seen on surveillance transbronchial biopsy.[1]

Lymphocytic bronchiolitis (LB), or grade B rejection, has also been identified as a risk factor for the development of BOS. A retrospective analysis of surveillance transbronchial biopsy samples from 299 patients found that the development of LB with a grade of B2 or higher increased the risk for both acute rejection and the development of BOS with an odds ratio of 3.3.[53] Others confirmed this finding by surveillance biopsies of 341 transplant recipients and noted that higher-grade LB is a risk factor for the development of BOS and death independent of acute vascular rejection, which raises questions regarding whether the grade A vascular rejection or grade B bronchiolitic rejection phenotype causes most of the changes seen with BOS.[54] However, this finding should be interpreted with caution in view of the known difficulties with the reliability of interpretation of surveillance biopsy specimens after transplantation.[55]

In addition to episodes of histologic rejection in the late phase after transplantation, antibody-mediated rejection based on donor-specific antibodies (DSAs) to human leukocyte antigens that are present before transplantation and occur de novo after transplantation has been linked with the development of BOS.[56] This connection is particularly true in patients with cystic fibrosis, who are noted to have a higher incidence of DSAs than occurs in those with other pretransplant diagnoses.[57] The incidence of DSAs after transplantation was as high as 56% in one study of 116 transplant recipients. Importantly, initiating treatment on the basis of the presence of DSAs may prevent the development of BOS.[58] As detection and classification of antibody-mediated rejection improve with the development of newer techniques, this link may play an expanding role in directing therapy.

Recent studies also point to possible autoimmune phenomena driving BOS that involve sensitization to collagen V, which is expressed in the epithelia of small airways, presumably in response to events that damage the epithelium and cause ischemia-reperfusion injury after transplantation.[59] To date, such studies have been based primarily on animal models.[60] However, at least one study examining peripheral blood mononuclear cells from transplant recipients found a correlation between increased collagen V reactivity and the incidence and increased severity of BOS.[61] Autoantibodies to K-α_1-tubulin, which are also found in small airways, have also been linked to profibrotic factors noted in OB.[62] These antibodies are thought to possibly be generated by an IL-17–driven response of helper T cells, but the mechanism of this process has not been fully defined.[61,63,64]

Nonalloimmune risk factors

In addition to factors related to the interplay between donor and recipient, other extrinsic risk factors for the development of BOS exist. One of these is primary graft dysfunction (PGD), a form of ischemia-reperfusion injury that usually occurs in the immediate posttransplant period and has been linked to high early morbidity and mortality.[65-67] Although PGD has not been correlated with the subsequent development of rejection, studies do point to a relationship between PGD and BOS, especially with more severe forms of the disease.[68-70] Whether early identification and intervention for PGD can attenuate risk for the subsequent development of BOS is unclear.

Gastroesophageal reflux disease (GERD), both acid and nonacid, is an important modifiable risk factor for BOS. Unfortunately, a significant percentage of lung transplant recipients are known to have GERD before transplantation, and the disease in many worsens after transplantation.[71-75] In one study of 120 transplant recipients, elevated bile acid levels in BAL fluid were correlated with shorter time until the development of BOS.[76] Patients with confirmed BOS have also been noted to have elevated levels of bile acid in other studies, and such levels have a negative impact on response to azithromycin.[77-79] Strategies to treat GERD can affect BOS, which is discussed in detail later in this chapter.

Viral infections may play a role in the pathogenesis of BOS; this is particularly in the case of cytomegalovirus (CMV), which can cause BOS in the nontransplant setting. In several studies CMV pneumonitis after transplantation was associated with the subsequent development of BOS.[44,47,80] In a cohort of 231 transplant recipients, the development of CMV pneumonitis within 6 months of a transplant significantly increased the risk for BOS and overall mortality.[81] CMV positivity in the donor organ also increased risk for the subsequent development of BOS.[82] Other studies investigating similar viruses, such as Epstein-Barr virus, have correlated viral load in peripheral blood with BOS, but this finding has been inconsistent.[83,84] Community-acquired viral infections, such as influenza and respiratory syncytial virus, have also been linked prospectively to the subsequent development of BOS, although studies focusing on the pediatric population have not replicated this finding.[85-88]

Like viral infections, bacterial and fungal infections have also been associated with the development of BOS. The bacterium *Pseudomonas aeruginosa* (PA) has been investigated the most, in part because of the population of patients with bronchiectasis, who are often infected or colonized with this pathogen before transplantation.[89,90] New colonization by PA after transplantation also increases the risk for BOS: in one study of 155 lung transplant recipients PA colonization preceded BOS in 78% of the patients in whom the disease developed.[91] *Aspergillus fumigatus* infection and colonization increase risk for the development of BOS as well.[92,93] In a review of 201 lung transplant recipients, detection of *Aspergillus* in BAL fluid significantly increased the risk for both the development of BOS and BOS-associated mortality independent of acute rejection.[94]

Other risk factors

The degree of BAL neutrophilia is correlated with the severity of BOS and is potentially a marker of response to specific therapies, such as azithromycin.[42,95] In a study of 63 transplant recipients who underwent surveillance BAL, an increased percentage of neutrophils predicted the onset of BOS within the following year.[15] This relationship has been confirmed in other studies with similar threshold percentages of neutrophils (16% to 24%) as a marker for the future development of disease.[16,96,97] BAL neutrophilia is also correlated with the development of early-onset BOS.[17] As discussed elsewhere in this chapter, neutrophils are now thought to drive the proinflammatory response that leads to pathologic OB, and neutrophilia has become a focus of investigation for treatment.

The type of transplant may have an effect on the subsequent development of BOS. In a review of 225 patients with a variety of diagnoses and comorbid conditions before transplantation, the rate of BOS was higher in the single–lung transplant population than in the double–lung transplant population (49% versus 32%) even after control for differences in baseline characteristics.[98] The same group examined a cohort of 221 patients with chronic obstructive pulmonary disease and found that patients who received a bilateral lung transplant had better long-term survival and freedom from BOS at 3 and 5 years than did their counterparts with a single-lung transplant.[99] However, this finding has not been replicated in patient populations with pulmonary hypertension.[100] Finally, it should be noted that medication noncompliance is often considered a risk factor for the development of BOS. This risk is probably due to the development of episodes of acute and chronic rejection as a consequence of lapses in immunosuppressive therapy, although this hypothesis has not been validated in large studies.[101]

APPROACH TO DIAGNOSIS AND MANAGEMENT OF BRONCHIOLITIS OBLITERANS SYNDROME

The following approach to BOS is based on current evidence and clinical consensus by lung transplant experts. The ISHLT/American Thoracic Society (ATS)/European Respiratory Society (ERS) clinical practice guidelines highlight the approach to patients with BOS (Figure 33.3).[1] These guidelines suggest that if a lung transplant recipient shows a decline in pulmonary function, further evaluation is warranted to identify potentially reversible causes of the decline. This evaluation should include a chest radiograph with or without an HRCT scan, primarily to evaluate for causes other than BOS (e.g., pneumonia, pulmonary edema, and native lung hyperinflation in single-lung transplants) in acknowledgment of the fact that radiographic imaging has not been shown to be either sensitive or specific for

the development of BOS. However, HRCT with expiratory views may support a diagnosis of BOS if findings such as air trapping, mosaic attenuation, bronchial wall thickening, and dilatation are present.[25-27]

In addition, bronchoscopy, BAL, and transbronchial biopsy should be performed. Like radiography, bronchoscopy is useful when looking for potential alternative causes of declining pulmonary function because the yield of transbronchial biopsy for OB is extremely low. The presence of BAL neutrophilia may be suggestive of the onset of BOS but is often nonspecific, especially in the setting of infection.[15-17,96,97] Bronchoscopy may also help in diagnosing other reversible causes of decreased pulmonary function, including the presence of infection, acute cellular rejection, acute antibody-mediated rejection, lymphocytic bronchiolitis, or other pulmonary infiltrative disease. However, it should be noted that in some instances, the presence of an acute reversible process may occur in conjunction with the development of BOS. As a result, it is recommended that aggressive treatment of an acutely reversible condition be undertaken and follow-up spirometry be performed to identify possible concurrent BOS.

In addition, in a patient with declining pulmonary function, the presence of circulating DSAs is suggestive of antibody-mediated rejection. The existence of characteristic histologic findings, complement deposition, or both on transbronchial biopsy will help confirm this diagnosis.[56-58] Finally, the presence of GERD should be ascertained because it may be a potentially reversible cause of declining pulmonary function.[102] Full pulmonary function tests or repeated spirometry should be performed in 3 weeks to show the persistent decline in FEV_1 required for the diagnosis of BOS.

PREVENTION AND TREATMENT OF BRONCHIOLITIS OBLITERANS SYNDROME

Prevention of BOS remains elusive, and no definitive evidence that any particular immunosuppressive regimen is superior in the prevention of BOS exists. Current therapies for prevention of BOS include treatment of known risk factors associated with BOS (e.g., infection, acute rejection, GERD) and modulation of immunosuppression with the use lymphocyte-depleting therapies. Retransplantation is a last-resort therapy for patients with refractory BOS in whom all other treatment has failed. Unfortunately, strategies for the prevention and treatment of BOS have been confounded by the lack of randomized controlled trials, as well as by limited understanding of the pathogenesis and natural history of BOS.

Treatment of acute cellular rejection (grade A) and lymphocytic bronchiolitis (grade B)

Current recommendations per the international ISHLT/ATS/ ERS clinical practice guidelines suggest that nonminimal

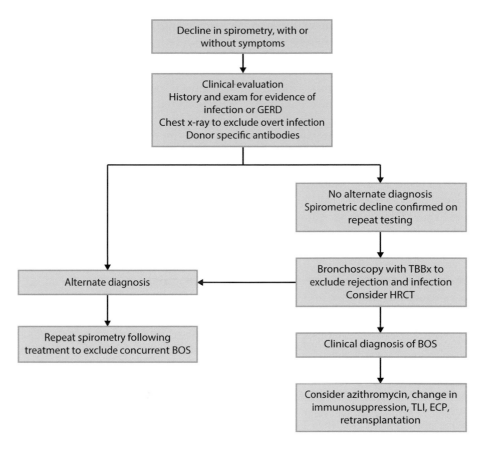

Figure 33.3 Diagnosis of bronchiolitis obliterans syndrome. BOS, bronchiolitis obliterans syndrome; ECP, extracorporeal photophoresis; GERD, gastroesophageal reflux; HRCT, high-resolution computed tomography; TBBx, transbronchial biopsy; TLI, total lymphoid irradiation.

acute cellular rejection (grade A rejection) and LB (grade B rejection) be treated to prevent the development of BOS.[1] These recommendations are based on previous studies demonstrating a strong association between acute cellular rejection and the subsequent development of BOS.[43-50] In addition, the presence of LB has been shown to be an independent risk factor for the development of BOS and should also be treated with augmented immunosuppression.[53-33] Detection and treatment of minimal (grade A1) rejection have been more controversial. Several recent publications have shown a connection between grade A1 rejection and BOS.[51,52] On the basis of these studies, the international ISHLT/ATS/ERS clinical practice guidelines recommend treating clinically significant grade A1 rejection. Although the guidelines note that the recommendations are conditional because they are based on very low quality evidence, a high value is nevertheless placed on treating this life-threatening complication after lung transplantation.[1]

IMMUNOSUPPRESSION

Once the diagnosis of BOS has made, it is important to recognize that no immunosuppressive regimen has been found to be superior for treating BOS. In addition, high-dose corticosteroids (prednisone, ≥ 30 mg/day) are not recommended for the early treatment of BOS because they have not been shown to improve lung function and are associated with significant adverse events.[1]

CONVERSION OF CYCLOSPORINE TO TACROLIMUS

Currently, immunosuppression after lung transplantation includes a calcineurin inhibitor (cyclosporine or tacrolimus), an antimetabolite (azathioprine or mycophenolate mofetil), and corticosteroids. Four randomized controlled trials have compared tacrolimus with cyclosporine.[103-106] Although the results of these studies are conflicting, overall they suggest that tacrolimus may be beneficial in decreasing the incidence of BOS. The most recent randomized multicenter trial comparing tacrolimus with cyclosporine in combination with mycophenolate mofetil and prednisone found a reduction in the incidence of BOS at 3 years (12% with tacrolimus and 21% with cyclosporine, $P = .037$) but did not show any difference in rates of acute rejection or survival.[105] In addition, an international multicenter study suggested that switching cyclosporine to tacrolimus after the onset of BOS may decrease the rate of decline in pulmonary function.[107] On the basis of these results, switching cyclosporine to tacrolimus in patients with BOS is reasonable.

AZITHROMYCIN

The correlation with BAL neutrophilia and other inflammatory markers with the presence of BOS has prompted investigation and use of macrolides as an anti-inflammatory therapy in this syndrome. The evidence that azithromycin is beneficial in both preventing and treating a subset of patients with BOS is increasing.[42,95] In a single-center, randomized controlled trial, Vos and colleagues randomly assigned 83 de novo lung transplant recipients to receive standard triple-drug immunosuppression with either azithromycin or placebo.[108] Patients who received azithromycin had a lower incidence of BOS at 2 years after their lung transplant (12.5%) than did those who received placebo (44.2%). The same patients also had higher FEV_1 values, reduced BAL neutrophilia, and decreased systemic inflammation. Several other studies have shown that adding azithromycin to standard immunosuppression may slow or even reverse the decline in pulmonary function in approximately one third of lung recipients with BOS.[42,95] This clinical condition has been termed *azithromycin-responsive allograft dysfunction*.[11] Its characteristics include the presence of BAL neutrophilia (neutrophil percentage >15%) and HRCT findings of peribronchiolar infiltrates and a tree-in-bud appearance.

Adverse events associated with azithromycin include gastrointestinal effects (e.g., nausea, dyspepsia and diarrhea, hearing loss, and the development of azithromycin-resistant organisms).[42,95,108] In addition, fatal cardiac arrhythmias associated with azithromycin have been described in other transplant recipient populations, but they have not been reported in the lung transplant population thus far.[109] Adverse events in the lung transplantation literature are described in less than 5% of patients and are most commonly secondary to gastrointestinal issues. In view of the current evidence, a trial of azithromycin, 250 mg three times weekly, in patients with an early onset of BOS is recommended.

Treatment of gastroesophageal reflux disease

GERD is highly prevalent both before and after lung transplantation and has recently been identified as a risk factor for the development of BOS.[74-79] In patients showing a decline in pulmonary function, further testing with pH monitoring/impedance testing of proximal esophageal motility should be performed to assess for GERD. Because medical therapy does not prevent GERD-associated injury to the lung allograft, which in turn leads to BOS, evaluation for surgical treatment with gastric fundoplication is recommended in all patients with evidence of GERD and declining pulmonary function.[1] One study showed that early gastric fundoplication (within 3 months after lung transplantation) has been associated with greater freedom from BOS and increased survival at 1 and 3 years after transplantation than seen in patients who did not undergo fundoplication, patients who underwent delayed fundoplication (>3 months), or patients without a history of GERD.[102] At the same center, antireflux surgery was associated with improved pulmonary function in a subset of patients who underwent fundoplication early in the course of BOS.[110] Complications from antireflux surgery have been reported to range from 5% to 25% and

include intraoperative complications (including bleeding and stomach perforation) and dysphagia.[102,109] In view of the improvement in the pulmonary function of lung recipients with GERD after antireflux surgery, it is recommended that lung transplant patients with BOS and GERD be evaluated for potential fundoplication. However, further studies are needed to determine the efficacy of antireflux surgery, identify the appropriate patient population, and establish the best time for the procedure.

Lymphocyte depletion

In patients with a progressive decline in FEV_1, lymphocyte depletion by various modalities, including augmentation of immunosuppression, total lymphoid irradiation (TLI), and photopheresis, may be considered. Augmentation of immunosuppression with the addition of cytolytic therapies such as antithymocyte globulin and alemtuzumab has been shown to stabilize lung function in a subset of patients with refractory BOS.[111-113] However, because these studies are single-center, retrospective case series, their results are limited. In addition, the adverse events and increased risk for infection that have been associated with augmentation of immunosuppression should be assessed when weighing the benefits and risks of using such therapies for the treatment of BOS.

In TLI, radiation is applied to the lymphatic areas to reduce the activity of lymphocytes in patients. The benefit of TLI in patients with refractory BOS has been evaluated in a few retrospective case series.[114-116] Overall, their results suggest a reduction in the decline of FEV_1 in a subset of patients with BOS. In general, initiation of TLI earlier in the course of BOS has been associated with greater response. However, because the current studies are small single-center retrospective case series, the overall benefit of TLI remains to be determined.

Extracorporeal photopheresis

Extracorporeal photopheresis (ECP) is a therapy that consists of incubating a patient's peripheral blood monocytes with 8-methoxypsoralen, irradiating the cells with ultraviolet light, and reinfusing them into the patient. This process has been shown to have immunomodulatory effects on peripheral blood monocytes and to decrease the rate of decline in patients with BOS. Meloni and colleagues found that patients with refractory BOS who were stabilized by ECP had higher levels of $CD4^+CD25^+$ regulatory T cells than did those who exhibited a decline in their pulmonary function, thus suggesting a potential mechanism by which ECP may benefit such patients.[117]

Several single-center case series have suggested that ECP may decrease the rate of decline in pulmonary function in patients with refractory BOS.[118,119] In a recent published series conducted in a single center over a 10-year period, Benden and colleagues found a decrease in the rate of decline in FEV_1 after implementation of ECP in 12 patients (112 mL/mo before ECP versus 12 mL/mo afterward).[120] In another larger series, Morrell and colleagues evaluated the effect of ECP in 60 patients with BOS throughout a 7-year period.[121] They also found an overall decrease in the decline in FEV_1 (116 mL/mo before ECP versus 29 mL/mo afterward). In some patients, ECP therapy increased pulmonary function. As is the case for many of the therapies for refractory BOS, the studies evaluating ECP are limited by their retrospective, nonrandomized, single-center designs. Further evaluation of all these therapies for refractory BOS should include a prospective randomized controlled study design to allow better understanding of their efficacy and safety.

Retransplantation

Retransplantation is a last-resort therapy for patients with BOS. Although only a small percentage of patients with BOS undergo retransplantation, the number has increased over the past decade. This increase has been due in part to implementation of the lung allocation system, which enables patients with rapidly progressive lung disease (including those with BOS) to receive priority during donor allocation. In addition, outcomes after retransplantation for BOS have improved continually over the past decade and are becoming similar to those after primary transplants. As a result, interest in considering retransplantation for BOS is increasing. However, important ethical considerations regarding retransplantation remain in connection with the shortage of donor organs and rising mortality while on the lung transplant waiting list.

Several observational studies and case series have evaluated the benefit of retransplantation in lung recipients with BOS. Overall, these studies suggest that patients who undergo retransplantation for BOS have better outcomes than do patients who have received a retransplant for other reasons, including PGD.[122-127] Outcomes after retransplantation for BOS are improving but still remain inferior to those after primary transplants. Rates of survival after a retransplant for BOS are 60% to 78% at 1 year, 53% to 64% at 2 years, and 44% to 61% at 5 years. The primary cause of mortality in patients undergoing retransplantation is infection, which occurs most commonly in the rejected retained lung allograft. The research suggests that retransplantation for a rejected lung allograft as a single-lung transplantation procedure may be beneficial in reducing the risk for infection in the retained allograft. Although the data are somewhat conflicting, in general, patients who undergo retransplantation for BOS appear to have a higher recurrence of BOS afterward.[128] Overall, given the high mortality in lung recipients with end-stage BOS, it is recommended that patients with BOS refractory to other medical therapies be referred for possible retransplantation.

CONCLUSION

OB/BOS remains a major cause of morbidity and mortality after lung transplantation. Progress in understanding this disease process has been increasing in recent years. Improved definition of BOS, further studies of its clinical indicators, and differentiation of its various phenotypes will assist in understanding its pathogenesis and, ultimately, in its treatment. Increasing evidence suggests that treatment of the risk factors for BOS (including acute rejection and GERD) may decrease its incidence and that therapies such as azithromycin and ECP provide some benefit in a subset of patients who have it. Although OB/BOS remains a devastating complication after lung transplantation, the prospects for better understanding and treatment of this disease are increasing.

REFERENCES

1. Meyer KC, Raghu G, Verleden GM, et al. An international ISHLT/ATS/ERS clinical practice guideline: Diagnosis and management of bronchiolitis obliterans syndrome. Eur Respir J 2014;44:1479-1503.
2. Boehler A, Kesten S, Weder W, Speich R. Bronchiolitis obliterans after lung transplantation: A review. Chest 1998;114:1411-1426.
3. Estenne M, Hertz MI. Bronchiolitis obliterans after human lung transplantation. Am J Respir Crit Care Med 2002;166:440-444.
4. Todd JL, Palmer SM. Bronchiolitis obliterans syndrome: The final frontier for lung transplantation. Chest 2011;140:502-508.
5. Burke CM, Theodore J, Dawkins KD, et al. Post-transplant obliterative bronchiolitis and other late lung sequelae in human heart-lung transplantation. Chest 1984;86:824-829.
6. Kramer MR, Stoehr C, Whang JL, et al. The diagnosis of obliterative bronchiolitis after heart-lung and lung transplantation: Low yield of transbronchial lung biopsy. J Heart Lung Transplant 1993;12:675-681.
7. Pomerance A, Madden B, Burke MM, Yacoub MH. Transbronchial biopsy in heart and lung transplantation: Clinicopathologic correlations. J Heart Lung Transplant 1995;14:761-773.
8. Cooper JD, Billingham M, Egan T, et al. A working formulation for the standardization of nomenclature and for clinical staging of chronic dysfunction in lung allografts. International Society for Heart and Lung Transplantation. J Heart Lung Transplant 1993;12:713-716.
9. Estenne M, Maurer JR, Boehler A, et al. Bronchiolitis obliterans syndrome 2001: An update of the diagnostic criteria. J Heart Lung Transplant 2002;21:297-310.
10. Kapila A, Baz MA, Valentine VG, et al. Reliability of diagnostic criteria for bronchiolitis obliterans syndrome after lung transplantation: A survey. J Heart Lung Transplant 2015;35:65-74.
11. Verleden GM, Raghu G, Meyer KC, et al. A new classification system for chronic lung allograft dysfunction. J Heart Lung Transplant 2014;33:127-133.

12. Christie JD, Edwards LB, Kucheryavaya AY, et al. The Registry of the International Society for Heart and Lung Transplantation: Twenty-ninth adult lung and heart-lung transplant report—2012. J Heart Lung Transplant 2012;31:1073-1086.

13. International Society for Heart & Lung Transplantation. http://ishlt.org. Accessed November 15, 2014.

14. Kennedy VE, Todd JL, Palmer SM. Bronchoalveolar lavage as a tool to predict, diagnose and understand bronchiolitis obliterans syndrome. Am J Transplant 2013;13:552-561.

15. Neurohr C, Huppmann P, Samweber B, et al. Prognostic value of bronchoalveolar lavage neutrophilia in stable lung transplant recipients. J Heart Lung Transplant 2009;28:468-474.

16. Reynaud-Gaubert M, Marin V, Thirion X, et al. Upregulation of chemokines in bronchoalveolar lavage fluid as a predictive marker of post-transplant airway obliteration. J Heart Lung Transplant 2002;21:721-730.

17. Scholma J, Slebos DJ, Boezen HM, et al. Eosinophilic granulocytes and interleukin-6 level in bronchoalveolar lavage fluid are associated with the development of obliterative bronchiolitis after lung transplantation. Am J Respir Crit Care Med 2000;162:2221-2225.

18. DiGiovine B, Lynch JP 3rd, Martinez FJ, et al. Bronchoalveolar lavage neutrophilia is associated with obliterative bronchiolitis after lung transplantation: Role of IL-8. J Immunol 1996;157:4194-4202.

19. Nelsestuen GL, Martinez MB, Hertz MI, et al. Proteomic identification of human neutrophil alpha-defensins in chronic lung allograft rejection. Proteomics 2005;5:1705-1713.

20. Ramirez AM, Nunley DR, Rojas M, Roman J. Activation of tissue remodeling precedes obliterative bronchiolitis in lung transplant recipients. Biomark Insights 2008;3:351-359.

21. Madill J, Aghdassi E, Arendt B, et al. Lung transplantation: Does oxidative stress contribute to the development of bronchiolitis obliterans syndrome? Transplant Rev 2009;23:103-110.

22. Madill J, Aghdassi E, Arendt BM, et al. Oxidative stress and nutritional intakes in lung patients with bronchiolitis obliterans syndrome. Transplant Proc 2009;41:3838-3844.

23. Riise GC, Andersson BA, Kjellstrom C, et al. Persistent high BAL fluid granulocyte activation marker levels as early indicators of bronchiolitis obliterans after lung transplant. Eur Respir J 1999;14:1123-1130.

24. Meyer KC, Raghu G, Baughman RP, et al. An official American Thoracic Society clinical practice guideline: The clinical utility of bronchoalveolar lavage cellular analysis in interstitial lung disease. Am J Respir Crit Care Med 2012;185:1004-1014.

25. Berstad AE, Aalokken TM, Kolbenstvedt A, Bjortuft O. Performance of long-term CT monitoring in diagnosing bronchiolitis obliterans after lung transplantation. Eur J Radiol 2006;58:124-131.

26. Collins J. Imaging of the chest after lung transplantation. J Thorac Imaging 2002;17:102-112.

27. Bankier AA, Van Muylem A, Knoop C, et al. Bronchiolitis obliterans syndrome in heart-lung transplant recipients: Diagnosis with expiratory CT. Radiology 2001;218:533-539.

28. Konen E, Gutierrez C, Chaparro C, et al. Bronchiolitis obliterans syndrome in lung transplant recipients: Can thin-section CT findings predict disease before its clinical appearance? Radiology 2004;231:467-473.

29. Lee ES, Gotway MB, Reddy GP, et al. Early bronchiolitis obliterans following lung transplantation: Accuracy of expiratory thin-section CT for diagnosis. Radiology 2000;216:472-477.

30. Leung AN, Fisher K, Valentine V, et al. Bronchiolitis obliterans after lung transplantation: Detection using expiratory HRCT. Chest 1998;113:365-370.

31. Fisher AJ, Gabbay E, Small T, et al. Cross sectional study of exhaled nitric oxide levels following lung transplantation. Thorax 1998;53:454-458.

32. Gabbay E, Walters EH, Orsida B, et al. Post–lung transplant bronchiolitis obliterans syndrome (BOS) is characterized by increased exhaled nitric oxide levels and epithelial inducible nitric oxide synthase. Am J Respir Crit Care Med 2000;162:2182-2187.

33. Van Muylem A, Knoop C, Estenne M. Early detection of chronic pulmonary allograft dysfunction by exhaled biomarkers. Am J Respir Crit Care Med 2007;175:731-736.

34. Brugiere O, Thabut G, Mal H, et al. Exhaled NO may predict the decline in lung function in bronchiolitis obliterans syndrome. Eur Respir J 2005;25:813-819.

35. Verleden GM, Dupont LJ, Van Raemdonck D, Vanhaecke J. Effect of switching from cyclosporine to tacrolimus on exhaled nitric oxide and pulmonary function in patients with chronic rejection after lung transplantation. J Heart Lung Transplant 2003;22:908-913.

36. Nathan SD, Ross DJ, Belman MJ, et al. Bronchiolitis obliterans in single-lung transplant recipients. Chest 1995;107:967-972.

37. Lama VN, Murray S, Lonigro RJ, et al. Course of FEV(1) after onset of bronchiolitis obliterans syndrome in lung transplant recipients. Am J Respir Crit Care Med 2007;175:1192-1198.

38. Brugiere O, Pessione F, Thabut G, et al. Bronchiolitis obliterans syndrome after single-lung transplantation: Impact of time to onset on functional pattern and survival. Chest 2002;121:1883-1889.

39. Sato M, Ohmori-Matsuda K, Saito T, et al. Time-dependent changes in the risk of death in pure bronchiolitis obliterans syndrome (BOS). J Heart Lung Transplant 2013;32:484-491.

40. Burton CM, Carlsen J, Mortensen J, et al. Long-term survival after lung transplantation depends on development and severity of bronchiolitis obliterans syndrome. J Heart Lung Transplant 2007;26:681-686.

41. Finlen Copeland CA, Snyder LD, Zaas DW, et al. Survival after bronchiolitis obliterans syndrome among bilateral lung transplant recipients. Am J Respir Crit Care Med 2010;182:784-789.

42. Gottlieb J, Szangolies J, Koehnlein T, et al. Long-term azithromycin for bronchiolitis obliterans syndrome after lung transplantation. Transplantation 2008;85:36-41.

43. Bando K, Paradis IL, Similo S, et al. Obliterative bronchiolitis after lung and heart-lung transplantation. An analysis of risk factors and management. J Thorac Cardiovasc Surg 1995;110:4-13; discussion 13-14.

44. Keller CA, Cagle PT, Brown RW, et al. Bronchiolitis obliterans in recipients of single, double, and heart-lung transplantation. Chest 1995;107:973-980.

45. El-Gamel A, Sim E, Hasleton P, et al. Transforming growth factor beta (TGF-beta) and obliterative bronchiolitis following pulmonary transplantation. J Heart Lung Transplant 1999;18:828-837.

46. Girgis RE, Tu I, Berry GJ, et al. Risk factors for the development of obliterative bronchiolitis after lung transplantation. J Heart Lung Transplant 1996;15:1200-1208.

47. Heng D, Sharples LD, McNeil K, et al. Bronchiolitis obliterans syndrome: Incidence, natural history, prognosis, and risk factors. J Heart Lung Transplant 1998;17:1255-1263.

48. Husain AN, Siddiqui MT, Holmes EW, et al. Analysis of risk factors for the development of bronchiolitis obliterans syndrome. Am J Respir Crit Care Med 1999;159:829-833.

49. Kroshus TJ, Kshettry VR, Savik K, et al. Risk factors for the development of bronchiolitis obliterans syndrome after lung transplantation. J Thorac Cardiovasc Surg 1997;114:195-202.

50. Sharples LD, McNeil K, Stewart S, Wallwork J. Risk factors for bronchiolitis obliterans: A systematic review of recent publications. J Heart Lung Transplant 2002;21:271-281.

51. Hopkins PM, Aboyoun CL, Chhajed PN, et al. Association of minimal rejection in lung transplant recipients with obliterative bronchiolitis. Am J Respir Crit Care Med 2004;170:1022-1026.

52. Hachem RR, Khalifah AP, Chakinala MM, et al. The significance of a single episode of minimal acute rejection after lung transplantation. Transplantation 2005;80:1406-1413.

53. Burton CM, Iversen M, Scheike T, et al. Is lymphocytic bronchiolitis a marker of acute rejection? An analysis of 2,697 transbronchial biopsies after lung transplantation. J Heart Lung Transplant 2008;27:1128-1134.

54. Glanville AR, Aboyoun CL, Havryk A, et al. Severity of lymphocytic bronchiolitis predicts long-term outcome after lung transplantation. Am J Respir Crit Care Med 2008;177:1033-1040.

55. Chakinala MM, Ritter J, Gage BF, et al. Reliability for grading acute rejection and airway inflammation after lung transplantation. J Heart Lung Transplant 2005;24:652-657.

56. Chalermskulrat W, Neuringer IP, Schmitz JL, et al. Human leukocyte antigen mismatches predispose to the severity of bronchiolitis obliterans syndrome after lung transplantation. Chest 2003;123:1825-1831.

57. Lobo LJ, Aris RM, Schmitz J, Neuringer IP. Donor-specific antibodies are associated with antibody-mediated rejection, acute cellular rejection, bronchiolitis obliterans syndrome, and cystic fibrosis after lung transplantation. J Heart Lung Transplant 2013;32:70-77.

58. Hachem RR, Yusen RD, Meyers BF, et al. Anti–human leukocyte antigen antibodies and preemptive antibody-directed therapy after lung transplantation. J Heart Lung Transplant 2010;29:973-980.

59. Weber DJ, Wilkes DS. The role of autoimmunity in obliterative bronchiolitis after lung transplantation. Am J Physiol Lung Cell Mol Physiol 2013;304:L307-L311.

60. Sumpter TL, Wilkes DS. Role of autoimmunity in organ allograft rejection: A focus on immunity to type V collagen in the pathogenesis of lung transplant rejection. Am J Physiol Lung Cell Mol Physiol 2004;286:L1129-L1139.

61. Burlingham WJ, Love RB, Jankowska-Gan E, et al. IL-17–dependent cellular immunity to collagen type V predisposes to obliterative bronchiolitis in human lung transplants. J Clin Invest 2007;117:3498-3506.

62. Goers TA, Ramachandran S, Aloush A, et al. De novo production of K-alpha1 tubulin-specific antibodies: Role in chronic lung allograft rejection. J Immunol 2008;180:4487-4494.

63. Gelman AE, Li W, Richardson SB, et al. Cutting edge: Acute lung allograft rejection is independent of secondary lymphoid organs. J Immunol 2009;182:3969-3973.

64. Lee Y, Awasthi A, Yosef N, et al. Induction and molecular signature of pathogenic TH17 cells. Nat Immunol 2012;13:991-999.

65. Christie JD, Carby M, Bag R, et al. Report of the ISHLT Working Group on Primary Lung Graft Dysfunction part II: Definition. A consensus statement of the International Society for Heart and Lung Transplantation. J Heart Lung Transplant 2005;24:1454-1459.

66. Christie JD, Kotloff RM, Ahya VN, et al. The effect of primary graft dysfunction on survival after lung transplantation. Am J Respir Crit Care Med 2005;171:1312-1316.

67. King RC, Binns OA, Rodriguez F, et al. Reperfusion injury significantly impacts clinical outcome after pulmonary transplantation. Ann Thorac Surg 2000;69:1681-1685.

68. Bharat A, Kuo E, Steward N, et al. Immunological link between primary graft dysfunction and chronic lung allograft rejection. Ann Thorac Surg 2008;86:189-195; discussion 196-197.

69. Bharat A, Narayanan K, Street T, et al. Early post-transplant inflammation promotes the development of alloimmunity and chronic human lung allograft rejection. Transplantation 2007;83:150-158.

70. Huang HJ, Yusen RD, Meyers BF, et al. Late primary graft dysfunction after lung transplantation and bronchiolitis obliterans syndrome. Am J Transplant 2008;8:2454-2462.

71. Basseri B, Conklin JL, Pimentel M, et al. Esophageal motor dysfunction and gastroesophageal reflux are prevalent in lung transplant candidates. Ann Thorac Surg 2010;90:1630-1636.

72. Fortunato GA, Machado MM, Andrade CF, et al. Prevalence of gastroesophageal reflux in lung transplant candidates with advanced lung disease. J Bras Pneum 2008;34:772-778.

73. Singer LG, Gould MK, Tomlinson G, Theodore J. Determinants of health utility in lung and heart-lung transplant recipients. Am J Transplant 2005;5:103-109.

74. Sweet MP, Herbella FA, Leard L, et al. The prevalence of distal and proximal gastroesophageal reflux in patients awaiting lung transplantation. Ann Surg 2006;244:491-497.

75. Young LR, Hadjiliadis D, Davis RD, Palmer SM. Lung transplantation exacerbates gastroesophageal reflux disease. Chest 2003;124:1689-1693.

76. D'Ovidio F, Mura M, Tsang M, et al. Bile acid aspiration and the development of bronchiolitis obliterans after lung transplantation. J Thorac Cardiovasc Surg 2005;129:1144-1152.

77. Blondeau K, Mertens V, Vanaudenaerde BA, et al. Gastro-oesophageal reflux and gastric aspiration in lung transplant patients with or without chronic rejection. Eur Respir J 2008;31:707-713.

78. D'Ovidio F, Mura M, Ridsdale R, et al. The effect of reflux and bile acid aspiration on the lung allograft and its surfactant and innate immunity molecules SP-A and SP-D. Am J Transplant 2006;6:1930-1938.

79. Mertens V, Blondeau K, Van Oudenhove L, et al. Bile acids aspiration reduces survival in lung transplant recipients with BOS despite azithromycin. Am J Transplant 2011;11:329-335.

80. Sundaresan S, Mohanakumar T, Smith MA, et al. HLA-A locus mismatches and development of antibodies to HLA after lung transplantation correlate with the development of bronchiolitis obliterans syndrome. Transplantation 1998;65:648-653.

81. Keenan RJ, Lega ME, Dummer JS, et al. Cytomegalovirus serologic status and postoperative infection correlated with risk of developing chronic rejection after pulmonary transplantation. Transplantation 1991;51:433-438.

82. Taylor DO, Edwards LB, Boucek MM, et al. Registry of the International Society for Heart and Lung Transplantation: Twenty-fourth official adult heart transplant report—2007. J Heart Lung Transplant 2007;26:769-781.

83. Engelmann I, Welte T, Fuhner T, et al. Detection of Epstein-Barr virus DNA in peripheral blood is associated with the development of bronchiolitis obliterans syndrome after lung transplantation. J Clin Virol 2009;45:47-53.

84. Manuel O, Kumar D, Moussa G, et al. Lack of association between beta-herpesvirus infection and bronchiolitis obliterans syndrome in lung transplant recipients in the era of antiviral prophylaxis. Transplantation 2009;87:719-725.

85. Gottlieb J, Schulz TF, Welte T, et al. Community-acquired respiratory viral infections in lung transplant recipients: A single season cohort study. Transplantation 2009;87:1530-1537.

86. Kumar D, Husain S, Chen MH, et al. A prospective molecular surveillance study evaluating the clinical impact of community-acquired respiratory viruses in lung transplant recipients. Transplantation 2010;89:1028-1033.

87. Liu M, Mallory GB, Schecter MG, et al. Long-term impact of respiratory viral infection after pediatric lung transplantation. Pediatr Transplant 2010;14:431-436.

88. Liu M, Worley S, Arrigain S, et al. Respiratory viral infections within one year after pediatric lung transplant. Transpl Infect Dis 2009;11:304-312.

89. Gottlieb J, Mattner F, Weissbrodt H, et al. Impact of graft colonization with gram-negative bacteria after lung transplantation on the development of bronchiolitis obliterans syndrome in recipients with cystic fibrosis. Respir Med 2009;103:743-749.

90. Gregson AL, Wang X, Weigt SS, et al. Interaction between *Pseudomonas* and CXC chemokines increases risk of bronchiolitis obliterans syndrome and death in lung transplantation. Am J Respir Crit Care Med 2013;187:518-526.

91. Botha P, Archer L, Anderson RL, et al. *Pseudomonas aeruginosa* colonization of the allograft after lung transplantation and the risk of bronchiolitis obliterans syndrome. Transplantation 2008;85:771-774.

92. Valentine VG, Gupta MR, Walker JE Jr, et al. Effect of etiology and timing of respiratory tract infections on development of bronchiolitis obliterans syndrome. J Heart Lung Transplant 2009;28:163-169.

93. Weigt SS, Copeland CA, Derhovanessian A, et al. Colonization with small conidia *Aspergillus* species is associated with bronchiolitis obliterans syndrome: A two-center validation study. Am J Transplant 2013;13:919-927.

94. Weigt SS, Elashoff RM, Huang C, et al. *Aspergillus* colonization of the lung allograft is a risk factor for bronchiolitis obliterans syndrome. Am J Transplant 2009;9:1903-1911.

95. Vos R, Vanaudenaerde BM, Ottevaere A, et al. Long-term azithromycin therapy for bronchiolitis obliterans syndrome: Divide and conquer? J Heart Lung Transplant 2010;29:1358-1368.

96. Reynaud-Gaubert M, Thomas P, Badier M, et al. Early detection of airway involvement in obliterative bronchiolitis after lung transplantation. Functional and bronchoalveolar lavage cell findings. Am J Respir Crit Care Med 2000;161:1924-1929.

97. Slebos DJ, Postma DS, Koeter GH, et al. Bronchoalveolar lavage fluid characteristics in acute and chronic lung transplant rejection. J Heart Lung Transplant 2004;23:532-540.

98. Hadjiliadis D, Davis RD, Palmer SM. Is transplant operation important in determining posttransplant risk of bronchiolitis obliterans syndrome in lung transplant recipients? Chest 2002;122:1168-1175.

99. Hadjiliadis D, Chaparro C, Gutierrez C, et al. Impact of lung transplant operation on bronchiolitis obliterans syndrome in patients with chronic obstructive pulmonary disease. Am J Transplant 2006;6:183-189.

100. Sundaresan S. The impact of bronchiolitis obliterans on late morbidity and mortality after single and bilateral lung transplantation for pulmonary hypertension. Semin Thorac Cardiovascular Surg 1998;10:152-159.

101. Bosma OH, Vermeulen KM, Verschuuren EA, et al. Adherence to immunosuppression in adult lung transplant recipients: Prevalence and risk factors. J Heart Lung Transplant 2011;30:1275-1280.

102. Cantu E 3rd, Appel JZ 3rd, Hartwig MG, et al. J. Maxwell Chamberlain Memorial Paper. Early fundoplication prevents chronic allograft dysfunction in patients with gastroesophageal reflux disease. Ann Thorac Surg 2004;78:1142-1151; discussion 1151.

103. Hachem RR, Yusen RD, Chakinala MM, et al. A randomized controlled trial of tacrolimus versus cyclosporine after lung transplantation. J Heart Lung Transplant 2007;26:1012-1018.

104. Keenan RJ, Konishi H, Kawai A, et al. Clinical trial of tacrolimus versus cyclosporine in lung transplantation. Ann Thorac Surg 1995;60:580-584; discussion 584-585.

105. Treede H, Glanville AR, Klepetko W, et al. Tacrolimus and cyclosporine have differential effects on the risk of development of bronchiolitis obliterans syndrome: Results of a prospective, randomized international trial in lung transplantation. J Heart Lung Transplant 2012;31:797-804.

106. Zuckermann A, Reichenspurner H, Birsan T, et al. Cyclosporine A versus tacrolimus in combination with mycophenolate mofetil and steroids as primary immunosuppression after lung transplantation: One-year results of a 2-center prospective randomized trial. J Thorac Cardiovasc Surg 2003;125:891-900.

107. Sarahrudi K, Estenne M, Corris P, et al. International experience with conversion from cyclosporine to tacrolimus for acute and chronic lung allograft rejection. J Thorac Cardiovasc Surg 2004;127:1126-1132.

108. Vos R, Vanaudenaerde BM, Verleden SE, et al. A randomised controlled trial of azithromycin to prevent chronic rejection after lung transplantation. Eur Respir J 2011;37:164-172.

109. Svanstrom H, Pasternak B, Hviid A. Use of azithromycin and death from cardiovascular causes. N Engl J Med 2013;368:1704-1712.

110. Hartwig MG, Anderson DJ, Onaitis MW, et al. Fundoplication after lung transplantation prevents the allograft dysfunction associated with reflux. Ann Thorac Surg 2011;92:462-468; discussion 468-469.

111. Cai J, Terasaki PI. Induction immunosuppression improves long-term graft and patient outcome in organ transplantation: An analysis of United Network for Organ Sharing registry data. Transplantation 2010;90:1511-1515.

112. Reams BD, Musselwhite LW, Zaas DW, et al. Alemtuzumab in the treatment of refractory acute rejection and bronchiolitis obliterans syndrome after human lung transplantation. Am J Transplant 2007;7:2802-2808.

113. Shyu S, Dew MA, Pilewski JM, et al. Five-year outcomes with alemtuzumab induction after lung transplantation. J Heart Lung Transplant 2011;30:743-754.

114. Diamond DA, Michalski JM, Lynch JP, et al. Efficacy of total lymphoid irradiation for chronic allograft rejection following bilateral lung transplantation. Int J Radiol Oncol Biol Phys 1998;41:795-800.

115. Fisher AJ, Rutherford RM, Bozzino J, et al. The safety and efficacy of total lymphoid irradiation in progressive bronchiolitis obliterans syndrome after lung transplantation. Am J Transplant 2005;5:537-543.

116. Verleden GM, Lievens Y, Dupont LJ, et al. Efficacy of total lymphoid irradiation in azithromycin non-responsive chronic allograft rejection after lung transplantation. Transplant Proc 2009;41:1816-1820.

117. Meloni F, Cascina A, Miserere S, et al. Peripheral CD4(+)CD25(+) TREG cell counts and the response to extracorporeal photopheresis in lung transplant recipients. Transplant Proc 2007;39:213-217.

118. Slovis BS, Loyd JE, King LE Jr. Photopheresis for chronic rejection of lung allografts. N Engl J Med 1995;332:962.

119. Villanueva J, Bhorade SM, Robinson JA, et al. Extracorporeal photopheresis for the treatment of lung allograft rejection. Ann Transplant 2000;5:44-47.
120. Benden C, Speich R, Hofbauer GF, et al. Extracorporeal photopheresis after lung transplantation: A 10-year single-center experience. Transplantation 2008;86:1625-1627.
121. Morrell MR, Despotis GJ, Lublin DM, et al. The efficacy of photopheresis for bronchiolitis obliterans syndrome after lung transplantation. J Heart Lung Transplant 2010;29:424-431.
122. Aigner C, Jaksch P, Taghavi S, et al. Pulmonary retransplantation: Is it worth the effort? A long-term analysis of 46 cases. J Heart Lung Transplant 2008;27:60-65.
123. Brugiere O, Thabut G, Castier Y, et al. Lung retransplantation for bronchiolitis obliterans syndrome: Long-term follow-up in a series of 15 recipients. Chest 2003;123:1832-1837.
124. Kawut SM, Lederer DJ, Keshavjee S, et al. Outcomes after lung retransplantation in the modern era. Am J Respir Crit Care Med 2008;177:114-120.
125. Novick RJ, Stitt LW, Al-Kattan K, et al. Pulmonary retransplantation: Predictors of graft function and survival in 230 patients. Pulmonary Retransplant Registry. Ann Thorac Surg 1998;65:227-234.
126. Osaki S, Maloney JD, Meyer KC, et al. Redo lung transplantation for acute and chronic lung allograft failure: Long-term follow-up in a single center. Eur J Cardiothorac Surg 2008;34:1191-1197.
127. Strueber M, Fischer S, Gottlieb J, et al. Long-term outcome after pulmonary retransplantation. J Thorac Cardiovasc Surg 2006;132:407-412.
128. Novick RJ, Schafers HJ, Stitt L, et al. Recurrence of obliterative bronchiolitis and determinants of outcome in 139 pulmonary retransplant recipients. J Thorac Cardiovasc Surg 1995;110:1402-1413; discussion 1413-1414.

34

Chronic lung allograft dysfunction other than bronchiolitis obliterans syndrome

STIJN E. VERLEDEN, ROBIN VOS, BART M. VANAUDENAERDE, AND GEERT M. VERLEDEN

Chronic lung allograft dysfunction (CLAD) is a relatively new term in the field of lung transplantation that was recently introduced because different phenotypes of chronic allograft rejection had been identified. For decades, the term *bronchiolitis obliterans syndrome* (BOS) has been used to reflect chronic rejection; clinically, it has been defined as a persistent, irreversible decline in forced expiratory volume in the first second of respiration (FEV_1) of at least 20% in comparison to the mean of the best two postoperative values in the absence of confounding factors such as acute rejection, infections, suture problems, or recurrence of native disease.[1] The pathologic correlate of BOS was considered to be the presence of obliterative bronchiolitis (OB) lesions, which is basically filling of the bronchiolar lumen with a collagenous matrix that leads to obstructive airflow limitation. Other typical characteristics have included refractoriness to treatment and the presence of neutrophilic airway inflammation.[1] As early as 1984, many remarkable findings in explanted lung specimens were described in one of the first publications on OB.[2] Indeed, a progressive restrictive ventilatory defect developed in three of five patients.[3,4] Moreover, in addition to the typical OB lesions, significant pleural fibrosis was found in two of five patients. Later reports described a combination of a restrictive pulmonary function defect and severe pulmonary infiltrates in patients with end-stage BOS that was confirmed by computed tomography (CT).[5] These findings alone illustrate that not all patients experiencing chronic rejection manifest a strictly obstructive ventilatory defect and that clinical and pathophysiologic alterations other than OB occur in rejected grafts.[3]

More recently, it became clear that in some lung transplant recipients with a diagnosis of BOS, pulmonary function can improve to the point where they no longer meet the criteria for a diagnosis of BOS (FEV_1 improved to a value above the 20% cutoff for a diagnosis of BOS), provided that a macrolide antibiotic (azithromycin or clarithromycin) is added to their therapeutic regimen.[6] Approximately 40% of patients can benefit from one of these drugs, which is contradictory to the earlier definition of BOS as being characterized by an irreversible decline in FEV_1.[6] Therefore, because the term *BOS* appeared to no longer cover the entire spectrum of chronic rejection, the term *CLAD* was introduced to cover all forms of allograft rejection (whether treatable or untreatable) with a pattern of restrictive, obstructive, or mixed pulmonary function. This chapter focuses on the forms of CLAD that do not fit the criteria for true BOS (obstructive lung disease, refractoriness to treatment, and presence of OB), as well as on the prevalence, diagnosis, characteristics, mechanism, and treatment of and risk factors for neutrophilic reversible allograft dysfunction (NRAD) and restrictive allograft syndrome (RAS), which are the two most frequent forms of CLAD following BOS. In addition, the need for and problems of adequate phenotyping are illustrated.

NEUTROPHILIC REVERSIBLE ALLOGRAFT DYSFUNCTION

History

The role of the neutrophil in BOS has been well established for more than 2 decades, with numerous studies showing an association between an elevated percentage of neutrophils in bronchoalveolar lavage (BAL) fluid and the development of BOS. Digiovine and colleagues and Riise and coworkers were the first to demonstrate a central role for neutrophils and the associated protein CXCL8/interleukin-8 (IL-8), which is a major neutrophil chemoattractant in the inflammatory response preceding BOS.[7-9] Even more convincing was a study showing that when the number of neutrophils increased, the severity of BOS also increased.[10] Based on this information, a number of studies attempted to define a cutoff to predict later development of BOS, which was determined to be between 16% and 24% depending on the study.[11-13]

However, the introduction of azithromycin caused a paradigm shift. Azithromycin is a neomacrolide antibiotic (also called an azalide) with a 15-membered macrolactone ring structure that is derived from *Streptomyces* species.[14]

It was first introduced into clinical practice to treat diffuse panbronchiolitis, for which it was used mainly because of its effect against *Pseudomonas*.[15] Later studies were able to show that azithromycin was beneficial in patients who suffered from cystic fibrosis and were chronically colonized with *Pseudomonas*.[16] At approximately the same time Gerhardt and colleagues published the first report demonstrating a 0.5-L improvement in FEV$_1$ in five of six patients with BOS who were treated with azithromycin (250 mg three times per week).[17] This pilot study was followed by several other smaller studies that all confirmed improvement in FEV$_1$ in a subset of patients with BOS.[18,19] The different studies have been summarized in a comprehensive review.[14] Administration of azithromycin to all 412 patients with BOS in all the retrospective studies led to an improvement in FEV$_1$ in 145 (35%) of them (mean increase, 7.6%). A representative example is presented in Figure 34.1. However, not all the studies have reported beneficial effects: in particular, one study failed to show any improvement in FEV$_1$ but did at least show stabilization of FEV$_1$, which is also of great value in patients with BOS.[20] Not all centers use azithromycin; instead, some use clarithromycin, another macrolide with comparable anti-inflammatory effects.[21] However, clarithromycin should be used with caution because of its

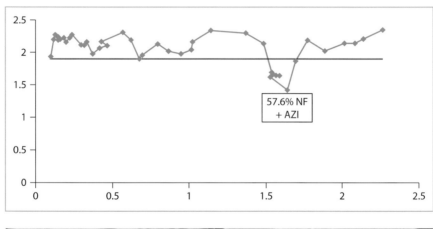

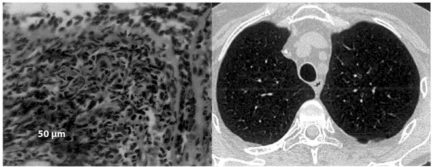

Figure 34.1 Top, Evolution of pulmonary function in a patient suffering from neutrophilic reversible allograft dysfunction (NRAD). Forced expiratory volume in the first second of respiration (FEV$_1$) was below the threshold for bronchiolitis obliterans syndrome (red line) for more than 3 weeks. Bronchoalveolar lavage was performed and showed a neutrophil percentage of 57.6%, after which the patient was given azithromycin. The patient's pulmonary function increased again and reached values similar to those before the NRAD episode. Bottom left, Lymphocytic infiltrate in the submucosa found at the time of diagnosis of azithromycin-responsive lymphocytic bronchiolitis. Bottom right, A representative computed tomography scan showing centrilobular nodules.

known effect on trough levels of calcineurin,[22] and its possible side effects, though limited, should also be borne in mind. Azithromycin remains an antibiotic that can cause bacterial resistance. Also, a slight increase in risk for cardiovascular death during treatment with azithromycin for 5 days has been noted[23]; in a young cohort, however, long-term treatment did not show any adverse cardiovascular events associated with macrolide treatment.[24] Rare reports of prolongation of the QT interval in patients undergoing azithromycin therapy do exist, but such risk appears to increase only in vulnerable patients.[25] The same statement holds true for cardiac arrhythmias: azithromycin does not generally increase the risk for arrhythmias, although extra caution should be exercised when azithromycin is used in patients with additional risk factors.[26] Furthermore, it seems that BAL neutrophilia can redevelop despite azithromycin therapy, in which case it may be associated with a renewed decline in FEV_1 similar to that with BOS but refractory to treatment. The prevalence and the significance of these findings remain to be established.

Prevalence and diagnosis

Why some patients respond to azithromycin treatment whereas others do not exhibit any observable effect is still a mystery. The first clue hinting at azithromycin's mechanism of action against BOS came in 2006: the main differences between the azithromycin responders and nonresponders in a cohort of 14 lung transplant patients were the total number of neutrophils and the percentage of neutrophils in their BAL fluid at the start of azithromycin treatment. A correlation between the increase in response in terms of FEV_1 and the percentage of neutrophils and CXCL8 mRNA in BAL fluid was seen. Additionally, azithromycin resulted in a decrease in the percentage of neutrophils in BAL fluid after 3 to 6 months of treatment.[27] These findings were later confirmed in a larger cohort, in which a threshold BAL neutrophil content of 20% was proved to be predictive of a response to azithromycin.[28] The observed discrepancies led to the proposal of a dichotomy in chronic rejection and the existence of two phenotypes. The azithromycin responders (an increase in FEV_1 of at least 10% after treatment) were characterized by a high percentage of BAL neutrophilia; a rather early posttransplant onset; coarse crackles and increased sputum production; and a tree-in-bud appearance, centrilobular nodules, and bronchiectasis on CT.[6] This condition was initially called NRAD and subsequently renamed *azithromycin-responsive allograft dysfunction* (ARAD).[29] A representative evolution of FEV_1 in a typical patient with NRAD or ARAD can be seen in Figure 34.1. On the other hand, azithromycin nonresponders showed no signs of airway inflammation and had a relatively late onset, as well as air trapping and mosaic attenuation visible on CT. Such patients were deemed to have fibroproliferative BOS.

Whether treatment with azithromycin should be initiated before the onset of BOS (preventive) or once FEV_1 starts to decrease (curative) remained an open question.

A randomized placebo-controlled trial in which patients' treatment was supplemented with azithromycin at discharge following lung transplantation provided the answer: chronic rejection was observed less frequently in the group receiving azithromycin than in the placebo group (12.5% versus 44%). Although no significant survival benefit was found, the mean FEV_1 value was higher whereas the level of C-reactive protein (as a marker of systemic inflammation) and percentage of neutrophils in BAL fluid remained lower in the azithromycin group throughout the entire study. The absence of a survival benefit is probably due to the fact that patients experiencing a 20% drop in FEV_1 were shifted to active open-label treatment with azithromycin, which resulted in an improvement in FEV_1 in 56% of patients and thus probably reduced mortality.[30] This study clearly demonstrated that the NRAD phenotype can be prevented with azithromycin.

Radiology and pathology

Because all the early studies of radiologic and pathologic findings in cases of CLAD were probably evaluating a mixture of different phenotypes, they should be interpreted with care. The main radiologic findings that have historically been associated with BOS are air trapping and mosaic attenuation on CT and evidence of OB in histopathologic analysis.[31,32] However, the existence of differences between patients with true BOS and those with NRAD or ARAD is very likely. Indeed, the pretreatment and posttreatment chest CT scans of 41 azithromycin-responsive lung transplant recipients were compared with those of 59 nonresponders. Centrilobular nodules (including a tree-in-bud appearance) were the typical hallmark distinguishing patients with NRAD or ARAD from nonresponsive patients; no differences in bronchus dilatation, air trapping, mucus plugging, or the other parameters studied were evident. However, after 3 to 6 months of azithromycin, all the abnormalities observed in the azithromycin responders improved. In contrast, the nonresponders showed improvement only in mucus plugging, centrilobular abnormalities, airway wall thickening, and ground-glass opacities; their other abnormalities (bronchial dilatation, consolidation, and air trapping) worsened.[33] For a representative example, see Figure 34.1.

The pathology of NRAD is not well known because it bears a good prognosis: patients respond to treatment very well, as a result of which material explanted during retransplantation or autopsy is not available for pathologic examination. Currently, however, NRAD and ARAD appear to possibly have a great deal of similarity to lymphocytic bronchiolitis (LB). The term *lymphocytic bronchiolitis* was introduced by the International Society for Heart and Lung Transplantation (ISHLT) to grade the degree of airway inflammation (which is graded as B0, B1R, and B2R, depending on severity of the lymphocytic infiltrate).[32] Clinically, LB has great importance because its severity is associated with an increased risk for BOS and death.[34]

Nonetheless, the similarities between LB and NRAD are striking. For instance, from an immunology standpoint, both conditions are characterized by BAL neutrophilia and lymphocytic airway inflammation that is evident by biopsy.[35] Chambers and coworkers demonstrated that lymphocytic airway inflammation similar to that observed in LB is present in the bronchial wall of patients with BOS (patients with possible NRAD).[36] The radiologic findings for the two diseases also bear great similarities: CT shows centrilobular nodules and a tree-in-bud pattern equally in LB and NRAD. Clinically, steroids appear to be ineffective against both LB and NRAD,[37] whereas azithromycin brings relief in both conditions. Indeed, after 3 months of treatment of LB with azithromycin, histologically identified lymphocytic airway inflammation and IL-8 levels, total and differential total cell counts (macrophages, neutrophils, and eosinophils), and levels of C-reactive protein and pro-inflammatory markers in BAL fluid decreased significantly from the moment of diagnosis.[37a] The idea that NRAD is a manifestation of LB that persists longer in transplanted lungs and thus leads to a progressive decline in FEV_1 seems plausible. However, adequate treatment with azithromycin reverses this airflow limitation. The long-term effect of such episodes of NRAD or LB remains to be established, but it appears to be deleterious in view of the negative impact of NRAD on survival.[38]

Mechanism

Whether the beneficial effect of azithromycin is the result of its antibiotic and antimicrobial effects or its anti-inflammatory effects remains a matter of debate. Its direct antibacterial effects include binding to the 50S ribosome subunit, which results in decreased protein synthesis, a decrease in *Pseudomonas aeruginosa* biofilm formation, and interaction with outer cellular membrane proteins. In addition to these direct effects, indirect antiviral and antibacterial effects, such as an increase in interferon-stimulated genes, a decrease in mucin, and an increase in acute degranulation and phagocytosis-associated burst have also been described.[14] Along with its antimicrobial effects, azithromycin also possesses a range of anti-inflammatory effects, which are considered to be even more important to its benefit in patients with NRAD. IL-17 probably plays a crucial part in the pathophysiology of NRAD; it is an important immunomodulatory mediator in many chronic respiratory diseases because of its role in the interplay between the innate and adaptive immune responses—a role that is based mainly on recruiting neutrophils via IL-8.[39] IL-17 has long been implicated in the pathophysiology of chronic rejection, as has been demonstrated by evidence in both animals and humans.[40,41] However, our own data indicate that such involvement seems to be specific to patients with NRAD or LB. Additional evidence in support of this hypothesis is a positive correlation between the numbers of IL-17–positive cells in the submucosa and neutrophils in BAL fluid.[42] Interestingly, IL-17 immunohistochemical staining showed

that azithromycin is able to reduce the number of IL-17–positive lymphocytes in the bronchial submucosa.[42] Other in vitro evidence has demonstrated that azithromycin can reduce IL-17–induced production of IL-8 via a reduction in activation of mitogen-activated protein kinase (MAPK) and secretion of 8-isoprostane from smooth muscle cells of the human airway,[43] as well as from airway epithelial cells.[44] In addition to this effect on IL-8, an inhibitory effect on granulocyte-macrophage colony-stimulating factor (GM-CSF), matrix metalloproteinase 2 (MMP-2), and MMP-9 has been shown.[44] In vivo studies examining the effect of azithromycin on lung transplant recipients are rare; however, one study showed a reduction in levels of serum IL-8, monocyte chemotactic peptide-1 (MCP-1), I-309, macrophage inflammatory protein-1α (MIP-1α), and tumor necrosis factor α (TNF-α) in patients treated with azithromycin.[45] Additionally, it has been shown that azithromycin treatment for 3 to 6 months significantly reduced levels of MMP-9, activated MMP-9, and gelatinase activity in BAL fluid. One surprising finding was that the aforesaid levels did not decrease to the levels of stable patients but instead remained significantly elevated. These findings provide proof that the remodeling is still "ongoing" and might indicate that preventive treatment is better than treatment once BOS is diagnosed,[46] and they might also help explain why despite showing an initial response of pulmonary function to treatment, patients who experience an episode of NRAD can still be expected to have a worse outcome versus patients who do not experience an episode of NRAD.[38] Another rather unexpected finding was that azithromycin may also inhibit angiogenesis, as was indicated by a study demonstrating azithromycin's ability to inhibit fibroblast growth factor 1 (FGF-1)- and FGF-2–induced production of vascular endothelial growth factor (VEGF) via inhibition of the p38 (MAPK) pathway in smooth muscle cells of the human airway.[47] A final study evaluated the expression of 32 different proteins in BAL fluid at the moment of diagnosis of NRAD and compared this expression with that in the classic form of BOS and in stable patients as control group. Concentrations of MCP-1, regulated on activation normal T-cell–expressed and secreted (RANTES), IL-1β, IL-8, tissue inhibitor of metalloproteinase 1 (TIMP-1), MMP-8, MMP-9, hepatocyte growth factor (HGF), myeloperoxidase, and bile acids were upregulated exclusively in the NRAD group; not a single mediator was expressed differently in the BAL fluid of patients with BOS than in the BAL fluid of stable patients.[48]

RESTRICTIVE ALLOGRAFT SYNDROME

History

A 1985 study of explanted lungs analyzed the pathophysiologic alterations in five heart-lung transplant recipients with progressive airflow limitation. Although varying degrees of OB were evident in all the lungs, diffuse increases in interstitial fibrosis were also noted in all the biopsy specimens, whereas the pleura was focally fibrotic and thickened.[4] These findings were later confirmed in both animal and human studies.[49] On the basis of these findings, two forms of BOS were identified: "pure bronchiolitis obliterans" and "bronchiolitis obliterans organizing pneumonia." The latter was characterized by focal and cellular bronchiolitis obliterans extending into the distal alveolar spaces.[2] Likewise, a 2006 study by Martinu and coworkers that reviewed pathologic alterations in lungs explanted at retransplantation showed the presence of varying degrees of OB, as well as interstitial fibrosis, in 2 of 12 patients. Imaging studies showed pleural thickening and interstitial infiltrates in 3 of 12 patients.[5] Even routine biopsies performed 2 years after lung transplantation provided evidence of the occurrence of interstitial abnormalities: the biopsy samples of 37% of the recipients showed signs of interstitial or focal fibrosis.[50] The aforesaid studies are all historical examples demonstrating parenchymal involvement in CLAD that is not present in classic obstructive BOS (in which alterations are present only within the airways, whereas the parenchyma is more or less normal). However, these findings had always been regarded as rare, unusual, and not fitting the definition of BOS, and further characterization and classification were never attempted. Only in the past few years have interest in and knowledge about patients with such complications emerged.

A joint project of the Toronto and Duke groups was the first attempt to identify the subgroup of patients experiencing restrictive pulmonary function. They described a novel form of upper lobe fibrosis in 13 of 686 (1.9%) patients. The diagnosis was made by radiology (upper lobe fibrosis); pathologic analysis demonstrated interstitial fibrosis and OB, and spirometry showed a mixed obstructive and restrictive pulmonary function defect.[51] The numbers were too low to allow a statement about the impact on long-term survival after diagnosis, however. The next attempt (by Woodrow and colleagues) made a distinction between patients suffering from "nonspecific" and "specific" CLAD.[52] Patients with "nonspecific" CLAD (35%) showed persistent infiltrates over a period of more than 6 months, whereas in those with "specific" CLAD (65%) infiltrates either were absent or resolved within 6 months. The researchers further subdivided patients in the latter group as having an obstructive (37%) or restrictive (28%) deficit in pulmonary function (determined on the basis of a decline in forced vital capacity (FVC) of at least 20%). Although the researchers were not able to demonstrate an effect on survival after diagnosis, their attempt was very valuable because it laid the foundation for later work on phenotyping of CLAD.

Prevalence and diagnosis

A seperate clinical phenotype was only introduced in 2011 when Sato and associates defined the RAS clinical phenotype of CLAD, which is characterized by restrictive rather than obstructive pulmonary function.[53] By using a cutoff decrease in total lung capacity (TLC) of at least 10% versus the baseline to define restrictive pulmonary function, they were able to identify the almost 30% of their total population of patients with CLAD who were suffering from RAS. Importantly, survival time after diagnosis was 1.5 years in the group with RAS versus 4 years in the group with BOS. These results were directly confirmed in a second, independent cohort of 72 patients, 20 (28%) of whom were suffering from RAS. Because TLC was not routinely measured, FVC and the FEV_1/FVC ratio were instead used to diagnose RAS. Because patients with RAS showed a simultaneous decrease in FVC and FEV_1, their FEV_1/FVC ratio remained normal or even above normal (as a result of which, a cutoff of 0.70 was used).[38] As in the previous study, patients with RAS had a worse prognosis than did those with BOS (median survival times of 8 and 36 months, respectively).[38] A final approach to distinguish patients with restrictive pulmonary function came from the Duke group, which used the decline in FVC at time of diagnosis of CLAD to classify patients as restrictive (best FEV_1/FVC, <0.80) or obstructive (best FEV_1/FVC, >0.80), and it was able to demonstrate that 65 (30%) of the 216 patients with CLAD showed a decrease in FVC at time of diagnosis of CLAD.[54] The median time of survival after a diagnosis of CLAD was significantly lower in patients showing a drop in FVC (309 days) than in patients with no drop in FVC (1070 days), thus confirming once again the poor prognosis of patients with restrictive pulmonary function. These three independent studies clearly show that restrictive pulmonary function is a problem that cannot be neglected because it is common (in 30% of patients with CLAD) and bears a very bad prognosis (with a survival time after diagnosis of approximately 1 year). Nonetheless, an internationally approved definition of RAS does not yet exist.

The clinical evolution of RAS is very difficult to predict; however, a stepwise pattern of regression appears to exist.[55] Patients with RAS experienced between one and four episodes of acute exacerbation that were associated with acute respiratory deterioration (a sudden drop in pulmonary function, evidence of diffuse alveolar damage [DAD] in biopsy samples, and patchy or diffuse ground-glass opacities with some consolidation on CT). Such acute exacerbation occurred in a period during which resolution of ground-glass opacities, progression of consolidation, interstitial reticular shadows, and traction bronchiectasis were frequently observed. In most patients such acute exacerbation will lead to death or urgent redo transplantation. A representative example of the evolution of pulmonary function is provided in Figure 34.2A.

Radiology and pathology

All the studies of RAS have confirmed that patients' CT scans will exhibit typical characteristics of interstitial fibrosis and some degree of pleural and septal thickening. The most common findings in patients with RAS have included interstitial opacities, traction bronchiectasis, architectural distortion, and ground-glass opacities.[53] In a cohort of 24 patients with RAS, changes in patients'

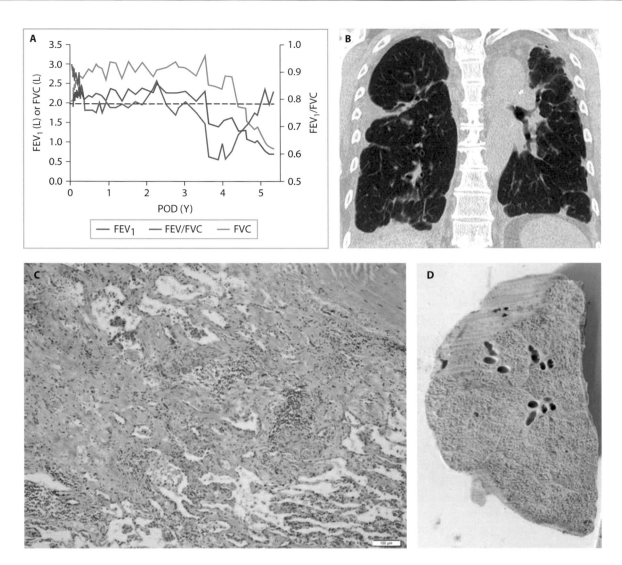

Figure 34.2 **(A)** Evolution of pulmonary function (forced expiratory volume in the first second of respiration [FEV$_1$], forced vital capacity [FVC], and FEV$_1$/FVC ratio) of a patient with a condition that was initially diagnosed as bronchiolitis obliterans syndrome (a decrease in FEV$_1$/FVC) but subsequently evolved into end-stage restrictive allograft syndrome (RAS) (increase in FEV$_1$/FVC >0.70). The dotted black line indicates the 20% threshold for a diagnosis of chronic lung allograft dysfunction. **(B)** Last available computed tomography scan before the same patient with RAS underwent retransplantation; the scan shows pleural and subpleural fibrosis and persistent infiltrates. **(C)** Histopathology of the explanted lung at retransplantation showing regions with dense alveolar fibrosis and extensive inflammation. **(D)** Coronal slice of a lung of a patient with RAS showing dense pleural and subpleural fibrosis.

CT scans were examined from the pre-CLAD time point (last CT scan before CLAD was diagnosed) to end-stage CLAD (last available CT scan). Remarkably, the CT scans of almost half of the patients already showed abnormalities at the pre-CLAD time point; however, this fact was not indicative of a worse outcome. The most prominent CT features at time of diagnosis of CLAD were the appearance of central and peripheral ground-glass opacities. The "evolution" of CT abnormalities after the diagnosis of CLAD included significant increases in (traction) bronchiectasis, central and peripheral consolidation, architectural deformation, volume loss, and hilus retraction, with almost all patients showing signs of these abnormalities.[56] None of the measured parameters were correlated with survival after diagnosis, however, which makes CT useful for diagnosis

but not a good tool for predicting survival after diagnosis. Figure 34.2B presents a typical CT scan showing end-stage RAS. Additionally, ^{18}F-fluorodeoxyglucose positron emission tomography may be helpful in diagnosing RAS and may even serve as prognostic tool because it allows observation of hypermetabolic activity in the subpleural region.[57] At the moment, however, further evidence supporting its diagnostic and eventual prognostic utility is lacking.

On histopathologic examination, the lungs of patients with RAS showed DAD, extensive alveolar fibrosis, thickened interlobular septa, and fibrotic visceral pleura.[53] Figure 34.2C shows the representative histology of a lung with RAS. Of note, OB lesions, the typical pathologic correlate of BOS, were also present in nearly all the lung specimens examined.[58] A parallel was drawn with idiopathic pleuroparenchymal fibroelastosis, which is a disease that is described primarily after allogeneic stem cell transplantation and characterized by upper lobe–predominant pleural and subpleural fibrosis. The same fibrosis is seen in some patients with RAS as end-stage lungs begin exhibiting more signs of an upper lobe–predominant disease than at the start of their disease.[56,58] A sharp demarcation between healthy and fibrotic zones is evident and often delineated by thickened septa. Interestingly, DAD that tended to merge with zones of fibroelastosis was also evident; hence, a biopsy finding of DAD was suggested to be one of the first findings of RAS. Indeed, late-onset DAD was very frequently observed before the diagnosis of RAS, whereas early-onset DAD was associated more with BOS.[59] How the recently proposed variant acute fibrinoid organizing pneumonia (AFOP) will fit into the conception of BOS and RAS is not entirely certain. The definition of AFOP is based primarily on histopathology and less on pulmonary function.[60] Histopathologic analysis of AFOP shows mainly open bronchioles with a peribronchiolar deposition of intra-alveolar loose fibrillary fibrin that fills the alveolar space and minimal presence of inflammatory infiltrates or interstitial thickening. From the standpoint of the relationship between radiologic findings and survival of patients with AFOP, however, numerous similarities with RAS exist. Indeed, ground-glass opacities and interlobular septal thickening are frequently observed, although survival after diagnosis is lower than that of patients with classic BOS (101 days versus 294 days). Moreover, pulmonary function was also mostly restrictive. However, no upper lobe–predominant disease in the lungs of patients with AFOP was reported, and DAD (which is typically observed in RAS) is histopathologically distinct from AFOP, both in nature and distribution. Future research will prove whether AFOP can stand on its own as a distinct phenotype of CLAD. The advantage of the biopsy-based definition is that it can be used in patients who are too sick to perform pulmonary function testing; however, its main disadvantage is that biopsies are sometimes non-diagnostic, invasive, and very difficult to perform in certain critically ill patients.

Risk factors and mechanism

The risk factors and mechanism of RAS remain elusive because no comprehensive studies have been performed to date. Women appeared to be more predisposed to the development of restrictive lung disease in one study,[54] and patients with RAS seemed to be younger in other studies,[38,53] but these patterns were not confirmed in the other studies.[54,60] Likewise, cytomegalovirus mismatch seemed to predispose recipients to RAS in one study but not in the others.[53] However, on the basis of the scarce existing reports, it seems that different kinds of inflammation may predispose recipients to RAS. Severe LB, which is the pathologic correlate of severe airway inflammation accompanied by lymphocytes in biopsy samples and neutrophils in BAL fluid,[35] appears to be the sole risk factor differentiating RAS from

BOS,[61] whereas BAL neutrophilia on days 90 and 720 after transplantation, acute rejection, *Pseudomonas* colonization, and pulmonary infection may be associated with predisposition to RAS just as they are linked to predisposition to classic BOS.[61] Another study showed that an episode of elevated BAL eosinophilia (defined as ≥2%) predisposed recipients to the later development of CLAD and, in particular, RAS.[62] Two additional studies demonstrated that late-onset DAD is a risk factor for RAS[53,63] and further established that as a potent chemoattractant for mononuclear cells, the CXCR3 axis plays a major role in this process. Indeed, concentrations of CXCL9, CXCL10, and CXCL11 (CXCR3 ligands) in BAL fluid were elevated at the moment of diagnosis of DAD, and persistent elevation of these chemokines proved to be predictive of the subsequent development of RAS.[63] Caution should be exercised when generalizing the results of these studies: most are single-center studies with small numbers of patients, and some risk factors found in some papers could not be confirmed in others. These limitations hint at coincidental findings that are a consequence of the single-center approach and do not reflect the actual risk factors in the general population of patients with RAS. Therefore larger, preferably multicenter studies would seem to be necessary to investigate possible risk factors in more detail.

The mechanism of RAS is largely unknown; no researchers have attempted to study it in depth and compare it with the mechanism of the well-known BOS type of rejection. However, analysis of mediators in the BAL fluid of patients with RAS at the time of diagnosis and comparison of the findings with those of analysis of BAL fluid from patients with BOS and stable patients have shown elevation of not just eosinophils but also neutrophils in patients with RAS. More detailed analysis demonstrated that levels of IL-1β, IL-1Rα, IL-6, IL-8/CXCL8, IP-10/CXCL10, MCP-1/CCL2, MIP-1α/CCL3, MIP-1β/CCL4, and VEGF were regulated differently in patients with RAS than in stable patients.[63a] Interestingly BAL IL-6, PARC/CCL18, IP-10/CXCL10, and eosinophilia were correlated with survival in patients with RAS after diagnosis and thus might prove to be important as clinical biomarkers. Alveolar alarmins are another interesting group of mediators that might be active in RAS. Levels of S100, which is an important proinflammatory protein, were higher in the BAL fluid of patients with RAS than in that of patients with BOS or stable patients.[64] Because we do not know the mechanism of RAS, no good biomarker is currently available. However, serum levels of KL-6 (a marker that is commonly used in identifying patients with interstitial pulmonary fibrosis [IPF] and has chemotactic, proliferative, and antiapoptotic effects on fibroblasts in vitro) are higher in patients with RAS than in patients with BOS.[65] The significance of this finding must be confirmed by larger series. However, on the basis of the aforementioned findings, it is difficult to point to one specific cell or pathway as the culprit in the development of RAS. Not only eosinophils, but also natural killer cells (CXCL10 and CXCL11) and B cells (IL-6) could be important mediators, but this hypothesis remains to be investigated. Thus, the evidence to date suggests that inflammation plays an important role and should therefore be a topic for future investigation.

Treatment

Because patients with RAS have a poor prognosis after diagnosis, research to identify adequate treatment is urgently needed. In this regard, several attempts to treat RAS or at least slow it down have already been made; however, most of the studies have been based on only one or a few patients. Given the fact that (as mentioned in the previous section) inflammation may play a very important role in RAS, depletion of T cells might be a means to treat it. Extracorporeal photophoresis (ECP) depletes the body of T cells by ex vivo treatment of white blood cells with a photoactive drug that is activated by ultraviolet light, thereby leading to cell apoptosis. Evidence supporting the use of ECP for therapy-resistant BOS is increasing; the largest prospective study included 51 patients, 61% of whom responded to treatment (defined as sustained stability of pulmonary function).[66] A recent study adequately phenotyped patients undergoing ECP and showed that in patients with RAS, ECP did not lead to stabilization of pulmonary function, which instead deteriorated further.[67] Conversely, patients with high BAL neutrophilia showed the best response to ECP treatment.

Another possible strategy to slow the development of RAS is to use pirfenidone, which is currently the first-line treatment of IPF and has been shown to slow the decline in FVC in patients with established IPF.[68] Pirfenidone's exact mechanism of action has not yet been determined, but it seems to be able to influence the production of transforming growth factor β (TGF-β), a main profibrotic molecule, and arrest the proliferation of fibroblasts,[69,70] which are two areas of interest in the study of RAS because extensive alveolar fibrosis is its main hallmark. After a first case report showing potential benefit of pirfenidone in slowing the development of BOS,[71] another case report demonstrated its potential to slow the development of RAS by demonstrating that the drug resulted in less pronounced decreases in FEV_1 and FVC and improvement in consolidation and ground-glass opacities on CT.[57] These findings require further confirmation in a larger population of patients with RAS.

Another drug that can be used is alemtuzumab (Campath-1H); it is an antagonist of CD52, a protein expressed on B cells, lymphocytes, dendritic cells, and monocytes. It was first used successfully in lung transplantation to treat recurrent episodes of therapy-refractory acute rejection but has also been used to treat BOS.[72,73] New evidence that it can likewise be used in the treatment of RAS is emerging. In a patient suffering from pulmonary chronic graft-versus-host disease, a disease with many similarities to chronic rejection after lung transplantation, consolidation zones and reticulonodular areas resolved after treatment.[74] Moreover, the oxygen saturation and chest radiography findings of a lung transplant patient who showed signs of RAS on CT (persistent ground-glass appearance

with interlobular septal thickening and focal consolidation) improved significantly after the administration of alemtuzumab, as did the same patient's pathologic signs (nonspecific diffuse interstitial inflammation and alveolar septal fibrosis).[75] Lung function in the three other patients described also improved significantly after treatment. These separate case reports demonstrate the great promise of Campath; however, its numerous known side effects, particularly in immunocompromised patients, and the associated risk for infection must be kept in mind. Therefore, more studies involving larger numbers of patients and more research are needed before the use of Campath is extended into general practice.

Retransplantation is a possible last-resort option; it is an accepted ultimate treatment option that can be offered to patients with end-stage chronic rejection. Mean survival after retransplantation is generally comparable to that after primary lung transplantation.[76] However, patients with RAS suffer from far worse 1- and 3-year survival rates compared to BOS patients.[76a]

PHENOTYPING CLAD: IS THE END NEAR?

A recent paper proposed a classification system for CLAD, according to which patients demonstrating a decrease in pulmonary function are classified on the basis of the cause of the decline in their pulmonary function.[29] When the cause of a failing allograft is known (e.g., persistent acute rejection, infection, anastomotic stricture, disease recurrence, pleural disease, diaphragm dysfunction, and native lung hyperinflation), patients should not be classified as having CLAD due to chronic rejection. Patients previously categorized as having NRAD or ARAD are also considered to have graft failure with a known cause and hence are no longer classified as having CLAD because adequate treatment exists and improves pulmonary function (which is contrary to the definition of CLAD). However, to exclude ARAD or NRAD as a cause of decline in the pulmonary function of patients in whom CLAD is suspected, azithromycin should be administered to them. The only two recognized subgroups of patients with CLAD (i.e., patients who are not responding to azithromycin treatment and have allograft failure with no known cause) are those with BOS (defined as a persistent decrease in FEV_1 of at least 20%) and those with RAS (defined as a persistent decrease in FEV_1 and FVC of at least 20%). Further research will indicate whether this definition of CLAD will stand or whether more phenotypes of RAS must be defined. In this respect, differences in radiologic findings may be identified given the fact that extensive apical pleural fibrosis develops in some patients whereas interstitial changes throughout the whole lung (albeit most apparently in the upper lobes) occur in others. BOS and RAS may also coexist, with BOS developing first in some patients (no decline in TLC) and a syndrome that is consistent with RAS (a decline in TLC ≥ 10%) and is characterized by interstitial infiltrates on high-resolution CT developing only later.

Table 34.1 Typical clinical characteristics of patients with NRAD/ARAD and RAS in comparison to those of patients with the conventional form of CLAD (BOS)

Characteristic	NRAD/ARAD	RAS	BOS
Inflammation (identified by BAL)	Neutrophilic airway inflammation	Eosinophils	No airway inflammation
Biopsy findings	Lymphocytic airway inflammation	Alveolar fibrosis, pleural thickening, OB	Constrictive bronchitis
Pulmonary function	Obstructive	Restrictive (decline in TLC >10%), increasing FEV_1/FVC index	Obstructive
Radiology	Bronchiectasis, airway wall thickening, mucus plugging, centrilobular nodules	Consolidation, reticular pattern, persistent infiltrate	Air trapping and mosaic attenuation
Treatment	Macrolides	Pirfenidone? Campath?	ECP? Re-LTx?
Survival	Very good	Very bad (±1 year)	Poor (±3 years)

Note: ARAD, azithromycin-responsive allograft dysfunction; BAL, bronchoalveolar lavage; BOS, bronchiolitis obliterans syndrome, CLAD, chronic lung allograft dysfunction; ECP, extracorporeal photophoresis; FEV_1/FVC, ratio of forced expiratory volume in the first second of respiration to forced vital capacity; NRAD, neutrophilic reversible allograft dysfunction; OB, obliterative bronchiolitis; RAS, restrictive allograft syndrome; ReLTx, repeat lung transplantation; TLC, total lung capacity.

Many questions remain. Do all the aforementioned conditions represent manifestations of chronic rejection, or are different pathophysiologic mechanisms involved? More importantly, will they affect patients' survival? What about other manifestations of chronic rejection, such as follicular bronchiolitis[77] or exudative bronchiolitis,[78] that do not strictly fit the definition of BOS or RAS? Indeed, follicular bronchiolitis, which is rare, seems to be a manifestation outside the scope of BOS and RAS. CT shows mild bronchiectasis but, more importantly, impressive bilateral centrilobular, reticulonodular opacities with mucus plugging but no infiltrates and very mild pleural thickening. Histologically, pronounced bronchus-associated lymphoid tissue that is homogeneously distributed within the lung (thus causing luminal obstruction) is observed. Exudative bronchiolitis is similarly a concern. Exudative bronchiolitis is diagnosed mainly by a CT scan showing thickening and inflammation of small airways, which appear as centrilobular nodules and branching lines (tree-in-bud pattern) that probably represent bronchioles impacted with inflammatory material and peribronchiolar inflammation. Although both conditions are rare, they do exist and cannot be classified at this time.

One must be aware that each lung transplantation patient has an individual posttransplant trajectory and not all patients may fit perfectly within a phenotype. For example, some patients with neutrophilia do not respond to azithromycin therapy, whereas other patients without neutrophilia do respond to it. Moreover, many possible confounding factors exist, thus making it difficult to phenotype each patient. Retrospective assessment is extremely difficult because an individual clinic may not yet be using azithromycin or routinely performing full pulmonary function testing (including measurement of TLC) and CT. Patients who received only a single-lung transplant are very difficult to assess because their native lung can have a big influence on the transplanted lung (for example, hyperinflation or further deterioration of the native lung). Moreover, patients with end-stage pulmonary disease are often colonized by

bacteria or fungi, which can also lead to an elevated level of airway neutrophilia, thereby making them difficult to classify within a certain phenotype. Some patients can also evolve from one phenotype to another with no clear cause or explanation; hence, care should always be taken when classifying patients at a given moment, and the evolution of their disease should be taken into account.

SUMMARY

Phenotyping of CLAD has very important implications for current clinical practice. A diagnosis of NRAD is established most easily by using BAL fluid, and such patients will benefit from azithromycin treatment (as per the definition) and have a very good prognosis. RAS is diagnosed by measuring TLC and by CT of the thorax; such patients have a dismal prognosis. Table 34.1 summarizes the typical characteristics of the different phenotypes of CLAD. Phenotyping of CLAD also has important scientific implications in view of the fact that most previous studies involved a mixed pool of patients suffering from BOS or RAS. Now, however, each phenotype is presumed to have its own characteristics and risk factors and possibly even different mechanisms, which suggests that accurate phenotyping is necessary for valid scientific research. Only by adequate phenotyping of patients can better long-term survival be achieved. The future probably lies with individualized therapy tailored to a patient's pattern of CLAD, which is probably the best hope for winning the ongoing battle against chronic rejection after lung transplantation and finally achieving long-term survival consistent with that after other solid-organ transplants.

REFERENCES

1. Estenne M, Maurer JR, Boehler A, et al. Bronchiolitis obliterans syndrome 2001: An update of the diagnostic criteria. J Heart Lung Transplant 2002;21:297-310.

2. Burke CM, Theodore J, Dawkins KD, et al. Post-transplant obliterative bronchiolitis and other late lung sequelae in human heart-lung transplantation. Chest 1984;86:824-829.

3. Abernathy EC, Hruban RH, Baumgartner WA, et al. The two forms of bronchiolitis obliterans in heart-lung transplant recipients. Hum Pathol 1991;22:1102-1110.

4. Yousem SA, Burke CM, Billingham ME. Pathologic pulmonary alterations in long-term human heart-lung transplantation. Hum Pathol 1985;16:911-923.

5. Martinu T, Howell DN, Davis RD, et al. Pathologic correlates of bronchiolitis obliterans syndrome in pulmonary retransplant recipients. Chest 2006;129:1016-1023.

6. Vanaudenaerde BM, Meyts I, Vos R, et al. A dichotomy in bronchiolitis obliterans syndrome after lung transplantation revealed by azithromycin therapy. Eur Respir J 2008;32:832-843.

7. DiGiovine B, Lynch JP, III, Martinez FJ, et al. Bronchoalveolar lavage neutrophilia is associated with obliterative bronchiolitis after lung transplantation: Role of IL-8. J Immunol 1996;157:4194-4202.

8. Riise GC, Williams A, Kjellstrom C, et al. Bronchiolitis obliterans syndrome in lung transplant recipients is associated with increased neutrophil activity and decreased antioxidant status in the lung. Eur Respir J 1998;12:82-88.

9. Riise GC, Andersson BA, Kjellstrom C, et al. Persistent high BAL fluid granulocyte activation marker levels as early indicators of bronchiolitis obliterans after lung transplant. Eur Respir J 1999;14:1123-1130.

10. Devouassoux G, Drouet C, Pin I et al. Alveolar neutrophilia is a predictor for the bronchiolitis obliterans syndrome, and increases with degree of severity. Transpl Immunol 2002;10:303-310.

11. Neurohr C, Huppmann P, Samweber B, et al. Prognostic value of bronchoalveolar lavage neutrophilia in stable lung transplant recipients. J Heart Lung Transplant 2009;28:468-474.

12. Reynaud-Gaubert M, Thomas P, Badier M, et al. Early detection of airway involvement in obliterative bronchiolitis after lung transplantation. Functional and bronchoalveolar lavage cell findings. Am J Respir Crit Care Med 2000;161:1924-1929.

13. Slebos DJ, Postma DS, Koeter GH, et al. Bronchoalveolar lavage fluid characteristics in acute and chronic lung transplant rejection. J Heart Lung Transplant 2004;23:532-540.

14. Vos R, Vanaudenaerde BM, Verleden SE, et al. Antiinflammatory and immunomodulatory properties of azithromycin involved in treatment and prevention of chronic lung allograft rejection. Transplantation 2012;94:101-109.

15. Kobayashi H, Ohgaki N, Takeda H. Therapeutic possibilities for diffuse panbronchiolitis. Int J Antimicrob Agents 1993;3(Suppl 1):S81-S86.

16. Saiman L, Marshall BC, Mayer-Hamblett N, et al. Azithromycin in patients with cystic fibrosis chronically infected with *Pseudomonas aeruginosa*: A randomized controlled trial. JAMA 2003;290:1749-1756.

17. Gerhardt SG, McDyer JF, Girgis RE, et al. Maintenance azithromycin therapy for bronchiolitis obliterans syndrome: Results of a pilot study. Am J Respir Crit Care Med 2003;168:121-125.

18. Verleden GM, Dupont LJ. Azithromycin therapy for patients with bronchiolitis obliterans syndrome after lung transplantation. Transplantation 2004;77:1465-1467.

19. Yates B, Murphy DM, Forrest IA, et al. Azithromycin reverses airflow obstruction in established bronchiolitis obliterans syndrome. Am J Respir Crit Care Med 2005;172:772-775.

20. Shitrit D, Bendayan D, Gidon S, et al. Long-term azithromycin use for treatment of bronchiolitis obliterans syndrome in lung transplant recipients. J Heart Lung Transplant 2005;24:1440-1443.

21. Benden C, Boehler A. Long-term clarithromycin therapy in the management of lung transplant recipients. Transplantation 2009;87:1538-1540.

22. Ibrahim RB, Abella EM, Chandrasekar PH. Tacrolimus-clarithromycin interaction in a patient receiving bone marrow transplantation. Ann Pharmacother 2002;36:1971-1972.

23. Ray WA, Murray KT, Hall K, et al. Azithromycin and the risk of cardiovascular death. N Engl J Med 2012;366:1881-1890.

24. Svanstrom H, Pasternak B, Hviid A. Use of azithromycin and death from cardiovascular causes. N Engl J Med 2013;368:1704-1712.

25. Parnham MJ, Haber VE, Giamarellos-Bourboulis EJ, et al. Azithromycin: Mechanisms of action and their relevance for clinical applications. Pharmacol Ther 2014;143:225-245.

26. Albert RK, Schuller JL. Macrolide antibiotics and the risk of cardiac arrhythmias. Am J Respir Crit Care Med 2014;189:1173-1180.

27. Verleden GM, Vanaudenaerde BM, Dupont LJ, Van Raemdonck DE. Azithromycin reduces airway neutrophilia and interleukin-8 in patients with bronchiolitis obliterans syndrome. Am J Respir Crit Care Med 2006;174:566-570.

28. Gottlieb J, Szangolies J, Koehnlein T, et al. Long-term azithromycin for bronchiolitis obliterans syndrome after lung transplantation. Transplantation 2008;85:36-41.

29. Verleden GM, Raghu G, Meyer KC, et al. A new classification system for chronic lung allograft dysfunction. J Heart Lung Transplant 2014;33:127-133.

30. Vos R, Vanaudenaerde BM, Verleden SE, et al. A randomised controlled trial of azithromycin to prevent chronic rejection after lung transplantation. Eur Respir J 2011;37:164-172.

31. Konen E, Gutierrez C, Chaparro C, et al. Bronchiolitis obliterans syndrome in lung transplant recipients: Can thin-section CT findings predict disease before its clinical appearance? Radiology 2004;231:467-473.

32. Stewart S, Fishbein MC, Snell GI, et al. Revision of the 1996 working formulation for the standardization of nomenclature in the diagnosis of lung rejection. J Heart Lung Transplant 2007;26:1229-1242.

33. de Jong PA, Vos R, Verleden GM, et al. Thin-section computed tomography findings before and after azithromycin treatment of neutrophilic reversible lung allograft dysfunction. Eur Radiol 2011;21:2466-2474.

34. Glanville AR, Aboyoun CL, Havryk A, et al. Severity of lymphocytic bronchiolitis predicts long-term outcome after lung transplantation. Am J Respir Crit Care Med 2008;177:1033-1040.

35. Vos R, Vanaudenaerde BM, Verleden SE, et al. Bronchoalveolar lavage neutrophilia in acute lung allograft rejection and lymphocytic bronchiolitis. J Heart Lung Transplant 2010;29:1259-1269.

36. Chambers DC, Hodge S, Hodge G, et al. A novel approach to the assessment of lymphocytic bronchiolitis after lung transplantation—transbronchial brush. J Heart Lung Transplant 2011;30:544-551.

37. Ross DJ, Marchevsky A, Kramer M, Kass RM. "Refractoriness" of airflow obstruction associated with isolated lymphocytic bronchiolitis/bronchitis in pulmonary allografts. J Heart Lung Transplant 1997,16.832-038.

37a. Vos R, Verleden SE, Ruttens D, et al. Azithromycin and the treatment of lymphocytic airway inflammation after lung transplantation. Am J Transplant 2014;(12):2736-2748.

38. Verleden GM, Vos R, Verleden SE, et al. Survival determinants in lung transplant patients with chronic allograft dysfunction. Transplantation 2011;92:703-708.

39. Vanaudenaerde BM, Verleden SE, Vos R, et al. Innate and adaptive interleukin-17–producing lymphocytes in chronic inflammatory lung disorders. Am J Respir Crit Care Med 2011;183:977-986.

40. Fan L, Benson HL, Vittal R, et al. Neutralizing IL-17 prevents obliterative bronchiolitis in murine orthotopic lung transplantation. Am J Transplant 2011;11:911-922.

41. Vanaudenaerde BM, De Vleeschauwer SI, Vos R, et al. The role of the IL23/IL17 axis in bronchiolitis obliterans syndrome after lung transplantation. Am J Transplant 2008;8:1911-1920.

42. Verleden SE, Vos R, Vandermeulen E, et al. Involvement of interleukin-17 during lymphocytic bronchiolitis in lung transplant patients. J Heart Lung Transplant 2013;32:447-453.

43. Vanaudenaerde BM, Wuyts WA, Geudens N, et al. Macrolides inhibit IL17-induced IL8 and 8-isoprostane release from human airway smooth muscle cells. Am J Transplant 2007;7:76-82.

44. Murphy DM, Forrest IA, Ward C, et al. Effect of azithromycin on primary bronchial epithelial cells derived from stable lung allografts. Thorax 2007;62;834.

45. Federica M, Nadia S, Monica M, et al. Clinical and immunological evaluation of 12-month azithromycin therapy in chronic lung allograft rejection. Clin Transplant 2011;25:E381-E389.

46. Verleden SE, Vandooren J, Vos R, et al. Azithromycin decreases MMP-9 expression in the airways of lung transplant recipients. Transpl Immunol 2011;25:159-162.

47. Willems-Widyastuti A, Vanaudenaerde BM, Vos, et al. Azithromycin attenuates fibroblast growth factors induced vascular endothelial growth factor via p38(MAPK) signaling in human airway smooth muscle cells. Cell Biochem Biophys 2013;67:331-339.

48. Verleden SE, Vos R, Mertens V, et al. Heterogeneity of chronic lung allograft dysfunction: Insights from protein expression in bronchoalveolar lavage. J Heart Lung Transplant 2011;30:667-673.

49. Haverich A, Dawkins KD, Baldwin JC, et al. Long-term cardiac and pulmonary histology in primates following combined heart and lung transplantation. Transplantation 1985;39:356-360.

50. Burton CM, Iversen M, Carlsen J, Andersen CB. Interstitial inflammatory lesions of the pulmonary allograft: A retrospective analysis of 2697 transbronchial biopsies. Transplantation 2008;86:811-819.

51. Pakhale SS, Hadjiliadis D, Howell DN, et al. Upper lobe fibrosis: A novel manifestation of chronic allograft dysfunction in lung transplantation. J Heart Lung Transplant 2005;24:1260-1268.

52. Woodrow JP, Shlobin OA, Barnett SD, et al. Comparison of bronchiolitis obliterans syndrome to other forms of chronic lung allograft dysfunction after lung transplantation. J Heart Lung Transplant 2010;29:1159-1164.

53. Sato M, Waddell TK, Wagnetz U, et al. Restrictive allograft syndrome (RAS): A novel form of chronic lung allograft dysfunction. J Heart Lung Transplant 2011;30:735-742.

54. Todd JL, Jain R, Pavlisko EN, et al. Impact of forced vital capacity loss on survival after the onset of chronic lung allograft dysfunction. Am J Respir Crit Care Med 2014;189:159-166.

55. Sato M, Hwang DM, Waddell TK, et al. Progression pattern of restrictive allograft syndrome after lung transplantation. J Heart Lung Transplant 2013;32:23-30.

56. Verleden SE, de Jong PA, Ruttens, D et al. Functional and computed tomographic evolution and survival of restrictive allograft syndrome after lung transplantation. J Heart Lung Transplant 2014;33:270-277.

57. Vos R, Verleden SE, Ruttens D, et al. Pirfenidone: A potential new therapy for restrictive allograft syndrome? Am J Transplant 2013;13:3035-3040.

58. Ofek E, Sato M, Saito T, et al. Restrictive allograft syndrome post lung transplantation is characterized by pleuroparenchymal fibroelastosis. Mod Pathol 2013;26:350-356.

59. Sato M, Hwang DM, Ohmori-Matsuda K, et al. Revisiting the pathologic finding of diffuse alveolar damage after lung transplantation. J Heart Lung Transplant 2012;31:354-363.

60. Paraskeva M, McLean C, Ellis S, et al. Acute fibrinoid organizing pneumonia after lung transplantation. Am J Respir Crit Care Med 2013;187:1360-1368.

61. Verleden SE, Ruttens D, Vandermeulen, E et al. Bronchiolitis obliterans syndrome and restrictive allograft syndrome: Do risk factors differ? Transplantation 2013;95:1167-1172.

62. Verleden SE, Ruttens D, Vandermeulen E, et al. Elevated bronchoalveolar lavage eosinophilia correlates with poor outcome after lung transplantation. Transplantation 2014;97:83-89.

63. Shino MY, Weigt SS, Li N, et al. CXCR3 ligands are associated with the continuum of diffuse alveolar damage to chronic lung allograft dysfunction. Am J Respir Crit Care Med 2013;188:1117-1125.

63a. Verleden SE, Ruttens D, Vos R, et al. Differential cytokine, chemokine and growth factor expression in phenotypes of chronic lung allograft dysfunction. Transplantation 2015;99(1):86-93.

64. Saito T, Liu M, Binnie M, et al. Distinct expression patterns of alveolar "alarmins" in subtypes of chronic lung allograft dysfunction. Am J Transplant 2014;14:1425-1432.

65. Ohshimo S, Bonella F, Sommerwerck U, et al. Comparison of serum KL-6 versus bronchoalveolar lavage neutrophilia for the diagnosis of bronchiolitis obliterans in lung transplantation. J Heart Lung Transplant 2011;30:1374-1380.

66. Jaksch P, Scheed A, Keplinger M, et al. A prospective interventional study on the use of extracorporeal photophoresis in patients with bronchiolitis obliterans syndrome after lung transplantation. J Heart Lung Transplant 2012;31:950-957.

67. Greer M, Dierich M, de Wall C, et al. Phenotyping established chronic lung allograft dysfunction predicts extracorporeal photophoresis response in lung transplant patients. Am J Transplant 2013;13:911-918.

68. Noble PW, Albera C, Bradford WZ, et al. Pirfenidone in patients with idiopathic pulmonary fibrosis (CAPACITY): Two randomised trials. Lancet 2011;377:1760-1769.

69. Dosanjh A, Ikonen T, Wan B, Morris RE. Pirfenidone: A novel anti-fibrotic agent and progressive chronic allograft rejection. Pulm Pharmacol Ther 2002;15:433-437.

70. Nakazato H, Oku H, Yamane S, et al. A novel anti-fibrotic agent pirfenidone suppresses tumor necrosis factor-alpha at the translational level. Eur J Pharmacol 2002;446:177-185.

71. Ihle F, von Wulffen W, Neurohr C. Pirfenidone: A potential therapy for progressive lung allograft dysfunction? J Heart Lung Transplant 2013;32:574-575.

72. Reams BD, Davis RD, Curl J, Palmer SM. Treatment of refractory acute rejection in a lung transplant recipient with Campath 1H. Transplantation 2002;74:903-904.

73. Reams BD, Musselwhite LW, Zaas DW, et al. Alemtuzumab in the treatment of refractory acute rejection and bronchiolitis obliterans syndrome after human lung transplantation. Am J Transplant 2007;7:2802-2808.

74. Ruiz-Arguelles GJ, Ruiz-Delgado GJ, Moreno-Ford V. Re: Alemtuzumab-induced resolution of pulmonary noninfectious complications in a patient with chronic graft-versus-host disease. Biol Blood Marrow Transplant 2008;14:1434-1435.

75. Kohno M, Perch M, Andersen E, et al. Treatment of intractable interstitial lung injury with alemtuzumab after lung transplantation. Transplant Proc 2011;43:1868-1870.

76. Kawut SM. Lung retransplantation. Clin Chest Med 2011;32:367-377.

76a. Verleden SE, Todd JL, Sato M, et al. Impact of CLAD phenotype on survival after lung retransplantation: A multicenter study. Am J Transplant 2015;15(8):2223-2230.

77. Vos R, Vanaudenaerde BM, De Vleeschauwer SI, et al. Follicular bronchiolitis: A rare cause of bronchiolitis obliterans syndrome after lung transplantation: A case report. Am J Transplant 2009;9:644-650.

78. McManus TE, Milne DG, Whyte KF, Wilsher ML. Exudative bronchiolitis after lung transplantation. J Heart Lung Transplant 2008;27:276-281.

35

Medical complications of lung transplantation

KEITH C. MEYER

INTRODUCTION

Although optimizing and maintaining lung allograft function is a primary focus of posttransplant patient management, lung transplant recipients are at considerable risk for the development of many complications other than allograft dysfunction. The diverse array of potential medical complications can not only become life-threatening and shorten posttransplant survival but also have a major impact on health status and quality of life. Ideally, serious posttransplant medical complications would be prevented or, if they were to occur, detected in timely fashion and treated promptly (Table 35.1).

At the time of transplantation many patients already have significant comorbid medical problems that require appropriate management and close monitoring (e.g., diabetes, osteoporosis, hyperlipidemia, systemic hypertension). Patients with cystic fibrosis (CF) may not only harbor antibiotic-resistant bacteria in their lungs but also usually have extensive paranasal sinus disease, gastrointestinal (GI) dysfunction and malnutrition, and impaired glucose metabolism or insulin-dependent diabetes when their transplant is performed. Older patients with idiopathic pulmonary fibrosis (IPF) may have significant degrees of frailty and sarcopenia; such patients also usually have significant gastroesophageal reflux (GER) and are at increased risk for microaspiration of refluxed gastric contents, especially if sleep-disordered breathing (SDB) is present as a comorbid condition. Patients with scleroderma are at particular risk for esophageal dysmotility and significant GER, which would predispose them to aspiration and allograft dysfunction after transplantation.

Regardless of the indication for lung transplantation, any of a plethora of posttransplant medical complications, including the following, may develop in recipients after a successful transplant[1]: cardiovascular dysfunction (e.g., systemic hypertension, cardiac rhythm disturbances), metabolic disturbances (e.g., hyperkalemia, hyperglycemia or diabetes, hyperlipidemia), osteopenia or osteoporosis, excessive weight gain or obesity, endocrine dysfunction, anemia, leukopenia, infection, GI complications (e.g., altered bowel motility, GER, biliary tract disease), neurologic complications (e.g., tremor, headache, seizure, memory loss), and malignancies such as posttransplant lymphoproliferative disease (PTLD) or other neoplasms (e.g., skin cancer, primary lung cancer). Additionally, immunosuppressive medications, especially calcineurin inhibitors (CNIs), must be monitored carefully to avoid adverse effects on kidney and bone marrow function. Drug-drug interactions are another important cause of complications, and treating physicians must be aware that many drugs interact with CNIs (metabolized by the hepatic cytochrome P-450 system), which virtually all recipients must take for life to prevent rejection. This chapter reviews medical complications associated with lung transplantation and provides strategies to facilitate the prevention, detection, and management of such complications.

CARDIOVASCULAR COMPLICATIONS

Systemic hypertension, cardiac rhythm disturbances, and venous thrombosis and thromboembolism are common posttransplant complications. Chronic use of corticosteroids, CNIs, and weight gain are strongly associated with hypertension, and it is estimated that systemic hypertension

Table 35.1 Potential medical complications following lung transplantation

- Cardiovascular complications
  - Systemic hypertension
  - Cardiac rhythm disturbances
  - Coronary artery disease
  - Venous thromboembolism
    - Deep venous thrombosis
    - Pulmonary embolism
- Renal dysfunction
  - Acute renal insufficiency
  - Chronic kidney disease
  - Electrolyte abnormalities
    - Hyperkalemia
    - Hypomagnesemia
- Gastrointestinal complications
  - Significant gastroesophageal reflux (may lead to microaspiration and CLAD)
  - Impaired motility
    - Bezoar formation (e.g., in patients with cystic fibrosis)
    - Esophageal dysmotility (e.g., in patients with scleroderma)
    - Intestinal obstruction
  - Biliary tract dysfunction
- Hematologic abnormalities
  - Anemia
  - Leukopenia
  - Thrombocytopenia
- Endocrine and metabolic complications
  - Steroid- or drug-induced diabetes
  - Hyperlipidemia
  - Excessive weight gain or obesity (may cause sleep-disordered breathing)
  - Gonadal dysfunction
- Musculoskeletal complications
  - Osteopenia and osteoporosis
  - Myopathy (e.g., corticosteroid induced)
- Neurologic complications
  - Seizure
  - CNS suppression (e.g., coma caused by tacrolimus)
  - Tremor
  - Memory loss
  - Peripheral neuropathy
- Malignancy
  - Posttransplant lymphoproliferative disease
  - Colon cancer (patients with cystic fibrosis are at increased risk)
  - Skin cancer
- Adverse drug reactions or effects
  - Immunosuppressive drugs (e.g., calcineurin inhibitor toxicity)
  - Drug-drug interactions (especially drugs metabolized via the CYP-450 system)
- Infection (bacterial, viral, fungal, mycobacterial, protozoan)
  - Early (e.g., lung allograft, native lung, ports, lines, catheters)
  - Subacute/late (e.g., allograft, native lung, extrapulmonary)
  - Chronic (e.g., bronchiectasis in the allograft or native lung)

Note: CLAD, chronic lung allograft dysfunction; CNS, central nervous system; CYP-450, cytochrome P-450.

requiring treatment will develop in up to 90% of solid-organ transplant recipients.[2,3] Hyperlipidemia (which frequently occurs as a side effect of chronic administration of immunosuppressive agents) is also eventually encountered in most patients,[4,5] and screening for hyperlipidemia (e.g., with a serum lipid panel) and systemic hypertension should be performed at reasonably frequent intervals because both systemic hypertension and dyslipidemia will eventually develop in most recipients. Interestingly, administration of statins to control hyperlipidemia has been associated with improved recipient survival and allograft function.[6]

Cardiac rhythm disturbances are commonly encountered early after transplantation.[7-10] Supraventricular tachycardia and atrial fibrillation may occur preoperatively and often subside within days but require treatment. β-Blockers, amiodarone, or both may prove useful to control or convert such tachydysrhythmias, and calcium channel blockers or β-blockers may be needed for chronic treatment of these conditions, as well as systemic hypertension. Occasionally, electrophysiologic evaluation and ablative approaches to suppress persistent, clinically significant rhythm disturbances may be required.

Venous thrombosis and thromboembolism are not infrequent events following lung transplantation,[11-17] and maintaining an adequate degree of clinical suspicion for such events is key to the detection of deep venous thrombosis and pulmonary embolism. Other potential complications include coronary artery disease (CAD), congestive heart failure, and peripheral vascular disease. Although the presence of nonsevere CAD is not a contraindication to lung transplantation,[18-20] patients with IPF appear to be at higher risk for CAD,[21,22] and although such recipients can do well and appear to be at relatively low risk for coronary artery occlusive events, they should be carefully monitored.

RENAL COMPLICATIONS

All recipients are at risk for the development of significant acute or chronic renal dysfunction over time.[23] Up to 65% of lung transplant recipients have been reported to have experienced at least one episode of acute kidney injury within the first weeks following transplantation,[24,25] and chronic kidney disease (CKD) that progresses to end-stage kidney disease and thus requires renal replacement therapy or renal transplantation can develop in a substantial number of patients.[25-29] Risk factors for the development of CKD following solid-organ transplantation include a low pretransplant level of kidney function, perioperative renal insults, requirement for prolonged mechanical ventilation, advanced age, female sex, diabetes mellitus, systemic hypertension, renal vasoconstriction caused by exposure to CNIs, and a diagnosis of pulmonary disease other than chronic obstructive pulmonary disease.[23,30]

CNIs can have adverse effects on renal tubular function, and nephrotoxicity is a well-recognized side effect of chronic CNI administration.[31,32] Acute kidney injury associated with CNI therapy results from decreased renal blood flow, which is in turn a consequence of vasoconstriction of the afferent and efferent renal arteries; it is often reversible with appropriate management. CNI nephrotoxicity may be accentuated by hemodynamic instability or concomitant use of other drugs that can cause nephrotoxicity and CKD. Surveillance and management of patients in whom posttransplant CKD develops should follow published guidelines,[33] and kidney transplantation can be considered for recipients in whom stage IV CKD develops and renal replacement therapy is required.[34] Electrolyte abnormalities are frequently encountered in transplant recipients and are largely a consequence of the effects of CNI therapy or other drugs on renal function. Hyperkalemia is the most common abnormality, but hypomagnesemia and hyponatremia may also occur. Additionally, secondary hyperparathyroidism may develop in patients with advanced CKD.

Management of CKD in transplant recipients should focus on keeping CNI levels as low as possible as long as immunosuppression remains adequate. When an acute decline in renal function occurs, CNI therapy should be withheld and adequate intravascular volume restored to allow recovery of renal function. Aggressive management of comorbid conditions that can also worsen renal function (systemic hypertension, diabetes, and hyperlipidemia) is likewise protective,[35] and renal function should be monitored frequently to allow early detection of declining kidney function.

GASTROINTESTINAL COMPLICATIONS

Excessive GER that is significantly worse than that observed in normal individuals and GER disease (GERD) are highly prevalent in patients with advanced lung disease[36-46]; in addition, this markedly excessive GER may persist, worsen, or appear de novo following transplantation. Refluxate reaching the proximal esophagus, reduced lower esophageal sphincter (LES) pressure, esophageal dysmotility, and prolonged gastric emptying are all highly prevalent in patients with end-stage lung disease (ESLD) at the time of referral for lung transplantation.[47] D'Ovidio and colleagues[36] evaluated 78 consecutive patients with ESLD who were referred for transplantation; they reported that 63% had typical GER symptoms: LES pressure was hypotensive in 72%; 33% had esophageal body dysmotility; 44% had delayed gastric emptying; and pH testing detected abnormal GER in 38%, with 20% having proximal GER discovered by pH probe monitoring (32% had increased DeMeester scores). Sweet and coworkers[39] evaluated GER in a cohort of 109 patients who were awaiting a lung transplant and found a hypotensive LES in 55%, esophageal dysmotility in 47%, distal GER in 68%, and proximal GER in 37%. In this cohort the presence of GER symptoms was not highly correlated with presence of the actual disease (sensitivity, 67%; specificity, 26%). Similarly, Fortunato and associates[42] reported that abnormal GER was highly prevalent in lung transplant candidates: abnormal esophageal manometry results (in 80%), LES hypotonia (80%), and abnormal esophageal manometry results (94%) were highly prevalent in patients with chronic obstructive pulmonary disease, and GER was documented in 50% of patients with bronchiectasis. Finally, Hoppo and colleagues[46] reported that laryngopharyngeal reflux was present in 31% of lung transplant candidates with ESLD.

An abnormal degree of GER, which places recipients at risk for microaspiration of refluxed gastroduodenal secretions, is also highly prevalent in lung transplant recipients and has been linked to posttransplant lung allograft complications, especially bronchiolitis obliterans syndrome (BOS). Hadjiliadis and coworkers[48] retrospectively evaluated 43 transplant recipients who had survived to 6 months after lung transplantation and found that 30 (69.8%) had abnormal total acid contact times during 24-hour pH monitoring. An expanded, retrospectively identified cohort of 128 lung transplant recipients was also reported by Davis and associates[49]; 93 (72.7%) of them were found to have abnormal GER by pH monitoring. A number of other studies have also shown a high prevalence of a significant degree of GER in lung transplant recipients.[37,50-54] Young and colleagues[55] evaluated pre– and post–lung transplant GER in 23 patients by 24-hour pH monitoring, esophageal manometry, and gastric-emptying assessments. The percentage of patients with abnormal acid contact times increased from 35% before lung transplantation to 65% afterward; this change was not correlated with alterations in esophageal or gastric motility. Notably, only 20% of lung transplant recipients with abnormal pH study results had symptoms of GER.

Penetration of refluxate into the lung may cause allograft dysfunction secondary to airway injury, increase susceptibility to infection, or trigger acute allograft rejection. Via pH-impedance testing Halsey and associates[56] detected nonacid reflux that was associated with diffuse alveolar damage, and in a cohort of 60 lung recipients, Shah and colleagues[57] found that GERD was associated with a significantly higher incidence of acute rejection episodes, as well as with earlier onset of acute rejection and a tendency toward multiple episodes. Hadjiliadis and coworkers[48] reported a negative correlation between increasing severity of acid reflux (as measured by 24-hour pH study) and posttransplant level of forced expiratory volume in the first second of respiration (FEV$_1$), and Molina and associates[58] reported that GERD was associated with an increased incidence of BOS in a cohort of 162 lung transplant recipients, although GERD did not appear to have an impact on survival. Additionally, King and team[52] reported that the presence of nonacid reflux (as measured by impedance testing) increased the risk for BOS nearly threefold. Aspiration of bile acid has been linked with increased risk for the development of BOS[50,59] and with allograft colonization by *Pseudomonas aeruginosa*[60]; abnormal GER has also been connected with the development of sensitization of T cells to collagen V,[61] which is a significant risk factor for the development of BOS.[62]

Because the presence of significant GER predisposes lung recipients to microaspiration of refluxate and has been associated with chronic lung allograft dysfunction (CLAD) resulting from BOS, centers should consider screening all candidates for significant GER, esophageal dysmotility, or both before transplantation to identify such abnormalities and determine how they should be managed before and after transplantation. Detection of pepsin and bile acids in bronchoalveolar lavage fluid may be particularly useful to identify patients at risk for GER-associated aspiration.[63] Patients with significant esophageal dysmotility (e.g., patients with scleroderma) are at particular risk for aspiration events[64-66] and will require adherence to protocols aimed at minimizing risk for aspiration following lung transplantation.[67] A number of investigations have demonstrated that antireflux surgery (ARS) can be performed safely in the pretransplant or posttransplant setting and may help prevent posttransplant complications such as BOS.[38,68] In addition, ARS has been reported to stabilize or even improve allograft function if significant reflux is found to be linked to evolving BOS.[46,49,69] These data suggest that ARS may be an appropriate intervention for at-risk patients or those with evolving CLAD associated with the presence of significant reflux, but outcomes of definitive randomized, prospective, adequately powered studies are not yet available.

Other GI complications include posttransplant ileus, gastroparesis and intestinal motility disorders (e.g., patients with CF or diabetes), bezoar formation (e.g., patients with CF), bleeding, liver disease or hepatobiliary complications (cholecystitis, significant biliary stasis, and ascending cholangitis, especially in patients with CF), pancreatitis, bowel infection (e.g., *Clostridium difficile* colitis), diverticulitis, diarrhea and constipation (frequently a complication of medications), colon cancer (especially in recipients with CF), and bowel perforation.[70-73] Any patient in whom diarrhea develops should be screened for *C. difficile* colitis, and it should be recognized that diarrhea may not develop in some patients with *C. difficile* colitis (in particular, those with CF). Older recipients are particularly at risk for diverticulitis and bowel perforation, and patients with CF are especially at risk for motility disorders, hepatobiliary dysfunction, *C. difficile* colitis, and colon cancer.

HEMATOLOGIC COMPLICATIONS

Because recipients must take many drugs chronically to maintain optimal immunosuppression and prevent infection (as well as drugs for other indications), they are susceptible to bone marrow dysfunction (anemia, leukopenia, and thrombocytopenia), and neutropenia can greatly increase risk for infection. Anemia is a commonly encountered problem that has multiple potential causes,[74] and a standardized approach to detect them should be undertaken. Drug combinations (e.g., a CNI plus a cytotoxic agent) may have additive effects on bone marrow suppression, whereas other drugs (e.g., ganciclovir or trimethoprim-sulfamethoxazole given for prophylaxis of infection) may impair marrow function and potentiate the effect of immunosuppressive drugs. In addition to bone marrow suppression caused by drugs (e.g., ganciclovir or valganciclovir) given for prophylaxis or treatment of cytomegalovirus infection, cytomegalovirus itself can also suppress bone marrow function.

METABOLIC AND ENDOCRINE COMPLICATIONS

Immunosuppressive medications, especially corticosteroids, can disrupt glucose metabolism and promote both obesity and new-onset diabetes mellitus; the incidence of diabetes in lung transplant recipients is 24.3% at 1 year and 33.5% at 5 years after transplantation.[75] Many patients already have diabetes when they undergo lung transplantation, and those who are diabetic at the time of transplantation have a higher risk for mortality than do those without diabetes. In addition to glucocorticoid and CNI use, factors such as older recipient age, body mass index (BMI) greater than 30 kg/m², and frequent episodes of acute rejection treated with high-dose corticosteroids are also associated with increased risk for diabetes.[76] Treatment thresholds for fasting glucose levels and hemoglobin A_{1C} levels have been recommended,[77] and early intervention may attenuate the increased risk for the development of infection, cardiovascular disease, or both.

Significant gonadal dysfunction can develop in both male and female recipients and lead to impotence in men and menstrual irregularities in premenstrual women.[78,79] Additionally, because hormonal deficiency secondary to hypogonadism may increase risk for the development of osteopenia and osteoporosis,[80] referral to an endocrinology consultant to weigh the risks versus benefits of hormone replacement therapy should be considered if hypogonadism is detected.[81,82]

MUSCULOSKELETAL COMPLICATIONS

Osteopenia and osteoporosis are highly prevalent in patients with advanced lung disease (especially in those with a low pretransplant BMI and previous corticosteroid therapy),[83-85] and recipients are at risk for accelerated bone demineralization after transplantation.[86-89] Although administration of corticosteroids and, to a lesser degree, other immunosuppressants is thought to be a major cause of posttransplant bone demineralization, other factors (such as reduced mobility or hypogonadism) also raise risk.[90] Bone loss appears to be particularly increased during the first few months following a transplant,[91-93] thus placing recipients at higher risk for new fractures that may significantly affect quality of life and allograft function. Supplemental calcium and vitamin D are recognized as basic therapies for prevention and treatment of osteoporosis,[88] and regular weight-bearing exercise may also be beneficial.[94] Additionally, hormone replacement therapy combined with calcium and vitamin D has been shown to decrease the decline in bone mineral density (BMD) in cardiac or liver transplant recipients.[95,96] However, hormone replacement therapy may increase the risk for other complications, and calcium and vitamin D alone appear to have little efficacy in preventing osteoporosis in lung transplant recipients.[91,97,98] Bisphosphonates are considered to be the most effective antiresorptive therapy and can reduce the fracture rate in transplant recipients[99-101];

such therapy may be particularly effective when started before transplantation (when patients are placed on the waiting list).[93] Dual-energy x-ray absorptiometry (DEXA) scanning should be performed before transplantation to evaluate BMD and fracture risk, and recipients should have BMD scanning performed on a regular basis (e.g., yearly) to allow decision making concerning preventive or therapeutic interventions and duration of therapy (e.g., bisphosphonates) for those with osteopenia or osteoporosis.

Other potential musculoskeletal complications include rhabdomyolysis, myopathy, osteonecrosis, and avascular necrosis. Chronic corticosteroid therapy is the major risk factor for myopathy and avascular necrosis, and chronic dosages should be kept at the lowest possible level while still maintaining efficacy. Additionally, frailty and sarcopenia (muscle loss associated with aging) may be significant issues for older patients, particularly older patients with IPF,[102] and the presence of significant frailty at the time of transplantation may indicate an increased risk for a poor outcome.[103]

NEUROLOGIC AND PSYCHIATRIC COMPLICATIONS

Various centers have reported a high incidence of significant acute and chronic neurologic complications following transplantation.[104-107] Mateen and colleagues[106] reported a 92% incidence of neurologic complications in a cohort of 123 recipients; the complications ranged from tremor, headache, confusion, and memory loss to seizure, delirium, encephalopathy (including coma), blindness, posterior reversible encephalopathy syndrome, complications of cerebrovascular disease (e.g., stroke), and peripheral neuropathy. Acute neurologic events can be severe and life-threatening, and they may be linked to CNI therapy (e.g., tremor, seizure, encephalopathy). Another serious complication that may occur is nervous system infection, and it may be unusual, resistant to therapy, or both.

Anxiety and depression are quite prevalent among lung transplant candidates,[108-110] and they can persist or possibly worsen following successful transplantation.[111-113] Individuals with persistent or new-onset psychological dysfunction are more likely to be nonadherent to recommended monitoring and medication regimens,[114] which may have a significant effect on posttransplant outcomes. The lung transplant team should include health psychology experts and social workers who can intervene when problems arise and assist patients with coping mechanisms both before and after lung transplantation.

MALIGNANCY

The incidence and prevalence of malignancy in solid-organ transplant recipients are significantly higher than in the general population, and lung and other solid-organ transplant recipients face an increased risk for the development of malignancy over time.[115-118] This increased risk is probably due to the chronic immunosuppressive therapies that recipients must take to avoid allograft rejection,[119] and the risks in some recipient cohorts may differ for one immunosuppressant to another.[120] Skin cancer is the most commonly seen neoplasm in transplant recipients, but a variety of other cancers may occur in them as well. Following skin cancer, PTLD is the next most common malignancy diagnosed in solid-organ and lung transplant recipients.[121,122] Epstein-Barr virus infection has been linked to the pathogenesis of certain forms of PTLD (especially B-cell lymphomas),[123-125] and Epstein-Barr virus seronegativity at the time of transplantation and intensive immunosuppression are among the risk factors for PTLD.[118,126] Mainstays of therapy for PTLD include a reduction in the intensity of immunosuppression and administration of rituximab,[127-129] and patients who have been successfully placed into remission and in whom advanced CLAD subsequently develops can do well following retransplantation.[130]

Other solid tumors that may arise in lung transplant recipients include lung cancer and GI malignancy. Belli and associates[131] reviewed 335 lung recipients and found that 6 explanted lungs had tumors and that cancer developed in the native lung of 6 single-lung recipients (all with a 20-pack-year smoking history). In addition, a significant incidence of posttransplant colon cancer and colonic polyps detected during screening colonoscopy has been described in lung transplant recipients with CF[132,133]; however, even patients with CF who have not received a transplant are at increased risk for bowel cancer.[134] Because no guidelines for cancer screening in the lung transplant recipient population currently exist, general cancer screening protocols should be followed. Furthermore, because skin cancers can be very aggressive in transplant recipients, frequent (e.g., yearly) evaluation by a dermatologist should be considered, and pretransplant or early posttransplant colon cancer screening should be contemplated for recipients with CF.

DRUG REACTIONS

Transplant recipients must be constantly monitored for adverse drug reactions, and many of the drugs used for maintenance immunosuppression can cause significant morbidity (Table 35.2). Prednisone therapy, especially if kept at high levels over time, can lead to numerous complications, including diabetes, significant weight gain and obesity (which may lead to SDB), myopathy, dyslipidemia, osteoporosis, psychological disturbance, and growth retardation (in children). Because CNIs, which are metabolized by hepatic cytochrome P-450 3A4 (CYP3A4), can cause very serious and potentially life-threatening reactions, their levels in the blood of patients taking them must be monitored frequently.[135,136] Similarly, drugs that inhibit mammalian target of rapamycin (mTOR) are also metabolized by CYP3A4, and mTOR inhibitors (sirolimus, everolimus) must also be monitored via testing of blood levels.[136] Mycophenolate can cause GI toxicity, with diarrhea being the most prominent symptom, and mycophenolate levels in peripheral blood can be obtained if toxicity is suspected. Drug-drug interactions

should always be considered when new drugs are initiated or chronic therapy is modified, and antifungal imidazoles (also metabolized by CYP3A4) in particular should never be given without adjustment of the immunosuppressant dose and close monitoring of CNI or mTOR levels if patients are receiving chronic CNI or mTOR therapy.

OTHER COMPLICATIONS

A number of additional, non–allograft-related medical complications may also occur. Non–allograft-related infectious complications include extrapulmonary infection (e.g., catheter-associated infection; infection of subcutaneous infusion ports, skin and soft tissue, and the paranasal sinuses; C. difficile colitis; diverticulitis; biliary tract infection), and non–allograft-related thoracic infection (e.g., infection in the native lung in single-lung recipients, chest wall incision, and pleural space). Additionally, recurrence of primary disease has been reported in patients with sarcoidosis, Langerhans cell histiocytosis, and lymphangioleiomyomatosis. Another comorbid condition that may develop is SDB, which is highly prevalent in non–transplant recipients with various forms of ESLD but may also arise following transplantation as a consequence of weight gain, advancing age, or both. Naraine and team[137] reported a 63% incidence of SDB (obstructive sleep apnea in 38% and central SDB in 25%) in a cohort of 24 recipients studied with polysomnography; of note, the group with SDB had higher BMIs and systemic hypertension. Malouf and coworkers[138] also found a high prevalence of SDB in lung transplant recipients; some instances were new-onset cases following transplantation. Because of the association between GER and obstructive sleep apnea, concern has been raised that SDB may promote GER, microaspiration, and the development of CLAD. However, Shepherd and colleagues[139] studied a small cohort of 14 recipients and did not find a significant relationship between the severity of GER or obstructive sleep apnea and the severity of bronchiolitis obliterans.

MONITORING AND TROUBLESHOOTING

If an acute posttransplant complication in a previously stable patient (e.g., infection) is suspected, a diagnosis must be aggressively sought and appropriate treatment (which may need to be empiric initially) started as soon as possible. Imaging studies (e.g., computed tomography, magnetic resonance imaging, ultrasound) can be invaluable in making a diagnosis, and recipients may benefit from early referral and, if needed, transfer to their lung transplant center for evaluation and treatment. When an acute illness develops in a recipient, drugs that can cause nephrotoxicity (especially CNIs) should be withheld or minimized while intravascular volume status is optimized to ensure adequate renal perfusion and kidney function and CNI drug levels are ascertained.

In addition to assessment of allograft status and pulmonary physiology, routine surveillance to detect and manage

Table 35.2 Potential complications and monitoring of immunosuppressive drug therapies

Drug	Mechanism of action	Metabolism and elimination	Major potential complications	Precautions and monitoring
Cyclosporine	Inhibits T-cell function (suppresses IL-2 signaling)	Metabolized via CYP3A4, excreted mainly via the biliary tract	Nephrotoxicity, hyperkalemia, hypomagnesemia, hypertension, CNS dysfunction (headache, tremor, seizure, coma, encephalopathy), hepatotoxicity	• Periodically monitor blood levels • Monitor renal function, potassium, CBC, blood pressure, glucose, lipids • Adjust dosing for renal insufficiency • Adjust dose if CYP3A4-metabolized or CYP3A4-inducing drugs are coadministered
Tacrolimus	Inhibits T-cell function (suppresses IL-2 signaling via FK506-binding proteins)	Metabolized via CYP3A4, excreted via the biliary tract	Nephrotoxicity, hyperkalemia, diabetes mellitus, cardiovascular (prolonged QT interval, hypertension, cardiomegaly), hypomagnesemia, neurologic (headache, tremor, insomnia, paresthesia, encephalopathy, coma), GI upset, anemia, thrombocytopenia	
Sirolimus	Inhibits mTOR (suppresses T cells and production of antibodies and cytokines)	Hepatic metabolism via CYP3A4, elimination via the biliary tract and feces	Dyslipidemia, hypertension, fever, infection, pain, GI upset, anemia, thrombocytopenia, pancytopenia, DVT/PE, pulmonary toxicity	• Monitor blood levels periodically • Monitor lipid profile during therapy • Monitor blood pressure and renal function
Everolimus	Everolimus forms a complex with FK506- binding protein complex, thus causing mTOR inhibition	Metabolized via CYP3A4 in the liver, elimination via feces	Dyslipidemia, hypertension, fever, infection, pain, GI upset, anemia, thrombocytopenia, pancytopenia, DVT/PE	• Avoid perioperative use (wound healing can be suppressed) • Evaluate respiratory symptoms (rule out pulmonary toxicity)
Mycophenolate	Blocks de novo guanosine nucleotide synthesis (inhibits nucleic acid synthesis, which impairs T- and B-cell responses)	Metabolized extensively via liver, eliminated via the kidney	Diarrhea, bone marrow suppression, PML (black box warning)	• Periodically monitor CBC • Blood level can be measured to assist in evaluation of possible GI toxicity
Azathioprine	Purine antagonist; may inhibit DNA, RNA, and protein synthesis	Metabolized via systemic and hepatic routes: eliminated via systemic, hepatic, and renal pathways	Leukopenia, pancreatitis, hepatitis, bone marrow suppression	• Periodically monitor CBC and liver function • Avoid coadministration of allopurinol • Check for thiopurine methyltransferase deficiency (avoid use if deficient) • Start with low dose (50 mg/day) and escalate gradually

Note: CBC, complete blood count; CNS, central nervous system; CYP3A4, cytochrone-P450 3A4; GI, gastrointestinal; DVT, deep venous thrombosis; IL-2, interleukin-2; mTOR, mammalian target of rapamycin; PE, pulmonary embolism; PML, progressive multifocal leukoencephalopathy.

posttransplant medical complications in the outpatient setting should include a comprehensive patient interview with a complete medication history to ensure compliance with treatment regimens, measurement of vital signs (especially to detect systemic hypertension), a careful physical examination, and testing of peripheral blood as appropriate (e.g., determination of CNI and mTOR inhibitor levels, a complete blood count, measurement of electrolyte levels, assessment of renal function) (Table 35.3). Intermittent monitoring of bone marrow function via a complete blood count with differential should be performed at regular intervals. Suggested approaches to problems that are commonly encountered in the outpatient setting are presented in Table 35.4.

SUMMARY

All lung transplant recipients are at risk for the development of serious medical complications following a successful transplant. As the survival of lung transplant recipients gradually improves, medical complications related to long-term exposure to immunosuppressive and other drugs, as well as the aging process (in older patients), are increasingly likely to occur. Quality of life and survival may be improved significantly by appropriate monitoring and screening to facilitate early detection of medical complications and prompt intervention when such complications are detected. Therefore, lung transplant physicians and other medical personnel who evaluate and manage lung transplant recipients must be aware of the many potential medical complications that can occur following successful lung transplantation. Frequent communication between health care personnel (e.g., transplant coordinators) and transplant recipients is of key importance in identifying many of the aforementioned problems in timely fashion. Clinical evaluation of recipients and laboratory testing (according to comprehensive monitoring and screening protocols) performed at appropriate intervals may detect medical complications at early stages, when they may be more amenable to therapy and therefore less likely to progress and become serious, life-threatening, and possibly refractory to treatment interventions.

Table 35.3 Suggested posttransplant outpatient screening for lung transplant recipients

Potential problem or potential/ established complication	Type of screening	Frequency of testing[a]
Normal or mildly abnormal kidney function: KDOQI stages 1 (GFR, ≥90 mL/min) or 2 (GFR, 60 to 89 mL/min)[b]	• Cr, BUN, U/A • Spot protein/Cr ratio (urine)	Every 6 months
Abnormal kidney function: KDOQI stage 3 (GFR, 30 to 59 mL/min)[b]	• Cr, BUN, U/A • Spot protein/Cr ratio (urine)	Every 2 to 3 months
Abnormal kidney function: KDOQI stage 4 (GFR, 15 to 29 mL/min)[b]	• Cr, BUN, U/A • Spot protein/Cr ratio (urine)	Monthly
Electrolyte abnormality	• Serum electrolytes (especially potassium, magnesium) • Others (e.g., calcium) as needed	Every 2 months or as indicated (usually combined with kidney function assessment)
Bone marrow suppression	• CBC with platelets	Every 2 to 3 months
Hyperlipidemia	• Lipid panel	Every 6 months
Gastrointestinal function	• Symptom review • Hepatic function (alkaline phosphatase, AST, ALT, bilirubin)	Every 3 to 6 months
Glucose intolerance or diabetes	• Fasting blood glucose and HbA_{1c}	Every 6 months
Osteopenia or osteoporosis	• Bone mineral density scan	Every 1 to 2 years
Cataract formation	• Eye examination	6 months after transplantation, then yearly
Malignancy (dermatologic)	• Skin examination	Every 3 or 6 months
Malignancy (female reproductive tract and breast)	• Gynecologic evaluation and mammography	Per current/institutional guidelines
Malignancy (prostate)	• Urologic evaluation (e.g., PSA)	Per current published or institutional guidelines

Note: AST, aspartate transaminase; ALT, alanine transaminase; BUN, blood urea nitrogen; CBC, complete blood count; Cr, creatinine; GFR, glomerular filtration rate; HbA_{1c}, hemoglobin A_{1c}; KDOQI, Kidney Disease Outcomes Quality Initiative; PSA, prostate-specific antigen; U/A, urinalysis.

[a] Protocols for specific testing and the frequency with which they are obtained should be determined by individual centers; some recipients may require more intensive and/or frequent testing for specific situations.

[b] If abnormal or worsening, rule out drug effect (e.g., calcineurin inhibitor renal toxicity).

Table 35.4 Troubleshooting for frequently encountered problems

Problem	Evaluation
Fever, cough, dyspnea	• Vital signs, pulse oximetry • Comprehensive history • Careful physical examination • Routine posteroanterior and lateral chest radiographs (additional imaging if indicated) • Spirometry
Rising blood pressure, hypertension	• Assess renal function • Consider drug effect (e.g., tacrolimus)
Rising creatinine, blood urea nitrogen	• Assess hydration status • Obtain blood levels of CNIs and electrolytes (especially potassium) • Urinalysis, nephrology consultation if needed
Hyperkalemia	• Assess renal function • Check levels of CNIs and other electrolytes (magnesium)
Diarrhea	• Consider infection (e.g., *Clostridium difficile* colitis, cryptosporidiosis) • Consider drug effect (e.g., mycophenolate)
Anemia	• Consider medication effect (e.g., combined effect of CNIs plus cytotoxic agent) • Rule out gastrointestinal or other bleeding • Check iron stores
Neutropenia	• Consider drug toxicity (adjust medications as appropriate) • Consider infection as cause (e.g., cytomegalovirus infection)

Note: CNIs, calcineurin inhibitors.

REFERENCES

1. Meyer KC. Lung transplantation: Chronic complications and management. In Vigneswaran WT, Garrity ER Jr, eds. Lung Transplantation. London: Informa Healthcare; 2010:357-374.
2. Zbroch E, Małyszko J, Myśliwiec M, et al. Hypertension in solid organ transplant recipients. Ann Transplant 2012;17:100-107.
3. Barbari A. Posttransplant hypertension: Multipathogenic disease process. Exp Clin Transplant 2013;11:99-108.
4. Silverborn M, Jeppsson A, Martensson G, et al. New-onset cardiovascular risk factors in lung transplant recipients. J Heart Lung Transplant 2005;24:1536-1543.
5. Yusen RD, Christie JD, Edwards LB, et al. International Society for Heart and Lung Transplantation. The Registry of the International Society for Heart and Lung Transplantation: Thirtieth adult lung and heart-lung transplant report—2013; focus theme: Age. J Heart Lung Transplant 2013;13:965-978.
6. Johnson BA, Iacono AT, Zeevi A, et al. Statin use is associated with improved function and survival of lung allografts. Am J Respir Crit Care Med 2003;167:1271-1278.
7. Henri C, Giraldeau G, Dorais M, et al. Atrial fibrillation after pulmonary transplantation: Incidence, impact on mortality, treatment effectiveness, and risk factors. Circ Arrhythm Electrophysiol 2012;5:61-67.
8. Azadani PN, Kumar UN, Yang Y, et al. Frequency of atrial flutter after adult lung transplantation. Am J Cardiol 2011;107:922-926.
9. Isiadinso I, Meshkov AB, Gaughan J, et al. Atrial arrhythmias after lung and heart-lung transplant. Effects on short-term mortality and the influence of amiodarone. J Heart Lung Transplant 2011;30:37-44.
10. Orrego CM, Cordero-Reyes AM, Estep JD, et al. Atrial arrhythmias after lung transplant: Underlying mechanisms, risk factors, and prognosis. J Heart Lung Transplant 2014;33:734-740.
11. Kroshus TJ, Kshettry VR, Hertz MI, Bolman RM 3rd. Deep venous thrombosis and pulmonary embolism after lung transplantation. J Thorac Cardiovasc Surg 1995;110:540-544.
12. Kahan ES, Petersen G, Gaughan JP, Criner GJ. High incidence of venous thromboembolic events in lung transplant recipients. J Heart Lung Transplant 2007;26:339-344.
13. Izbicki G, Bairey O, Shitrit D, et al. Increased thromboembolic events after lung transplantation. Chest 2006;129:412-416.
14. Yegen HA, Lederer DJ, Barr RG, et al. Risk factors for venous thromboembolism after lung transplantation. Chest 2007;132:547-553.

15. Burns KE, Iacono AT. Pulmonary embolism on postmortem examination: An underrecognized complication in lung transplant recipients? Transplantation 2004;77:692-698.

16. Krivokuca I, van de Graaf EA, van Kessel DA, et al. Pulmonary embolism and pulmonary infarction after lung transplantation. Clin Appl Thromb Hemost 2011;17:421-424.

17. Schulman LL, Anandarangam T, Leibowitz DW, et al. Four-year prospective study of pulmonary venous thrombosis after lung transplantation. J Am Soc Echocardiogr 2001;14:806-812.

18. Choong CK, Meyers BF, Guthrie TJ, et al. Does the presence of preoperative mild or moderate coronary artery disease affect the outcomes of lung transplantation? Ann Thorac Surg 2006;82:1038-1042.

19. Zanotti G, Hartwig MG, Castleberry AW, et al. Preoperative mild-to-moderate coronary artery disease does not affect long-term outcomes of lung transplantation. Transplantation 2014;97:1079-1085.

20. Jones RM, Enfield KB, Mehrad B, Keeley EC. Prevalence of obstructive coronary artery disease in patients undergoing lung transplantation: Case series and review of the literature. Catheter Cardiovasc Interv 2014;84:1-6.

21. Nathan SD, Basavaraj A, Reichner C, et al. Prevalence and impact of coronary artery disease in idiopathic pulmonary fibrosis. Respir Med 2010;104:1035-1041.

22. Izbicki G, Ben-Dor I, Shitrit D, et al. The prevalence of coronary artery disease in end-stage pulmonary disease: Is pulmonary fibrosis a risk factor? Respir Med 2009;103:1346-1349.

23. Bloom RD, Reese PP. Chronic kidney disease after nonrenal solid-organ transplantation. J Am Soc Nephrol 2007;18:3031-3041.

24. Wehbe E, Duncan AE, Dar G, et al. Recovery from AKI and short-and long-term outcomes after lung transplantation. Clin J Am Soc Nephrol 2013;8:19-25.

25. Jacques F, El-Hamamsy I, Fortier A, et al. Acute renal failure following lung transplantation: Risk factors, mortality, and long-term consequences. Eur J Cardiothorac Surg 2012;41:193-199.

26. Pham PT, Slavov C, Pham PC. Acute kidney injury after liver, heart, and lung transplants: Dialysis modality, predictors of renal function recovery, and impact on survival. Adv Chronic Kidney Dis 2009;16:256-267.

27. Esposito C, De Mauri A, Vitulo P, et al. Risk factors for chronic renal dysfunction in lung transplant recipients. Transplantation 2007;84:1701-1703.

28. Mason DP, Solovera-Rozas M, Feng J, et al. Dialysis after lung transplantation: Prevalence, risk factors and outcome. J Heart Lung Transplant 2007;26:1155-1162.

29. Wehbe E, Brock R, Budev M, et al. Short-term and long-term outcomes of acute kidney injury after lung transplantation. J Heart Lung Transplant 2012;31:244-251.

30. Rocha PN, Rocha AT, Palmer SM, et al. Acute renal failure after lung transplantation: Incidence, predictors and impact on perioperative morbidity and mortality. Am J Transplant 2005;5:1469-1476.

31. Canales M, Youssef P, Spong R, et al. Predictors of chronic kidney disease in long-term survivors of lung and heart-lung transplantation. Am J Transplant 2006;6:2157-2163.

32. Robinson PD, Shroff RC, Spencer H. Renal complications following lung and heart-lung transplantation. Pediatr Nephrol 2013;28:375-386.

33. KDOQI clinical practice guidelines and clinical practice recommendations for diabetes and chronic kidney disease. Am J Kidney Dis 2007;49:S12-S154.

34. Ojo AO, Held PJ, Port FK, et al. Chronic renal failure after transplantation of a nonrenal organ. N Engl J Med 2003;349:931-940.

35. Bloom RD, Doyle AM. Kidney disease after heart and lung transplantation. Am J Transplant 2006;6:671-679.

36. D'Ovidio F, Singer LG, Hadjiliadis D, et al. Prevalence of gastroesophageal reflux in end-stage lung disease candidates for lung transplant. Ann Thorac Surg 2005;80:1254-1261.

37. Button BM, Roberts S, Kotsimbos TC, et al. Gastroesophageal reflux (symptomatic and silent): A potentially significant problem in patients with cystic fibrosis before and after lung transplantation. J Heart Lung Transplant 2005;24:1522-1529.

38. Linden PA, Gilbert RJ, Yeap BY, et al. Laparoscopic fundoplication in patients with end-stage lung disease awaiting transplantation. J Thorac Cardiovasc Surg 2006;131:438-446.

39. Sweet MP, Herbella FA, Leard L, et al. The prevalence of distal and proximal gastroesophageal reflux in patients awaiting lung transplantation. Ann Surg 2006;244:491-497.

40. Sweet MP, Patti MG, Leard LE, et al. Gastroesophageal reflux in patients with idiopathic pulmonary fibrosis referred for lung transplantation. J Thorac Cardiovasc Surg 2007;133:1078-1084.

41. Gasper WJ, Sweet MP, Hoopes C, et al. Antireflux surgery for patients with end-stage lung disease before and after lung transplantation. Surg Endosc 2008;22:495-500.

42. Fortunato GA, Machado MM, Andrade CF, et al. Prevalence of gastroesophageal reflux in lung transplant candidates with advanced lung disease. J Bras Pneumol 2008;34:772-778.

43. Blondeau K, Dupont LJ, Mertens V, et al. Gastro-oesophageal reflux and aspiration of gastric contents in adult patients with cystic fibrosis. Gut 2008;57:1049-1055.

44. Sweet MP, Patti MG, Hoopes C, et al. Gastro-oesophageal reflux and aspiration in patients with advanced lung disease. Thorax 2009;64:167-173.

45. Blondeau K, Pauwels A, Dupont L, et al. Characteristics of gastroesophageal reflux and potential risk of gastric content aspiration in children with cystic fibrosis. J Pediatr Gastroenterol Nutr 2010;50:161-166.

46. Hoppo T, Jarido V, Pennathur A, et al. Antireflux surgery preserves lung function in patients with gastroesophageal reflux disease and end-stage lung disease before and after lung transplantation. Arch Surg 2011;146:1041-1047.

47. Meyer KC, Maloney JD. Gastroesophageal reflux in lung transplantation. In Meyer KC, Raghu G, eds. Gastroesophageal Reflux and the Lung. New York: Humana Press; 2012.

48. Hadjiliadis D, Duane Davis R, Steele MP, et al. Gastroesophageal reflux disease in lung transplant recipients. Clin Transplant 2003;17:363-368.

49. Davis RD Jr, Lau CL, Eubanks S, et al. Improved lung allograft function after fundoplication in patients with gastroesophageal reflux disease undergoing lung transplantation. J Thorac Cardiovasc Surg 2003;125:533-542.

50. D'Ovidio F, Mura M, Tsang M, et al. Bile acid aspiration and the development of bronchiolitis obliterans after lung transplantation. J Thorac Cardiovasc Surg 2005;129:1144-1152.

51. Robertson AG, Ward C, Pearson JP, et al. Longitudinal changes in gastro-oesophageal reflux from 3 months to 6 months after lung transplantation. Thorax 2009;64:1005-1007.

52. King BJ, Iyer H, Leidi AA, Carby MR. Gastroesophageal reflux in bronchiolitis obliterans syndrome: A new perspective. J Heart Lung Transplant 2009;28:870-875.

53. Davis CS, Shankaran V, Kovacs EJ, et al. Gastroesophageal reflux disease after lung transplantation: Pathophysiology and implications for treatment. Surgery 2010;148:737-744.

54. Blondeau K, Mertens V, Vanaudenaerde BA, et al. Gastro-oesophageal reflux and gastric aspiration in lung transplant patients with or without chronic rejection. Eur Respir J 2008;31:707-713.

55. Young LR, Hadjiliadis D, Davis RD, Palmer SM. Lung transplantation exacerbates gastroesophageal reflux disease. Chest 2003;124:1689-1693.

56. Halsey KD, Wald A, Meyer KC, et al. Non-acidic supraesophageal reflux associated with diffuse alveolar damage and allograft dysfunction after lung transplantation: A case report. J Heart Lung Transplant 2008;27:564-567.

57. Shah N, Force SD, Mitchell PO, et al. Gastroesophageal reflux disease is associated with an increased rate of acute rejection in lung transplant allografts. Transplant Proc 2010;42:2702-2706.

58. Molina EJ, Short S, Monteiro G, et al. Symptomatic gastroesophageal reflux disease after lung transplantation. Gen Thorac Cardiovasc Surg 2009;57:647-653.

59. Blondeau K, Mertens V, Vanaudenaerde BA, et al. Nocturnal weakly acidic reflux promotes aspiration of bile acids in lung transplant recipients. J Heart Lung Transplant 2009;28:141-148.

60. Vos R, Blondeau K, Vanaudenaerde BM, et al. Airway colonization and gastric aspiration after lung transplantation: Do birds of a feather flock together? J Heart Lung Transplant 2008;27:843-849.

61. Bobadilla JL, Jankowska-Gan E, Xu Q, et al. Reflux-induced collagen type V sensitization: Potential mediator of bronchiolitis obliterans syndrome. Chest 2010;138:363-370.

62. Burlingham WJ, Love RB, Jankowska-Gan E, et al. IL-17–dependent cellular immunity to collagen type V predisposes to obliterative bronchiolitis in human lung transplants. J Clin Invest 2007;117:3498-3506.

63. Reder NP, Davis CS, Kovacs EJ, Fisichella PM. The diagnostic value of gastroesophageal reflux disease (GERD) symptoms and detection of pepsin and bile acids in bronchoalveolar lavage fluid and exhaled breath condensate for identifying lung transplantation patients with GERD-induced aspiration. Surg Endosc 2014;28:1794-1800.

64. Marie I, Dominique S, Levesque H, et al. Esophageal involvement and pulmonary manifestations in systemic sclerosis. Arthritis Rheum 2001;45:346-354.

65. Patti MG, Debas HT, Pellegrini CA. Esophageal manometry and 24-hour pH monitoring in the diagnosis of pulmonary aspiration secondary to gastroesophageal reflux. Am J Surg 1992;163:401-406.

66. Savarino E, Bazzica M, Zentilin P, et al. Gastroesophageal reflux and pulmonary fibrosis in scleroderma. A study using pH-impedance monitoring. Am J Respir Crit Care Med 2009;179:408-413.

67. Fisichella PM, Jalilvand A. The role of impaired esophageal and gastric motility in end-stage lung diseases and after lung transplantation. J Surg Res 2014;186:201-206.

68. Gasper WJ, Sweet MP, Golden JA, et al. Lung transplantation in patients with connective tissue disorders and esophageal dysmotility. Dis Esophagus 2008;21:650-655.

69. Cantu E 3rd, Appel JZ 3rd, Hartwig MG, et al. Maxwell Chamberlain Memorial Paper. Early fundoplication prevents chronic allograft dysfunction in patients with gastroesophageal reflux disease. Ann Thorac Surg 2004;78:1142-1151.

70. Gautam A. Gastrointestinal complications following transplantation. Surg Clin North Am 2006;86:1195-1206.

71. Lee JT, Kelly RF, Hertz MI, et al. Clostridium difficile infection increases mortality risk in lung transplant recipients. J Heart Lung Transplant 2013;32:1020-1026.

72. Egressy K, Jansen M, Meyer KC. Recurrent Clostridium difficile colitis in cystic fibrosis: An emerging problem. J Cyst Fibros 2013;12:92-96.

73. Meyer KC, Francois ML, Thomas HK, et al. Colon cancer in lung transplant recipients with CF: Increased risk and results of screening. J Cyst Fibros 2011;10:366-369.

74. Modrykamien A. Anemia post-lung transplantation: Mechanisms and approach to diagnosis. Chron Respir Dis 2010;7:29-34.

75. Trulock EP, Christie JD, Edwards LB, et al. Registry of the International Society for Heart and Lung Transplantation: Twenty-fourth official adult lung and heart-lung transplantation report—2007. J Heart Lung Transplant 2007;26:782-795.

76. Ollech JE, Kramer MR, Peled N, et al. Post-transplant diabetes mellitus in lung transplant recipients: Incidence and risk factors. Eur J Cardiothorac Surg 2008;33:844-848.

77. Wilkinson A, Davidson J, Dotta F, et al. Guidelines for the treatment and management of new-onset diabetes after transplantation. Clin Transplant 2005;19:291-298.

78. Barry JM. Treating erectile dysfunction in renal transplant recipients. Drugs 2007;67:975-983.

79. Heneghan MA, Selzner M, Yoshida EM, et al. Pregnancy and sexual function in liver transplantation. J Hepatobil 2008;49:507-519.

80. Stein E, Shane E. Secondary osteoporosis. Endocrinol Metab Clin N Am 2003;32:115-134.

81. Hoppé E, Bouvard B, Royer M, et al. Is androgen therapy indicated in men with osteoporosis? Joint Bone Spine 2013;80:459-465.

82. Rozenberg S, Vandromme J, Antoine C. Postmenopausal hormone therapy: Risks and benefits. Nat Rev Endocrinol 2013;9:216-227.

83. Gluck O, Colice G. Recognizing and treating glucocorticoid-induced osteoporosis in patients with pulmonary disease. Chest 2004:125:1859-1876.

84. Caplan-Shaw CE, Arcasoy SM, Shane E, et al. Osteoporosis in diffuse parenchymal lung disease. Chest 2006;129:140-146.

85. Stephenson A, Jamal S, Dowdell T, et al. Prevalence of vertebral fractures in adults with cystic fibrosis and their relationship to bone mineral density. Chest 2006;130:539-544.

86. Aris RM, Neuringer IP, Weiner MA, et al. Severe osteoporosis before and after lung transplantation. Chest 1996;109:1176-1183.

87. Maurer JR. Metabolic bone disease in lung transplant recipients. In Lynch JP III, Ross DJ, eds. Lung and Heart-Lung Transplantation. New York: Taylor & Francis Group, 2006.

88. Maalouf NM, Shane E. Osteoporosis after solid organ transplantation. J Clin Endocrinol Metab 2005;90:2456-2465.

89. Kulak CA, Cochenski Borba VZ, Kulak J, Ribeiro Custódio M. Osteoporosis after solid organ transplantation. Minerva Endocrinol 2012;37:221-231.

90. Cohen A, Shane E. Osteoporosis after solid organ and bone marrow transplantation. Osteoporos Int 2003;14:617-630.

91. Spira A, Gutierrez C, Chaparro C, et al. Osteoporosis and lung transplantation: A prospective study. Chest 2000;117:476-481.

92. Julian BA, Laskow DA, Dubovsky J, et al. Rapid loss of vertebral mineral density after renal transplantation. N Engl J Med 1991;325:544-550.

93. Cahill BC, O'Rourke MK, Parker S, et al. Prevention of bone loss and fracture after lung transplantation: A pilot study. Transplantation 2001;72:1251-1255.

94. Braith RW, Conner JA, Fulton MN, et al. Comparison of alendronate vs alendronate plus mechanical loading as prophylaxis for osteoporosis in lung transplant recipients: A pilot study. J Heart Lung Transplant 2007;26:132-137.

95. Isoniemi H, Appelberg J, Nilsson CG, et al. Transdermal oestrogen therapy protects postmenopausal liver transplant women from osteoporosis. A 2-year follow-up study. J Hepatol 2001;34:299-305.

96. Stempfle HU, Werner C, Echtler S, et al. Prevention of osteoporosis after cardiac transplantation: A prospective, longitudinal, randomized, double-blind trial with calcitriol. Transplantation 1999;68:523-530.

97. Ferrari SL, Nicod LP, Hamacher J, et al. Osteoporosis in patients undergoing lung transplantation. Eur Respir J 1996;9:2378-2382.

98. Shane E, Papadopoulos A, Staron RB, et al. Bone loss and fracture after lung transplantation. Transplantation 1999;68:220-227.

99. Henderson K, Eisman J, Keogh A, et al. Protective effect of short-term calcitriol or cyclical etidronate on bone loss after cardiac or lung transplantation. J Bone Miner Res 2001;16:565-571.

100. Trombetti A, Gerbase MW, Spiliopoulos A, et al. Bone mineral density in lung-transplant recipients before and after graft: Prevention of lumbar spine post-transplantation-accelerated bone loss by pamidronate. J Heart Lung Transplant 2000;19:736-743.

101. Chauhan V, Ranganna KM, Chauhan N, et al. Bone disease in organ transplant patients: Pathogenesis and management. Postgrad Med 2012;124:80-90.

102. Meyer K. Management of interstitial lung disease in elderly patients. Curr Opin Pulm Med 2012;18:483-492.

103. Hook JL, Lederer DJ. Selecting lung transplant candidates: Where do current guidelines fall short? Expert Rev Respir Med 2012;6:51-61.

104. Goldstein LS, Haug MT 3rd, Perl J 2nd, et al. Central nervous system complications after lung transplantation. J Heart Lung Transplant 1998;17:185-191.

105. Zivković SA, Jumaa M, Barisić N, McCurry K. Neurologic complications following lung transplantation. J Neurol Sci 2009;280:90-93.

106. Mateen FJ, Dierkhising RA, Rabinstein AA, et al. Neurological complications following adult lung transplantation. Am J Transplant 2010;10:908-914.

107. Shigemura N, Sclabassi RJ, Bhama JK, et al. Early major neurologic complications after lung transplantation: Incidence, risk factors, and outcome. Transplantation 2013;95:866-871.

108. Barbour KA, Blumenthal JA, Palmer SM. Psychosocial issues in the assessment and management of patients undergoing lung transplantation. Chest 2006;129:1367-1374.

109. Dobbels F, Verleden G, Dupont L, et al. To transplant or not? The importance of psychosocial and behavioural factors before lung transplantation. Chron Respir Dis 2006;3:39-47.

110. Myaskovsky L, Dew MA, Switzer GE, et al. Avoidant coping with health problems is related to poorer quality of life among lung transplant candidates. Prog Transplant 2003;13:183-192.

111. Fusar-Poli, Lazzaretti M, Ceruti M, et al. Depression after lung transplantation: Causes and treatment. Lung 2007;185:55-65.

112. Dew MA, DiMartini AF. Psychological disorders and distress after adult cardiothoracic transplantation. J Cardiovasc Nurs 2005;20:S51-S66.

113. Goetzmann L, Ruegg L, Stamm M, et al. Psychosocial profiles after transplantation: A 24-month follow-up of heart, lung, liver, kidney and allogeneic bone-marrow patients. Transplantation 2008;86:662-668.

114. De Geest S, Dobbels F, Fluri C, et al. Adherence to the therapeutic regimen in heart, lung, and heart-lung transplant recipients. J Cardiovasc Nurs 2005;20:S88-S98.

115. Buell JF, Gross TG, Woodle ES. Malignancy after transplantation. Transplantation 2005;80(Suppl 2):S254-S264.

116. Amital A, Shitrit D, Raviv Y, et al. Development of malignancy following lung transplantation. Transplantation 2006;81:547-551.

117. Zafar SY, Howell DN, Gockerman JP. Malignancy after solid organ transplantation: An overview. Oncologist 2008;13:769-778.

118. Metcalfe MJ, Kutsogiannis DJ, Jackson K, et al. Risk factors and outcomes for the development of malignancy in lung and heart-lung transplant recipients. Can Respir J 2010;17:e7-e13.

119. Penn I. Post-transplant malignancy: The role of immunosuppression. Drug Saf 2000;23:101-113.

120. Wimmer CD, Angele MK, Schwarz B, et al. Impact of cyclosporine versus tacrolimus on the incidence of de novo malignancy following liver transplantation: A single center experience with 609 patients. Transpl Int 2013;26:999-1006.

121. Al-Mansour Z, Nelson BP, Evens AM. Post-transplant lymphoproliferative disease (PTLD): Risk factors, diagnosis, and current treatment strategies. Curr Hematol Malig Rep 2013;8:173-183.

122. Kremer BE, Reshef R, Misleh JG, et al. Post-transplant lymphoproliferative disorder after lung transplantation: A review of 35 cases. J Heart Lung Transplant 2012;31:296-304.

123. Wheless SA, Gulley ML, Raab-Traub N, et al. Post-transplantation lymphoproliferative disease: Epstein-Barr virus DNA levels, HLA-A3, and survival. Am J Respir Crit Care Med 2008;178:1060-1065.

124. Baldanti F, Rognoni V, Cascina A, et al. Post-transplant lymphoproliferative disorders and Epstein-Barr virus DNAemia in a cohort of lung transplant recipients. Virol J 2011;8:421.

125. Nourse JP, Jones K, Gandhi MK. Epstein-Barr virus–related post-transplant lymphoproliferative disorders: Pathogenetic insights for targeted therapy. Am J Transplant 2011;11:888-895.

126. Saueressig MG, Boussaud V, Amrein C, et al. Risk factors for post-transplant lymphoproliferative disease in patients with cystic fibrosis. Clin Transplant 2011;25:E430-E436.

127. Jagadeesh D, Woda BA, Draper J, Evens AM. Post transplant lymphoproliferative disorders: Risk, classification, and therapeutic recommendations. Curr Treat Options Oncol 2012;13:122-136.

128. Zimmermann H, Trappe RU. Therapeutic options in post-transplant lymphoproliferative disorders. Ther Adv Hematol 2011;2:393-407.

129. Knoop C, Kentos A, Remmelink M, et al. Post-transplant lymphoproliferative disorders after lung transplantation: First-line treatment with rituximab may induce complete remission. Clin Transplant 2006;20:179-187.

130. Johnson SR, Cherikh WS, Kauffman HM, et al. Retransplantation after post-transplant lymphoproliferative disorders: An OPTN/UNOS database analysis. Am J Transplant 2006;6:2743-2749.

131. Belli EV, Landolfo K, Keller C, et al. Lung cancer following lung transplant: Single institution 10 year experience. Lung Cancer 2013;81:451-454.

132. Meyer KC, Francois ML, Thomas HK, et al. Colon cancer in lung transplant recipients with CF: Increased risk and results of screening. J Cyst Fibros 2011;10:366-369.

133. Billings JL, Dunitz JM, McAllister S, et al. Early colon screening of adult patients with cystic fibrosis reveals high incidence of adenomatous colon polyps. J Clin Gastroenterol 2014;48:85-88.

134. Maisonneuve P, Marshall BC, Knapp EA, Lowenfels AB. Cancer risk in cystic fibrosis: A 20-year nationwide study from the United States. J Natl Cancer Inst 2013;105:122-129.

135. Meyer KC, Decker C, Baughman R. Toxicity and monitoring of immunosuppressive therapy used in systemic autoimmune diseases. Clin Chest Med 2010;31:565-588.

136. Baughman RP, Meyer KC, Nathanson I, et al. Executive summary: Monitoring of nonsteroidal immunosuppressive drugs in patients with lung disease and lung transplant recipients: American College of Chest Physicians evidence-based clinical practice guidelines. Chest 2012;142:1284-1288.

137. Naraine VS, Bradley TD, Singer LG. Prevalence of sleep disordered breathing in lung transplant recipients. J Clin Sleep Med 2009;5:441-447.

138. Malouf MA, Milrose MA, Grunstein RR, et al. Sleep-disordered breathing before and after lung transplantation. J Heart Lung Transplant 2008;27:540-546.

139. Shepherd KL, Chambers DC, Gabbay E, et al. Obstructive sleep apnoea and nocturnal gastroesophageal reflux are common in lung transplant patients. Respirology 2008;13:1045-1052.

36

Malignancy following lung transplantation

KATHERINE M. VANDERVEST AND MARTIN R. ZAMORA

INTRODUCTION

Evidence of an increased risk for malignancy in recipients of solid-organ transplants has been well established. Multiple large population-based studies have suggested that the incidence of de novo development of cancer in transplant recipients is at least twice that in the general population,[1,2] and a meta-analysis of five retrospective investigations reported a threefold higher cancer risk in transplant recipients.[3] Despite the current recognition that along with chronic rejection, neoplastic disease is a leading cause of late transplant mortality,[4] the compendium of interrelated factors linked to malignant transformation remains incompletely understood. Data on cancer prevalence in the setting of transplantation are limited because of heterogeneity among investigations, small study cohorts, registries' dependence on voluntary reporting, and limited duration or follow-up. Analyses also support the existence of some variance in tumor type according to the organ transplanted.[1,4]

Although the evidence on lung and heart-lung allograft recipients is more limited than that on individuals with other solid-organ implants, thoracic organ recipients have been shown to have the highest relative risk for malignancy in the postoperative period.[2,4] To date, four national population-based studies have included a cohort of lung allograft recipients. A Swedish study reviewed 117 lung transplant recipients and reported an increased risk for non-Hodgkin lymphoma (NHL) in allografts other than kidneys.[5] Lung or heart-lung transplant recipients accounted for 5% of a U.K. cohort in which the rates of malignancy by type of organ transplanted were compared. The overall risk for cancer was greatest for lung transplant recipients, with nonmelanoma

skin cancer (NMSC) being the most common type. NHL was also found to occur at a higher rate in recipients of cardiothoracic transplants.[2] The spectrum of cancer risk was further examined in recipients of solid-organ transplants in the United States from 1987 through 2008. As in the U.K. study, the standardized incidence ratio (SIR) for cancer in the U.S. study was highest in lung transplant recipients (SIR = 6.13; 95% confidence interval = 5.18 to 7.21) despite the small percentage of lung patients included in the study.[1] The only investigation to include lung and heart-lung transplant cases exclusively was a single-institution experience from Australia. Its authors reported a sevenfold higher risk for malignancy in cardiothoracic transplant recipients, with lymphoproliferative, head and neck, and lung cancer comprising the most common diagnoses.[6]

This chapter discusses the malignancies encountered most frequently in lung and heart-lung transplant recipients and the effect of immunosuppression on cancer development. Risk factors for carcinoma are also addressed. Finally, we highlight potential strategies for prevention and treatment of cancer.

EFFECTS OF IMMUNOSUPPRESSANT THERAPY ON MALIGNANCY

The risk for malignancy secondary to immunosuppressant therapy after lung transplantation remains an area of controversy. Although the increased incidence of cancer since the 1950s has generally coincided with the evolution of immunosuppressant medications, the data supporting an increased risk for cancer specific to any one immunosuppressant drug are equivocal. The calcineurin inhibitors (CNIs) cyclosporine

(CYA) and tacrolimus (TAC) prevent T-cell–dependent immune responses, including the generation of Epstein-Barr virus (EBV)-specific cytotoxic T lymphocytes. Limiting T-cell response and leaving B-cell proliferation unregulated may be correlated with an increased rate of posttransplant lympho-proliferative disorder (PTLD) in lung transplant recipients. Israel Penn noted that the rate of lymphoma development in transplant recipients receiving CYA-based regimens was 15% higher than in those receiving maintenance care with azathioprine (AZA) or cyclophosphamide.[7] However, this increased risk associated with CYA was later attributed to concomitant risk factors.[8] Other current series also do not corroborate a higher risk for lymphoma with CYA than with other immunosuppressant drugs.[9-11] A review of the Australia and New Zealand Dialysis and Transplant Registry showed no difference in the rate of development before and after the introduction of CYA.[9] Even less evidence on the potential risk for the development of PTLD associated with taking TAC is available; the strongest connection between it and risk for malignancy occurs in pediatric transplant recipients.[10,12,13] The increasing implementation of multidrug treatment programs may also place solid-organ transplant recipients at greater risk for PTLD. An analysis of the large Collaborative Transplant Study database reported a 1.5-fold higher relative risk for PTLD during the first year after a transplant when triple-drug therapy is used than when AZA or CYA is administered alone.[11] Higher rates of occurrence of lymphoma have also been observed in non–renal transplant recipients, who are generally treated with more potent immunosuppressant regimens.

Treatment with the leukocyte-reducing monoclonal antibody OKT3 and polyclonal antithymocyte globulin has been shown to be correlated with a significant risk for the development of PTLD.[10,11,14,15] Use of these biologic agents for induction or antirejection therapy, particularly above a threshold aggregate dose, has been associated with higher risk for lymphoma during the first year after transplantation. The same relationship does not hold true for the anti-CD25 monoclonal antibody basiliximab, which inhibits interleukin-2 (IL-2) receptors.[10,14]

The risk for PTLD may actually be decreased with use of the antimetabolite mycophenolate mofetil (MMF). A study by Cherikh and colleagues reported a significantly lower risk for PTLD and graft loss with MMF maintenance immunosuppression than with AZA.[14] However, multiple studies in renal transplant recipients[13] and one investigation in heart transplant recipients[16] revealed no difference in the incidence of early-onset PTLD in patients receiving MMF. The potential for a lower rate of occurrence of PTLD with MMF may be due to its inhibitory effects on B-cell proliferation.

A connection between specific immunosuppressant therapy and increased risk for skin cancer after transplantation has not been strongly established. Although it has been suggested that AZA and CYA may play a role in cutaneous carcinogenesis, clear-cut evidence of an elevated risk for NMSC has not been proved. A study of NMSC in renal transplant recipients indicated that the incidence of malignancy at 3 months did not differ between those receiving AZA and those receiving MMF or between those taking CYA and those taking TAC.[2] Other investigations have reported more convincing data supporting a correlation between skin cancer and overall aggressiveness of the immunosuppressive regimen. A retrospective study by Glover and coworkers reported that the use of three- versus two-drug immunosuppressive therapy raised the incidence of NMSC from 29 to 48 cases per 1000 person-years.[17] Antifungal medications administered in conjunction with more powerful immunosuppressant therapy have also been associated with the development of NMSC. Multiple investigations in lung transplant recipients have demonstrated a statistically significant elevated risk for squamous cell skin cancer with prolonged use of voriconazole.[18,19]

A category of immunosuppressive medications that may actually have antineoplastic effects in solid-organ transplant recipients is the mammalian target of rapamycin (mTOR) inhibitors. Their protective effects were supported by a large meta-analysis of the United Network for Organ Sharing (UNOS) database, which concluded that the use of mTOR inhibitors such as sirolimus (SRL) may reduce the occurrence of malignancy, particularly skin cancer.[3] Complete regression of Kaposi sarcoma (KS) in transplant recipients who have been transitioned to SRL from CNI-based therapy has also been described in multiple case reports.[20,21] Yakupoglu and associates additionally reported a lower rate of skin tumors in kidney transplant recipients receiving SRL and CYA with or without prednisone than in those receiving CYA and AZA with or without prednisone therapy. The same study found that the incidence of PTLD was more than 50% lower in patients treated with SRL and CYA plus prednisone than in those receiving a combination of TAC and MMF.[22] The mechanism of cancer prevention by mTOR inhibitors is believed to be multifactorial. Such agents block tumor angiogenesis by diminishing transforming growth factor β and vascular endothelial growth factor signal transduction. SRL has also been shown to induce cellular apoptosis independent of p53 and can enhance E-cadherin contact-dependent interactions, thereby impeding metastatic progression.[22] Furthermore, mTOR inhibitors can disrupt the intracellular signaling pathways that are vital for malignant transformation and cellular proliferation.[23]

ONCOGENIC VIRUSES

Many types of cancer that occur with greater frequency in solid-organ transplant populations have been shown to have a viral etiology. Malignancies linked to viral infections include PTLD; NHL; Hodgkin disease; KS; cervical cancer; cancer of the vulva, vagina, penis and anus; cancer of the oral cavity and oropharynx; and liver cancer. All human oncogenic viruses have the ability to establish persistent latent infections in their host. When the balance of immune control is altered following organ transplantation, viral replication and expansion of infected cells become unregulated, thus leading to malignant conversion. One of the strongest connections between tumor viruses and immunodeficiency-associated cancer occurs between EBV and PTLD.[1,4,8,10,13,24,25] Although many studies report that EBV proteins are present in most tissue affected by PTLD, the specific role of EBV in the pathogenesis of PTLD remains unclear. In vivo, EBV-infected B cells can adopt four different latency patterns that are defined by the differential expression of several proteins, including EBV nuclear antigens, EBV-encoded RNA, and latent membrane proteins. In PTLD, EBV typically exhibits type III latency, which involves six EBV nuclear antigens, two EBV-encoded RNAs, and three latent membrane proteins.[25,26] In immunocompetent individuals, type III latency proteins are targeted by cytotoxic T lymphocytes, which proficiently eliminate B-cell immortalization by the virus. However, in immunosuppressed transplant recipients, the EBV latency proteins are left unchecked and can drive the development of polyclonal B-cell proliferation. In addition to promoting the disruption of B- and T-cell balance by immunosuppressant medications, EBV proteins can also stimulate several immunoregulatory cytokines. The cytokine IL-10, which is often present in serum of patients with PTLD, can prevent T-cell recognition of EBV-infected B cells through suppression of HLA class II antigen presentation.[25] It also blocks cytotoxic T-cell stimulation by inhibition of IL-2 production. Through continued unopposed B-cell growth, polyclonal proliferation can progress to monoclonal lymphoma. Because T-cell inhibition clearly plays a role in the occurrence of PTLD, therapies focused on T cell augmentation, including an overall reduction in immunosuppression and adoptive transfer of autologous EBV-specific cytotoxic T cells, may be efficacious in the management of PTLD.

Cytomegalovirus (CMV) is also believed to play a role in the development of PTLD. Lung transplant recipients with a mismatched CMV status have been shown to be at increased risk for PTLD.[27] CMV may act indirectly in the development of PTLD by preventing stimulation of the tumor suppressor gene p53.[28,29] Active CMV disease also increases the probability of rejection, which requires intensification of immunosuppression and diminished activity of cytotoxic T cells. Thus, antiviral medications (acyclovir and ganciclovir) may be useful in the treatment of PTLD by preventing or eliminating CMV.

Another virus with oncogenic potential is human herpesvirus 8 (HHV-8). Its connection to KS was confirmed in 1994,[30] and data from numerous cohort and case-control studies have since validated this association.[26] HHV-8 induces tumor development through transformation of endothelial cells. The virus modifies the expression of the transcription factor Prox-1, podoplanin, and vascular endothelial growth factor receptor 3, thereby leading to extended survival, growth factor independence, and loss of contact inhibition in endothelial cells.[31] Multiple viral proteins have also been reported to have tumorigenic capability, but the exact role of these proteins in the establishment of KS remains undetermined. HHV-8 is present in infected tissue and can also be seen in normal skin from patients with KS. Detection of the virus, as well as anti–HHV-8 antibody titers in peripheral blood, may be correlated with stage and progression of the cancer.[26,32]

Scientific evidence has also supported a relationship between human papillomavirus (HPV) and anogenital and oropharyngeal cancer. Malignancies of the anogenital region account for 2.8% of cancer in transplant recipients, in whom the incidence of such cancer is 30 to 100 times greater than in the general population.[30,33] The risk is higher in women and the mean interval between transplantation and diagnosis is 7 years.[30] Several HPV subtypes have oncogenic potential, but HPV-16 carries the most risk for cancer. Studies have suggested that a significant part of HPV's tumor-inducing capability is due to the viral proteins E6 and E7. The protein E6 promotes cancer growth by mediating degradation of the tumor suppressor gene p53 and thus inhibiting p53-dependent and p53-independent apoptosis.[26] E7 targets the retinoblastoma tumor suppressor protein, which assists in regulation of the cell cycle. Silencing of both these tumor suppressor components can also impede normal DNA repair and thereby lead to genetic mutations in HPV-infected cells and a heightened chance of malignant transformation.[26,34]

POSTTRANSPLANT LYMPHOPROLIFERATIVE DISORDER

PTLD was first described in renal transplant recipients in 1968.[35] The advent of modern immunosuppressant therapy has been correlated with an increase in the incidence of these malignancies during the past few decades. Recent population-based studies indicate that PTLD is the most common malignancy within the first year after a transplant.[1,7,10] Lung transplantation is associated with the highest risk for the development of PTLD: 20% versus 0.8% in renal transplants, 1.8% in heart transplants, and 4.6% in heart-lung transplant recipients.[36] The risk may be even greater in pediatric transplant recipients, in whom PTLD accounts for 52% of cancer.[36] Children may be at increased risk because they are more likely to be seronegative for EBV and thus acquire a primary infection.[10,13,36] Adults with pretransplant EBV seronegativity also have a 10- to 75-fold higher incidence of PTLD than do EBV-seropositive recipients.[13,15,27] Additional risk factors for PTLD have also been described; they include extremes of age, CMV mismatch status or CMV disease, episodes of acute rejection, and pre-existing chronic immune stimulation (as is seen in recipients with underlying autoimmune disease).[13,24]

PTLD encompasses a spectrum of disease ranging from polyclonal B-cell hyperplasia to monoclonal malignant B-cell lymphoma. Most of these illnesses occur as a result of T- or null-cell proliferation. The pathogenesis in most cases is believed to be due to antigenic stimulation of EBV-infected B cells, which leads to unregulated proliferation in the usual posttransplant T-cell immunosuppressed state.[13,37] The B cells selectively transform from an initial polyclonal population into a monoclonal subset, and after further cytogenetic mutation, they become a malignant entity. Cytokines are also believed to play an important role in the development of PTLD: data demonstrate increased IL-4, IL-6, and IL-10 expression in early and aggressive cases of PTLD.[13]

Correlations of specific immunosuppressants and the overall level of immunosuppression to the development of PTLD have also been suggested. However, the data regarding a direct link between individual medications and the occurrence of PTLD are conflicting. The strongest evidence for an association exists for the use of induction agents in all age groups and TAC in pediatric transplant recipients. Polyclonal antilymphocyte antibodies and the monoclonal lymphocyte-depleting antibody OKT3 have been shown to be correlated with an increased incidence of PTLD within the first year after transplantation.[10,13] OKT3 can inhibit cytotoxic T lymphocytes and stimulate inflammatory cytokines and thus lead to unopposed infection of B lymphocytes by EBV.[13] An investigation by Walker and colleagues reported a 500-fold greater risk for the development of PTLD in recipients who were EBV negative, were CMV mismatched, and received OKT3.[27] However, nonlymphocyte-depleting monoclonal antibodies such as basiliximab do not appear to impart an increased risk. Although the issue of risk for the development of PTLD and use of TAC or CNIs in adults remains controversial, the evidence supporting an increased risk for PTLD when TAC is administered to pediatric transplant recipients is stronger.[10,12,13] Despite publications indicating these connections, many still believe that the net state and duration of immunosuppression are what dictate probability of the development of PTLD. This impression is supported by the higher incidence of PTLD in lung transplant patients, who receive some of the strongest immunosuppressant regimens prescribed for solid-organ transplant recipients.[11,38]

In lung transplant recipients PTLD primarily affects the allograft, which is probably due to its lymphoid-rich environment. Histopathologic examination remains the "gold standard" for diagnosis of PTLD. Cytologic specimens are tested for clonality and EBV status. Although no disease-specific staging system exists, consensus reports recommend that a modification of the Ann Arbor staging classification system for NHL be applied to PTLD to provide a uniform reference scheme for the relationship of tumor burden to outcome.[24] Serologic testing has been shown to be of limited value in transplant recipients.[13,24] Immunosuppressed transplant patients may fail to produce detectable antibody responses, and the level of viral burden is often not correlated with the measured viral titers.[24,36] Clinical manifestations are also unreliable because patients can exhibit a spectrum of signs and symptoms ranging from asymptomatic disease to prominent B symptoms (fever, night sweats, and weight loss). Posttransplant NHL also differs from NHL in the general population in terms of disease distribution. Extranodal and central nervous system involvement are more frequent in transplant recipients.[7,10]

Evidence-based guidelines for the treatment of PTLD in lung transplant recipients remain to be determined. The recommendations regarding management are based on data from case reports or small cohorts of patients. Larger prospective studies are required to further validate treatment options. The therapeutic evidence supporting initial reduction of immunosuppressant therapy is the strongest. Spontaneous regression of disease following a reduction in the level of immunosuppression without concomitant therapy has been described in 25% to 50% of transplant patients.[39-44] This strategy is most effective in early-onset PTLD or in patients with an infectious mononucleosis–like illness. In lung transplant recipients, in whom higher levels of immunosuppression are required to preserve graft function and diminish risk of rejection, concurrent treatment strategies earlier in the course of disease may be prudent. Anecdotal reports of success with several treatment agents have been published, although the efficacy of the individual therapies is uncertain because most are seldom used without additional interventions.

Antiviral medications (acyclovir and ganciclovir) have been used alone or as an adjuvant therapy for PTLD.[24,45] Such drugs may work by preventing the recruitment of B cells into the lymphoproliferative process. Intravenous immunoglobulin (IVIG) has also been used to treat PTLD by potentially inhibiting new infection of cells or antibody-mediated cytotoxicity.[24,39] Achieving remission with interferon alfa (IFN-α), which demonstrates inherent antiviral and antiproliferative activity in addition to activity as a helper T cell type 1–associated cytokine, has also been attempted.[12] IFN-α therapy has yielded remission rates as high as 70%, but issues with infection, allograft rejection, and disease relapse have resulted in disease-free survival rates of less than 50%.[45]

More recent approaches to the treatment of PTLD have focused on immunotherapy with anti–B-cell antibodies. The first treatment attempts were made with antibodies against CD21 and CD24. Although use of these biologics resulted in a long-term disease-free survival rate of 55%,[46] they are no longer available for administration in the United States. The anti-CD20 antibody rituximab is the newest therapeutic target under investigation for PTLD. Even though its relatively low toxicity profile makes rituximab (Rituxan) an attractive first-line agent, published data on its effectiveness differ. In a study that investigated only five patients, including one heart-lung transplant recipient, rituximab resulted in a 58% remission rate.[47] Benkerrou and team reported a rate of response to rituximab of 65% with an 18% relapse rate.[46] In one of the largest evaluations of rituximab's efficacy, the overall response rate was only 44%, with more than half of the patients progressing or dying during the investigation.[48]

Cytotoxic chemotherapy for resistant cases has been implemented less frequently because of the high risk for neutropenic and septic complications. Anthracycline-based regimens have been noted to achieve a remission rate as high as 69% in patients with B-cell tumors.[24] Additional experimental approaches to treatment of PTLD include adoptive transfer of autologous EBV-specific cytotoxic T lymphocytes and use of anti–IL-6 antibodies.[24] Surgical debulking of focal tumors to reduce complications and localized radiotherapy for certain tumors, such as central nervous system lesions, are nonpharmacologic options reserved for specific cases. Standardized recommendations for managing response to treatment are lacking. Monitoring of EBV load during treatment may be helpful, although values are not necessarily correlated with disease burden and some patients may be EBV negative. Measurement of serum IL-4 and IL-10 has been suggested for evaluating response of PTLD to therapy, but the specific levels at which therapeutic intervention is appropriate still need to be determined.[49,50]

Survival outcomes in solid-organ transplant patients with lymphoma variants of PTLD have traditionally been poor, particularly in patients with late-onset PTLD. Reported 1-year mortality rates for renal and heart transplant patients with lymphoma have been as high as 40% to 50%,[10] and the risk for death in patients who do not respond to initial treatment approaches may be as high as 90%.[45] However, lung transplant recipients with lymphomas restricted to their allografts have experienced more favorable survival rates. Factors that have been associated with treatment failure include EBV negativity, monoclonal disease, late-onset PTLD, and central nervous system involvement. Defective expression of the B-cell surface proteins CD21 and CD24, as well as BCL6 gene mutations in transformed lymphocytes, have also been suggested to inhibit response to treatment on a molecular level.[24,39]

CUTANEOUS MALIGNANCIES

Nonmelanoma skin carcinoma

The most common cancer after lung transplantation is NMSC. Squamous cell carcinoma (SCC) and basal cell carcinoma (BCC) account for 90% to 95% of all skin malignancies in transplant recipients. Risk for the development of SCC is at least 65 times greater than that in the general population, and the incidence of BCC increases 10-fold.[30,51] Whereas BCC predominates in immunocompetent individuals, the ratio of SCC to BCC in solid-organ transplant recipients is inverted and equals 4:1.[30,51] The average time from transplantation to diagnosis is 8 years for those who received transplants at the age of 40 years as opposed to only 3 years for those who received transplants after the age of 60.[30] In addition to age, several other risk factors for the development of NMSC exist, including ethnicity (the highest risk is in whites), male sex, cumulative ultraviolet (UV) exposure, fair skin, carcinogen exposure, and history of radiation therapy.[4,51] The intensity and duration of immunosuppression also have a major influence on the occurrence and progression of cancer. An investigation by Wisgerhof and associates estimated the cumulative incidence of NMSC after transplantation to be 3% at 5 years, 9% at 10 years, 24% at 20 years, and up to 40% after 30 years.[52] Analyses of renal transplant recipients have reported that a cutaneous malignancy will be diagnosed in 50% or more

of white transplant recipients.[53-55] Although the chance of NMSC has been shown to increase proportionally to the potency and duration of immunosuppression, the data indicating an increased risk related to specific immunosuppressant agents are equivocal. Infection with both oncogenic (HPV-16 and HPV-18) and nononcogenic (HPV-6 and HPV-11) variants is also thought to be a risk factor for the development of NMSC. Perhaps the strongest independent predictor of posttransplant NMSC is a history of pretransplant NMSC.[4]

SCC is typically a more aggressive lesion in transplant recipients, with deeper infiltration into adjacent tissue, a higher probability of perineural and lymphatic invasion, and higher rates of metastatic disease than in the general population.[51] Recurrence rates are also significantly increased in transplant recipients. Lindelöf and colleagues reported that 25% of patients with SCC will have a second lesion within 13 months and 50% will have a second lesion within 3.5 years.[56] Another study reported that 13.4% of cases of NMSC are local recurrences (usually within the first year) and that 5% to 8% of them metastasize (usually within the second year).[57]

Because of the potentially rapid progression of NMSC, it is imperative that lung transplant recipients receive routine preventive care, proactive treatment, and close follow-up. Starting at the time of pretransplant evaluation, patients should receive repeated and strict education on the dangers of UV exposure and the absolute necessity for protection from sun exposure. In view of the lack of standardized guidelines for skin surveillance, individual risk assessments can be beneficial in determining the appropriate schedule for skin checks by dermatology. For low-risk patients with no history of skin cancer, a yearly skin evaluation is sufficient. For recipients with numerous risk factors, a 6- or 12-month visit to a dermatologist is advised, and for patients with any history of NMSC or precancerous lesions, a 3- or 6-month evaluation is warranted.

Management of skin carcinoma in transplant recipients depends on the type of lesion and its extent. Precancerous lesions or very superficial NMSC may be treated with cyclic topical therapies, such as cryotherapy, 5-fluorouracil, imiquimod, topical retinoid, and photodynamic therapy. More infiltrative but uncomplicated instances of SCC and BCC require prompt excision or Mohs micrographic surgery with histologic examination to verify clear margins and determine tumor stage. Adjuvant radiation therapy is often recommended if lymph node infiltration or extracapsular spread is present. Chemotherapy with bleomycin, fluorouracil, and cisplatin is generally reserved for metastatic disease.[30] Multiple novel therapies are under investigation. One such agent is cetuximab, an endothelial growth factor receptor inhibitor that is used for metastatic SCC in the head and neck. Another is ingenol mebutate, a topical medication for treating actinic keratosis.[51]

A critical component of slowing tumor progression and managing recurrence is tapering or adjusting immunosuppressant regimens. Achieving a balance between decreasing

NMSC aggressiveness and preventing allograft rejection with immunosuppressant titration is difficult, particularly in lung transplant recipients, who require higher drug levels to prevent rejection. Specific medications such as CYA and AZA have been reported to be more likely to promote malignant transformation. Consideration should be given to preferentially lowering levels of CYA or replacing it with alternative drugs (such as TAC, MMF, or both) that have less potent cancer-causing properties. mTOR inhibitors (SRL or everolimus) are also believed to have antineoplastic effects and can be used in combination with CNIs to lower CNI levels.

The general response to treatment of advanced NMSCs is poor, as a result of which morbidity and mortality are high. Prognostic indicators for poor outcomes include a history of pretransplant skin cancer, multiple tumors, cephalic location, presence of extracutaneous tumors, old age, and heavy exposure to UV sunlight.[30]

Melanoma

The incidence of melanoma following solid-organ transplantation is much lower than that of NMSC. Melanoma accounts for 6.2% of skin cancer in adult transplant recipients and for 15% in pediatric patients.[58] Despite the decreased occurrence of melanoma, transplant recipients still have more than twice the chance of receiving a diagnosis of melanoma than do members of the general population.[4,59] Risk factors for the development of melanoma include advanced age, male sex, and white race. Patients with a history of melanoma before transplantation may have a risk for recurrence as high as 20%, even if the primary lesion occurred more than a decade before engraftment.[58] The average time to diagnosis of melanoma after transplantation is 5 years.[55,58] Malignant lesions require extensive surgical excision to ensure clear margins and, possibly, biopsy of a sentinel lymph node, depending on the histologic features of the primary tumor.

As with NMSC, reducing the level of immunosuppression is a first-line management strategy. The prognosis for survival is based on several factors, including depth of invasion (reported as Breslow thickness or Clark level), presence of ulceration, lymph node involvement, mitoses, and distant metastasis.[60] Outcomes for solid-organ transplant recipients with melanoma are not well defined; the evidence is based on case reports or small case series. The Skin Care in Organ Transplant Patients Europe (SCOPE) study[61] and an investigation by Dapprich and coworkers[62] both suggested that transplant patients with more superficial tumors (<2 mm thick) had survival rates similar to those of a national sample of immunocompetent individuals with melanoma. A statistically significant decrease in the survival of transplant recipients with stage T3 or higher malignant melanoma was reported in the SCOPE study.[61] Lower cause-specific survival rates of malignant melanoma in transplant recipients were further supported in a retrospective review of 724 cases, in which overall survival was worse in transplant recipients regardless of Breslow thickness or Clark level. However, transplant recipients with thicker melanomas (Cark level III or IV or Breslow thickness of 1.5 to 3 mm) had a significantly higher cause-specific mortality rate.[60]

Miscellaneous cutaneous cancer

In a very small percentage of lung and other solid-organ transplant recipients, types of skin cancer other than NMSC and melanoma are diagnosed. The most frequently diagnosed cancer within this group of uncommon cutaneous malignancies is KS, the incidence of which in transplant recipients is 80- to 500-fold higher than in the general population.[51,63,64] It usually appears within the first 2 years after transplantation, and men are affected three times more often than women. An association between KS and HHV-8 was first reported in 1994. The global prevalence rates of HHV-8 appear to be correlated with the ethnic specificities of KS. The incidence of the disease is 0.5% in Western countries, where most recipients of solid-organ allografts are seronegative for HHV-8, versus 5.3% in regions of Africa, where more than half the population has had previous exposure to HHV-8.[65] KS lesions are found on the skin and mucous membranes in 90% of transplant recipients; visceral involvement is observed in 30% of kidney and 50% of cardiac or liver transplant recipients.[30] Localized disease can be treated with surgery, cryotherapy, lasers, or topical retinoids. Widespread lesions may require high-dose radiation therapy or systemic chemotherapy with agents such as doxorubicin, vinblastine, bleomycin, and cisplatin.[30,51] Successful use of antiviral drugs (acyclovir and ganciclovir) in vivo has not been reliably established. Lowering immunosuppression is also a hallmark of therapy. mTOR inhibitors, used either together with or instead of CNI-based regimens, have been shown to have efficacy in achieving remission from KS while reducing the risk for graft rejection.[66] Survival rates depend on the extent of disease, but a review of KS by Euvrard and colleagues described a survival rate of 90% at 1 year for cutaneous disease and 70% for visceral involvement. The 5-year survival rate was estimated to be 69%.[30]

Sarcomas other than KS are rarely described in transplant recipients. In a review of national and international solid-organ transplant registries, a 1.7% incidence of mixed and soft tissue sarcomas (which is higher than the 1% occurrence rate in immunocompetent individuals) was observed.[67] Several histologic types of sarcoma, including fibrosarcoma, leiyomyosarcoma, malignant fibrous histiocytoma, angiosarcoma, rhabdomyosarcoma, chondrosarcoma, osteosarcoma, Ewing sarcoma, spindle cell sarcoma, and liposarcoma, have been described. Malignant lesions occur most commonly in the head and neck region, and most are high grade at the time of diagnosis. Treatment usually consists of wide local incision with adjuvant chemotherapy, radiation therapy, or both. A published review of 27 cases of sarcoma in transplant recipients revealed that 40% involved cancer that was metastatic at the time of discovery, the rate of recurrence rate was 30%, and the 5-year survival rate was low (25%).[68]

Two additional malignancies with skin involvement that are uncommon in transplant recipients are neuroendocrine skin (i.e., Merkel cell) carcinoma and cutaneous lymphoma. Merkel cell carcinoma is characterized by nonspecific nodular growths and high rates of lymph node metastases. Mohs surgery with wide excisional margins is the first step in therapy. Chemotherapy with possible radiation treatment is implemented when evidence of lymph node involvement is present. The prognosis is poor, with a mortality rate of 56% at 2 years as opposed to 25% to 35% in nonimmunosuppressed patients.[30] Cutaneous lymphoma can be of B- or T-cell origin. B-cell variants appear as single or multiple papules that may be ulcerated. Clinical manifestations of T-cell lymphoma are heterogeneous and can include mycosis fungoides, erythroderma, or hemorrhagic lesions, often with generalized lymphadenopathy. As for other cutaneous malignancy, the mainstays of treatment are surgical excision, radiotherapy, chemotherapy, and reduction in immunosuppression.[69] Because many B-cell tumors are positive for EBV, the use of IFN-α and acyclovir has also been attempted but shown limited success.[69] Overall survival outcomes are worse for T-cell lymphoma.

SOLID-ORGAN TUMORS

Just as virally driven cancer has been proved to occur much more frequently in transplant recipients, some solid-organ malignancy also has a higher incidence in allograft recipients. Primary lung cancer is the third most common cancer (following PTLD and NMSC) in lung transplant recipients.[1,70] Two retrospective studies have suggested that the risk for bronchogenic carcinoma in single-lung transplant recipients is between 5% and 7% versus 0% in bilateral lung transplant recipients.[71,72] In addition to single-lung transplant recipient status, risk factors for lung cancer included increasing age, significant smoking history, and underlying diagnosis of chronic obstructive pulmonary disease. Most of the lung tumors were non–small cell cancer that developed in the native lung. Both investigations additionally reported that bronchogenic carcinoma in lung transplant recipients was more aggressive and characterized by a higher frequency of recurrence and mortality rates between 67% and 75%.[71,72] Other recent studies have also suggested that colorectal cancer is more common in transplant patients than in the general population.[71,74] Like posttransplant lung cancer, colorectal neoplasm in transplant recipients carries decreased 5-year survival rates and survival outcomes, which become even lower with more advanced cancer stages.[73,74] A 2004 study of the Australian and New Zealand registry data additionally suggested that cancer of the esophagus, liver, thoracic organs, bone, urogenital tract, and endocrine organs occurs at a higher rate than anticipated in the general population.[73]

Although prostate and breast cancer are the second most common types of cancer in American men and women, respectively, they do not demonstrate an increased incidence in solid-organ transplant recipients.[1,2,4,70] In fact, breast cancer has been suggested to occur in recipients at lower rates than in the general population.[1,70] The diagnosis of cervical cancer is also uncommon in lung transplant recipients. The evidence suggesting a comparable incidence of these malignancies is unclear, which may in part be related to more aggressive national preventive screening programs. Despite the fact that rates of development of breast, prostate, and cervical cancer in transplant recipients are similar to those in the general population, the survival outcomes in each of these respective patient groups differ. Cancer in transplant recipients is diagnosed more often at advanced stages of malignancy, and the tumors appear to be more aggressive, which may be connected with the use of immunosuppressive medications. Solid-organ transplantation has also been identified as a negative risk factor for survival, with higher mortality rates for all cancer stages regardless of tumor type.[73,75]

POSTTRANSPLANTATION MANAGEMENT OF RISK FOR MALIGNANCY

Understanding the increased risk for the development of cancer in transplant recipients, recognizing the factors involved, and identifying the types of cancer that are more common after a transplant will not only enable providers to better educate transplant candidates about the procedure but will also give them parameters to consider when attempting to minimize recipients' risk for the development of malignancy postoperatively. For example, patients with seronegative EBV status or other reasons for a heightened risk for PTLD may benefit from routine monitoring of EBV antibodies and titers. An individualized stratification of risk for the development of skin cancer following transplantation could be used to determine recommended intervals between skin examination. Transplant patients must also be educated regarding the probability of skin cancer development after transplantation and the necessity for protection from harmful UV radiation. Recipients with a history of HPV infection may warrant more frequent gynecologic examinations. Earlier detection of lung cancer may also be possible with yearly thoracic computed tomography in single-lung transplant recipients with emphysema-related lung disease or a smoking history of greater than 50 pack-years. Because of the increased incidence of colorectal cancer in transplant recipients, more frequent colonoscopy should also be considered.

Perhaps one of the most pivotal cancer prevention–related goals of posttransplant management is to attain the optimal balance between allograft rejection and reduction in immunosuppressant therapy. Although advances in transplant pharmacology have led to improved survival outcomes, newer multidrug therapy has also increased cancer rates. Consideration should be given to implementing risk minimization strategies, particularly in higher-risk recipients such as those older than 60 years and those with a history of cancer before transplantation. Approaches to reducing risk for the development of cancer should include avoidance of lymphocyte-reducing monoclonal antibodies and long-term use of voriconazole for antifungal prophylaxis. Use of MMF and SRL in treatment regimens may also offer an advantage in terms of inhibition of malignancy. Individualizing treatment and surveillance plans on the basis of estimated risk for the development of cancer may help reduce malignant complications following lung transplantation.

CONCLUSION

Lung and other solid-organ transplant recipients experience an overall increased risk for malignancy after transplantation. Like bronchiolitis obliterans syndrome, cancer remains one of the leading causes of chronic posttransplant mortality. The intricate compilation of factors influencing the development of neoplasms in the setting of transplantation is incompletely understood, although evidence supports a significant role for intensity and duration of immunosuppression in their development. Advancing age, genetic susceptibility, infection by viral agents, history of tobacco smoking, and exposure to carcinogens are also believed to play varying roles in the genesis of cancer. Understanding the increased risk for and pathogenesis of the types of cancer that are prevalent in transplant recipients could allow uniform screening and surveillance guidelines in the postoperative period.

REFERENCES

1. Engles EA, Pfeiffer RM, Fraumeni JF, et al. Spectrum of cancer risk among U.S. solid organ transplant recipients. JAMA 2011;306:1891-1901.
2. Collett D, Mumford L, Banner NR, et al. Comparison of the incidence of malignancy in recipients of different types of organs: A UK registry audit. Am J Transplant 2010;10:1889-1896.
3. Grulich AE, van Leeuwen MT, Falster MO, Vajdic CM. Incidence of cancers in people with HIV/AIDS compared with immunosuppressed transplant recipients: A meta-analysis. Lancet 2007;370:59-67.
4. Vajdic CM, van Leeuwen MT. Cancer incidence and risk factors after solid organ transplantation. Int J Cancer 2009;125:1747-1754.
5. Adami J, Gäbel H, Lindelöf B, et al. Cancer risk following organ transplantation: A nationwide cohort study in Sweden. Br J Cancer 2003;89:1221-1227.
6. Roithmaier S, Haydon AM, Loi S, et al. Incidence of malignancies in heart and/or lung transplant recipients: A single-institution experience. J Heart Lung Transplant 2007;26:845-849.
7. Penn I. Cancers complicating organ transplantation. N Engl J Med 1990;323:1767-1769.
8. Penn I. Cancers in cyclosporine-treated vs azathioprine treated patients. Transplant Proc 1996;86:876-878.
9. Sheil AGR, Disney APS, Mathew TH, et al. Lymphoma incidence, cyclosporine, and the evolution and major impact of malignancy following organ transplantation. Transplant Proc 1997;29:825-827.
10. Opelz G, Döhler B. Lymphomas after solid organ transplantation: A collaborative transplant study report. Am J Transplant 2003;4:222-230.
11. Opelz G, Henderson R. Incidence of non-Hodgkin lymphoma in kidney and heart transplant recipients. Lancet 1993;342:1514-1516.
12. Dharnidharka VR, Sullivan EK, Stablein DM, et al. Risk factors for posttransplant lymphoproliferative disorder (PTLD) in pediatric kidney transplantation: A report of the North American Pediatric Renal Transplant Cooperative Study (NAPRTCS). Transplantation 2001;71:1065-1068.
13. Cockfield SM. Identifying the patient at risk for post-transplant lymphoproliferative disorder. Transpl Infect Dis 2001;3:70-78.
14. Cherikh WS, Kauffman HM, McBride MA, et al. Association of the type of induction immunosuppression with posttransplant lymphoproliferative disorder, graft survival, and patient survival after primary kidney transplantation. Transplantation 2003;76:1289-1293.
15. Swinnen LJ, Costanzo-Nordin MR, Fisher SG et al. Increased incidence of lymphoproliferative disorder after immunosuppression with the monoclonal antibody OKT3 in cardiac transplant recipients. N Engl J Med 1990;323:1723-1728.
16. Kobashigawa J, Miller K, Renlund D, et al. Randomized active-controlled trial of mycophenolate mofetil in heart transplant recipients. Transplantation 1998;66:507-515.
17. Glover MT, Deeks JJ, Raftery MJ, et al. Immunosuppression and risk of non melanoma skin cancer in renal transplant recipients. Lancet 1997;349:398.
18. Feist A, Lee R, Osborne S, et al. Increased incidence of cutaneous squamous cell carcinoma in lung transplant recipients taking long-term voriconazole. J Heart Lung Transplant 2012;31:1177-1181.
19. Singer JP, Boker A, Metchnikoff C, et al. High cumulative dose exposure to voriconazole is associated with cutaneous squamous cell carcinoma in lung transplant recipients. J Heart Lung Transplant 2012;31:694-699.
20. Campistol JM, Gutierrez-Dalmau A, Torregrosa JV. Conversion to sirolimus: A successful treatment for posttransplantation Kaposi's sarcoma. Transplantation 2004;77:760-762.
21. Stallone G, Schena A, Infante B, et al. Sirolimus for Kaposi's sarcoma in renal-transplant recipients. N Engl J Med 2005;352:1317-1323.
22. Yakupoglu YK, Buell JF, Woodle S, et al. Individualization of immunosuppressive therapy. III. Sirolimus associated with a reduced incidence of malignancy. Transplant Proc 2006;38:358-361.

23. Geissler EK. The impact of mTOR inhibitors on the development of malignancy. Transplant Proc 2008;40:S32-S35.

24. Preiksaitis JK, Keay S. Diagnosis and management of posttransplant lymphoproliferative disorder in solid-organ transplant recipients. Clin Infect Dis 2001;33(Suppl 1):S38-S46.

25. Tanner JE, Alfieri C. The Epstein-Barr virus and post-transplant lymphoproliferative disease: Interplay of immunosuppression, EBV, and the immune system in disease pathogenesis. Transpl Infect Dis 2001;3:60-69.

26. Schulz TF. Cancer and viral infections in immunocompromised individuals. Int J Cancer 2009;125:1755-1763.

27. Walker RC, Marshall WF, Strickler JG, et al. Pretransplantation assessment of the risk of lymphoproliferative disorder. Clin Infect Dis 1995;20:1346-1353.

28. Wang J, Belcher JD, Marker PH, et al. Cytomegalovirus inhibits p53 nuclear localization signal function. J Mol Med 2001;78:642-647.

29. Labalette M, Queyrel V, Masy E, et al. Implication of cyclosporine in up-regulation of Bcl-2 expression and maintenance of CD8 lymphocytosis in cytomegalovirus-infected allograft recipients. Transplantation 1995;59:1714-1723.

30. Euvrard S, Kanitakis J, Claudy A. Skin cancers after organ transplantation. N Engl J Med 2003;348:1681-1691.

31. Carroll PA, Brazeau E, Lagunoff M. Kaposi's sarcoma-associated herpesvirus infection of blood endothelial cells induces lymphatic differentiation. Virology 2004;328:7-18.

32. Pellet C, Chevret S, Francès C, et al. Prognostic value of quantitative Kaposi sarcoma–associated herpesvirus load in posttransplantation Kaposi sarcoma. J Infect Dis 2002;186:110-113.

33. Penn I. Cancers of the anogenital region in renal transplant recipients: Analysis of 65 cases. Cancer 1986;58:611-616.

34. Munger K, Basile JR, Duensing S, et al. Biological activities and molecular targets of the human papillomavirus E7 oncoprotein. Oncogene 2001;20:7888-7898.

35. Penn I, Hammond W, Brettschneider L, Starzl TE. Malignant lymphomas in transplantation patients. Transplant Proc 1969;1:106-112.

36. Gao SZ, Chaparro SV, Perlroth M, et al. Post-transplantation lymphoproliferative disease in heart and heart-lung transplant recipients: 30-year experience at Stanford University. J Heart Lung Transplant 2003;22:505-514.

37. Birkeland SA. Chronic antigenic stimulation from the graft as a possible oncogenic factor after renal transplantation. Scand J Urol Nephrol 1983;17:355-359.

38. Nalesnik MA, Makowska L, Starzl T. The diagnosis and treatment of posttransplant lymphoproliferative disorders. Curr Probl Surg 1988;25:371-472.

39. Andreone P, Gramenzi A, Lorenzini S, et al. Posttransplantation lymphoproliferative disorders. Arch Intern Med 2003;163:1997-2004.

40. Starzl TE, Nalesnik MA, Porter KA, et al. Reversibility of lymphomas and lymphoproliferative lesions developing under cyclosporine-steroid therapy. Lancet 1984;1:584-587.

41. Penn I. Immunosuppression: A contributory factor in lymphoma formation. Clin Transplant 1992;6:214-219.

42. Salloum E, Cooper DL, Howe G, et al. Spontaneous regression of lymphoproliferative disorders in patients treated with methotrexate for rheumatoid arthritis and other rheumatic diseases. J Clin Oncol 1996;14:1943-1949.

43. Rinde-Hoffman D, Dintron G, Ferguson J, et al. Lymphoproliferative disorder early after cardiac transplantation. Am J Cardiol 1991;68:1724-1725.

44. Swinnen LJ, Mullen GM, Carr TJ, et al. Aggressive treatment for postcardiac transplant lymphoproliferation. Blood 1995;86:3333-3334.

45. Orjuela M, Gross TG, Cheung YK, et al. A pilot study of chemoimmunotherapy (cyclophosphamide, prednisone, and rituximab) in patients with post-transplant lymphoproliferative disorder following solid organ transplantation. Clin Cancer Res 2003;9:3945s-3952s.

46. Benkerrou M, Jais JP, Leblond V, et al. Anti–B-cell monoclonal antibody treatment of severe posttransplant B-lymphoproliferative disorder: Prognostic factors and long-term outcome. Blood 1998;92:3137-3147.

47. Zilz ND, Olson LJ, McGregor CG. Treatment of post-transplant lymphoproliferative disorder with monoclonal CD20 antibody (rituximab) after heart transplantation. J Heart Lung Transplant 2001;20:770-772.

48. Choquet S, Leblond V, Herbrecht R, et al. Efficacy and safety of rituximab in B-cell post-transplantation lymphoproliferative disorders: Results of a prospective multicenter phase 2 study. Blood 2006;107:3053-3057.

49. Birkeland SA, Bendtzen K, Moller B, et al. Interleukin-10 and posttransplant lymphoproliferative disorder after kidney transplantation. Transplantation 1999;67:876-881.

50. Faro A, Kurland G, Michaels MG, et al. Interferon-alpha affects the immune response in post-transplant lymphoproliferative disorder. Am J Respir Crit Care Med 1996;153:1442-1447.

51. Bangash HK, Colegio OR. Management of non-melanoma skin cancer in immunocompromised solid organ transplant recipients. Curr Treat Options Oncol 2012;13:354-376.

52. Wisgerhof HC, van der Geest LG, de Fijter JW, et al. Incidence of cancer in kidney-transplant recipients: A long-term cohort study in a single center. Cancer Epidemiol 2011;35:105-111.

53. Webb MC, Compton F, Andrews PA, Koffman CG. Skin tumours posttransplantation: A retrospective analysis of 28 years' experience at a single centre. Transplant Proc 1997;29:828-830.

54. Hartevelt MM, Bavinck JN, Kootte AMM, et al. Incidence of skin cancer after renal transplantation in the Netherlands. Transplantation 1990;49:506-509.

55. Bouwes-Bavinck JN, Hardie DR, Green A, et al. The risk of skin cancer in renal transplant recipients in Queensland, Australia: A follow-up study. Transplantation 1996;61:715-721.

56. Lindelöf B, Sigurgeirsson B, Gäbel H, Stern RS. Incidence of skin cancer in 5356 patients following organ transplantation. Br J Dermatol 2000;143:513-519.

57. Martinez JC, Otley CC, Stasko T, et al. Defining the clinical course of metastatic skin cancer in organ transplant recipients: A multicenter collaborative study. Arch Dermatol 2003;139:301-306.

58. Penn I. Malignant melanoma in organ allograft recipients. Transplantation 1996;61:274-278.

59. Buell JF, Hanaway MJ, Thomas M, et al. Skin cancer following transplantation: The Israel Penn International Transplant Tumor Registry experience. Transplant Proc 2005;37:962-963.

60. Brewer JD, Christenson LJ, Weaver AL. Malignant melanoma in solid transplant recipients: Collection of database cases and comparison with surveillance, epidemiology, and end results data for outcome analysis. Arch Dermatol 2011;147:790-796.

61. Matin RN, Mesher D, Proby CM, et al. Melanoma in organ transplant recipients: Clinicopathological features and outcome in 100 cases. Am J Transplant 2008;8:1891-1900.

62. Dapprich DC, Weenig RH, Rohlinger AL, et al. Outcomes of melanoma in recipients of solid organ transplant. J Am Acad Dermatol 2008;59:405-417.

63. Woodle E, Hanaway M, Buell J, et al. Kaposi's sarcoma: An analysis of the U.S. and international experiences from the Israel Penn International Transplant Tumor Registry. Transplant Proc 2001;33:3660-3661.

64. Jenkins FJ, Hoffman LJ, Liegey-Dougall A. Reactivation of and primary infection with human herpesvirus 8 among solid organ transplant recipients. J Infect Dis 2002;185:1238-1243.

65. Cattani P, Capuano M, Graffeo R, et al. Kaposi's sarcoma associated with previous human herpesvirus 8 infection in kidney transplant recipients. J Clin Microbiol 2001;39:506-508.

66. Campistol JM, Eris J, Oberbauer R, et al. Sirolimus therapy after early cyclosporine withdrawal reduces the risk for cancer in adult renal transplantation. J Am Soc Nephrol 2006;17:581-589.

67. Penn I. Sarcomas in organ allograft recipients. Transplantation 1995;60:1485-1491.

68. Husted TL, Buell JF, Hanaway MJ, et al. De novo sarcomas in solid organ transplant recipients. Transplant Proc 2002;34:1786-1787.

69. Mozzanica N, Cattaneo A, Fracchiolla N, et al. Posttransplantation cutaneous B-cell lymphoma with monoclonal Epstein-Barr virus infection, responding to acyclovir and reduction in immunosuppression. J Heart Lung Transplant 1997;16:964-968.

70. Hall EC, Pfeiffer RM, Segev DL, et al. Cumulative incidence of cancer after solid organ transplantation. Cancer 2013;119:2300-2308.

71. Dickson RP, Davis D, Rea JB, et al. High frequency of bronchogenic carcinoma after single-lung transplantation. J Heart Lung Transplant 2006;25:1297-1301.

72. Minai OA, Shah S, Mazzone P, et al. Bronchogenic carcinoma after lung transplantation: Characteristics and outcomes. J Thorac Oncol 2008;3:1404-1409.

73. Buell JF, Gross TG, Woodle ES. Malignancy after transplantation. Transplantation 2005;80:S254–S264.

74. Buell JF, Papaconstantinou HT, Skalow B, et al. De novo colorectal cancer: Five-year survival is markedly lower in transplant recipients compared with the general population. Transplant Proc 2005;37:960-961.

75. Miao Y, Everly JJ, Gross TG, et al. De novo cancers arising in organ transplant recipients are associated with adverse outcomes compared with the general population. Transplantation 2009;87:1347-1359.

Quality of life following lung transplantation

NATHAN M. MOLLBERG AND MICHAEL S. MULLIGAN

INTRODUCTION

Patients with advanced or end-stage lung failure suffer from decreased health-related quality of life (HRQoL) as a result.[1,2] Although long-term outcomes of lung transplantation have improved over the past 2 decades, they continue to lag behind those of kidney and heart transplant recipients. Ever-increasing health care costs have brought added scrutiny to treatments such as lung transplantation, which can be costly and have poor long term outcomes. Therefore, demonstrating effectiveness of treatment in terms of enhancing quality of life (QoL) has become increasingly important. Although numerous studies have reported enhanced QoL after lung transplantation, the quality of their methodology has varied. This chapter focuses on the current state of knowledge regarding QoL after lung transplantation and identifies opportunities for future research in this area.

VALIDATED INSTRUMENTS FOR MEASURING QUALITY OF LIFE

The validity and performance of instruments measuring HRQoL in lung transplant recipients have been evaluated in only a handful of studies. Stavem and colleagues administered three instruments to 31 lung transplant recipients and 15 candidates to assess their reliability and validity[3]: the St. George's Respiratory Questionnaire (SGRQ), which is a lung-specific health status instrument; the 36-item Short-Form (SF-36), which is a general measure; and the Hospital Anxiety and Depression Scale (HADS). All three instruments demonstrated reliability with an internal consistency (Cronbach's coefficient α) ranging between 0.77 and 0.95. The associations between dimensions related to physical and mental health among the instruments were high, thus demonstrating validity as well. A second study evaluating the SF-36 also demonstrated good internal consistency and discriminant validity.[4]

The Health Utilities Index (HUI) consists of two systems (HUI2 and HUI3) that include a generic comprehensive health status classification system and a generic HRQoL utility scoring system. Santana and coworkers evaluated the HUI3 and compared clinician-based predictions with observed correlations.[5] The authors were able to demonstrate that the HUI3 performed largely as anticipated. A qualitative approach to measuring HRQoL by using patient narratives demonstrated that patients often have feelings that cannot be measured by quantitative methods (e.g., feelings regarding the donor and their family), as well as issues that may affect responses to standard instruments (e.g., the sense of responsibility that comes with receiving a valuable commodity such as a donated organ).[6]

DETERMINANTS OF QUALITY OF LIFE

Development of bronchiolitis obliterans syndrome

The published literature has consistently demonstrated that loss of graft function is associated with a decrease in QoL scores. Smeritschnig and colleagues administered the

SGRQ, SF-36, and HADS to 104 lung transplant recipients in a cross-sectional manner and demonstrated that the development of bronchiolitis obliterans syndrome (BOS) was strongly associated with poorer HRQoL.[7] Two studies evaluated the effect of the development of BOS on HRQoL longitudinally and demonstrated similar findings.[8,9] Physical functioning and energy were the domains most influenced by the development of BOS, which affected recipients' ability to perform activities of daily living and their subsequent HRQoL. One study, which evaluated only patients who survived at least 55 months after transplantation, demonstrated significant improvements on most dimensions of the Nottingham Health Profile (NHP), with more patients able to walk without dyspnea at approximately 43 months after transplantation.[10] Subsequently, however, patients experienced more dyspnea, anxiety, and depression and a lower sense of well-being. These changes coincided with the development of complications associated with immunosuppressant medications and BOS. A number of other studies have also reported that BOS is strongly associated with a decrease in HRQoL. However, such studies often fail to adjust for potential confounders and simply compare changes in HRQoL in patients with and without BOS. In addition, many of the instruments used (e.g., the NHP) have not been formally validated for lung transplant recipients.

Single-lung versus bilateral lung transplantation

A few studies have assessed the effect of the type of lung transplant (single versus bilateral) performed on postoperative QoL. Anyanwu and colleagues administered the EQ-5D, a generic instrument from the EuroQol Group that assigns utility values to health in five different domains, to 109 single-lung and 79 bilateral lung transplant recipients.[11] Utility values 3 years after transplantation were 0.61 for single- and 0.82 for bilateral lung transplant recipients; the values for bilateral transplant recipients were consistently superior to those for single-lung recipients. In addition, problems in all five domains were more frequent in single-lung recipients. However, the remaining published literature demonstrates either conflicting results or no difference at all in HRQoL among patients undergoing single-lung as opposed to bilateral lung transplantation.

Pretransplant diagnosis

Vasiliadis and coworkers administered the SF-36 to 71 lung transplant recipients and used multivariate analysis to model each of the eight health domains as a function of individual determinants associated with lung transplantation.[12] After adjusting for a number of variables, the authors reported that lung transplant recipients with cystic fibrosis had significantly higher scores in almost every domain than did recipients with other diagnoses. Other studies have substantiated these results, with patients who have

cystic fibrosis scoring higher on the sections devoted to social role functioning and emotional role functioning after transplantation than did patients with other diagnoses.[2,7] In addition, improvements in energy and mobility have consistently been demonstrated. Because patients with cystic fibrosis are more likely to be attending school or working than are those in other pretransplant diagnostic categories, the improvement in QoL may be a result of an improved ability to resume pretransplant activities other than those of daily living.

Development of symptoms

A symptom-focused questionnaire to evaluate the impact of symptoms on QoL was administered to 287 lung transplant recipients.[13] Patients who experienced symptoms (tremor and hirsutism being the most common) were more likely to report decreased QoL in all dimensions than were those without such symptoms. Although the results of a number of other studies have similarly demonstrated an association between the development of symptoms and decreased QoL, a number of other factors need to be considered. The development of symptoms related to medications is also strongly associated with patients taking "drug holidays" as a result, as well as with the development of BOS.[14,15] It may be that as medication-related symptoms develop in patients, they become more prone to the development of BOS as a result of lack of compliance with immunosuppressants. As already mentioned, the development of BOS is also associated with decreased HRQoL scores and may be confounding for the studies evaluating the effect of medication-related symptoms on QoL.

Employment status

Few studies have evaluated the relationship between pretransplant or posttransplant employment status in lung transplant patients and QoL. The percentages of patients who are working at the time of transplantation that have been reported in the literature vary greatly. A study from Germany measured the employment status of 88 lung transplant recipients over time and its relationship with QoL scores.[16] Although none of the patients were working before transplantation, 25% reported full-time employment 1 year afterward, and returning to work was associated with increased QoL scores in a number of domains. Professional reintegration was an independent predictor of QoL and remained so at each time point examined for 5 years after transplantation. Reporting on employment status has been confounded by differences in terminology, including whether patients identify themselves as "having a job" as opposed to actually working at the time of transplantation.[17] Returning to paid employment is associated with younger age and, consequently, may affect the QoL of patients with cystic fibrosis more than that of patients with other conditions.

COMPARISONS OF QUALITY OF LIFE BEFORE AND AFTER LUNG TRANSPLANTATION

Kugler and colleagues conducted a prospective longitudinal study to evaluate QoL in 88 lung transplant recipients who survived at least 1 year.[16] The authors administered the SF-36 before transplantation, 6 and 12 months thereafter, and then yearly between 24 and 60 months after transplantation. They demonstrated that lung transplantation resulted in significant improvement in QoL, with the greatest improvement occurring in the first year after transplantation. Although only 55% (48/88) of patients provided responses at 5 years after transplantation, the improvement in QoL persisted for at least that time. A number of other studies have reported differences in QoL before and after transplantation; however, the results are difficult to interpret because the studies are plagued by small cohorts or methodologic flaws related to comparison of patients listed for transplantation with different patients who had already undergone the procedure. Despite these flaws, lung transplantation has consistently been shown to improve QoL overall. Specifically, the physical health and functioning domains have typically demonstrated the largest changes from before transplantation to afterward. Although other domains, such as pain, mental health, and emotional well-being, have not been reported to change significantly, the scores for them are comparable to the normative population scores.

QUALITY OF LIFE AS A PREDICTOR OF SURVIVAL

The data regarding pretransplant QoL as a predictor of posttransplant survival are conflicting. Squier and colleagues evaluated 74 patients who were listed for lung transplantation (49 of whom eventually underwent transplantation) by providing each with a quality of well-being score.[18] The authors found that patients with a higher baseline quality of well-being score had a significantly better survival rate than did those with lower scores. Time on the waiting list was entered as a time-dependent covariate and was not a significant predictor of survival. Unfortunately, the survival analysis was unadjusted and potential bias cannot be accounted for. Vermeulen and coworkers administered the NHP to 200 patients who were listed for lung transplantation; it was given at 3-month intervals from the time of listing through 7 months after transplantation and at 6-month intervals thereafter.[19] When the authors used an adjusted analysis, they found no significant association between pretransplant QoL and subsequent posttransplant survival.

EFFECTS OF MENTAL HEALTH AND SOCIAL SUPPORT ON QUALITY OF LIFE

Symptoms of depression and anxiety are highly prevalent in patients awaiting a transplant and in lung transplant recipients. Although the poor survival and physical functioning of patients with end-stage lung failure contribute to these symptoms, those who experience them before transplantation are more likely to still have them afterward,[20] thus indicating that poor coping mechanisms, rather than patients' perception of their health and disease alone, also play a significant role. A number of studies have demonstrated that patients demonstrate significant declines in the symptoms of both depression and anxiety after lung transplantation.[20,21] Although these declines in symptoms coincide with improvements in QoL scores, their importance as determinants of QoL is uncertain.[21] The International Society of Heart and Lung Transplantation considers inadequate social support an absolute contraindication to transplantation.[22] This view is due in part to the arduous posttransplant regimen with which patients must comply and the emotional and tangible support required by recipients. A single study demonstrated that patients who perceived higher levels of social support reported higher QoL scores.[23] In addition, the level of social support has been associated not only with recipient QoL but also with long-term outcomes.[23,24]

LONGITUDINAL ASSESSMENT OF EFFECTS ON QUALITY OF LIFE AFTER LUNG TRANSPLANTATION

Myaskovsky and colleagues administered the SF-36 to 112 lung transplant recipients (who survived for at least 1 year) at 2, 7, and 12 months after transplantation.[23] The greatest gains in QoL scores occurred in the first 6 months in the domains of role-emotional, physical functioning, and social functioning. Scores at 1 year after transplantation were not significantly different from those at 6 months but remained stable. In another study the HUI3 was administered to 43 patients during the pretransplant period and then at 3 and 6 months after transplantation.[20] Once again, the greatest gains occurred in the earlier assessment, with scores subsequently stabilizing but remaining significantly higher than the pretransplant level. A number of other studies have also consistently reported that the greatest gains in QoL scores occur early in the posttransplant period, after which they stabilize or decline slightly (but never below pretransplant levels).[25] Unfortunately, few studies have evaluated the persistence of QoL scores beyond 1 year.

QUALITY OF LIFE OF TRANSPLANT RECIPIENTS' CAREGIVERS

As mentioned earlier, the role of caregivers in the long-term outcomes of lung transplant recipients is only recently becoming appreciated. In a recent study the SF-36 was administered to 134 caregivers of lung transplant recipients to assess predictors of caregiver QoL and whether caregiver QoL affected recipient survival.[26] By using an adjusted analysis, the authors demonstrated that greater caregiver burden predicted poorer caregiver QoL at 1 year after transplantation. In addition, recipients whose caregivers had lower perceived general health at 1 year after transplantation showed significantly poorer long-term survival rates. It may be that if caregivers' health and wellness decrease, the amount of support that they are able to provide affects their ability to help recipients maintain compliance with the posttransplant regimen.

COST-EFFECTIVENESS AND QUALITY OF LIFE

In an era of ever-increasing demands that health care dollars be used efficiently, demonstrating cost-effectiveness is becoming more and more a necessity as new technologies and therapies evolve. The quality of any study on this topic depends on the outcome assumptions used and the QoL data available. Unfortunately, only a single U.S. study attempting to demonstrate the cost-effectiveness of lung transplantation has been published in the last 20 years. Ramsey and coworkers from the University of Washington performed a pilot study comparing the costs and outcomes of lung transplants in 25 patients with those of 24 wait-listed patients.[27] Charges for transplant patients were considerably more than those for wait-listed patients. Although the researchers were able to demonstrate that utility scores were significantly higher for the patients who received a transplant than for those on the waiting list, the life expectancy of the transplant recipients was not greater than that of the wait-listed patients, and the incremental cost of transplantation per quality-adjusted life year gained for the transplant recipients was $176,817. Hence, although lung transplantation was an effective treatment, it was costly as well. The last 2 decades have seen improvements in outcomes for lung transplant recipients but also increases in cost. Thus, the cost-effectiveness of lung transplantation has yet to be elucidated.

POTENTIAL THERAPIES TO IMPROVE QUALITY OF LIFE

Another question that has been considered is whether QoL can be improved through therapeutic intervention. In a German study to determine the effect of inpatient rehabilitation on HRQoL 60 lung transplant recipients who had survived at least 1 year were randomly assigned to undergo inpatient rehabilitation or outpatient physiotherapy.[28] Both groups experienced significant improvement in cardiopulmonary function that was correlated with increases in QoL scores, thus indicating that a structured rehabilitation program (whether inpatient or outpatient) has the potential to increase recipients' QoL. Two other studies assessed the impact of ongoing outcome measurements on the QoL of lung transplant recipients. A Canadian study randomly assigned 213 patients to complete the HUI2 and HUI3 during outpatient clinic visits.[29] Those in the treatment group had their results reviewed by their clinician, whereas those in the control group did not. Although the results suggested

that clinician feedback resulted in increased patient-clinician communication, no significant difference in changes in patient management between the two groups was found. In another study from the United States, 30 transplant recipients were randomly assigned either to use a handheld computer-based device to record, review, and report health data or to perform standard self-care.[30] Patients who had been randomly assigned to use the device had significantly greater measures of self-care and QoL than did those who received standard care.

AREAS FOR RESEARCH ON QUALITY IMPROVEMENT

Although the existing data have consistently demonstrated that lung transplantation increases QoL for recipients, research on QoL after lung transplantation is characterized by a number of methodologic flaws that can be addressed. Collaborations between institutions could increase cohort sizes and thus the generalizability of results. Prospective longitudinal designs that include multivariate analyses would better demonstrate the impact of the treatment on recipients' QoL and how long the changes may persist. Using validated instruments that include both general and disease-specific components would allow comparison across populations (the general instrument) and determination of the impact of the treatment on QoL scores (the disease-specific instrument). Another important aspect for authors to consider is the conceptual and operational definitions of QoL that are being used and the framework in which they will be applied. Because no universal definition of QoL exists, study authors must provide a conceptual definition so that the concept of QoL can be understood. For example, one study defined QoL as "a sense of well-being, satisfaction, and happiness with the important aspects of one's life." The operational definition then indicated how the conceptual definition would be measured. This definition has implications for the type of tool to be used because many contain either single-dimensional or multidimensional and either generic or disease-specific designs. Finally, the interdependence of the QoL of both the recipient and the caregiver must be considered. An ideal study would include administration of QoL instruments to both recipient and caregiver at each time point to identify changes in QoL in one that affect the other.

REFERENCES

1. Eskander A, Waddell TK, Faughnan ME, et al. BODE index and quality of life in advanced chronic obstructive pulmonary disease before and after lung transplantation. J Heart Lung Transplant 2011;30:1334-1341.
2. Ramsey SD, Patrick DL, Lewis S, et al. Improvement in quality of life after lung transplantation: A preliminary study. The University of Washington Medical Center Lung Transplant Study Group. J Heart Lung Transplant 1995;14:870-877.

3. Stavem K, Bjortuft O, Lund MB, et al. Health-related quality of life in lung transplant candidates and recipients. Respiration 2000;67:159-165.

4. Feurer ID, Moore DE, Speroff T, et al. Refining a health-related quality of life assessment strategy for solid organ transplant patients. Clin Transplant 2004;18(Suppl 12):39-45.

5. Santana M-J, Feeny D, Johnson J, et al. Assessing the use of health-related quality of life measures in the routine clinical care of lung-transplant patients. Qual Life Res 2010;19:371-379.

6. Festle MJ. Qualifying the quantifying: Assessing the quality of life of lung transplant recipients. Oral Hist Rev 2002;29:59-86.

7. Smeritschnig B, Jaksch P, Kocher A, et al. Quality of life after lung transplantation: A cross-sectional study. J Heart Lung Transplant 2005;24:474-480.

8. Van den Berg J, Geertsma A, van Der BW, et al. Bronchiolitis obliterans syndrome after lung transplantation and health-related quality of life. Am J Respir Crit Care Med 2000;161:1937-1941.

9. Vermeulen KM, Groen H, van der Bij W, et al. The effect of bronchiolitis obliterans syndrome on health related quality of life. Clin Transplant 2004;18:377-383

10. Vermeulen KM, Ouwens JP, van der Bij W, et al. Long-term quality of life in patients surviving at least 55 months after lung transplantation. Gen Hosp Psychiatry 2003;25:95-102.

11. Anyanwu AC, McGuire A, Rogers CA, Murday AJ. Assessment of quality of life in lung transplantation using a simple generic tool. Thorax 2001;56:218-222.

12. Vasiliadis HM, Collet JP, Poirier C. Health-related quality-of-life determinants in lung transplantation. J Heart Lung Transplant 2006;25:226-233.

13. Kugler C, Fischer S, Gottlieb J, et al. Health-related quality of life in two hundred-eighty lung transplant recipients. J Heart Lung Transplant 2005;24:2262-2268.

14. Kugler C, Fischer S, Gottlieb J, et al. Symptom experience after lung transplantation: Impact on quality of life and adherence. Clin Transplant 2007;21:590-596.

15. Lanuza DM, McCabe M, Norton-Rosko M, et al. Symptom experiences of lung transplant recipients: Comparisons across gender, pretransplantation diagnosis, and type of transplantation. Heart Lung 1999;28:429-437.

16. Kugler C, Tegtbur U, Gottlieb J, et al. Health-related quality of life in long-term survivors after heart and lung transplantation: A prospective cohort study. Transplantation 2010;90:451-457

17. Lanuza DM, Norton N, McCabe M, Garrity ER. Lung transplant patients' quality of life and symptom experiences. Circulation 1997;96(Suppl 1):440.

18. Squier HC, Ries AL, Kaplan RM, et al. Quality of well-being predicts survival in lung transplantation candidates. Am J Respir Crit Care Med 1995;152:2032-2036.

19. Vermeulen KM, TenVergert EM, Verschuuren EA, et al. Pre-transplant quality of life does not predict survival after lung transplantation. J Heart Lung Transplant 2008;27:623-627.

20. Santana MJ, Feeny D, Jackson K, et al. Improvement in health-related quality of life after lung transplantation. Can Respir J 2009;16:153-158.

21. Limbos MM, Joyce DP, Chan CK, Kesten S. Psychological functioning and quality of life in lung transplant candidates and recipients. Chest 2000;118:408-416.

22. Orens JB, Estenne M, Arcasoy S, et al. International guidelines for the selection of lung transplant candidates: 2006 update—a consensus report from the Pulmonary Scientific Council of the International Society for Heart and Lung Transplantation. J Heart Lung Transplant 2006;25:745-755.

23. Myaskovsky L, Dew MA, McNulty ML, et al. Trajectories of change in quality of life in 12-month survivors of lung or heart transplant. Am J Transplant 2006;6:1939-1947.

24. Mollberg NM, Farjah F, Howell E, et al. The impact of primary caregivers on long-term outcomes after lung transplantation. Paper presented at the 34th Annual Meeting of the International Society of Heart and Lung Transplantation, April 11, 2014, San Diego, CA.

25. Kugler C, Strueber M, Tegtbur U, et al. Quality of life 1 year after lung transplantation. Prog Transplant 2004;14:331-336.

26. Myaskovsky L, Posluzny DM, Schulz R, et al. Predictors and outcomes of health-related quality of life in caregivers of cardiothoracic transplant recipients. Am J Transplant 2012;12:3387-3397.

27. Ramsey SD, Patrick DL, Albert RK, et al. The cost-effectiveness of lung transplantation. A pilot study. University of Washington Medical Center Lung Transplant Study Group. Chest 1995;108:1594-1601.

28. Ihle F, Neurohr C, Huppmann P, et al. Effect of inpatient rehabilitation on quality of life and exercise capacity in long-term lung transplant survivors: A prospective, randomized study. J Heart Lung Transplant 2011;30:912-919.

29. Santana MJ, Feeny D, Johnson J, et al. Assessing the use of health-related quality of life measures in the routine clinical care of lung-transplant patients. Qual Life Res 2010;19:371-379.

30. DeVito Dabbs A, Dew MA, Myers B, et al. Evaluation of a hand-held, computer-based intervention to promote early self-care behaviors after lung transplant. Clin Transplant 2009;23:537-545.

Future of Lung Transplantation

38

Future therapies in lung transplantation

ELIZABETH A. LENDERMON AND JOHN F. MCDYER

Despite the many advances in the field of lung transplantation, the average time of survival after a transplant is only 5.5 years and has not improved significantly over the past 2 decades.[1] Chronic rejection in the form of bronchiolitis obliterans syndrome (BOS) remains the primary limitation to long-term survival in lung transplant recipients.[1] Medical management after lung and other solid-organ transplants has thus far been characterized by nonspecific suppression of T-cell responses to antigens. Calcineurin inhibitor therapy revolutionized the world of organ transplantation in the 1970s and clearly impairs T-cell responses to alloantigen to some degree, thereby resulting in decreased acute cellular rejection (ACR). However, it also results in impaired T-cell responses to infectious pathogens and fails to prevent chronic rejection. Induction of tolerance remains the "holy grail" of transplant immunology because it would result in immune recognition of alloantigen coupled with the lack of an inflammatory response to that antigen specifically. That tolerance is an active immune process requiring not only the absence of certain cellular events but also the presence of others is becoming increasingly clear. In addition to induction of tolerance, the ability to direct immunosuppressive therapy in a manner targeted toward suppression of specific alloantigen responses would be ideal therapeutically. In many ways, the field of lung transplantation stands to benefit most from these potential advances in transplant pharmacotherapy because chronic rejection has a greater impact on the survival of lung allografts than on that of other transplanted solid organs, such as the heart, liver, or kidney. For this reason, novel immunologic therapies for use in transplantation may be best tested in lung transplant recipients, and it is critical that transplant pulmonologists explore such therapies in an effort to improve long-term outcomes in such patients.

COSTIMULATION BLOCKADE

T-cell activation, proliferation, and differentiation require more than one signal. In addition to antigen-specific binding of T-cell receptors to the antigen presented by the major histocompatibility complex (MHC) on antigen-presenting cells (APCs), costimulatory signals also occur via engagement of other surface proteins on T cells with proteins on APCs. These costimulatory signals facilitate optimal T-cell activation and processes that lead to an effective T-cell response (Figure 38.1). Blocking these costimulatory signals at the time of engagement of T-cell receptors results in anergy, a process during which antigen-specific T cells are rendered nonresponsive when they encounter antigen.[2] For this reason, drugs have been developed to block such costimulatory signals. Here, we focus on the two most studied pathways, CD28-B7 and CD154-CD40.

CD28-B7 pathway (abatacept and belatacept)

CD28 belongs to the immunoglobulin superfamily and is expressed on the surface of T cells. It binds to B7.1 (CD80) and B7.2 (CD86) on APCs to facilitate T-cell activation and proliferation. Specifically, interaction between CD28 and

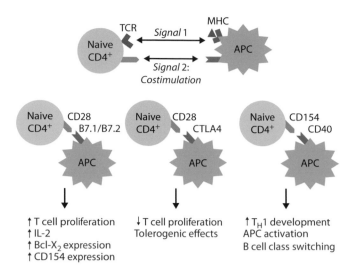

Figure 38.1 Select costimulatory pathways targeted by existing pharmacotherapy directed at inducing tolerance in solid-organ transplantation. APC, antigen-presenting cell; IL-2, interleukin 2; MHC, major histocompatibility complex; TCR, T-cell receptor.

B7 results in increased T-cell proliferation, production of interleukin-2 [IL-2], expression of the antiapoptotic protein Bcl-xL, and increased expression of CD154 (discussed later) on T cells. Blocking these effects would seemingly be desirable in terms of allograft acceptance. However, in addition to binding CD28, B7 (CD80/CD86) is also able to bind with higher avidity and affinity to CTLA4 on T cells. This interaction, in contrast to the interaction between CD28 and B7, inhibits T-cell proliferation and has peripheral tolerogenic effects, the mechanisms of which are not fully understood. CTLA4 expression is induced in activated T cells (presumably as a negative feedback mechanism), and it is expressed constitutively in certain regulatory T cells. Blocking the tolerogenic effects of interaction of CTLA4 with B7 is not desirable from the standpoint of allograft acceptance. However, the implications of interaction between CTLA4 and B7 were not known when the initial attempts to block CD28-B7 began.

To effectively block interaction of CD28 and B7 without consequent agonistic effects, the extracellular portion of CTLA4 was fused to a mutated Fc portion of human IgG1 to create CTLA4Ig (abatacept [Orencia]). Because CTLA4 binds to B7 with higher avidity and affinity than to CD28, CTLA4Ig competes with CD28 for binding. CTLA4Ig alone or in combination with other stimulation blockade has been shown in several experimental rodent transplant models to result in improved allograft acceptance.[3-9] Notably, CTLA4Ig in combination with anti-CD154 has been demonstrated to improve lung allograft acceptance in mouse orthotopic lung transplantation.[10] However, in at least some models, donor-specific transfusion appears to be required for durable tolerance.[11] Abatacept was approved for use in patients with rheumatoid arthritis in 2006. Because abatacept unfortunately did not effectively improve allograft acceptance in nonhuman primate renal transplant recipients,

the second-generation drug belatacept, which demonstrates improved affinity for B7, was developed. Belatacept was approved for use in renal transplantation in 2011, and it has shown some favorable effects in clinical studies of renal transplant patients.

Belatacept has been shown to be effective as backbone immunosuppression in renal transplant recipients when used in combination with steroids and mycophenolate mofetil.[12,13] In clinical studies, it is associated with superior renal allograft function despite an increased incidence of episodes of ACR. Unfortunately, belatacept also appears to be associated with an increased risk for the development of posttransplant lymphoproliferative disorder, including that with central nervous system involvement (especially in Epstein-Barr virus–negative transplant recipients). Interestingly, patients who received higher doses of belatacept had more episodes of ACR, thus raising the possibility that blockade of the negative costimulatory signal between CTLA4 and B7 is occurring more substantially at these higher doses and is in fact deleterious. Therefore, the role of belatacept in organ transplantation remains undefined.

No clinical trials have evaluated the effects of belatacept as backbone immunosuppressive therapy in lung transplant recipients even though it has been used as such. Although the safety and efficacy of belatacept in lung transplant recipients remain unclear, at our center we have used belatacept in selected patients who were completely unable to tolerate calcineurin inhibitor therapy.

CD154-CD40 (anti-CD154 and ASKP1240/anti-CD40 monoclonal antibodies)

CD154 (CD40L) is a protein that belongs to the tumor necrosis factor (TNF) superfamily and is expressed on the surface of activated CD4+ T cells. It binds to CD40 on APCs to effect activation in these cells, as well as on B cells, in which case binding is necessary for immunoglobulin class switching. In addition, interaction between CD154 and CD40 has been shown to be important for the development of the type 1 helper T-cell (Th1) responses[14,15] that are critical in transplant rejection. In multiple experimental transplant models (both rodents and nonhuman primates), blockade of the CD154-CD40 pathway via use of a monoclonal antibody (mAb) against CD154 at the time of transplantation has been shown to result in improved allograft acceptance.[16-19] Multiple mechanisms of anti-CD154–induced allograft acceptance appear to exist. Early animal studies examining anti-CD154 in combination with CTLA4Ig revealed an important role for activation-induced cell death.[20,21] Subsequent studies demonstrated that anti-CD154 therapy provided an infectious tolerance that is now attributable to regulatory T cells.[22-24] In a mouse orthotopic transplant model, use of anti-CD154 alone at the time of transplantation resulted in abrogation of allospecific CD4+ and CD8+ effector cytokine responses, a massive increase in the population of regulatory T cells in the allograft, and improved allograft acceptance.[25] Therefore, it is clear that anti-CD154 therapy has many desirable tolerogenic effects in animal models.

Unfortunately, CD154 is also expressed on platelets. A nondepleting, humanized IgG1 anti-CD154 mAb (toralizumab) and a fully human IgG1 anti-CD154 mAb (AB1793) were designed for clinical trials; their use resulted in unexpected thromboembolic events attributed to platelet activation.[26] For this reason, focus has switched to antibody therapy directed at CD40 to block the CD154-CD40 pathway. A human anti-CD40 mAb lacking cytotoxicity (ASKP1240) prolonged allograft survival in nonhuman primates that underwent renal transplantation.[27,28] Currently, a phase II clinical trial comparing the safety and efficacy of ASKP1240 (in addition to basiliximab induction, prednisone, and mycophenolate mofetil) with that of tacrolimus (NCT01780844) in renal transplant patients is under way.

In summary, the role of blockade of the CD154-CD40 pathway in organ transplantation also remains undefined at this moment. However, blocking both the CD154-CD40 and CD28-B7 pathways has been the mainstay of inducing tolerance in animal models for many years. For this reason, anti-CD40 is a particularly promising therapy. Whether blocking the CD28-B7 pathway along with the CD154-CD40 pathway is necessary to effect durable allograft acceptance in transplant patients or whether the resultant blockade of the negative costimulation signal via CTLA4 particularly impairs regulatory T-cell responses that may be beneficial for allograft acceptance remains unclear.

CYTOKINE-TARGETED THERAPY

Anticytokine therapy is a far from new concept that has evolved to be the mainstay of therapy in patients with moderate to severe autoimmune disease such as rheumatoid arthritis and Crohn's disease. Its goal is to block a particular immune response characterized by the cytokine contributing to a disease state but not all immune responses. The success with several agents, including infliximab (Remicade) and etanercept (Enbrel), both of which block TNF-α in autoimmune disease, has sparked great interest in the development of new anticytokine therapies for autoimmune and inflammatory disease states. Because rejection of transplanted organs is characterized by the production of effector cytokines, such therapies could potentially be used in transplantation as well. Of note, two anticytokine agents, basiliximab and daclizumab, are already being widely used for induction in lung and other solid-organ transplantation. Both are mAbs that target the receptor for IL-2 (CD25) and are being widely used for induction of immunosuppressive therapy.

Tumor necrosis factor α inhibitors (infliximab, adalimumab, and etanercept)

TNF-α is a cytokine involved in systemic inflammation and one of a group of cytokines that can stimulate the acute-phase reaction. Although originally described as being produced by macrophages, it can also be produced by CD4+ and CD8+ lymphocytes, B lymphocytes, and natural killer cells. It plays an essential role in host defense against viruses and sepsis, as well against malignancies. Dysregulation of TNF-α has been implicated in a variety of autoimmune diseases, including inflammatory bowel disease and rheumatoid arthritis. Importantly, TNF-α has also been implicated in the pathogenesis of ACR and graft-versus-host disease (GVHD).

To target the detrimental effects of TNF-α on autoimmune disease states, several drugs have been developed to inhibit binding of TNF-α to its receptor. Infliximab is a humanized, chimeric mAb that is directed against TNF-α, and adalimumab is a fully human mAb with the same target. Both are approved by the Food and Drug Administration for the treatment of rheumatoid arthritis, psoriatic arthritis and psoriasis, ankylosing spondylitis, Crohn's disease, and ulcerative colitis. Etanercept is a fusion protein that inhibits TNF-α activity by serving as a soluble receptor. It was created by fusion of the TNF receptor to the Fc portion of an IgG1 molecule. Etanercept has been approved by the Food and Drug Administration for treatment of rheumatoid arthritis, psoriatic arthritis and psoriasis, and ankylosing spondylitis.

Because TNF-α is recognized as a mediator of tissue damage in ACR, use of TNF-α inhibitors in transplantation has attracted interest. In renal transplantation, patients in whom acute rejection develops have been shown to have higher serum levels of TNF-α than do those in whom it does not.[29] Several studies in animal models of cardiac transplantation have also demonstrated a favorable effect of TNF-α blockade on vasculopathy,[30,31] and anti–TNF-α therapy (alone or in combination with cyclosporine) has been found to prolong cardiac allograft survival in rats.[32,33] In addition, inhibition of TNF-α has been shown to ameliorate intestinal GVHD.[34] Despite the absence of clinical studies indicating the safety and efficacy of TNF-α inhibitor therapy in solid-organ transplant recipients, etanercept has been used in conjunction with antithymocyte globulin for the treatment of patients with steroid-refractory GVHD and has provided a higher response rate than tacrolimus and antithymocyte globulin alone.[35] In summary, the evidence is certainly sufficient to warrant further investigation of TNF-α inhibitors in solid-organ transplantation, including lung transplantation.

To date, no studies have investigated the effects of TNF-α inhibitors on lung transplant patients. One study of heterotopic tracheal transplantation in mice showed some attenuation of obliterative airway disease with anti–TNF-α therapy.[36] In our studies involving a fully MHC-mismatched model of mouse orthotopic lung transplantation, TNF-α has not been the dominant cytokine detected during ACR.[25] Nonetheless, it may still play a critical role in rejection and may break through standard immunosuppressive therapy. If it does have such an effect in even some patients, several ways to selectively block the TNF-α response that have been well studied in autoimmune disease now exist. For this reason, further studies in lung transplant patients to define the role of TNF-α, particularly in refractory rejection, are necessary.

Anti–interleukin-17 (secukinumab, ixekizumab, and brodalumab)

IL-17 was not discovered until 1993 and is now known to be produced by a special subset of helper T cells, Th17 cells. IL-17 has the potent ability to recruit neutrophils, and it plays a role in host defense against extracellular bacteria and fungi (notably mucocutaneous candidiasis), as well as in pathogenic inflammation in disease such as rheumatoid arthritis. Because of its role in rheumatoid arthritis, several mAbs against IL-17 have been developed.

Several lines of evidence suggest that IL-17 plays an important role in BOS in lung transplant recipients. A recent study in a minor MHC-mismatched, mouse orthotopic lung transplant model showed that neutralization of IL-17 prevented the development of obliterative bronchiolitis lesions.[37] In addition, a cross-sectional study that compared bronchoalveolar lavage fluid from lung transplant recipients with BOS to that of recipients without BOS revealed increased levels of IL-17 mRNA and increased IL-17–skewing cytokine mRNA, including IL-23 in patients with BOS.[38] Although CD4+ Th17 cells have classically been thought to be the major source of IL-17, CD8+ Th17 cells can also produce IL-17 and have been shown to be the major source of IL-17 in T-bet–deficient mice experiencing acute rejection after orthotopic lung transplantation (data not published) and in lung transplant patients with lymphocytic bronchiolitis.[39] Together, these studies provide evidence that IL-17 may indeed play an important role in lung allograft rejection and obliterative bronchiolitis. Therefore, anti–IL-17 therapy is an intriguing concept in lung transplantation. In fact, lung allografts may be more susceptible to IL-17–mediated injury than are other allografts, given the predilection for Th17 cells at mucosal surfaces.

Secukinumab (Novartis) is a fully human IgG1 mAb that binds with high affinity and selectivity to human IL-17A, thereby resulting in effective neutralization. Initial studies in patients with rheumatoid arthritis had favorable results, which prompted a phase II clinical trial in patients who failed to achieve the primary end point; nonetheless, it did demonstrate safety and suggested the possibility of efficacy. A phase III trial in patients with rheumatoid arthritis is currently under way, and in a phase III trial it demonstrated efficacy against psoriasis. Ixekizumab (Lilly) is a humanized IgG4 mAb against IL-17A that has also been evaluated in phase II clinical trials in patients with rheumatoid arthritis, although current development efforts are focused on its use in patients with psoriasis and psoriatic arthritis. Finally, brodalumab (Amgen) is a fully human IgG2 anti–IL-17RA (the IL-17 receptor) mAb. Although it failed to demonstrate efficacy in a phase II clinical trial in patients with rheumatoid arthritis, it did provide positive results in phase II and III clinical trials in patients with psoriasis. None of these three agents have been tested in organ transplantation to date. However, given the aforementioned evidence suggesting a role of IL-17 specifically in lung transplant rejection and obliterative bronchiolitis, they should be considered possible therapeutic options for both treatment and prevention of BOS in lung transplant patients. Importantly, how current immunosuppressive regimens potentially affect the IL-17 axis remains completely unclear.

THERAPIES DIRECTED AT ANTIBODY-MEDIATED REJECTION

Antibody-mediated rejection (AMR) is increasingly being recognized as a significant risk factor for BOS, although its definition in the lung transplant community remains controversial. Increasing evidence connects the formation of anti-HLA antibodies, particularly donor-specific antibodies (DSAs), to chronic rejection. DSAs have a reported incidence of 10% to 40% in lung transplant patients, and DSAs both precede and are associated with an increased risk for the development of BOS.[40-43] Furthermore, pretransplant sensitization in lung transplant recipients has been found to be correlated with worse survival.[44] In addition, other studies have shown that DSAs are associated with severe or recurrent ACR and lymphocytic bronchiolitis, two forms of cellular rejection that are major risk factors for the development of BOS.[45,46] Moreover, detection of DSAs with or without an association with clinical AMR in lung transplant recipients is particularly difficult to treat and is linked with higher morbidity and mortality.[47] Thus, DSAs are emerging as a formidable challenge in lung transplantation. To date, little agreement exists regarding screening or when and how to initiate therapy.

For patients with clinical AMR, treatment aims to decrease DSA levels, inhibit the effects of anti-donor antibodies on the allograft, or both. Plasma exchange (PE) and intravenous immune globulin (IVIG) have been the mainstays of therapy. PE directly removes circulating antibodies.[48,49] By binding to inhibitory F_c receptors and blocking activating Fc receptors, IVIG not only inhibits antibody production but also appears to inhibit activation of innate immunity and possibly modulate pathogenic antibody effects through anti-idiotypic binding and interference with complement activation.[50] In addition, many centers use rituximab, a chimeric mAb against CD20 that targets CD20+ B cells for depletion. Recent evidence has shown that elimination of DSAs by using IVIG therapy alone or in combination with rituximab decreases the risk for the development of BOS that is faced by lung transplant recipients with persistence of DSAs. Recently, however, concerns have been raised regarding the fact that plasma cells, which are important producers of DSAs, do not express CD20 and thus are not affected by rituximab therapy.

Plasma cell–directed therapeutic approaches are under investigation for the treatment of AMR by using a class of drugs called proteasome inhibitors (PIs). Currently, PIs such as bortezomib are being used to treat multiple myeloma and AMR because they are the only agents that directly deplete antibody-producing cells.[51,52] By inhibiting protein degradation in the proteasome, PIs inhibit the activation of nuclear factor κ B, alter the balance of cell cycle proteins, and cause the accumulation of misfolded proteins in the endoplasmic reticulum of cells with active protein synthesis, thereby leading to cell cycle arrest and apoptosis.[53,54] Bortezomib was used to effectively treat six renal transplant patients with combined refractory AMR and ACR; it stably reduced DSAs by at least 50%.[55] A single cycle of bortezomib alone was as effective as bortezomib combined with PE and IVIG or rituximab in reducing de novo DSAs.[56] Of 11 patients who received bortezomib alone, 4 had a 50% decrease in DSAs, whereas 7 had complete remission (which lasted more than 2 years in 3 of the 7).[56] Patients with stable complete remission had lower serum creatinine levels at 14 months than did those with DSA relapse, thus adding credence to the notion that successful treatment of DSAs may alter outcome. Importantly, PIs appear to be well tolerated, and neither overall IgG levels nor IgG levels in response to childhood immunizations were changed.[51,57] The relatively specific loss of DSAs after the administration of PIs may be related to the fact that they primarily affect the most active antibody responses, with residual DSAs binding to the allograft. Interestingly, recent evidence in vitro indicates that PIs also induce B-cell apoptosis in addition to affecting plasma cells.[58]

Experience with PI therapy in lung transplantation to reduce the impact of DSAs is very limited. However, a study to investigate the new generation PI carfilzomib, which binds irreversibly to the proteasome, is under way at our center. Carfilzomib has been effective in treating patients with multiple myeloma in whom bortezomib treatment has failed, and it exhibits a better safety profile, specifically with less neuropathy.[59-61]

CELLULAR THERAPY

Increasing recognition that tolerance is a process involving active cellular processes and that immunoregulation plays a central role in allograft acceptance has led to the exploration of many forms of therapy involving transfer of cells that mediate allograft acceptance into allograft recipients. Such therapy is in the early stages of development and is inherently more complicated than drug therapy because of the complexity of cells. However, the basic science supporting its advancement is progressing, and its potential impact on translational medicine is significant.

Regulatory T cells

Regulatory T cells are CD4+CD25+Foxp3+ cells that suppress immune responses against both self-antigens and foreign antigens. That such cells play a major role in both the induction and maintenance of transplant tolerance has become clear. In a mouse model of cardiac transplantation in which recipients were treated with anti-CD154 therapy to induce allograft acceptance, allospecific regulatory T cells from cardiac allograft recipients were adoptively transferred into skin graft recipients and shown to prevent CD8+ cell–mediated skin graft rejection.[24] In view of this finding, it is easy to hypothesize that regulatory T cells could be given to transplant recipients to effect tolerance. In mouse orthotopic lung transplantation, allograft acceptance in the setting of anti-CD154 therapy is very clearly accompanied by markedly increased allograft regulatory T cells.[25] In addition, lung transplant recipients with BOS have been shown to have lower levels of regulatory T cells in their peripheral blood than do those without BOS.[62] However, regulatory T cells are difficult to expand in vitro, are small in number in peripheral blood, would need to maintain function with expansion, and may need to be able to recognize alloantigen to effectively suppress antiallograft responses. Given the increasing recognition of the plasticity of T cells, whether cells differentiated in vitro will maintain this phenotype and function in vivo remains unclear. Thus, the fate of adoptive regulatory cell therapy in transplantation remains difficult to predict. However, experts believe that such cell therapy will be viable for testing in the near future.

Tolerogenic dendritic cells

Dendritic cells are bone marrow–derived professional APCs. That such cells are capable of effecting immune responses has long been understood; now, however, their ability to effect tolerance is also clear. Dendritic cells are quite plastic and can be manipulated to become what are now referred to as *tolerogenic dendritic cells*. Compelling data in rodent transplant models have demonstrated the ability of tolerogenic dendritic cells generated in vitro to induce donor-specific tolerance. Rapamycin-conditioned host dendritic cells that are pulsed with donor antigen and administered before transplantation prolong cardiac allograft survival indefinitely.[63] In addition, dendritic cells that are conditioned with the active form of vitamin D_3 and mycophenolate mofetil induce tolerance of pancreatic islet grafts.[64] In both these examples, the tolerogenic effects of dendritic cells are associated with induction of regulatory T cells. It is hypothesized that tolerogenic dendritic cells drive regulatory T-cell expansion and that regulatory T cells maintain tolerogenicity in dendritic cells.[65] Therefore, dendritic cells also show great promise in translational work directed at induction of tolerance in human transplant patients.

Mesenchymal stem cells

The mesenchymal stem cell was originally described by Friedenstein and coworkers in the 1960s and 1970s. They noted nonhematopoietic stem cells in plated bone marrow that adhered to Petri dishes and had the ability to grow colonies from a single cell. It is now known that mesenchymal stem cells can also be derived from other sources, including umbilical cord, liver, and adipose tissue. These fibroblastoid cells not only have significant proliferative capacity but are also plastic and nonimmunogenic. Because of such properties and their immunomodulatory capacity, their use in transplantation has been explored. In a model of renal transplantation in mice, autologous mesenchymal stem cells given before transplantation were shown to localize to lymphoid tissue, enhance allograft survival, and induce regulatory T cells.[66,67] In addition, a clinical trial in which autologous bone marrow–derived mesenchymal stem cells were administered to 105 renal transplant patients before reperfusion and 2 weeks after transplantation demonstrated a significantly decreased incidence of acute rejection, improved renal function, and reduced incidence of infection after 1 year.[68] Mesenchymal stem cell therapy has been established to be safe, but further studies are needed to determine its long-term efficacy with regard to allograft acceptance.

Combined hematopoietic stem cell and organ transplantation

Several clinical case reports have demonstrated durable renal allograft acceptance in the absence of immunosuppressive therapy in patients who were previously treated with myeloablative bone marrow transplantation (BMT) from the same donor.[69-72] However, that myeloablation and full donor chimerism may not be necessary for induction of durable solid-organ allograft tolerance with BMT is becoming clear. An association between the development of mixed lymphohematopoietic chimerism after nonmyeloablative BMT and tolerance of a solid-organ allograft from the same donor has clearly been demonstrated in multiple models of transplantation in rodents and large animals.[73-78] In 1999, Spitzer and colleagues reported the first intentional induction of mixed lymphohematopoietic chimerism after a nonmyeloablative preparative regimen to treat multiple myeloma and establish renal allograft tolerance.[79] In their research, a preparative regimen consisting of cyclophosphamide, antithymocyte globulin, thymic irradiation, and initiation of cyclosporine was used before BMT, which was immediately followed by renal transplantation. Cyclosporine was continued initially but gradually tapered off by day 73 after transplantation. By day 147, despite two donor lymphocyte infusions for a graft-versus-tumor effect, the level of donor $CD3^+$ and $CD3^-$ cells found was less than 1%, but renal function nonetheless remained normal until at least day 174 after transplantation, thus suggesting donor alloantigen tolerance. This finding is consistent with data in nonhuman primates suggesting that even transient donor chimerism is sufficient for donor-specific tolerance of renal grafts.[77] A clinical trial examining the use of combined BMT and renal transplantation in patients with multiple myeloma and end-stage renal disease (NCT00854139) is currently under way, and whether durable allograft acceptance in the absence of immunosuppression is established will be of particular importance to the field of transplant immunology.

A case study demonstrating the successful use of sequential lung transplantation and BMT in a pediatric patient to treat advanced lung disease secondary to bronchiectasis in the setting of combined immunodeficiency disease was published in 2015.[80] Bone marrow for the patient described was harvested from a 5/10 HLA-matched donor at the time of lung transplantation and stored. First, the lung transplant was performed with standard immunosuppressive therapy and basiliximab induction. The bone marrow was depleted of T and B cells. Three months after the lung transplant, the patient began preparation for BMT by taking hydroxyurea, one dose of alemtuzumab, antithymocyte globulin, and one dose of thiotepa and receiving one fraction of total body irradiation with lung shielding. The protocol described in the report resulted in 100% donor chimerism (unlike in the case described earlier). Tacrolimus was discontinued 16 months after BMT, and the patient remained well and with good lung allograft function. Thus, despite its significant immediate-term risks, BMT is yet another option that could potentially improve lung allograft survival and result in induction of tolerance, thereby allowing cessation of immunosuppression. Whether 100% donor chimerism is necessary to achieve durable allograft acceptance in lung transplantation remains unclear.

CONCLUSION

In summary, despite the many unknowns that remain with regard to the exact cellular mechanisms and molecular pathways involved in lung allograft rejection and induction of tolerance, one thing is known very well: survival of lung allografts is less than optimal at this time. However, a multitude of potentially beneficial therapeutic options continue to arise as research continues and more is learned about the alloimmune response. With commitment to ongoing research and translational studies involving the use of novel techniques to more eloquently manipulate the immune response to alloantigen, there is no reason to believe that this problem cannot be solved.

REFERENCES

1. Yusen RD, Christie JD, Edwards LB, et al. The Registry of the International Society for Heart and Lung Transplantation: Thirtieth Adult Lung and Heart-Lung Transplant Report—2013; focus theme: Age. J Heart Lung Transplant 2013;32:965-978.
2. Jenkins MK, Schwartz RH. Antigen presentation by chemically modified splenocytes induces antigen-specific T cell unresponsiveness in vitro and in vivo. J Exp Med 1987;165:302-319.
3. Pearson TC, Alexander DZ, Winn KJ, et al. Transplantation tolerance induced by CTLA4-Ig. Transplantation 1994;57:1701-1706.
4. Lin H, Bolling SF, Linsley PS, et al. Long-term acceptance of major histocompatibility complex mismatched cardiac allografts induced by CTLA4Ig plus donor-specific transfusion. J Exp Med 1993;178:1801-1806.

5. Baliga P, Chavin KD, Qin L, et al. CTLA4Ig prolongs allograft survival while suppressing cell-mediated immunity. Transplantation 1994;58:1082-1090.

6. Turka LA, Linsley PS, Lin H, et al. T-cell activation by the CD28 ligand B7 is required for cardiac allograft rejection in vivo. Proc Natl Acad Sci U S A 1992;89:11102-11105.

7. Larsen CP, Elwood ET, Alexander DZ, et al. Long-term acceptance of skin and cardiac allografts after blocking CD40 and CD28 pathways. Nature 1996;381:434-438.

8. Lakkis FG, Konieczny BT, Saleem S, et al. Blocking the CD28-B7 T cell costimulation pathway induces long term cardiac allograft acceptance in the absence of IL-4. J Immunol 1997;158:2443-2448.

9. Lenschow DJ, Zeng Y, Thistlethwaite JR, et al. Long-term survival of xenogeneic pancreatic islet grafts induced by CTLA4Ig. Science 1992;257:789-792.

10. Okazaki M, Sugimoto S, Lai J, et al. Costimulatory blockade-mediated lung allograft acceptance is abrogated by overexpression of Bcl-2 in the recipient. Transplant Proc 2009;41:385-387.

11. Sayegh MH, Zheng XG, Magee C, et al. Donor antigen is necessary for the prevention of chronic rejection in CTLA4Ig-treated murine cardiac allograft recipients. Transplantation 1997;64:1646-1650.

12. Vincenti F, Charpentier B, Vanrenterghem Y, et al. A phase III study of belatacept-based immunosuppression regimens versus cyclosporine in renal transplant recipients (BENEFIT study). Am J Transplant 2010;10:535-546.

13. Durrbach A, Pestana JM, Pearson T, et al. A phase III study of belatacept versus cyclosporine in kidney transplants from extended criteria donors (BENEFIT-EXT study). Am J Transplant 2010;10:547-557.

14. Grewal IS, Xu J, Flavell RA. Impairment of antigen-specific T-cell priming in mice lacking CD40 ligand. Nature 1995;378:617-620.

15. McDyer JF, Goletz TJ, Thomas E, et al. CD40 ligand/CD40 stimulation regulates the production of IFN-gamma from human peripheral blood mononuclear cells in an IL-12– and/or CD28-dependent manner. J Immunol 1998;160:1701-1707.

16. Elster EA, Xu H, Tadaki DK, et al. Primate skin allotransplantation with anti-CD154 monotherapy. Transplant Proc 2001;33:675-676.

17. Hancock WW, Sayegh MH, Zheng XG, et al. Costimulatory function and expression of CD40 ligand, CD80, and CD86 in vascularized murine cardiac allograft rejection. Proc Natl Acad Sci U S A 1996;93:13967-13972.

18. Markees TG, Phillips NE, Noelle RJ, et al. Prolonged survival of mouse skin allografts in recipients treated with donor splenocytes and antibody to CD40 ligand. Transplantation 1997;64:329-335.

19. Kirk AD, Burkly LC, Batty DS, et al. Treatment with humanized monoclonal antibody against CD154 prevents acute renal allograft rejection in nonhuman primates. Nat Med 1999;5:686-693.

20. Wells AD, Li XC, Li Y, et al. Requirement for T-cell apoptosis in the induction of peripheral transplantation tolerance. Nat Med 1999;5:1303-1307.

21. Li Y, Li XC, Zheng XX, et al. Blocking both signal 1 and signal 2 of T-cell activation prevents apoptosis of alloreactive T cells and induction of peripheral allograft tolerance. Nat Med 1999;5:1298-1302.

22. Graca L, Honey K, Adams E, et al. Cutting edge: Anti-CD154 therapeutic antibodies induce infectious transplantation tolerance. J Immunol 2000;165:4783-4786.

23. Taylor PA, Noelle RJ, Blazar BR. CD4(+)CD25(+) immune regulatory cells are required for induction of tolerance to alloantigen via costimulatory blockade. J Exp Med 2001;193:1311-1318.

24. van Maurik A, Herber M, Wood KJ, Jones ND. Cutting edge: CD4+CD25+ alloantigen-specific immunoregulatory cells that can prevent CD8+ T cell–mediated graft rejection: Implications for anti-CD154 immunotherapy. J Immunol 2002;169:5401-5404.

25. Dodd-o JM, Lendermon EA, Miller HL, et al. CD154 blockade abrogates allospecific responses and enhances CD4(+) regulatory T-cells in mouse orthotopic lung transplant. Am J Transplant 2011;11:1815-1824.

26. Sidiropoulos PI, Boumpas DT. Lessons learned from anti-CD40L treatment in systemic lupus erythematosus patients. Lupus 2004;13:391-397.

27. Imai A, Suzuki T, Sugitani A, et al. A novel fully human anti-CD40 monoclonal antibody, 4D11, for kidney transplantation in cynomolgus monkeys. Transplantation 2007;84:1020-1028.

28. Aoyagi T, Yamashita K, Suzuki T, et al. A human anti-CD40 monoclonal antibody, 4D11, for kidney transplantation in cynomolgus monkeys: Induction and maintenance therapy. Am J Transplant 2009;9:1732-1741.

29. Maury CP, Teppo AM. Raised serum levels of cachectin/tumor necrosis factor alpha in renal allograft rejection. J Exp Med 1987;166:1132-1137.

30. Clausell N, Molossi S, Sett S, Rabinovitch M. In vivo blockade of tumor necrosis factor-alpha in cholesterol-fed rabbits after cardiac transplant inhibits acute coronary artery neointimal formation. Circulation 1994;89:2768-2779.

31. Wollin M, Abele S, Bruns H, et al. Inhibition of TNF-alpha reduces transplant arteriosclerosis in a murine aortic transplant model. Transpl Int 2009;22:342-349.

32. Imagawa DK, Millis JM, Seu P, et al. The role of tumor necrosis factor in allograft rejection. III. Evidence that anti-TNF antibody therapy prolongs

allograft survival in rats with acute rejection. Transplantation 1991;51:57-62.

33. Bolling SF, Kunkel SL, Lin H. Prolongation of cardiac allograft survival in rats by anti-TNF and cyclosporine combination therapy. Transplantation 1992;53:283-286.

34. Brown GR, Lindberg G, Meddings J, et al. Tumor necrosis factor inhibitor ameliorates murine intestinal graft-versus-host disease. Gastroenterology 1999;116:593-601.

35. Kennedy GA, Butler J, Western R, et al. Combination antithymocyte globulin and soluble TNFalpha inhibitor (etanercept) +/- mycophenolate mofetil for treatment of steroid refractory acute graft-versus-host disease. Bone Marrow Transplant 2006;37:1143-1147.

36. Smith CR, Jaramillo A, Lu KC, et al. Prevention of obliterative airway disease in HLA-A2–transgenic tracheal allografts by neutralization of tumor necrosis factor. Transplantation 2001;72:1512-1518.

37. Fan L, Benson HL, Vittal R, et al. Neutralizing IL-17 prevents obliterative bronchiolitis in murine orthotopic lung transplantation. Am J Transplant 2011;11:911-922.

38. Vanaudenaerde BM, De Vleeschauwer SI, Vos R, et al. The role of the IL23/IL17 axis in bronchiolitis obliterans syndrome after lung transplantation. Am J Transplant 2008;8:1911-1920.

39. Verleden SE, Vos R, Vandermeulen E, et al. Involvement of interleukin-17 during lymphocytic bronchiolitis in lung transplant patients. J Heart Lung Transplant 2013;32:447-453.

40. Sundaresan S, Mohanakumar T, Smith MA, et al. HLA-A locus mismatches and development of antibodies to HLA after lung transplantation correlate with the development of bronchiolitis obliterans syndrome. Transplantation 1998;65:648-653.

41. Jaramillo A, Smith MA, Phelan D, et al. Development of ELISA-detected anti-HLA antibodies precedes the development of bronchiolitis obliterans syndrome and correlates with progressive decline in pulmonary function after lung transplantation. Transplantation 1999;67:1155-1161.

42. Palmer SM, Davis RD, Hadjiliadis D, et al. Development of an antibody specific to major histocompatibility antigens detectable by flow cytometry after lung transplant is associated with bronchiolitis obliterans syndrome. Transplantation 2002;74:799-804.

43. Snyder LD, Wang Z, Chen DF, et al. Implications for human leukocyte antigen antibodies after lung transplantation: A 10-year experience in 441 patients. Chest 2013;144:226-233.

44. Hadjiliadis D, Chaparro C, Reinsmoen NL, et al. Pretransplant panel reactive antibody in lung transplant recipients is associated with significantly worse post-transplant survival in a multicenter study. J Heart Lung Transplant 2005;24(Suppl 7):S249-S254.

45. Girnita AL, McCurry KR, Iacono AT, et al. HLA-specific antibodies are associated with high-grade and persistent-recurrent lung allograft acute rejection. J Heart Lung Transplant 2004;23:1135-1141.

46. Girnita AL, Duquesnoy R, Yousem SA, et al. HLA-specific antibodies are risk factors for lymphocytic bronchiolitis and chronic lung allograft dysfunction. Am J Transplant 2005;5:131-138.

47. Witt CA, Gaut JP, Yusen RD, et al. Acute antibody-mediated rejection after lung transplantation. J Heart Lung Transplant 2013;32:1034-1040.

48. Jordan S, Cunningham-Rundles C, McEwan R. Utility of intravenous immune globulin in kidney transplantation: Efficacy, safety, and cost implications. Am J Transplant 2003;3:653-664.

49. Jordan SC, Vo AA, Tyan D, et al. Current approaches to treatment of antibody-mediated rejection. Pediatr Transplant 2005;9:408-415.

50. Jordan SC, Vo AA, Peng A, et al. Intravenous gammaglobulin (IVIG): A novel approach to improve transplant rates and outcomes in highly HLA-sensitized patients. Am J Transplant 2006;6:459-466.

51. Perry DK, Burns JM, Pollinger HS, et al. Proteasome inhibition causes apoptosis of normal human plasma cells preventing alloantibody production. Am J Transplant 2009;9:201-209.

52. Woodle ES, Alloway RR, Girnita A. Proteasome inhibitor treatment of antibody-mediated allograft rejection. Curr Opin Organ Transplant 2011;16:434-438.

53. Walsh RC, Alloway RR, Girnita AL, Woodle ES. Proteasome inhibitor–based therapy for antibody-mediated rejection. Kidney Int 2012;81:1067-1074.

54. Mohty M, Brissot E, Savani BN, Gaugler B. Effects of bortezomib on the immune system: A focus on immune regulation. Biol Blood Marrow Transplant 2013;19:1416-1420.

55. Everly MJ, Everly JJ, Susskind B, et al. Bortezomib provides effective therapy for antibody- and cell-mediated acute rejection. Transplantation 2008;86:1754-1761.

56. Everly MJ, Terasaki PI, Trivedi HL. Durability of antibody removal following proteasome inhibitor–based therapy. Transplantation 2012;93:572-577.

57. Everly MJ, Terasaki PI, Hopfield J, et al. Protective immunity remains intact after antibody removal by means of proteasome inhibition. Transplantation 2010;90:1493-1498.

58. Mulder A, Heidt S, Vergunst M, et al. Proteasome inhibition profoundly affects activated human B cells. Transplantation 2013;95:1331-1337.

59. Vij R, Siegel DS, Jagannath S, et al. An open-label, single-arm, phase 2 study of single-agent carfilzomib in patients with relapsed and/or refractory multiple myeloma who have been previously treated with bortezomib. Br J Haematol 2012;158:739-748.

60. Siegel DS, Martin T, Wang M, et al. A phase 2 study of single-agent carfilzomib (PX-171-003-A1) in patients with relapsed and refractory multiple myeloma. Blood 2012;120:2817-2825.

61. Jagannath S, Vij R, Stewart AK, et al. An open-label single-arm pilot phase II study (PX-171-003-A0) of low-dose, single-agent carfilzomib in patients with relapsed and refractory multiple myeloma. Clin Lymphoma Myeloma Leuk 2012;12:310-318.

62. Meloni F, Vitulo P, Bianco AM, et al. Regulatory CD4+CD25+ T cells in the peripheral blood of lung transplant recipients: Correlation with transplant outcome. Transplantation 2004;77:762-766.

63. Turnquist HR, Raimondi G, Zahorchak AF, et al. Rapamycin-conditioned dendritic cells are poor stimulators of allogeneic CD4+ T cells, but enrich for antigen-specific Foxp3+ T regulatory cells and promote organ transplant tolerance. J Immunol 2007;178:7018-7031.

64. Gregori S, Casorati M, Amuchastegui S, et al. Regulatory T cells induced by 1 alpha,25-dihydroxyvitamin D3 and mycophenolate mofetil treatment mediate transplantation tolerance. J Immunol 2001;167:1945-1953.

65. Thomson AW, Turnquist HR, Zahorchak AF, Raimondi G. Tolerogenic dendritic cell–regulatory T-cell interaction and the promotion of transplant tolerance. Transplantation 2009;87(Suppl 9):S86-S90.

66. Casiraghi F, Azzollini N, Cassis P, et al. Pretransplant infusion of mesenchymal stem cells prolongs the survival of a semiallogeneic heart transplant through the generation of regulatory T cells. J Immunol 2008;181:3933-3946.

67. Casiraghi F, Azzollini N, Todeschini M, et al. Localization of mesenchymal stromal cells dictates their immune or proinflammatory effects in kidney transplantation. Am J Transplant 2012;12:2373-2383.

68. Tan J, Wu W, Xu X, et al. Induction therapy with autologous mesenchymal stem cells in living-related kidney transplants: A randomized controlled trial. JAMA 2012;307:1169-1177.

69. Sayegh MH, Fine NA, Smith JL, et al. Immunologic tolerance to renal allografts after bone marrow transplants from the same donors. Ann Intern Med 1991;114:954-955.

70. Jacobsen N, Taaning E, Ladefoged J, et al. Tolerance to an HLA-B,DR disparate kidney allograft after bone-marrow transplantation from same donor. Lancet 1994;343:800.

71. Sorof JM, Koerper MA, Portale AA, et al. Renal transplantation without chronic immunosuppression after T cell–depleted, HLA-mismatched bone marrow transplantation. Transplantation 1995;59:1633-1635.

72. Dey B, Sykes M, Spitzer TR. Outcomes of recipients of both bone marrow and solid organ transplants. A review. Medicine (Baltimore) 1998;77:355-369.

73. Colson YL, Wren SM, Schuchert MJ, et al. A nonlethal conditioning approach to achieve durable multilineage mixed chimerism and tolerance across major, minor, and hematopoietic histocompatibility barriers. J Immunol 1995;155:4179-4188.

74. Sharabi Y, Sachs DH. Mixed chimerism and permanent specific transplantation tolerance induced by a nonlethal preparative regimen. J Exp Med 1989;169:493-502.

75. de Vries-van der Zwan A, Besseling AC, de Waal LP, Boog CJ. Specific tolerance induction and transplantation: A single-day protocol. Blood 1997;89:2596-2601.

76. Gammie JS, Li S, Zeevi A, et al. Tacrolimus-based partial conditioning produces stable mixed lymphohematopoietic chimerism and tolerance for cardiac allografts. Circulation 1998;98(Suppl 19):II163-II168; discussion II168-II169.

77. Kawai T, Cosimi AB, Colvin RB, et al. Mixed allogeneic chimerism and renal allograft tolerance in cynomolgus monkeys. Transplantation 1995;59:256-262.

78. Kimikawa M, Sachs DH, Colvin RB, et al. Modifications of the conditioning regimen for achieving mixed chimerism and donor-specific tolerance in cynomolgus monkeys. Transplantation 1997;64:709-716.

79. Spitzer TR, Delmonico F, Tolkoff-Rubin N, et al. Combined histocompatibility leukocyte antigen–matched donor bone marrow and renal transplantation for multiple myeloma with end stage renal disease: The induction of allograft tolerance through mixed lymphohematopoietic chimerism. Transplantation 1999;68:480-484.

80. Szabolcs P, Buckley R, Davis RD. Tolerance and alloimmunity after sequential lung and bone marrow transplantation from an unrelated cadaveric donor. J Allergy Clin Immunol 2015;135:567-570.

39

New horizons in lung transplantation

JASON M. LONG AND WICKII T. VIGNESWARAN

End-stage lung disease is the third leading cause of death in the United States and a major health care challenge.[1] Lung transplantation is the only definitive treatment of end-stage lung disease, and it has been increasingly successful as a therapy that improves the quality and quantity of life for selected patients.[2] Only a minority of patients can benefit from it, however, because of the lack of acceptable donor organs. The largest source of donor lungs is donation after neurologic determination of death. Unfortunately, the number of lungs suitable for transplantation is low, thus leading to a disappointing procurement rate. An average of only 1700 lung transplant procedures are performed in the United States each year. The lack of donor lungs has been the impetus to create new tools to evaluate and potentially treat extended criteria lungs with ex vivo lung perfusion (EVLP), as well as to search for alternative lung sources, including donors who die after withdrawal of care and victims of sudden death (non–heart-beating donors [NHBDs]), bioengineering of whole lungs, and creation of artificial (mechanical) lungs. These emerging ideas and breakthroughs will probably contribute to the future of lung transplantation.

EVALUATION AND TREATMENT OF EXTENDED CRITERIA LUNGS WITH EX VIVO LUNG PERFUSION

One common strategy to maximize the use of lungs obtained after neurologic determination of death is to adopt extended criteria that fall outside the guidelines set by the International Society for Heart and Lung Transplantation (ISHLT).[3] Additionally, a systematic approach to the use of NHBDs after cardiac death creates a larger pool of donor organs from a source that is currently underutilized in the United States.[4] A variety of techniques have been used in this setting, depending on the exact nature of the organ source as described by the Maastricht category.[5] A major challenge in using extended criteria donor organs and NHBDs is the difficulty assessing which lungs can be used safely. Graft quality is generally measured by gas exchange and lung compliance. The evaluation process is performed before and during lung procurement—traditionally, while the lung is functioning within the deleterious physiologic milieu of a brain-dead donor. EVLP is a new technique that allows careful visual inspection of explanted lungs, measurement of hemodynamic and ventilatory parameters, and evaluation of gas exchange after procurement in a controlled environment.[6] EVLP is advantageous because the system provides an opportunity for recruitment and reexpansion of atelectatic lungs and permits effective bronchial clearing of secretions, removal of clots in the pulmonary circulation, and direct transfer of all ventilator volume and pressure settings to the lungs without interference by the immobile chest wall and diaphragm. EVLP allows differentiation between "good" and "bad" donor lungs in the pool of organs from extended criteria donors and NHBDs when graft function is questionable, thus resulting in outcomes equivalent to those with standard criteria donor lungs.[7]

RESUSCITATION AND OPTIMIZATION OF DONOR LUNGS

Part of the success of EVLP lies in the use of a buffered extracellular solution with an optimal colloid osmotic pressure, such as the lung perfusate that was developed by Steen and colleagues and is sold commercially as Steen solution.[8] Steen's group has used a normothermic ex vivo circuit for evaluation of pig and human NHBDs with subsequent successful clinical transplantation and survival.[9] Steen solution is believed to be hyperoncotic and to dehydrate edematous lung tissue. "Therapeutic" manipulation of the effect of the milieu of EVLP on donor lungs may provide additional success in the future. The initial success with ex vivo evaluation provided the foundation for further research that made it possible to extend normothermic ex vivo perfusion to allow preservation or repair of poorly functioning lungs, which in turn has now become an area of much interest and research.

Cypel and colleagues developed an ex vivo circuit that is based on perfusion and ventilation strategies and allows successful 12-hour normothermic ex vivo perfusion with stable pulmonary vascular resistance, airway pressure, and lung oxygenation capacity without induction of edema.[10] This platform allows ex vivo assessment, treatment, and perhaps pharmacologic or molecular therapeutic repair of injured donor lungs. Potential pharmacologic applications of the normothermic circuit include using it with hyperosmotic perfusates, as well as for administration of β-adrenergic drugs to accelerate removal of lung edema, intratracheal instillation of terbutaline to enhance clearance of fluid in the air space, use of fibrinolytics to help remove pulmonary emboli, and perfusion of the lung with high-dose antibiotics to help sterilize pneumonia.[11-13] Andreasson and coworkers investigated the effect of normothermic perfusion on the infectious burden in human donor lungs considered unusable for transplantation by adding high-dose, empirical, broad-spectrum antimicrobial agents to the perfusate.[14] Thirteen of 18 lungs had positive cultures, with the bacterial loads significantly decreasing after EVLP.[14] Yeast load increased when no antifungal treatment was given but was reduced when prophylactic antifungal treatment was added to the circuit.[15] Six lungs were ultimately transplanted into patients, all of whom survived until discharge from the hospital (although one patient died 11 months after transplantation).[14] Others have investigated agents administered during EVLP that might improve lung compliance. Arginase, which is a regulator of nitric oxide synthesis, can influence pulmonary compliance. George and coworkers have demonstrated that early administration of the novel nebulized arginase inhibitor 2-(S)-amino-6-boronohexanoic acid resulted in a transient increase in dynamic compliance.[15]

Another area of investigation is preconditioning grafts to reduce ischemia-reperfusion injury, which is a major cause of primary graft dysfunction and early mortality. Levels of the proinflammatory cytokine interleukin-8 (IL-8), as well as the ratio of IL-6 to IL-10, have been correlated with early graft failure.[16,17] When Yeung and colleagues transfected pig lungs with adenovirus encoding IL-10 either in vivo or while the lungs were on EVLP for 12 hours, those in the EVLP group showed superior function.[18] Next, human lungs that had been deemed not transplantable clinically were transfected, after which they demonstrated improved functional quality, increased oxygenation, decreased vascular resistance, improved cell-to-cell interaction, and a shift from a proinflammatory to an anti-inflammatory cytokine environment following 12 hours of EVLP.[19,20]

A beneficial side effect of EVLP is that it permits extension of organ ischemic time, thereby allowing long-distance procurements that were not possible before. This potential benefit of ex vivo technology was demonstrated by Wigfield and coworkers in a study in which a marginal donated lung was transported from a donor center in the midwestern United States to the organ repair center of the University of Toronto Lung Transplant Program and back to the recipient center.[21] This process extended the ischemic time to 15 hours and 20 minutes and served as the first case in support of conceptualizing and operationalizing a regional organ assessment and repair center (ARC)-based approach.

It is conceivable that in the near future, EVLP will be used as a platform for assessment, repair, and modification of organs that are of marginal quality and meet extended rather than standard donor criteria or when the best tissue match is in a geographically distant area.[22] With this approach, donor organs could be optimally assessed and evaluated in a regional ARC after procurement and static cold storage.[22] The organs could then be transported to the ARC, at which they would be evaluated and treated, and if deemed transplantable, they would then be allocated to the most suitable recipient in national or international fashion.[22]

EXPANDING THE ROLE OF LUNGS FROM NON–HEART-BEATING DONORS: SUDDEN DEATH VICTIMS

Increasing awareness that brainstem death is detrimental to the lung has led to investigation and use of NHBDs. Interest in recovering lungs from Maastricht category III donors, which involves elective withdrawal of ventilator support and results in death by asphyxia and cardiac arrest, has been growing. In the United States, the practice of transplantation of lungs obtained as a result of donation after cardiac death is still limited to only a few transplant centers; however, it is used more widely elsewhere. With more recent publications and communication of better experience, more centers are successfully adopting transplantation of lungs obtained via donation after cardiac death. Uncontrolled donors in Maastricht categories I and II remain a large untapped source of NHBDs. Egan and colleagues demonstrated that lungs remain viable for substantial periods after circulatory arrest and death because unlike the cells of other solid organs, lung cells do not rely on perfusion for cellular respiration. Oxygen is supplied via alveoli, air spaces, and bronchi.[23] Egan also demonstrated that cadaveric lungs could be retrieved from NHBDs in a canine model after death and safely transplanted.[23,24] Furthermore, simple maneuvers, such as ventilating the cadaver with oxygen after death, increased the "window" for recovery from NHBDs after death to 4 hours.[24] The number of Maastricht category I NHBDs in the United States is very large: more than 750,000 per year.[25] If only a small fraction (5%, which equates to 35,000) of sudden death victims' lungs could be retrieved and assessed for lung transplantation, the impact would be enormous.

In Europe and Australia, NHBDs already account for roughly 20% of transplants, a percentage that is far greater than that in the United States.[26,27] Such transplants have demonstrated that with carefully managed donors, the outcome is at least equivalent to that with organs from brain-dead donors. Novel ideas, including dual-temperature multiorgan recovery after circulatory death, may also decrease warm ischemic time for the abdominal extrarenal organs and increase their procurement rate.[29] In Sweden, Steen and associates developed an ex vivo perfusion system to allow objective assessment of the donor lung, and they performed the first transplant of a lung from an uncontrolled donor in 2000.[30] A few years later, a group from Madrid worked within an existing protocol for whole body perfusion of category I and II donors and reported successful lung retrieval and transplantation with results acceptable from the standpoints of both mid- and long-term survival and the rate of development of bronchiolitis obliterans syndrome but with higher rates of primary graft dysfunction.[31,32] Egan and colleagues have implemented a National Institutes of Health–funded phase II study to demonstrate success transplanting lungs after retrieval from uncontrolled NHBDs (Maastricht categories I and II) and EVLP assessment under the hypothesis that this new donor source and EVLP will provide not only many more lungs but, ultimately, lungs better than those currently being transplanted. The role of EVLP in management of extended criteria donors is still evolving, and it will probably become an important technique for increasing the number of lungs available for transplantation in the future.[28]

WHOLE LUNG TISSUE ENGINEERING

Currently, lung transplantation is the only definitive treatment of end-stage lung disease; however, its clinical impact is limited by the need for immunosuppression and by the shortage of donor organs. Postoperatively, one in three lung recipients will experience at least one episode of acute rejection in the first year, with half of those receiving a transplant surviving almost 6 years, and if alive at 1 year, half this cohort will have preserved graft function for up to 8 years.[2] Thanks to recent advances in tissue engineering and regenerative medicine, the development of alternative strategies to address end-organ failure, the shortage of donor organs, and chronic rejection has begun.

Bioartificial lung engineering aims to regenerate the broad spectrum of specialized tissue of native lungs—conducting airways, vasculature, and gas exchange tissue—in a three-dimensional physiologic context. Currently, bioartificial lung engineering relies on the interaction of lung progenitor cells with their native niches incorporated into complex scaffolds to recapitulate tissue formation.[33] The functional unit of the lung is the air-blood interface between the epithelium and endothelium. This interface must have a minimal diffusion length to allow efficient gas exchange between the alveoli and pulmonary capillaries. Physiologic gas exchange also depends on hierarchical branching airways and vascular networks, both of which allow efficient ventilation and perfusion.[33] The vascular network must resist thrombosis and possess barrier function sufficient to prevent flooding of the alveoli with blood or blood components.

Central to successful creation of a bioartificial lung is the engineering of its interstitial surfaces as a scaffold where the vital function of gas exchange takes place. To date, most progress in producing lung scaffolds has been due to decellularization of excised lungs, which are treated with detergents and enzymes to remove all cellular components of the tissue.[34] This approach yields a nonimmunogenic scaffold while preserving the lung's inherent architecture,[33,34] and it permits using not only human lungs as scaffolds but also xenogeneic scaffolds, such as decellularlized pig lungs.[35] A bioartificial lung must perform adequately and remain viable after implantation when the scaffold is seeded with appropriate cell types in numbers sufficient to line the airway lumina with epithelial cells and the pulmonary vasculature[30] with endothelial cells. Epithelial cells provide mucociliary clearance of the airways, whereas endothelial cells downregulate the thrombogenic response of blood platelets to the extracellular matrix and scaffolding.[36]

Two groups have been successful in regenerating functional lung tissues. Petersen and coworkers, as well as Ott and colleagues, successfully implanted engineered lungs that exchanged gas for several hours.[36,37] Both groups seeded acellular lung matrices with varying cell populations and cultured them in a bioreactor for approximately 1 week. Petersen and colleagues[36] used neonatal rat lung epithelium and microvascular endothelium, whereas Ott and associates[37] used a combination of human umbilical cord endothelial cells and rat fetal lung cells. The bioengineered lungs were then transplanted into syngeneic rats via left thoracotomy.[36,37] The engineered lungs became perfused with blood and inflated with air; blood gas analysis revealed that the lungs were effective in exchanging oxygen and carbon dioxide.[36,37]

Despite these milestones, significant challenges and hurdles remain and must be overcome before a bioengineered lung can be successfully transplanted into a human recipient. Re-creation of the natural architecture and structural properties of the native lung must be improved to obtain a scaffold with sufficient gas exchange capability, and a substrate appropriate for attachment and proliferation of cells must be provided. Determination of the exact kinds and numbers of cells sufficient to ensure that the bioartificial lung remains functional and viable is still a work in progress.[34] Creation of an effective source of the large numbers of differentiated cells required for seeding is another problem.[34] Extensive preclinical testing in small and large animal models is necessary. Clinical trials must adhere to strict ethical guidelines. As mentioned earlier, because of the shortage of human donors, tissue-engineered lungs may eventually require biologic scaffolds of animal origin or even completely artificial scaffolds.

ARTIFICIAL LUNG AND LUNG SUPPORT DEVICES

Because the demand for donor organs in lung transplantation continues to exceed the current supply, artificial lungs have been proposed as a bridge or alternative to lung transplantation. Patients with end-stage lung disease often suffer from life-threatening hypoxemia, hypercapnia, and respiratory acidosis despite maximal ventilator support. The only option for such patients is extracorporeal gas exchange. Several studies have shown that long-term extracorporeal membrane oxygenation (ECMO) can be used to bridge patients to lung transplantation. However, cannulation and the ECMO circuit could make pretransplant rehabilitation more difficult than would use of an artificial lung. The use of ECMO in adults with end-stage lung disease is generally limited to a run time of approximately 2 weeks, at which point the incidence of clinically relevant complications (e.g., blood element activation, hemolysis, and platelet consumption necessitating transfusion and leading to a systemic inflammatory response and organ system failure) increases significantly. Venovenous ECMO provides exchange of respiratory gases but does little to support right ventricular failure resulting from pulmonary hypertension associated with late-stage respiratory failure. Additionally, patients with pulmonary arterial hypertension often experience acute decompensation and suffer from low cardiac output despite preserved oxygenation and elimination of carbon dioxide. Venoarterial ECMO can provide tissue perfusion and right ventricular unloading, but support for the typically long waiting time before lung transplantation remains a problem. Thanks to advances in cannula development and ambulatory ECMO support as a bridge to transplantation, both have been used with increasing success.

A new clinical approach to this problem involves the use of a paracorporeal artificial lung. Via thoracotomy or sternotomy, blood is diverted from the pulmonary artery into a low-resistance artificial lung and returned to the left atrium, thus bypassing the native lungs. Blood flow is generated by the native cardiac output produced by the right ventricle, which obviates the need for a mechanical blood pump. Flow is parallel with the native pulmonary circulation and serves to decompress a heart failing because of right-sided pressure overload. Relative flow is determined by the comparative resistance of the extracorporeal circuit and the native pulmonary resistance. This approach has been tested in short- and long-term animal models and used clinically.[38-40]

The Novalung iLA (interventional lung assist) (Novalung GmbH, Hechingen, Germany), which is presented in Figure 39.1, is a low-resistance lung assist device designed for pulsatile blood flow with tight diffusion membranes and a protein matrix coating. It is driven by cardiac output and therefore does not require assistance from an extracorporeal pump. The iLA has been applied in a variety of clinical situations, such as severe chest trauma, pneumonia, adult respiratory distress syndrome, and airway obstruction. It has also been investigated with success as a bridge to lung

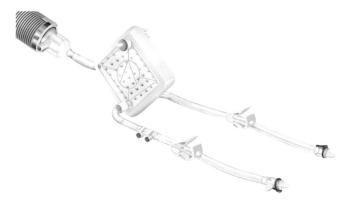

Figure 39.1 The Novalung iLA (interventional lung assist) membrane ventilator.

transplantation in patients with end-stage lung disease in case reports with short-term follow-up.[41-43] The device is not currently available for clinical use in the United States; however, it is available in Europe. To implant the iLA, the femoral artery and the contralateral femoral vein should be evaluated with ultrasound to identify and assess the diameter of the vessels. The cannula chosen should allow a residual lumen of 30%. Typically, the arterial cannula has a size of 12 to 15 French and the venous cannula is two French sizes larger. The vessels are subsequently cannulated via the Seldinger technique.

Interest in engineering artificial lungs that not only provide gas exchange, blood flow, and cardiac output but also allow ambulation, rehabilitation, and improved quality of life has been increasing. Such benefits have been demonstrated previously with ECMO[44]; however, conventional ECMO is labor intensive, traumatic to blood elements, and limited by its bulky complicated circuit. Recent devices in animals that may have a direct impact on use of the artificial lung as a bridge to recovery, transplantation, or destination therapy have been tested. The University of Michigan group has examined the use of a paracorporeal transthoracic artificial lung in parallel with the native lung, which offers the benefits of a single heart-driven pulmonary artery–left atrium shunt without the need for a separate blood pump.[45] The MC3 Biolung (MC3, Ann Arbor, Michigan), which is shown in Figure 39.2, was used as a total artificial lung device in sheep. Inflow was created with an end-to-side anastomosis to the pulmonary artery, and outflow was created with an anastomosis to the left atrium—both via an anterolateral thoracotomy and resection of the fourth rib. An animal model of pulmonary hypertension was created by injecting Sephadex beads into the pulmonary circulation via a central catheter for 60 days. The team used infusions of dobutamine in dosages of 0, 2, and 5 μg/kg/min as a surrogate for exercise in sheep with and without pulmonary hypertension in addition to progressive banding of the pulmonary artery to divert increasing amounts of blood flow through the artificial lung circuit until 90% of the cardiac output was diverted. The effects on right ventricular strain and other hemodynamic measurements were measured. Mild hemodynamic compromise with increased right ventricular strain was observed

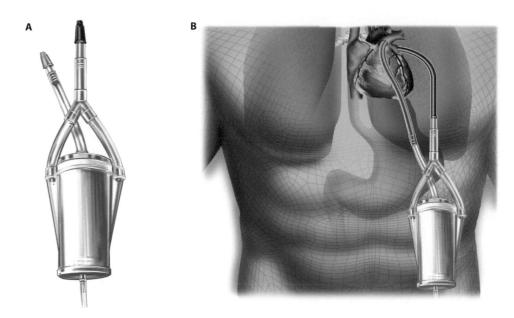

Figure 39.2 **(A)** MC3 BioLung. **(B)** Insertion through the left chest. The inflow cannula is from the pulmonary artery and the outflow cannula is attached to the left atrium.

at the highest blood flow rates and the highest dobutamine concentration. The study demonstrated that at levels consistent with mild exercise, however, the artificial lung could be well tolerated. The downsides with this model are the need for central cannulation, risk for thrombosis or air embolism, and variable amount of flow through the device depending on resistance in the pulmonary circuit.

Zwischenberger and colleagues recently published their results with a percutaneous ambulatory paracorporeal artificial lung (PAL) system in healthy sheep for up to 4 weeks.[46,47] The PAL system includes a compact low-resistance gas exchanger and compact centrifugal pump that form a simple and short paracorporeal circuit. Inflow and outflow are established via single-site venous cannulation with an Avalon Elite bicaval dual-lumen cannula. Postoperatively, the sheep were moved into a metabolic cage and transferred to an intensive care unit. The gas exchanger was secured on the sheep's back, and the CentriMag pump was hung on a weight-balanced pulley, which allowed the sheep to move freely along with the PAL system, thereby achieving in-cage ambulation and guaranteeing circuit security. A total of 15 gas exchangers were tested in 11 animals. The PAL system allowed the sheep to remain awake and alert after surgery, stand and sit freely, and eat and drink at will, thus obviating the need for artificial feeding. All the sheep had stable hemodynamics throughout the experimental period, with no need for inotropic medicine. In this study 11 animals were maintained on support for up to 24 days.

Expanding the pool of donor lungs is necessary to increase the number of lungs transplanted, and use of extended donor criteria and lungs from NHBDs, as well as optimization of lung function via EVLP, are major strategies that continue to advance this field. Currently, ambulatory ECMO and paracorporeal lung support are short-term mechanical bridges for lung transplant recipients. Wide and increasing use of these technologies and advances are expected in the near future. Truly artificial lungs with total or partial gas exchange devices pose many challenges for the future. Advances in stem cell technology, three-dimensional (3D) printing, and tissue engineering will help overcome some of these challenges. Thus, we can say that improved lung replacement is on the horizon.

REFERENCES

1. Murphy S, Xu J, Kochanek K. Deaths: Final data for 2010. Natl Vital Stat Rep 2013;61:1-118.
2. Yusen RD, Edwards LB, Kucheryavaya AY, et al. The Registry of the International Society for Heart and Lung Transplantation: Thirty-first adult lung and heart-lung transplant report—2014; focus theme: Retransplantation. J Heart Lung Transplant 2014;33:1009-1024.
3. Orens JB, Boehler A, de Perrot M, et al. A review of lung transplant donor acceptability criteria. J Heart Lung Transplant 2003;22:1183-1200.
4. Dark JH. Lung transplantation from the non–heart beating donor. Transplantation 2008;86:200-201.
5. Kootstra G, Daemen JH, Oomen AP. Categories of non–heart-beating donors. Transplant Proc 1995;27:2893-2894.
6. Yeung JC, Cypel M, Waddell TK, et al. Update on donor assessment, resuscitation, and acceptance criteria including novel techniques—non–heart-beating donor lung retrieval and ex vivo donor lung perfusion. Thorac Surg Clin 2009;19:261-274.
7. Cypel M, Yeung JC, Liu M, et al. Normothermic ex vivo lung perfusion in clinical lung transplantation. N Engl J Med 2011;364:1431-1440.

8. Steen S, Liao Q, Wierup PN, et al. Transplantation of lungs from non–heart-beating donors after functional assessment ex vivo. Ann Thorac Surg 2003;76:244-252.

9. Wierup P, Haraldsson A, Nilsson F, et al. Ex vivo evaluation of nonacceptable donor lungs. Ann Thorac Surg 2006;81:460-466.

10. Cypel M, Yeung JC, Hirayama S, et al. Technique for prolonged normothermic ex vivo lung perfusion. J Heart Lung Transplant 2008;27:1319-1325.

11. Frank JA, Briot R, Lee JW, et al. Physiological and biochemical markers of alveolar epithelial barrier dysfunction in perfused human lungs. Am J Physiol Lung Cell Med Physiol 2007;293:L52-L59.

12. Ware LB, Fang X, Wang Y, et al. Selected contribution: Mechanisms that may stimulate the resolution of alveolar edema in the transplanted human lung. J Appl Physiol 2002;93:1869-1874.

13. Brown CR, Brozzi NA, Vakil N, et al. Donor lungs with pulmonary embolism evaluated with ex vivo lung perfusion. ASAIO J 2012;58:432-434.

14. Andreasson A, Karamanou DM, Perry JD, et al. The effect of ex vivo lung perfusion on microbial load in human donor lungs. J Heart Lung Transplant 2014;33:910-916.

15. George TJ, Arnaoutakis GJ, Beaty CA, et al. A physiologic and biochemical profile of clinically rejected lungs on a normothermic ex vivo lung perfusion platform. J Surg Res 2013;183:75-83.

16. Fisher AJ, Donnely SC, Hirani N, et al. Elevated levels of interleukin-8 in donor lungs is associated with early graft failure after lung transplantation. Am J Respir Crit Care Med 2001;163:259-265.

17. Kaneda H, Waddell TK, de Perrot M, et al. Pre-implantation multiple cytokine mRNA expression analysis of donor lung grafts predicts survival after lung transplantation in humans. Am J Transplant 2006;6:544-551.

18. Yeung JC, Wagnetz D, Cypel M, et al. Ex Vivo adenoviral vector gene delivery results in decreased vector associated inflammation pre– and post–lung transplantation in the pig. Mol Ther 2012;20:1204-1211.

19. Cypel M, Rubacha M, Hirayama S, et al. Ex-vivo repair and regeneration of damaged human donor lungs. J Heart Lung Transplant 2008;27(Suppl 2):S180.

20. Cypel M, Liu M, Rubacha M, et al. Functional repair of human donor lungs by IL-10 gene therapy. Sci Transl Med 2009;1:1-9.

21. Wigfield CH, Cypel M, Yeung J, et al. Successful emergent lung transplantation after remote ex vivo perfusion optimization and transportation of donor lungs. Am J Transplant 2012;12:2838-2844.

22. Whitson BA, Black SM. Organ assessment and repair centers: The future of transplantation is near. World J Transplant 2014;4:40-42.

23. Egan TM, Lambert CJ Jr, Reddick R, et al. A strategy to increase the donor pool: Use of cadaver lungs for transplantation. Ann Thorac Surg 1991;52:1113-1120.

24. Ulicny KS Jr, Egan TM, Lambert CJ Jr, et al. Cadaver lung donors: Effect of preharvest ventilation on graft function. Ann Thorac Surg 1993;55:1185-1191.

25. Hoyert DL, Kung HC, Smith BL. Deaths: Preliminary data for 2003. Natl Vital Stat Rep 2005;53:1-48.

26. Saxena P, Zimmet AD, Snell G, et al. Procurement of lungs in transplantation following donation after circulatory death: The Alfred technique. J Surg Res 2014;192:642-646.

27. Johnson RJ, Bradbury LL, Martin K, et al. Organ donation and transplantation in the UK—the last decade: A report from the UK National Transplant Registry. Transplantation 2014;97(Suppl 1):S1-S27.

28. Cypel M, Keshavjee S. Strategies for safe donor expansion: Donor management, donations after cardiac death, ex-vivo lung perfusion. Curr Opin Organ Transplant 2013;18:513-517.

29. Oniscu GC, Siddique A, Dark J. Dual temperature multi-organ recovery from a Maastricht category III donor after circulatory death. Am J Transplant 2014;14:2181-2186.

30. Steen S, Sjoberg T, Pierre L, et al. Transplantation of lungs from a non–heart-beating donor. Lancet 2001;17:825-829.

31. Gomez de Antonion D, Marcos R, Laporta R, et al. Results of clinical lung transplant from uncontrolled non–heart beating donors. J Heart Lung Transplant 2007;26:529-534.

32. Gomez-de-Antonio D, Campo-Canaveral JL, Crowley S, et al. Clinical lung transplantation from uncontrolled non–heart-beating donors revisited. J Heart Lung Transplant 2012;31:349-353.

33. Song JJ, Ott HC. Bioartificial lung engineering. Am J Transplant 2012;12:283-288.

34. Lemon G, Lim ML, Ajalloueian F, Macchiarini P. The development of the bioartificial lung. Br Med Bull 2014;110:35-45.

35. Badylak SF. Xenogeneic extracellular matrix as a scaffold for tissue reconstruction. Transpl Immunol 2004;12:367-377.

36. Petersen TH, Calle EA, Zhao L, et al. Tissue-engineered lungs for in vivo implantation. Science 2010;329:538-541.

37. Ott HC, Clippinger B, Conrad C, et al. Regeneration and orthotopic transplantation of a bioartificial lung. Nat Med 2010;16:927-933.

38. Haft JW, Montoya P, Alnajjar O, et al. An artificial lung reduces pulmonary impedance and improves right ventricular efficiency in pulmonary hypertension. J Thorac Cardiovasc Surg 2001;122:1094-1100.

39. Strueber M, Hoeper MM, Fischer S, et al. Bridge to thoracic organ transplantation in patients with pulmonary arterial hypertension using a pumpless lung assist device. Am J Transplant 2009;9:853-857.

40. Cambioni D, Phillipp A, Arlt M, et al. First experience with a paracorporeal artificial lung in humans. ASAIO J 2009;55:304-306.

41. Fischer S, Simon AR, Welte T, et al. Bridge to lung transplantation with the novel pumpless interventional lung assist device NovaLung. J Thorac Cardiovasc Surg 2006;131:719-723.

42. Strueber M, Hoeper MM, Fischer S, et al. Bridge to thoracic organ transplantation in patients with pulmonary arterial hypertension using a pumpless lung assist device. Am J Transplant 2009;9:853-857.

43. Bartosik W, Egan JJ, Wood AE. The Novalung interventional lung assist as bridge to lung transplantation for self-ventilating patients—initial experience. Interact Cardiovasc Thorac Surg 2011;13:198-200.

44. Garcia JP, Iacono A, Kon ZN, Griffith BP. Ambulatory extracorporeal membrane oxygenation: A new approach to bridge-to-lung transplantation. J Thorac Cardiovasc Surg 2010;139:e137-e139.

45. Akay B, Reoma JL, Camboni D, et al. In-parallel artificial lung attachment at high flows in normal and pulmonary hypertension models. Ann Thorac Surg 2010;90:259-265.

46. Zhou X, Wang D, Sumpter R, et al. Long-term support with an ambulatory percutaneous paracorporeal artificial lung. J Heart Lung Transplant 2012;31:648-654.

47. Zwischenberger, JB, Alpard, SK, Artificial lungs: A new inspiration. Perfusion 2002;17:253-268.

Index

Note: Page numbers followed by f, t, and b indicate figures, tables, and boxes, respectively.